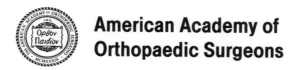

**American Academy of
Orthopaedic Surgeons**

Weapons of Mass Casualties and Terrorism Response
Handbook

Charles Stewart MD FACEP

JONES AND BARTLETT PUBLISHERS
Sudbury, Massachusetts
BOSTON   TORONTO   LONDON   SINGAPORE

Jones and Bartlett Publishers

World Headquarters
40 Tall Pine Drive
Sudbury, MA 01776
978-443-5000
info@jbpub.com
www.jbpub.com

Jones and Bartlett Publishers Canada
6339 Ormindale Way
Mississauga, Ontario L5V 1J2
Canada

Jones and Bartlett Publishers International
Barb House, Barb Mews
London W6 7PA
United Kingdom

Jones and Bartlett's books and products are available through most book-stores and online booksellers. To contact Jones and Bartlett Publishers directly, call 800-832-0034, fax 978-443-8000, or visit our website www.jbpub.com.
Substantial discounts on bulk quantities of Jones and Bartlett's publications are available to corporations, professional associations, and other qualified organizations. For details and specific discount information, contact the special sales department at Jones and Bartlett via the above contact information or send an email to specialsales@jbpub.com.

Production Credits

Chief Executive Officer: Clayton Jones
Chief Operating Officer: Don W. Jones, Jr.
President, Higher Education and Professional Publishing: Robert W. Holland, Jr.
V.P., Design and Production: Anne Spencer
V.P., Sales and Marketing: William Kane
V.P., Manufacturing and Inventory Control: Therese Connell
Publisher, Public Safety Group: Kimberly Brophy
Managing Editor: Carol Brewer

American Academy of Orthopaedic Surgeons

Editorial Credits
Chief Education Officer: Mark W. Wieting
Director, Department of Publications: Marilyn L. Fox, PhD
Managing Editor: Barbara A. Scotese

Associate Editor: Janet Morris
Production Editor: Jenny McIsaac
Senior Photo Researcher: Kimberly Potvin
Director of Marketing: Alisha Weisman
Cover Design: Kristin Ohlin
Text Design: Anne Spencer
Printing and Binding: Courier Company
Cover Printing: John Pow Company

ISBN: 0-7637-2425-4

Library of Congress Cataloging-in-Publication Data
Stewart, Charles E. (Charles Edward), 1947-
    Weapons of mass casualties and terrorism response handbook / AAOS and Charles Stewart.
        p. ; cm.
    Includes index.
    ISBN 0-7637-2425-4 (hardcover)
    1. Terrorism—Health aspects—Handbooks, manuals, etc. 2. Weapons of mass destruction—Health aspects—Handbooks, manuals, etc.
    [DNLM: 1. Biological Warfare. 2. Chemical Warfare. 3. Disaster Planning. 4. Bioterrorism. 5. Emergency Medical Services. 6. Emergency Medical Technicians. WA 295 S849w 2006] I. American Academy of Orthopaedic Surgeons. II. Title.
    RC88.9.T47.S744 2006
    363.34'97—dc22
                                                2005005147
Additional photo credits appear on page 286, which constitutes a continuation of the copyright page.

Printed in the United States of America
09 08 07 06 05   10 9 8 7 6 5 4 3 2 1

BRIEF CONTENTS

CONTENTS

PREVIEW

The *Weapons of Mass Casualties and Terrorism Response Handbook* is the ultimate resource on weapons of mass destruction for all levels of emergency care providers, covering emergency care of injuries and illnesses resulting from weapons of mass casualties.

Comprehensive information geared to both prehospital and in-hospital providers, with all text pertaining to inhospital providers distinctly marked

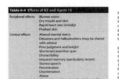

Separate 4-color insert containing full-color photos of medical symptoms

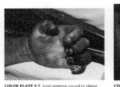
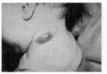
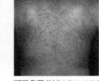
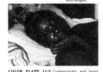

Six different boxed features throughout the text:

- **Incidents in Terrorism**—providing background on terrorist events involving weapons of mass casualties
- **Incidents Involving Chemicals**—providing background on non-terrorist incidents involving chemicals
- **Incidents Involving Biological Agents**—providing background on non-terrorist incidents involving biological agents
- **Incidents Involving Toxins**—providing background on events involving toxins
- **Incidents Involving Radiation**—providing background on events involving radiation
- **Incidents Involving Power**—providing background on events involving power supply

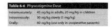
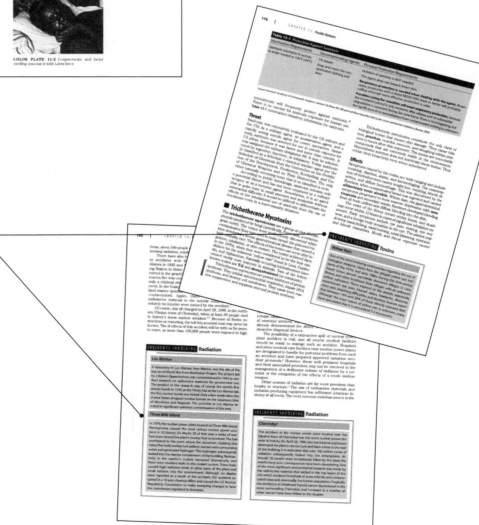

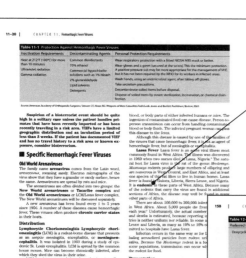

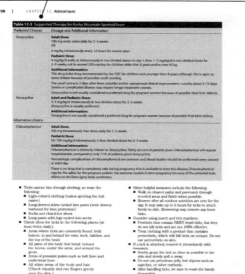

Vocabulary terms are bolded and defined throughout the text and a glossary provides ready-reference to key terms

Tables outlining protection methods, toxin exposure routes, effects, suggested therapies, and medication doses

In-text photos and illustrations depicting examples of autoinjectors, antidote kits, dispersal methods and tools, protective gear, and mass casualty incidents

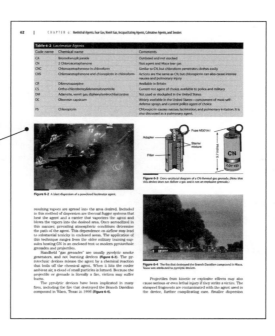

ACKNOWLEDGMENTS

Contributors

This was a massive effort spanning over 5 years. Many, many people read, commented, and helped with these chapters. Significant contributions were made by:

George Bizzigotti, PhD
Mitretek Systems, Inc.
Falls Church, VA

Kim Blake, RN

Bryan E. Bledsoe, DO FACEP
Adjunct Professor, Emergency Medicine
The George Washington University Medical Center
Washington, DC

R. Ranger Dorn
Ventura County Fire Department

Donell Harvin, MPH, MPA, NREMT-P
NYC EMS
New York, NY

Guy Haskell, PhD, NREMT-P
Director, Emergency Medical and Safety Services Consultants
Paramedic, Bedford Regional Medical Center EMS

Colleen Hayes, MBA, RN, EMT-P
Chief Executive Officer of Vertical Villages, Inc. and Editor-in-Chief of EMSvillage.com

Dexter W. Hunt, MEd, EMT-P
The Hunt Group
Boise, ID

Lou Jordan
Public Information Officer, Fire Police Officer, Union Bridge (MD) Fire Department

Kaylan Lyndell-Lees, EMT
Charles Stewart & Associates

Paul M. Maniscalco PhD(c), MPA, EMT-P
Adjunct Assistant Professor The George Washington University School of Medicine and Health Sciences; Deputy Chief, FDNY, EMS Command (ret.)

Louis N. Molino, Sr, CET
FF/NREMT-B/FSI/EMSI
Technical Editor, Industrial Fire World
Fire Protection Consultant/Training Specialist, Fire and Safety Specialists, Inc.

Michelle R. Mulberry, RN, BSN
Asst. Nurse Manager, Emergency Dept
United Medical Center, Cheyenne, WY
Capt., Wyoming Air National Guard

Robert G. Nixon, MBA, EMT-P
President, LifeCare Medical Training
Auburn, MA
Manager, Clinical Education and Domestic Preparedness
American Medical Response
New Haven, CT

Kenneth Phillips, PAC

Norm Rooker, EMT-P
Chief, Ouray County EMS

David Spiro, EMT-P
Director of Public Relations and Development
Blackfriars Theatre
Rochester, NY
Former Director of Pre-Hospital Care, St. Mary's Hospital of Brooklyn
Former QA/QI Coordinator, Catholic Medical Centers of New York (Now St. Vincent's/ Catholic Medical Centers.)

Bob Stewart, EMT-P
Regional Medical Response System Director
Lawton, OK

M. Kathleen Stewart, MSCIS, MSLA, EMT
Charles Stewart & Associates

Reviewers

Richard Alcorta, MD
State EMS Director
Maryland Institute for Emergency Medical Services Systems
Baltimore, MD

Daniel Doherty, NREMT-P
Captain, Albany Fire Department
Albany, NY

Bill Doss, Paramedic/Firefighter
Miami Township Fire and EMS
Clermont County, OH

Kim A. Jones, RN, EMT
Emergency Management, Leadership, Education, and
Development
Norco, CA

Paul J. Kapsar Jr, RN, MSN, CRNP
Instructor, Disaster and Mass Casualty Care
University of Pittsburgh School of Nursing
Pittsburgh, PA

Gene LaFavor, REMT-P
Lycoming County Department of Public Safety
Montoursville, PA

John L. Morrissey, NREMT-P
New York State Department of Health EMS Bureau
Syracuse, NY

Ronald L. Owsianny, NREMT-B
Milwaukee Area Technical College
Milwaukee, WI

Joe Pishioneri, Special Services Officer, DS II
Chemical, Impact, and Electronic Weapons Specialist
Lane County Sheriff's Office
Eugene, OR

Stephanie Raby, RN
Riverside County Department of Public Health
Riverside, CA

John Rinard
Texas Engineering Extension Service
College Station, TX

Dennis L. Rubin
Fire Chief
City of Atlanta Department of Fire
Atlanta, GA

Dr. Raymond Schleif, MMSc, ScD, NREMT
Training Institute for Medical Emergencies and Rescue
Staten Island, NY

Special Thanks

Janet Morris, Elizabeth Peterson, Scarlett Stoppa, Kimberly Potvin, Carol Brewer, Donnell Harvin, Kim Brophy . . . and the rest of the crew at Jones and Bartlett who advised, guided, edited, cajoled, and slugged it out with me about the book!

And, of course, my very most sincere thanks to my dearest, Kathleen Stewart, who read every single word of this book—several times—contributed thoughts to most of the chapters, and wrote the bulk of the chapter bearing her name . . . Without her, I'd be lost . . . and very lonely.

Introduction

■ Introduction

Chemical and biological weapons are weapons of terror and intimidation more than they are lethal weapons. They cause panic out of proportion to the casualties that they produce.

This is a book about weapons of mass casualties. Although many authors lump chemical and biological weapons with nuclear weapons and conventional terrorism as weapons of mass destruction, weapons of mass casualties do not necessarily cause mass destruction as well. There was little destruction associated with the many casualties resulting from the incident in **Bhopal**, India, the influenza epidemic of 1915 and 1916, smallpox, **Lassa fever**, or even the anthrax releases in 1979 and 2001. Instead of causing mass destruction, these weapons cause fearsome casualties, society-paralyzing panic, and emergency situations that may overwhelm all available medical facilities and surviving providers, but these weapons may be chosen particularly because they avoid any significant destruction of property.

The **Aum Shinrikyo** experience in the Tokyo subway showed that at least 70% of casualties presenting to the emergency departments had no symptoms of nerve agent exposure and were discharged. Israel experienced a similar pattern in response to Iraqi scud attacks. Any American experience is quite likely to produce similar "noncasualty" figures, as patients flock to emergency departments to get checked.

The events of September 11, 2001, in New York City and Washington, DC, and the spread of anthrax in the US postal system have brought home the threat of bioterrorism. The terrorists who engineered September 11 have studied in depth the abilities of chemical and biological agents to wreak havoc on the innocent. For these terrorists, the possession of chemical weapons is close at hand. In 1997, Secretary of Defense William Cohen identified Libya, Iraq, Iran, and Syria as countries that were aggressively seeking nuclear, biological, and chemical weapons. Indeed, Iraq and Iran have already used chemical weapons on each other and on the Kurdish population.

Chemical warfare is not a pleasant topic, but the potential of chemical warfare agents should be of overwhelming concern to civilian emergency physicians and prehospital providers. As General Pershing warned after World War I, ". . . the effect is so deadly to the unprepared that we can never afford to neglect the question."

Although a wide range of chemical weapons has been used in prior conflicts, government-sponsored education has concentrated on the small number of agents developed by the

INCIDENTS INVOLVING Chemicals

Bhopal, India

The crowded city of Bhopal, India, was the site of one of the most tragic accidental mass gas exposures in history. On December 3, 1984, a holding tank at the Union Carbide pesticide factory overheated and exploded. As a result, 65 gases, including hydrogen cyanide and methyl isocyanate, were released into the environment. Over 5,000 people were killed in the three days immediately following the explosion, and thousands more have died of exposure since. Even to this day, the survivors have been left with a number of devastating symptoms, ranging from neurologic disorders and early cataracts to panic attacks and depression.

INCIDENTS IN Terrorism

Aum Shinrikyo

A deadly nerve gas attack by a nonmilitary group occurred at the hands of the Aum Shinrikyo cult, a Japanese doomsday sect. During the height of the morning rush hour on March 25, 1995, Aum Shinrikyo members deposited plastic sacks of cult-produced **sarin** in a crowded Tokyo subway. The sarin, a highly volatile nerve agent originally developed in Nazi Germany, quickly evaporated and spread within the subway. Twelve people died as a result of the attacks, and over 5,000 were evaluated in emergency departments. Aum Shinrikyo also orchestrated another sarin gas release in Matsumoto, Japan, in June of 1994. The Matsumoto attack left 7 people dead and over 200 injured.

September 11, 2001

On the morning of September 11, 2001, followers of Osama bin Laden orchestrated one of the most devastating acts of terrorist violence the modern world has ever seen. Members of bin Laden's Al Qaeda network hijacked four passenger aircraft. At 8:46 AM, United Airlines Flight 11 hit the North Tower of the World Trade Center in New York City; 17 minutes later, United Airlines Flight 175 crashed into the South Tower. Also that morning, American Airlines Flight 77 crashed into the Pentagon, and United Airlines Flight 93 went down over rural Pennsylvania. As a result of the hijackings, more than 3,000 people lost their lives, two of the largest US cities suffered substantial physical damage, and an entire nation became tragically aware of the frightening reality of terrorism.

military that are thought to be useful to an aggressor or terrorist. Much money and effort has been allocated to deter and detect the use of these military agents, as well as to develop antidotes for and protection against them should they be used. These agents may be considered

likely terrorist agents because they have been well studied, discussed, and warned about by the media and the government alike. As such, they could easily provoke a significant panic response from the public and possibly the government.

This review will cover a wider spectrum of potential terrorist agents (including agents the military has discarded as being outmoded but that still may wreak havoc on an unprepared populace).

■ History

Poison gases have been used as early as 423 BC when burning wax, pitch, and sulfur were used in wars between the Athenians and Spartans.[1] The smoke from the burning mixture was introduced into a fort through a hollowed-out log. The Greeks continued to develop burning chemical mixtures and invented **Greek fire** during the seventh century AD. This burning mixture floated on water and lent itself to naval engagements.

The development of modern inorganic and organic chemistry during the 18th, 19th, and early 20th centuries generated both an interest in the ethics of using chemical warfare and an interest in chemicals as weapons. This interest ranged from a proposal to use burning ships laden with sulfur (the British Admiralty quashed this idea as being "against the rules of warfare") to chlorine-filled shells to be used by the Union against the Confederacy (not employed but obviously quite workable).

The European states signed the Treaty of the Hague in 1899, a vaguely worded agreement that excluded the use of ammunition containing poisonous gases. Despite this treaty, chemical warfare was used extensively in World War I by both sides, with devastating effects against unprepared and unprotected troops **(Figure 1-1)**.[2] **Sulfur mustard**, for example, caused five times as many casualties as either high explosives or shrapnel.[3] These agents were more incapacitating than lethal, however, with death from chemical weapons found in only 7% of casualties. This is about four times lower than the death-to-casualty ratio that is common with conventional munitions.

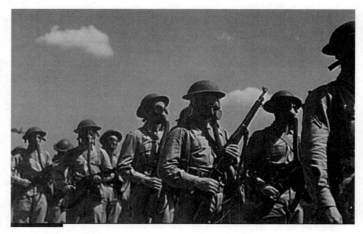

Figure 1-1 US military training in gas masks circa 1917.

Popular belief maintains that chemical weapons were first launched by the Imperial German Army in the form of chlorine gas against the Allies on April 22, 1915 at Ypres, Belgium.[4] In actuality, both sides used chemical weapons extensively in the months preceding this assault. In fact, several belligerents in World War I used shells filled with irritants from nearly the start of World War I. The French first used shells filled with **ethyl bromoacetate** in August 1914, less than one month into the war. The French then used **chloroacetone** in the French arsenal in November 1914. On October 27, 1914, the Germans at Neuve-Chappelle used the "Ni-Schrapnell" 105-mm shell, which consisted of lead balls embedded in powdered o-dianisidine chlorosulfonate. On January 31, 1915, at Boloimow, the Germans introduced 150-mm shells filled with "T-Stoff," a mixture of brominated aromatics including xylyl bromide, xylylene bromide, and benzyl bromide. All of these compounds are extreme irritants capable of severely limiting the effectiveness of unprotected troops.[5]

It should be no surprise that heavily industrialized Germany made the first large-scale use of these weapons of mass casualties. During the time of World War I, Germany had a large scientific base of both theoretical and applied chemistry and the capacity to mass-produce these chemicals.

During World War II, no chemical agents were used in combat, but the Germans used chemical weapons extensively in the genocidal killing of millions of Jews. The Italians sprayed **phosgene** and **mustard gas** on parts of Ethiopia from 1935 to 1936. The Japanese used mustard gas when invading China in 1938. In addition, both Russia and the Allies built extensive stocks of many different chemical agents for possible use during the conflict. These stocks remain in stockpiles today in various stages of decomposition **(Figure 1-2)**.

Not all of these stockpiles are known. Over 40,000 tons of chemical weapons are stored in officially declared military depots in Russia. The declared stockpile consists of 32,200 tons of nerve gases and 7,700 tons of **Lewisite** (a blister-forming agent similar to mustard and discussed in detail in Chapter 5 on vesicant agents), but there is evidence that mustard gas and other mixtures have also been stored. Thousands of other chemical bombs may be found in abandoned and uncharted weapons dumps.[6] The allies discarded 32,000 tons of mustard shells in the North Sea. These munitions are decomposing and occasionally surface and cause injuries to seamen in the area.

The Iraqis have shown a particular interest in chemical weapons **(Figure 1-3)**. They built "nylon" bombs and tricresyl-phosphate bombs. As noted earlier, both sides used mustard gas in the Iran–Iraq conflict from 1980 to 1988. The Iraqis also used typhus, cholera, and mycotoxins. All of these were used both against Iran and internally against the Kurds. Perhaps their worst weapon was a combination bomb with a mix of hydrogen cyanide, mustard gas, and nerve gas. This had a 60% fatality rate when used against the Kurds in 1985.[7]

It is obvious that despite active attempts of many countries to outlaw production of these agents, they are available in large quantities. Because some potential military adversaries continue to maintain large stocks of these agents and train under realistic conditions with these agents, it is likely that they will be used in future conflicts.

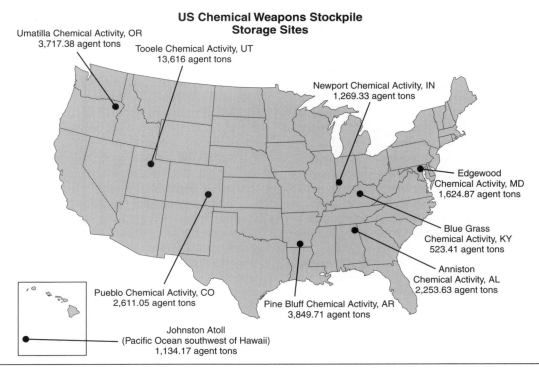

US Chemical Weapons Stockpile Storage Sites

Umatilla Chemical Activity, OR
3,717.38 agent tons

Tooele Chemical Activity, UT
13,616 agent tons

Newport Chemical Activity, IN
1,269.33 agent tons

Edgewood Chemical Activity, MD
1,624.87 agent tons

Blue Grass Chemical Activity, KY
523.41 agent tons

Anniston Chemical Activity, AL
2,253.63 agent tons

Pueblo Chemical Activity, CO
2,611.05 agent tons

Pine Bluff Chemical Activity, AR
3,849.71 agent tons

Johnston Atoll
(Pacific Ocean southwest of Hawaii)
1,134.17 agent tons

Figure 1-2 US chemical weapons stockpile storage sites.

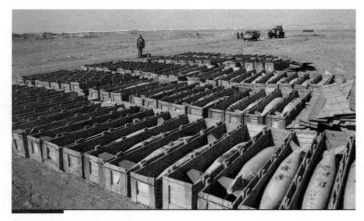

Figure 1-3 Iraqi chemical weapons.

Terrorist Actions

Important to the EMS professional, physician, and the poison control center is the possibility that a terrorist group might employ these agents. Even though the military has control of the agents in most countries, it is quite possible that terrorist groups could gain access to them. It is also within the realm of possibility that a state sponsor could simply give some terrorist groups these weapons. In addition, chemical warfare agents are easily synthesized from readily available chemicals. Terrorist operations, such as Aum Shinrikyo, can simply make their own. Osama bin Laden, the leader of at least one major terrorist group (Al Qaeda), has announced on television that he has stockpiles of both nuclear and chemical weapons, has demonstrated use of chemical agent research on animals, and has advocated the use of chemical agents. Although events in 2001 in Afghanistan have diminished this as a probability, Al Qaeda's use of these agents in terrorist acts remains a distinct possibility.

As noted earlier, history suggests that in military settings chemical weapons injure far more people than they kill. On the Western Front in World War I, it took an average of one ton of chemical agent to kill a single soldier. Only 2% to 3% of those exposed to gas in World War I actually died. Overall, gas was responsible for no more than 5% of casualties in the war. In Iraq's war against Iran, 27,000 Iranians were exposed to gas and only 265 died through March 1987.

It makes sense that chemical weapons tend to injure rather than kill in military settings, because it takes massive amounts of chemical agents to produce military casualties in open areas with any reliability. Maximizing military casualties with chemical agents has occupied scores of scientists in multiple countries and has proven to be a formidable task. Even with the nerve agents, the amount of chemical needed to produce heavy casualties in an unprotected population in a 1-km^2 open area is measured in tons. Clearly, even state-sponsored terrorists are unlikely to be able to import or manufacture military chemicals in this quantity.

Chemical warfare was very successfully used as a terror weapon by the military in World War I to instill confusion and panic among the enemy prior to an offensive. It was an effective psychological weapon when used in this fashion. This panic was created even among trained soldiers who were equipped with the best protection of the times and were expecting a chemical weapon attack. When the nonlethal tearing agents were used, they caused as much panic in World War I as the dreaded mustard gas.

One can look at the Japanese experience to see the results of a similar attack in an unprepared public. The two episodes of sarin exposure in Japan in 1994 and 1995 resulted in relatively few casualties yet still caused extreme panic in the public. There is no question that terrorists can easily use chemical or biological weapons to cause this kind of terror among civilians.

A problem in enlisting military planners as consultants in planning for an EMS response to terrorist events is that military planners tend to think of delivery of these weapons in military terms—as efficient operations involving large quantities of agents. However, the small-scale use of an agent would be effective in that it would cause widespread fear and panic. This panic was quite evident during the subway attack in Tokyo and during the 1996 Olympic bombing (which was completely conventional) in Atlanta.

The multiple pronouncements and counter-pronouncements associated with anthrax letter hoaxes prior to the 2001 anthrax letters is a very good example of this military thinking. Military planners assured government leaders (prior to the anthrax letters) that it was very difficult to build the technology to disseminate anthrax spores and cause any significant damage. These planners felt that anthrax would come from a state entity or state-sponsored terrorist movement and would involve the use of large amounts of high-quality (military-grade) agents. Perhaps the most famous assumption was the one offered by the Secretary of Defense on ABC-TV's *This Week*. Holding a 5-lb bag of sugar, the secretary indicated that such a quantity of anthrax would be needed to kill half the population of Washington, DC.

In one sense, the Secretary was absolutely correct; only a very small amount was needed to cause a monumental incident. As a consequence to the anthrax letters in 2001, the postal system was markedly degraded and the populace frightened with only a few letters and less than an ounce of anthrax spores. The media coverage of our governmental leaders and their uncoordinated responses during the 2001 anthrax letter investigations did little to assuage a frightened public.

An underlying presumption of many planners is that the United States will be attacked on a much grander scale. Strangely enough, the military's own research shows that small-scale attacks can be quite effective. Research such as the experiment in which lightbulbs were filled with harmless spores and dropped into the subway system in New York City in the 1960s clearly shows that a small amount of these agents can be rapidly and widely disseminated without the advantage of high-level technology or large quantities of agents.

Chemical agents can be quite effective in small quantities if used in relatively closed areas with significant

The Washington, DC Snipers

In October 2002, the Washington, DC area was the scene of a terrifying string of random shootings. After killing ten people and injuring three others, John Mohammed and his stepson, John Lee Malvo, were arrested at a rest stop. The pair allegedly used a .223 caliber Bushmaster XM-15 rifle to prey on their unsuspecting victims. Mohammed and Malvo are also being investigated for a number of other shootings in various parts of the country.

civilian traffic. Tunnels, subways, metro trains, auditoriums, sports arenas, and theaters are all potential targets for military or improvisational chemical agents. Mustard gas and nerve agents can persist for long periods and could suspend the use of airports, water supplies, bridges, and even highways. If released in a large building or stadium, the residual effects of these agents could render the building or stadium unusable for decades.

Governmental security planners should not be surprised if very small quantities of lethal agents are used in terrorist operations again. A likely scenario is that of a small amount of a common agent released in an area that evokes the maximum amount of public response and terror, such as the Japanese experience in the Tokyo subway. As the Japanese Aum Shinrikyo incident clearly showed, high technology and military-grade agents are simply not needed to make a substantial impact on the populace, the media, and law enforcement. Simultaneous releases of small amounts of agent in disparate parts of the country would provoke widespread panic and would cause a rapid overtaxation of chemically-trained and biologically-trained law enforcement experts and local supplies. As the experience with two snipers in the Washington, DC area showed, two terrorists can easily paralyze a widespread metropolitan area's law enforcement resources.

Manufacture of these lethal agents in small quantities is not difficult and does not take much chemical knowledge beyond college level chemistry. Theoretically, **precursor chemicals** are controlled, and defense analysts assure us that the federal government monitors every teaspoonful of potential weapons material. In actual fact, diversion of small quantities of these chemicals is easy, and at least one writer has obtained (by mail order) all of the chemicals needed to manufacture a small quantity of sarin.[8] The federal restrictions only apply when large quantities trigger an investigation or when the chemicals are destined for export. Modern pesticide-producing plants can manufacture nerve agents, while **ethylene** and **sulfurated petrochemicals** may be combined in the **Levinstein process** to produce sulfur mustard gas.[9]

If mass quantities of chemicals are to be used in a terrorist incident, it is likely that the terrorist will turn to the use of precursors or industrial chemicals to produce improvisational chemical warfare agents. There is a wide range of chemicals that the military considers unsuitable for use as chemical warfare agents that have significant application as agents of terrorism. With high volatility, readily available industrial compounds like phosgene, chlorine, hydrogen sulfide, and hydrogen cyanide could be used effectively in a confined area such as a subway or building. Releases of ammonia and chlorine in the civilian world have forced the evacuation of hundreds of families in recent times. The devastation of Bhopal, India from the accidental release of toxic gas on an unprepared civilian population has been well chronicled. With the exception of the use of cyanide, phosgene, and chlorine in World War I, none of these gases has a military application or designation.

Because these agents are shipped on our railways in tank cars and on our highways in tank trucks, there is a very real possibility that these agents could be diverted for a terrorist operation. An act of sabotage on a tank car or tank truck in a downtown middle-American city could rapidly discharge tons of potentially lethal chemicals. Fire fighter and hazardous materials crews are simply not trained to mitigate the sudden deliberate release of excessive amounts of vapor by explosive devices, along with potential booby-trapping and subsequent secondary explosions. Furthermore, if a few snipers were stationed in appropriate locations around the release, the fire fighters and law enforcement officers would not only be ineffective, they would likely become casualties. In theory, the tragedy at Bhopal could be brought to the US homelands as an act of terrorism.

The recent use of toxic chemical agents in the Tokyo and other Japanese subways mandates chemical preparedness by civilian medical providers **(Figure 1-4)**. The chemical tragedy at Bhopal should convince any reluctant emergency provider and physician that preparedness is necessary, even when no terrorists are involved **(Figure 1-5)**.

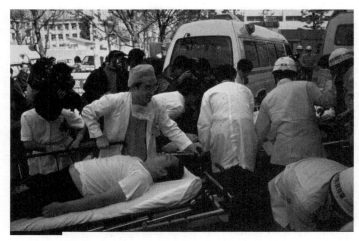

Figure 1-4 Evacuation of a Tokyo subway casualty.

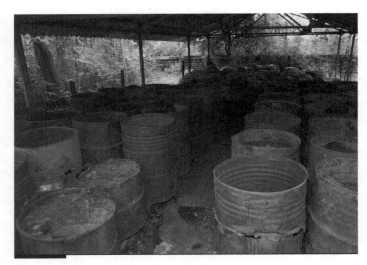

Figure 1-5 Abandoned Bhopal chemical factory.

■ Terminology

Chemical agents may come in a solid, liquid, or gaseous form, depending on the temperature. Most military chemical agents are dispersed as liquids or an aerosol (very small particles or droplets in a gas). Tear gas, for example, is not a gas at all, but an aerosolized solid. Mustard gas is also not a gas, but a liquid that may or may not evaporate (again, depending on the temperature). Remember that a vapor is the gaseous form of a substance that exists at a lower temperature than the boiling point of the gas. Sarin, with a vapor pressure close to that of water, will evaporate and generally be a vapor or *true* nerve gas.

Another method of chemical agent classification is whether the agent is **persistent** or **nonpersistent**. Persistency is used to describe how long an area remains contaminated at a level of toxicity that is dangerous to humans after a chemical agent has been employed. Thus, an agent is called persistent if the area in which it was used remains contaminated for about a day or more. Some persistent chemical agents such as mustard and **VX** do not easily evaporate and tend to render terrain or property unusable until they are dispersed or decontaminated.

Volatility and persistence are inversely related. A substance is more volatile if it evaporates quickly. A nonpersistent or volatile agent disperses quickly, sometimes in a matter of minutes or hours. Lewisite, cyanide, ammonia, chlorine, tearing agents, and sarin are nonpersistent agents. Nonpersistent agents present less risk of contamination to EMS or hospital providers. (These generalizations are subject to temperature, wind, and some surface characteristics.)

To make a nonpersistent agent persistent, thickeners can be added. As a result of the additional chemical additive, the agent becomes more difficult to destroy by certain means. In general, the more persistent an agent is, the more decontamination is required. Such agents will present significant dangers to the EMS providers at the scene of the initial contamination and may well cause contamination of ambulances and even emergency departments.

There are also some specific terms regarding dose that should be noted. The **LD$_{50}$**, or median lethal dose, represents the dose of a drug that will be fatal to 50% of the population. A counterpart exists for incapacitating agents: the **ID$_{50}$**, or median incapacitating dose, represents the dose that will incapacitate 50% of the population. Lastly, the **ED$_{50}$**, or median effect dose, represents the dose that will have an effect on 50% of the population.

Since the concept of dose applies only to injected, absorbed, or ingested chemicals, another term was devised for inhalation agents. This is the concentration time product, or **C•t**, often simply expressed as Ct. C•t refers to the agent concentration (usually measured in milligrams per cubed meter) multiplied by the time of exposure in minutes. Exposure of a concentration of 10 **mg/m^3** of **tabun** for 5 minutes results in a C•t of 50 mg•min/m^3. Exposure of a concentration of 5 mg/m^3 of tabun for 10 minutes also results in a C•t of 50 mg•min/m^3. For almost all chemical vapors and gases, the C•t associated with a specific biological effect is relatively constant even though the concentration and time may vary (within some limits). This means that a 10-minute exposure to 5 mg/m^3, a 5-minute exposure to 10 mg/m^3, and a 1-minute exposure to 50 mg/m^3 will all have about the same effect on the unprotected patient.

The EC•t$_{50}$, IC•t$_{50}$, and LC•t$_{50}$ correspond to the ingested ED$_{50}$, ID$_{50}$, and LD$_{50}$ respectively. The concentration time product does not take respiratory rate and depth into account. The exercising person will have a different exposure than the sedentary person. This difference may be significant at lower concentrations, but at high concentrations, there may be little difference between the two subjects.

■ Recognizing the Presence of Chemical Agents

Early identification of a terrorist event is critical to the protection of emergency providers and enhances the ability of these providers to save the lives of those affected by the attack. This early identification requires rapid analysis of clues from the environment, scrutiny of 9-1-1 calls, and close attention to indicators noted by law enforcement officers, fire fighters, EMS responders, and other knowledgeable observers.

In the Environment

The emergency responder must always be aware of the environment. If the emergency responder finds dead or dying animals in the area, the use of chemical agents should be suspected **(Figure 1-6)**. Chemicals that injure humans will usually affect animals, although sometimes in different ways and at different rates than humans. If animals seem to be dying at the same time without obvious cause, this suggests a chemical attack. Birds and small mammals are often more sensitive indicators than humans. (In the past, miners carried canaries into the mines as crude detectors of toxic gas.)

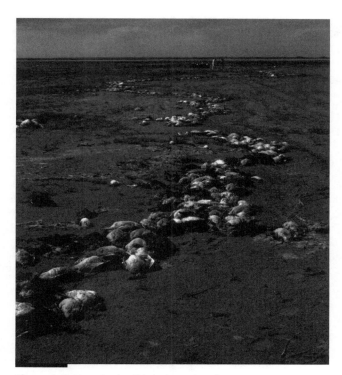

Figure 1-6 Mass death of birds due to botulism.

Likewise, multiple dead insects or the absence of insects may be a clue that chemical agents are in the area. Most of the chemical agents used as weapons against humans will also kill insects. Remember that the nerve agents were developed from pesticide research and may act so rapidly that large numbers of dead insects may be seen on the ground.

Dead plants may also be a clue that a toxic chemical is present. Some toxic chemicals will rapidly destroy plant life, so unusual patterns of dead grass, flowers, and the like may indicate dissemination of chemical warfare agents. This is usually a late finding, however, and may not be as helpful as mass deaths of insects and animals.

9-1-1 Calls

The first source of information about a terrorist event is likely to be emergency calls to 9-1-1. 9-1-1 operators may be alerted by any of the following:

- Numerous calls reporting similar signs or symptoms (often from a contiguous area)
- A large volume of calls reporting sick or injured people with no apparent cause
- Calls with symptoms indicative of a chemical agent exposure (such as drooling; tearing; shortness of breath; difficulty breathing; irritations of the eyes, nose, and throat; and reddening, burning, itching, or blistering of the skin)

Casualties

When an emergency provider notes a large number of casualties with similar symptoms, deployment of a chemical agent should be suspected. The release of a chemical agent will usu-

ally produce a group of casualties at locations near the release. Those who were closer or have had increased exposure would be expected to have the earliest and worst symptoms, while those on the periphery would have relatively minor symptoms. Exceptions to this are the mustard agents and some pulmonary agents (such as phosgene and PFIB). Due to the 4- to 6-hour latent period between exposure and the appearance of symptoms for mustard and these pulmonary agents, it is possible that casualties would appear in the emergency department over a period of several hours. These patients may initially complain of relatively minor symptoms.

The emergency provider should be aware that any sudden increase in the following nonspecific syndromes might indicate low-level exposure to a chemical agent.

- Sudden unexplained weakness in a previously healthy individual
- Hypersecretion syndrome such as drooling, tearing, diarrhea
- Eye pain and difficulty focusing
- Irritation of eyes, nose, throat, and membranes
- Skin reactions such as burns, redness, blisters or vesicles, itching, and sloughing

The emergency provider should also be aware that chemical agents may cause casualties in a distinctive pattern. Chemicals that have been disseminated as vapors or aerosols will move with the wind or air currents. Usually these chemicals will produce a sequential appearance of casualties as successive victims are exposed to the chemical agent in the air current. Although this may be most common in a release outside, release in a building will also follow the airflow within the structure.

Chemicals disseminated as vapors or aerosols inside a structure will affect those entering the structure, while those who remain outside of the structure will be spared. Those who spend only a short time in the structure would likely have the least symptoms. A good example of this was found in the pattern of those people exposed to sarin vapor in the Tokyo subway in 1995.

Other Signs of Chemical Agents
Odors

Odors should be considered unreliable detectors of chemical agents. Not only are many toxic chemicals unidentifiable by any distinctive odor, but also those that do produce a noticeable odor may not be noticed until toxins have already taken effect. Nonetheless, some agents do have distinctive odors. If the emergency provider does encounter an unusual odor, the provider should stay away from the area until the scene has been evaluated with appropriate detection devices and appropriate protective gear is available (and worn by those entering).

Unexplained Material or Equipment

If the provider finds unexplained liquid droplets or puddles (for example, inside an auditorium or shopping mall or where no sprinkling activity has occurred), this may be an indication that a chemical weapon has been deployed. Likewise, unexplained dust or powders may be an indicator of chemical agent use.

Spraying activity in inappropriate areas should also trigger an investigation. There would be no reason for a crop duster to fly over a residential area or for a lawn service to deploy a sprayer in a parking lot. Additionally, if the EMS provider finds abandoned spraying or dusting equipment, it should be investigated.

Explosive devices that seem to misfire or explode weakly and scatter liquids or solids may represent the deployment of a chemical agent with explosives. The liquid or solid may be a chemical agent. Bomb disposal responders in such a case should be appropriately garbed for a chemical agent attack.

Discarded antidote injectors or personal protective equipment (PPE), such as masks, gloves, and suits, may indicate the need for an investigation of the area. Containers with hazardous materials labels or stickers, pressurized gas cylinders, or containers of liquids in inappropriate locations would also indicate possible use of an agent.

Remember, in any incident involving a chemical or an explosive device, there may be additional devices set for later times to injure emergency responders and law enforcement personnel.

■ References

1. Hu H, Fine J, Epstein P, et al: Tear gas: Harassing agent or toxic chemical weapon? *JAMA* 1989;262:660-664.
2. Eckert WG: Mass deaths by gas or chemical poisoning. *Am J Forens Med Path* 1991;12:119-125.
3. Clark R: *The Silent Weapons*. New York, NY, David McKay, 1968.
4. *Gas Shell Bombardment of Ypres*. London, Public Record Office, July 12-13, 1917.
5. History of Chemical Warfare page. Mitretek Systems Web site. Available at: http://www.mitretek.org/home.nsf/Homeland Security/HistChemWar (accessed March 3, 2003).
6. Hoffman D: Cold war report: Russia's forgotten chemical weapons. WashingtonPost.com; August 16, 1998.
7. Heyndrickx A: Chemical warfare injuries. *Lancet* 1991;337:430.
8. Musser G: Better killing through chemistry. *Scientific American*, http://www.sciam.com/explorations/2001/110501sarin/index.html (accessed February 19, 2002).
9. Murphy S: Chemical warfare: The present position. *Med War* 1985;1:31-39.

Cyanide and Other Tissue Toxins

■ Introduction

The "blood agents" or tissue toxins act by destroying the ability of the blood and tissues to carry or process oxygen. Cyanide is the prototype agent in this group. These agents have long been considered a threat for use in terrorism. Cyanide compounds were used as adulterants in packages of Tylenol analgesic in 1982 in the Chicago area.[1] Cyanide-laced drinks were used for the mass suicide of the Reverend Jim Jones' People's Temple in Guyana in 1978.[2] Cyanide gas precursor compounds were found in several subway restrooms in Tokyo following the release of sarin in Tokyo in 1995.[3] Though unconfirmed, cyanide may have been added to the explosives used in the first attack in 1993 on the World Trade Center in New York City.[4]

■ Cyanide

Cyanide (CN) was identified by the Swedish chemist Scheele in 1782. **Hydrogen cyanide** (HCN) is a colorless liquid whose vapor is lighter than air and dissipates rapidly. The fastest route of poisoning is through inhalation **(Table 2-1)**. Both gaseous and liquid hydrogen cyanide, as well as cyanide salts in solution, can also be absorbed through the skin or ingested.

Cyanide gas is famous as the lethal agent used for executions in many states. Hydrogen cyanide is usually included among the agents of chemical weapons produced to cause general poisoning. Compounds containing cyanide have been stocked by some nations for use as chemical warfare agents.

Cyanide was used in World War I, but, because it is lighter than air and is highly volatile, it did not prove to be as successful as chlorine. The tissue toxins were abandoned as war agents during World War I because they were considered to be too volatile in open air and required high concentrations for effectiveness. Furthermore, the munitions delivering them were crude, and protection against their effects was too simple. However, it has been reported that hydrogen cyanide was used by Iraq in the war against Iran and against the Kurds in northern Iraq during the 1980s. During World War II, a form of hydrogen cyanide (Zyklon B) was used in the Nazi gas chambers.[5]

The NATO military designators for the cyanide compounds used in warfare are as follows:
- AC (hydrogen cyanide [HCN])
- CK (cyanogen chloride [CNCL])

INCIDENTS IN Terrorism

Cyanide-Laced Tylenol Capsules

In 1982, terror was infused into the minds of American consumers after seven Chicago-area residents died from taking Extra-Strength Tylenol capsules that had been injected with a massive dose of cyanide. Each Tylenol capsule was found to be laced with 65 mg of cyanide, which is thousands of times greater than the minimal amount of the poison needed to kill a person. No one has ever been convicted of this crime.

The 1993 World Trade Center Bombing

Eight years before the September 11, 2001, terrorist attacks demolished the World Trade Center towers, another terrorist act inflicted substantial damage to the Twin Towers and the psyche of a complacent United States. On February 26, 1993, the World Trade Center was rocked by a blast on the second floor of the parking basement, killing 6 people and injuring 1,000 more. The homemade explosive device, which was placed in the back of a rented van, was made of more than one ton of fertilizer-based explosives. In 1994, four men with ties to terrorist organizations were convicted of the bombing.

INCIDENTS INVOLVING Chemicals

The Jim Jones Massacre

Perhaps no case of intentional cyanide poisoning is more widely known than the horrific incident that occurred in Jonestown, Guyana. Led by the charismatic Jim Jones, the People's Temple religious sect had moved to French Guyana after coming under heavy scrutiny in the United States. In 1978, Congressman Leo Ryan and a team of investigators and reporters visited Jonestown to investigate alleged human rights violations at the hands of Jones. Ryan's group, including a number of People's Temple defectors, was ambushed at an airstrip, leaving Ryan, three reporters, and one defector dead. Hours after the ambush, Jones urged his followers to commit suicide and compelled them to drink Kool-Aid soft drink laced with cyanide. Those sect members who refused were either shot or injected with the poison. In all, over 900 people, including Jones, died.

The military incorrectly calls cyanide a blood agent, implying that the action is in the blood when it is, in fact, in the tissues.

Dissemination

These agents may be delivered by munitions from artillery, mortars, bombs, or simply released from canisters. The preferred way to deliver cyanide is by large munitions, because

Table 2-1 Hydrogen Cyanide Toxicity by Inhalation	
Concentration (mg/m³)	Effect
300	Immediately lethal
200	Lethal after 10 minutes
150	Lethal after 30 minutes
120–150	Highly dangerous (fatal) after 30–60 minutes
50–60	Endurable for 20 minutes to 1 hour without effect
20–40	Minimal symptoms after several hours

Adapted from: Ivarsson U, Nilsson H, Santesson J, eds. A *FOA briefing book on chemical weapons—threat, effects, and protection*, No. 16. Umeå, National Defence Research Establishment, 1992.

smaller weapons will not provide the concentration needed for lethal effect. Like all of the chemical warfare agents, the area of action is dependent on weather and wind. As noted earlier, cyanide is not at all persistent and dissipates rapidly.

Sources

Industry in the United States manufactures over 300,000 tons of hydrogen cyanide each year **(Figure 2-1)**. These cyanides are used in chemical processes, **electroplating**, mineral extraction, dye manufacture, printing, photography, and agriculture.

This agent can be readily found in tank cars in large amounts **(Figure 2-2)**. Although it was not found to be particularly effective as a chemical warfare agent in World War I, it could be more useful to terrorists for dissemination in a confined area or enclosed space.

Cyanide is also found in the burning fumes of x-ray film, wool, silk, nylon, paper, **nitriles**, rubber, urethanes, polyurethane, and other plastics. Cigarette smoke contains cyanide, and cyanide levels found in blood are two to three times higher in smokers than in nonsmokers. As a product of combustion, cyanide is commonly mixed with **isocyanates**, which are intense respiratory irritants. The reaction is often limited by temperature.

The effects of cyanide and carbon monoxide (both found in fires) are additive. Both agents contribute to tissue

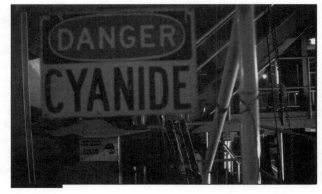

Figure 2-1 Cyanide is manufactured for use in various industries.

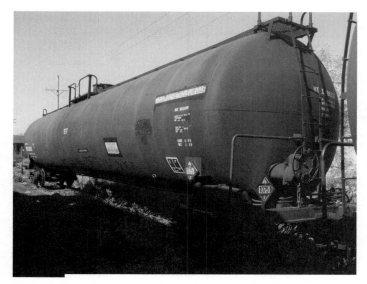

Figure 2-2 Cyanide is readily found in tank cars in large amounts.

Table 2-2 Adult Lethal Doses of Hydrogen Cyanide	
Lethal dose by inhalation	0.5 mg/kg
Lethal dose by ingestion	50 mg
Lethal dose by skin contamination	100 mg/kg

Adapted from: Cyanide AC, CK. United States Army Medical Research Institute of Chemical Defense: Medical Management of Chemical Casualties Handbook, Third Edition available at http://www.vnh.org/CHEMCASU/03Cyanide.html (accessed January 22, 2004).

Lethal hydrogen cyanide doses for various transmission routes are shown in **Table 2-2**.

Symptoms

Despite its reputation in fiction, cyanide is the least toxic of the lethal chemical agents. The symptoms of cyanide poisoning are relatively nonspecific. Inhalation of cyanide agents may cause the following reactions:

1. Dryness and burning of the throat
2. **Air hunger**
3. **Hyperpnea**
4. Tachycardia
5. Audible gasping respirations (in extreme exposures)
6. **Apnea**
7. Seizures and coma
8. Cardiovascular collapse

Early symptoms may include dryness and burning of the throat and air hunger. In small doses, headache, confusion, anxiety, dizziness, nausea, palpitations, tachycardia, tachypnea, and combativeness may all be found.

The most significant clinical manifestations of cyanide poisoning are cerebral and cardiac. In large doses, bradycardia, bradypnea, coma, gasping respirations, apnea, and rapid death may all be common manifestations. High concentrations of cyanide may also cause a gasping reflex. (An audible gasp is thought to be characteristic of extreme exposure to hydrogen cyanide.) High concentrations of cyanide also indirectly stimulate the release of epinephrine with subsequent tachycardia and hypertension. This is followed in 15 to 30 seconds by the onset of convulsions. Respiratory activity stops in 2 to 3 minutes and cardiac activity stops several minutes later.

The initial diagnosis of severe cyanide poisoning is difficult. Cyanide poisoning is an uncommon cause of the clinical presentation of coma, shock, seizures, and metabolic acidosis. The provider should be suspicious of acute cyanide intoxication if the patient has had an abrupt collapse without apparent cause and subsequently does not respond well to oxygen administration.

It should be noted that this sudden collapse that appears to be resistant to oxygen therapy may also be a characteristic response to high levels of nerve agent. Nerve agent exposure may cause **miosis** (contraction of the pupils) and increased nasal, oral, and ocular secretions. Cyanosis is more common with nerve agents than with cyanide exposure. Nerve agent exposure is discussed in detail in Chapter 3.

The diagnosis of hydrogen cyanide poisoning is difficult without a history of exposure. Particularly in the field,

hypoxia by different mechanisms. Many fire-related fatalities are caused by one or both of these chemicals.

Its high volatility and the fact that it is lighter than air makes hydrogen cyanide difficult to use as a terrorist agent, because there are problems in achieving sufficiently high concentrations outdoors. On the other hand, the concentration of hydrogen cyanide may rapidly reach lethal levels if it is released in a confined space. Potassium cyanide poisoning of food and water supplies is an ancient terrorist tactic.

Mechanism of Action

The human body can tolerate low levels of cyanide without harm. Indeed, some cyanide is normally present in the human body. This means that the same amount of cyanide that could kill if administered over a few minutes may be fully metabolized by the body if administered over several hours.

The most important toxic effect of hydrogen cyanide is the interruption of the aerobic cellular metabolism, which causes cellular hypoxia. This leads to a profound lactic acidosis as the body attempts to use anaerobic metabolism, which is less efficient. Subsequent central nervous system, respiratory, and myocardial depressions complicate the picture.

Inhaled hydrogen cyanide can be quite lethal. Exposure to 140 **ppm** for 60 minutes or 1500 ppm for 3 minutes has an estimated 50% mortality rate. For inhalation of large doses of cyanide, the toxic effect of cyanide depends on both the concentration of cyanide in the air inhaled and duration of exposure (C•t). In high concentrations, the C•t determines a specific relationship between the inhaled dose and the effect. The median lethal dose is about 2500 mg•min/m³, and the lethal dose for the most resistant individuals is about twice this level. At low concentrations, the C•t does not apply, because the body can metabolize and thereby detoxify small amounts of cyanide.

without laboratory support, these agents are difficult to identify. There are no specific physical findings that would implicate cyanide. The odor of almonds may be present, but about 50% of people are unable to smell the odor of cyanide.[6]

Cyanide toxicity should be considered in all smoke inhalation victims with central nervous system or cardiovascular findings.[7,8] Poisoning with cyanide should be considered in terrorist events precipitated by conventional explosives or incendiary agents.

Detection and Laboratory Testing

Chemical agent detection equipment such as the **M256A1** can be used to test the environment if such devices are readily available. Unfortunately, these devices often are not available in time.

There is no readily available test that can be performed in "real time" by medical personnel to confirm cyanide poisoning while trying to treat an acutely poisoned patient. **Spectrophotometry** and **gas chromatography** are tools for the pathologist, but not the clinician. A new **semiquantitative assay** that uses calorimetric test strips may improve the laboratory evaluation of hydrogen cyanide poisoning.[9] Before any cyanide level is correlated with a clinical appearance, the elapsed time since the exposure and since the specimen was obtained must be considered.

Arterial blood gases will often show a metabolic acidosis, with normal oxygenation and calculated hemoglobin saturation. Venous gases will show the same pattern, because the oxygen will not be used up at the tissues. Venous blood often looks arterial in color. The measured arterial oxygen saturation will be decreased, while the calculated saturation will be normal.[10]

This picture of an abnormal hemoglobin and less than adequate saturation is found commonly in only four poisons. The **toxidrome** includes cyanide, carbon monoxide, **hydrogen sulfide**, and **methemoglobin**. Methemoglobin and carboxyhemoglobin are easily measured. Hydrogen sulfide and cyanide are treated in a similar manner. Cyanide levels should be obtained in all cases. An elevated anion gap metabolic acidosis may exist but is not diagnostic.

Treatment

There is no worldwide consensus for treatment of cyanide intoxication. The definitive treatment of cyanide intoxication differs in various countries, but only one method is approved for use in the United States.

In moderate and severe cyanide intoxication, the clinical outcome is dependent on both the severity of the exposure and the delay before treatment is started. The success of therapy of acute cyanide intoxication depends primarily on the speed with which the cellular oxygen utilization is restored. Since hypoxia is a major component of this agent's toxicity, cerebral hypoxia and subsequent **encephalopathy** is common in severely poisoned casualties.

The patient should be immediately removed from the contaminated atmosphere. Early use of a protective mask for the patient will also prevent further inhalation. The removal of any liquid on skin or clothing should be performed as soon as possible. The patient's clothing should be removed once the patient has been moved to a safe environment to prevent liquid cyanide from releasing vapors or being absorbed by the patient.

The mainstays of treatment are oxygenation and ventilation. Oxygenation should be a part of supportive care for all patients suspected of cyanide intoxication. There is strong evidence that some patients who have ceased breathing will survive when appropriate respiratory support is given. If the patient still has intact circulation, then airway support and antidote therapy may be lifesaving. Lack of an antidote should not preclude the treatment of these patients with airway support and ventilation. Contaminated clothing must be removed and the skin washed.

Therapy beyond the basics is controversial and includes the classic Lilly cyanide kit, **hyperbaric oxygenation**, and massive doses of vitamin B_{12}. Lilly Research Laboratories has ceased making the Lilly cyanide kit. Today, the cyanide antidote kit is available from one source, Taylor Pharmaceuticals (formerly Pasadena Research Laboratories). For a while, the replacement was called the Pasadena kit after the company that manufactured it. In this text, we will call it the cyanide antidote kit **(Color plate 2-1)**.[11]

Contents of kit:
- Two 10-mL ampules of sodium nitrite—300 mg in 2 mL
- Two 50-mL vials of sodium thiosulfate—12.5 g in 50 mL
- Twelve ampules of amyl nitrite inhalant—5 mg in 0.3 mL
- One sterile 10-mL syringe with needle
- One stomach tube
- One sterile 60-mL syringe
- One sterile needle
- One nonsterile 60-mL syringe
- One tourniquet
- One set of instructions for the treatment of cyanide poisoning

Cyanide Antidote Kit

The US military currently advocates the use of nitrites and thiosulfate for treatment of cyanide intoxication. Sodium nitrite (10 mL of 3% solution) is used intravenously followed by sodium thiosulfate (50 mL of 25% solution). This is the only US-approved antidote to cyanide intoxication.

The cyanide antidote kit is not generally available in bulk stock in hospitals. It is not generally a prehospital drug. Even if it is available in **prepositioned medical supplies**, there is a significant chance that the majority of patients will be beyond saving or in no further need of therapy before these prepositioned stocks can be released, moved, and distributed.

Proposed in the 1930s by Chen and associates, intentional production of methemoglobin in the body is used to treat cyanide poisoning.[12] **Methemoglobinemia** is produced by inhalation of **amyl nitrite** followed by intravenous administration of sodium nitrite. About 30% methemoglobinemia is considered optimum, and the levels should be kept below 40%.

Treatment begins with sodium nitrite, which relieves the symptoms, followed by sodium thiosulfate, which enables the kidneys to excrete the toxin. The standard initial dose of 3% sodium nitrite solution is 10 mL, which is equivalent to one of the two sodium nitrite vials in the cyanide antidote kit. The initial dose of sodium thiosulfate is 50 mL, which is equivalent to one of the sodium thiosulfate vials in the cyanide antidote kit. A second dose of each antidote may be given of up to half of the original dose, if the clinician feels that this is appropriate. In cases where nitrites and the subsequent formation of methemoglobinemia may be dangerous, thiosulfate together with oxygen may be appropriate.

In patients with mixed gas exposure, induction of methemoglobinemia may induce tissue hypoxia. Too rapid administration of the sodium nitrite may cause vasodilation and hypotension. Instructions are supplied in the cyanide kits and should be followed explicitly.

Use of the Cyanide Antidote in Pediatric Patients Therapy with nitrites is not harmless, and the doses given to an adult can be fatal in children.[13] Treatment of children affected by cyanide intoxication must be individualized and based on body weight and hemoglobin concentration **(Table 2-3)**. The dose of sodium nitrite for children is 10 mg/kg immediately and 5 mg/kg repeated within 30 minutes if necessary. If the hemoglobin of the child is less than 12 gm/100 mL, a smaller amount of sodium nitrite should be used.

When less than the full adult dose of sodium nitrite is given, 5 mL of 25% sodium thiosulfate should be given for every 1 mL of 3% sodium nitrite.

Hyperbaric Oxygenation

Hyperbaric oxygenation may be the ideal adjunct to nitrite therapy **(Color plate 2-2)**. Hyperbaric oxygenation will mitigate concern about methemoglobinemia formed by nitrite administration. In the case of a mixed gas inhalation, carbon monoxide will be effectively displaced from hemoglobin and will allow higher levels of nitrite to be used. Hyperbaric oxygen therapy should not be considered as a replacement of the chemical treatments, however, because of the deleterious effects that can be caused by a delay in treatment. Hyperbaric oxygen therapy is unlikely to be available in the event of a terrorist attack with cyanide, because available chambers generally have the capacity for only a few patients at most.

Hydroxycobalamin

Hydroxycobalamin (vitamin B_{12a}) is the drug of choice for life-threatening anemia due to vitamin B12 deficiency and is approved by the FDA. Hundreds of thousands of doses are used yearly in the United States.

Hydroxycobalamin has been used at higher doses to prevent cyanide toxicity from prolonged administration of **sodium nitroprusside** as well as in the acute treatment of cyanide poisoning for over 40 years **(Color plates 2-3 and 2-4)**.[14-19] This agent reacts directly with the cyanide and does not form methemoglobin.

Hydroxycobalamin appears to be a preferable antidote for patients suffering from another concurrent gas exposure such as carbon monoxide and is used by prehospital providers on a protocol basis for the treatment of smoke inhalation in France.[20] There has been only limited experimental use in the United States to date, but more than 40 years of experience are documented in the French literature.[21,22]

For uncertain reasons, hydroxycobalamin is only rarely used in the United States for treatment of cyanide intoxication.[23] A dose of at least 4 grams in the adult is needed to neutralize a lethal amount of cyanide.[24,25] It is not currently available in the United States in the appropriate strength. (Current available formulation in the United States would require a minimum of 4000 1-mL [1-mg] ampules to be given for an appropriate dose.)

Hydroxycobalamin treatment is essentially devoid of complications. Some patients will develop urticaria, but this is rare. Tachycardia and hypertension have been occasionally reported in high-dose therapy. Transient pink discoloration of the mucous membranes, skin, and urine occurs in most patients immediately after the administration of hydroxycobalamin. This discoloration fades over 24 to 48 hours as the drug is eliminated through the urine.[26]

When made available, hydroxycobalamin may be the most appropriate antidote for children exposed to cyanide. Even when given the full adult dose, no toxic effects have been observed.

Dicobalt-EDTA

Cobalt salts have been proven to be effective in treating cyanide poisoning.[27] One such cobalt-based antidote available in Europe is **dicobalt-EDTA (Figure 2-3)**, sold as **Kelocyanor**.[28,29] This drug provides an antidote effect more quickly than the formation of methemoglobin, but a clear superiority to methemoglobin formation has not been demonstrated.

	Initial dose of NaNO$_2$ (mg/kg)	Initial dose of 3% NaNO$_2$ solution (mL/kg)	Initial dose of 25% sodium thiosulfate (mL/kg)
Hemoglobin			
7.0	5.8	0.19	0.95
8.0	6.6	0.22	1.10
9.0	7.5	0.25	1.25
10.0	8.3	0.27	1.35
11.0	9.1	0.30	1.50
12.0	10.0	0.33	1.65
13.0	10.8	0.36	1.80
14.0	11.6	0.39	1.95

Table 2-3 Pediatric Sodium Nitrite (NaNO$_2$) Doses

Adapted from: Comprehensive Review of Emergency Medicine 83 notes on cyanide intoxication by Guzzardi, L.

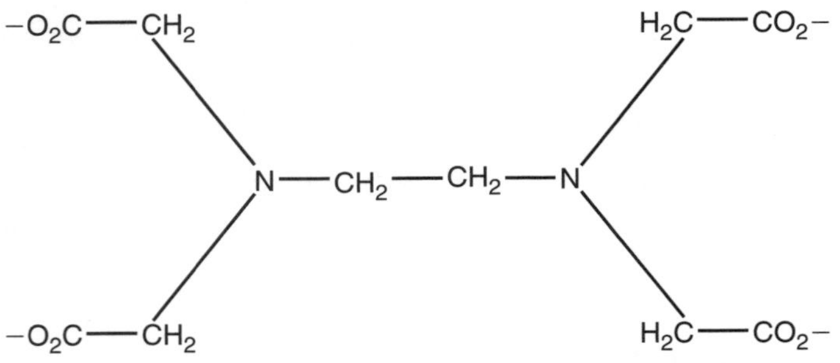

Figure 2-3 Dicobalt-EDTA molecule.

Dicobalt-EDTA does cause a significant hypertension and may cause arrhythmias if no cyanide is present when it is given. Patients may experience vomiting and periorbital edema after administration. Deaths have been noted after this drug was administered, and severe toxicity from cobalt can occur even after the patient recovers from the cyanide intoxication.[30,31]

Kelocyanor and hydroxycobalamin may be given together.[32] Hall and Rumack studied 10 French patients who were given combinations of thiosulfate and hydroxycobalamin and felt that this combination had some additive effect.[33]

4-DMAP

4-Dimethylaminophenol (4-DMAP) is a methemoglobin-forming compound with proven effects against cyanide.[34] The Germans proposed 4-DMAP as a more rapid antidote than nitrites, with lower toxicity. It is used currently by the German military and civilian population. Intravenous injection of 3 mg/kg of 4-DMAP will produce 15% methemoglobin levels within 1 minute.[35] As with the cyanide antidote kit, 4-DMAP must be used with thiosulfate.

IM injections of 4-DMAP may cause pain, fever, and elevated muscle enzymes and may cause necrosis in the area of injection. In some patients, extremely high levels of methemoglobin may be rarely seen.

Other agents that are similar methemoglobin-forming compounds with protective effects against cyanide include **p-aminoheptanoylphenone** (PAHP), **p-aminopropiophenone** (PAPP) and **p-aminooctanoylphenone** (PAOP).[36] PAHP may be the safest of the group. These agents reduce cyanide levels within red blood cells. PAPP in particular has an enhanced effect in the presence of thiosulfate.

Personal Protection

Cyanide is readily absorbed by inhalation as well as through the skin and mucous membranes. All first-line rescuers should be adequately protected before entering a confined area. Rescuers should wear Level A protective gear to avoid intoxication during rescue attempts. Structural fire fighter turnout gear is inadequate even with self-contained breathing apparatus (SCBA), because the hydrogen cyanide gas diffuses through the fabrics and can be absorbed through the skin.[37] Because this agent diffuses into clothing, full de-contamination of seriously exposed casualties, including the isolation of clothing and personal effects, is necessary. Medical providers who are decontaminating patients should wear Level B protection or higher.

■ Arsine

Arsine (SA) is a highly toxic, colorless gas with a mild garlic-like odor. It is water soluble and is readily absorbed by inhalation. Arsine is widely used as a **dopant** in the manufacture of semiconductors and is widely available. Arsine may also be generated during smelting, welding, soldering, galvanizing, and refining.

Exposure to 250 ppm is rapidly lethal. Exposure to 25–50 ppm for 30 minutes can also be fatal. Arsine binds to hemoglobin and causes **hemolysis**. It is also thought to liberate intracellular arsenic or bind to **sulfhydryl groups** essential for respiration.

Arsine is appropriately classified as a blood agent by the military. This agent actually causes significant hemolysis and subsequent kidney damage. Initial symptoms often begin 2 to 24 hours after inhalation. The initial symptoms may be headache, malaise, weakness, and dyspnea. The patient may complain of abdominal pain, nausea, and vomiting. These acute symptoms are followed in 4 to 6 hours by hematuria. Jaundice may be seen after 24 hours. The toxidrome of abdominal pain, hematuria, and jaundice is characteristic of arsine poisoning, though many patients will not have all three signs. Acute exposure to high concentrations of arsine may result in pulmonary edema.

Physical examination is usually unhelpful. The acute examination of the patient with significant toxicity may be indistinguishable from any of the pulmonary agents described later. In later stages, the patient may have yellow-bronze skin and **hepatomegaly** (enlargement of the liver).

Laboratory examination shows a picture of hemolytic anemia with elevated plasma hemoglobin and **hemoglobin-uria**. A history of exposure to arsine and plasma hemoglobin of more than 1.5% would confirm the diagnosis of arsine poisoning. Arsenic levels in serum and urine are not helpful in management of the acute patient, but will corroborate the diagnosis.

Treatment

Prehospital care of the patient exposed to arsine is supportive. The ABCs should be monitored at all times, and effective oxygenation should be maintained at all times. Extra care should be taken to limit the patient's physical activity, as this can severely worsen the patient's symptoms and course.

The definitive treatment is exchange transfusion and renal dialysis. Hemolysis may continue for up to 4 days after dialysis, because not all arsenic will be removed by dialysis. Death usually results from renal failure.

Personal Protection

Protection against these agents should be Level A, if possible. Decontamination activities may be conducted in Level B protection. Since arsine presents a vapor hazard, the patient's clothing should be removed to prevent **outgassing**.

Table 2-4 Summary of Tissue Toxins

Name	Code name	CAS number*	Appearance	Odor	Route of exposure
Cyanide	CN	74-90-8	Powder (dropped into acid to become liquid)	N/A	Inhalation, absorption, ingestion
Hydrogen cyanide	HCN, AC	74-90-8	Colorless liquid that readily evaporates. Gas is lighter than air.	Slight bitter almond odor, not always detectable	Inhalation, absorption, ingestion
Arsine	SA	7784-42-1	Colorless gas	Mild garliclike odor	Inhalation
Cyanogen chloride	CK	506-77-4	Colorless liquid, colorless gas	Pungent, biting odor (often unnoticed due to effects on mucous membranes)	Inhalation

*CAS stands for the unique chemical abstracts service number for each known chemical. Using the CAS, specific chemical information such as the chemical formula and known physical properties can be researched.

Cyanogen Chloride

Cyanogen chloride (CK) is a colorless, highly volatile liquid with a pungent, biting odor. The odor will often be unnoticed because of the agent's irritating effects on the mucous membranes.

Cyanogen chloride has similar action to that of hydrogen cyanide. It interferes with the use of oxygen by the body tissues. It is not lethal at lower concentrations, but it also possesses potent pulmonary irritant and **lacrimator effects**. The late effects are similar to those seen with cyanide.

Cyanogen chloride will cause irritation to the eyes, nose, and airway like the riot-control agents discussed later. This action is considered to be of little military importance compared to its tissue effects. Cyanogen chloride irritates the respiratory tract in a manner similar to phosgene. The patient will develop marked lacrimation, **rhinorrhea**, and bronchial secretions. Cyanogen chloride causes pulmonary edema much faster than in phosgene poisoning.

Cyanogen chloride is considered a nonpersistent agent and is used as a quick-acting casualty agent. Although cyanogen chloride evaporates quickly, the vapors may persist in heavily wooded areas under the right conditions.

Treatment

Prehospital therapy of patients who are exposed to cyanogen chloride consists of symptomatic hemodynamic support and effective oxygenation. The cyanide antidote kit should be used as soon as possible with these patients. Seizures should be controlled with usual agents such as benzodiazepines.

Decontamination

Patients may be decontaminated with soap and water and the removal of all clothing. A significant risk attributed to cyanogen chloride is that, in high concentrations, it quickly breaks down the filters in a military protective mask. For this reason, a terrorist may consider it as a mass-casualty agent. The EMS provider should use Level A personal protection (with self-contained breathing apparatus). Level B personal protection (with self-contained breathing apparatus or supplied air breathing apparatus) may be appropriate for decontamination activities. Protective masks are simply inadequate for this agent. Filtration devices, including powered filtration devices, may be rendered unsafe by exposure to this agent.

Summary

A summary of the tissue toxins is provided in **Table 2-4.**

References

1. Wolnick KA, Fricke FL, Bonnin E, et al: The Tylenol tampering incident: Tracing the source. *Anal Chem* 1984;56:466A-470A, 474A.
2. Sidell FR, Takafuji ET, Franz DR (eds): *Medical Aspects of Chemical and Biological Warfare.* Washington, DC, Office of the Surgeon General, Department of the Army, 1997.
3. Sidell FR, Takafuji ET, Franz DR (eds): *Medical Aspects of Chemical and Biological Warfare.* Washington, DC, Office of the Surgeon General, Department of the Army, 1997.
4. Brennan RJ, Waeckerle JF, Sharp TW, et al: Chemical warfare agents: Emergency medical and emergency public health issues. *Ann Emerg Med* 1999;34:191-204.
5. Baskin SI: Zyklon, in La Cleur W. (ed): *Encyclopedia of the Holocaust.* New Haven, CT, Yale University Press, 1998.
6. Anonymous: Recommendations for protecting human health against potential adverse effects of long term exposure to low doses of chemical warfare agents. *MMWR* 1988;37:72-74.
7. Baud FJ, Barriot P, Toffis V, et al: Elevated blood cyanide concentrations in victims of smoke inhalation. *NEJM* 1991;325:1761-1766.
8. Bermudez RM, Cabrera CA: Treatment of burns. *NEJM* 1997;336:1392-1393.
9. Fligner CL, Luthi R, Linkaityte-Weiss E, et al: Paper strip screening method for detection of cyanide in blood using CYANTESMO test paper. *Am J Forensic Med Pathol* 1992;13:81-84.
10. Hall AH, Rumack BH: Clinical toxicology of cyanide. *Ann Emerg Med* 1986;15:1067-1074.
11. Sauer SW: Hydroxocobalamin: Improved public health readiness for cyanide disasters. *Ann Emerg Med* 2001;37(6):635-641.
12. Chen KK, Rose CL, Clowes GHA: Methylene blue, nitrites, and sodium thiosulfate against cyanide poisoning. *Proc Exp Biol Med* 1933;31:250-252.

13. Berlin CM Jr: The treatment of cyanide poisoning in children. *Pediatrics* 1970;46:793-796.

14. Cottrell JE, Casthely P, Brodie JD, et al: Prevention of nitroprusside-induced cyanide toxicity with hydroxycobalamin. *N Engl J Med* 1978;298:809-811.

15. Graham DL, Laman D, Theodore J, Robin ED: Acute cyanide poisoning complicated by lactic acidosis and pulmonary edema. *Arch Intern Med* 1977;137:1051-1055.

16. Way JL, Sylvester D, Morgan RL, et al: Recent perspectives on the toxicodynamic basis of cyanide antagonism. *Fundam Appl Toxicol* 1984;4:S231-S239.

17. Mushett C: Antidotal efficacy of vitamin B$_{12a}$ (hydroxocobalamin) in experimental cyanide poisoning. *Proc Soc Exp Biol Med* 1952;81:234-237.

18. Hall AH, Rumack BH: Hydroxycobalamin/sodium thiosulfate as a cyanide antidote. *J Emerg Med* 1987;5:115-121.

19. Bismuth C, Baud FJ, Djeghout H, et al: Cyanide poisoning from propionitrile exposure. *J Emerg Med* 1987;5:191-195.

20. Sauer SW: Hydroxocobalamin: Improved public health readiness for cyanide disasters. *Ann Emerg Med* 2001;37(6):635-641.

21. Jouglard J, Fagot G, Deguigne B, et al: L'intoxication cyanhydrique aigue et son traitement d'urgence. *Marseille Medicale* 1971;9:571-575.

22. Cottrell JE, Casthely P, Brodie JD, et al: Prevention of nitroprusside-induced cyanide toxicity with hydroxocobalamin. *NEJM* 1978;298:809-811.

23. Litovitz TL, Klein-Schwartz W, Caravati EM, et al: 1998 annual report of the American Association of Poison Control Centers Toxic Exposure Surveillance System. *Am J Emerg Med* 1999;17:425-487.

24. Houeto P, Buneux F, Galliot-Guilley M, et al: Pharmacokinetics of hydroxocobalamin in smoke inhalation victims. *J Toxicol Clin Toxicol* 1996;34:397-404.

25. Houeto P, Buneux F, Galliot-Guilley M, et al: Monitoring of cyanocobalamin and hydroxocobalamin during treatment of cyanide intoxication. Letter. *Lancet* 1995;246:1706-1707.

26. Houeto P, Buneux F, Galliot-Guilley M, et al: Pharmacokinetics of hydroxocobalamin in smoke inhalation victims. *J Toxicol Clin Toxicol* 1996;34:397-404.

27. Evans CL: Cobalt compounds as antidotes for hydrocyanic acid. *Br J Pharmacol* 1964:23:455-475.

28. Vogel SN, Sultan TR, Ten Eyck RP: Cyanide poisoning. *Clin Toxicol* 1981;18:367-383.

29. Hillman B, Bardhan KD, Bain JTB: The use of dicobalt edetate (Kelocyanor) in cyanide poisoning. *Postgrad Med J* 1974:50:171-174.

30. Rose CL, Worth RM, Kikuchi K, Chen KK: Cobalt salts in acute cyanide poisoning. *Proc Soc Exp Biol Med* 1965;120:780-783.

31. Reynolds JEF, Prasad AB (eds): Dicobalt edetate (1033-p), in *Martindale: The Extra Pharmacopoeia*, ed 28. London, England, Pharmaceutical Press, 1982, p 382.

32. Bismuth C, Cantineau J, Pontal P, et al: Priorite de l'oxygenation dans l'intoxication cyanhydrique. *J Toxicol Med* 1984;4:107-121.

33. Hall AH, Rumack BH: Hydroxycobalamin/sodium thiosulfate as a cyanide antidote. *J Emerg Med* 1987;5:115-121.

34. Weger NP: Treatment of cyanide poisoning with 4-DMAP: Experimental and clinical overview. *Fundam Appl Toxicol* 1983;3:387-396.

35. Kiese M, Weger N: Formation of ferrihaemoglobin with aminophenols in the human for the treatment of cyanide poisoning. *Eur J Pharmacol* 1969;7:97-105.

36. Vick JA, Froehlich H: Treatment of cyanide poisoning. *J Toxicol Clin Exp* 1988;25:125-138.

37. Lam KK, Lau FL: An incident of hydrogen cyanide poisoning. *Am J Emerg Med* 2000;18:172-175.

Nerve Agents

■ Introduction

Since World War II, nerve agents have played a dominant role in chemical warfare planning by military strategists and tacticians. Nerve agents are supertoxic compounds that produce convulsions and rapid death. The vast majority of nerve agents are classified as **organophosphorus chemicals,** although the carbamates also act in a similar fashion. Although many organophosphorus compounds are highly toxic, only a limited number of them have the physical properties that give them military utility. In general, nerve agents are 100 to 1,000 times more poisonous than organophosphorus pesticides.[1]

Nerve agents developed in four generations: first-generation agents—the G agents; second-generation agents—the V agents; third-generation agents—the binary and trinary agents (such as GB-2); and fourth-generation agents—Novichok agents and possibly the carbamate chemicals. Nerve agents formerly researched and produced by the United States include the **G agents** and the **V agents**.

■ History

G Agents

The first three agents, the so-called G agents, are highly toxic compounds that were developed between World War I and World War II. Since 1934, Gerhard Schrader had been in charge of a program to develop new types of insecticides, which eventually led to the preparation of tabun.[2] In January 1937, Schrader was the first to observe the effects of nerve agents on human beings when he and a laboratory assistant began to experience miosis (pupillary contraction) and shortness of breath as a result of their exposure to tabun vapor in the laboratory.[3]

In 1935, in compliance with Nazi law, a sample of tabun was sent to the chemical warfare section of the Army Weapons Office. In May 1937, Schrader was asked to give a demonstration of tabun at Berlin-Spandau. After seeing this demonstration, Colonel Rüdringer, head of the German Army chemical warfare section, ordered the construction of new laboratories for the further investigation of tabun and related organophosphate compounds.

In 1938, a second potent organophosphate nerve agent was developed. This agent, sarin, was named for its four developers: *S*chrader, *A*mbrose, *R*üdringer, and van der *Lin*de.

The Germans started to manufacture tabun and sarin at several sites, including Dyernfurth, Spandau, and Falkenhagen. The plants designed to manufacture these agents took an extraordinarily long time to begin production because the chemical reactions were so corrosive to the equipment. Vessels were lined with silver or quartz and piping was double walled, with air circulating between the two walls. Workers were equipped with respirators and clothing made from a rubber/cloth/rubber sandwich; the clothing was discarded after the 10th wearing. Despite these precautions, over 300 accidents occurred during early production, and at least 10 workers died.

On May 11, 1943, the British captured a German chemist who had worked at the main Army chemical warfare research laboratory in Spandau. The prisoner gave the British detailed information on tabun, including its code name (Trilon 83), the chemical reactions by which it was produced, its effects, the German doctrine for its use, and the known methods of defense against it. This was compiled into an **MI9 intelligence report** on July 3, 1943.

In 1944, Dr. Richard Kuhn synthesized **soman** for the German military. However, soman was not known to have been produced by the Germans in deployable quantities.

In early 1945, Dyernfurth was abandoned as the Russians advanced. During the retreat, tons of liquid nerve agents were simply poured into the Oder River. The plant was rigged for demolition, but the Russians surrounded the plant before it could be destroyed. The Luftwaffe was then ordered to bomb the plant, but they also failed to destroy it. It is believed that the Russians captured both the full-scale tabun plant and the pilot sarin plant intact. The Russians later captured the nearly complete full-scale sarin plant at Falkenhagen.

V Agents

In 1952, Dr. Ranjit Ghosh, a chemist at the plant protection laboratories of the British firm Imperial Chemical Industries, investigated new pesticides to replace DDT. Dr. Ghosh developed the first of the V agents.

In 1954, Imperial Chemical Industries put one of these agents on the market as an insecticide named Amiton. It was soon withdrawn as being too toxic for use around humans. Another more persistent nerve agent, VX, evolved from this research and the research of Swedish Dr. Lars-Erik Tammelin. The Russians obtained the chemical formula for VX but not the molecular structure of the agent and subsequently developed a similar agent, usually called V-gas.

Military development of V agents was conducted by the United States, Great Britain, and the Soviet Union **(Figure 3-1)**. Each of these states implemented large-scale production of a V agent in the 1960s. In the 1980s and 1990s Iraq produced V agents in moderate quantities and used VX (or possibly V-gas) against the Iranians.

Deployment of the Agents
Military

Although the Nazis possessed these agents during World War II, they were never used by the German military. The only known military use of nerve agents was in the Iran–Iraq

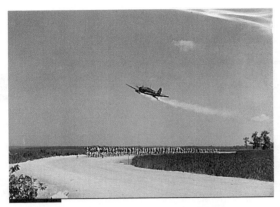

Figure 3-1 US military plane spraying tear gas in a training area. This same equipment could easily deliver many other chemical agents.

War in the 1980s. Iraq's use of chemical weapons caused relatively few deaths, but inspired panic among Iranian troops, disorganized formations, made defense more difficult, and encumbered the troops.

Terrorist

Nerve agents were brought to the public's attention by the Aum Shinrikyo cult in 1994 and 1995 when it employed sarin as a terrorist weapon, first in Matsumoto, Japan, and then in the Tokyo subway system. Aum Shinrikyo was found to have a well-developed production facility that was capable of making sarin in significant quantities.

In the Aum Shinrikyo cult's second use of sarin, five plastic bag containers of sarin were placed on three of Tokyo's subway lines in 1995, with dispersal accomplished only by evaporation. In all, 5,000 to 6,000 people were exposed; 3,227 were evaluated in emergency departments; 493 were admitted to hospitals; and 12 people died as a result of this terrorist exposure. Two of those killed were deputy station masters who attempted to clean up the sarin with paper towels and plastic bags, despite having no respiratory or barrier protection. Arguably, their sacrifice prevented other deaths.

The concentration within the rail cars with the containers was high, but the agent was not spread well through the subway system, and most exposures were mild. Of the ambulance personnel taking care of these victims, 135 developed symptoms and 33 were hospitalized. Many of the hospital staff also required treatment, but none required hospitalization. Neither ambulance personnel nor hospital staff had any chemical weapon protection.

In 1996, the US government acknowledged that troops operating during the Gulf War in 1991 were potentially exposed to nerve agents. This reportedly occurred after an Iraqi chemical weapons depot was destroyed at Khamisiyah.[4]

■ Mechanism of Action

Organophosphate nerve agents act by first binding with and then irreversibly inactivating **acetylcholinesterase**, producing a toxic accumulation of **acetylcholine** at **muscarinic**, **nicotinic**, and central nervous system (CNS)

synapses.[5-7] Carbamates have the same mechanism of action, but the binding and inactivation of acetylcholinesterase is reversible. The muscarinic receptors are found in the smooth muscles, exocrine glands, and the central nervous system. The nicotinic receptors are found in the skeletal muscles.

Acetylcholine normally causes activation of these receptors as a result of a nerve impulse and is then destroyed by acetylcholinesterase. When a nerve agent inactivates acetylcholinesterase, the acetylcholine continues to interact with the receptor and stimulates it uncontrollably **(Color plate 3-1)**. Persistent stimulation leads to muscle fatigue.

Routes of Exposure

Nerve agents are normally liquid. These liquids may be vaporized, aerosolized, or spread by droplets. The Russians have adapted SCUD missiles to splatter these agents with a small explosive charge. Other dissemination mechanisms can vary from being crude to sophisticated. Examples include the following:

- Evaporation of the liquid (This was the method used in the Tokyo subway.)
- Blower or fan to aid in the evaporation process and to aid in the spread of the agent vapor
- Introduction into a building ventilation system
- Explosive device (The larger the explosion, the more agent will be destroyed. Military munitions often use a burster or limited explosive device to break apart the agent container. Any artillery or mortar capable of delivering a chemical munition is suitable.)
- Pressurized spray release (Many aerosol sprayers can be adapted to deliver nerve agents.)

Delivery patterns are dependent on the munition, capacity of the chemical container, and weather patterns. Delivery patterns indoors are dependent on the munition and on airflows from heating and air-conditioning.

Nerve agents may enter the body through inhalation, ingestion, and absorption. The exposure route is dictated by the volatility of the agent. Volatile agents such as sarin enter the body through inhalation of gaseous vapors and absorption through mucous membranes.

The time of onset of a nerve agent's effects is related to the route of entry into the body. Symptoms appear much more slowly from absorption through the skin than from respiratory exposure. This is because the lungs contain a large surface area and numerous blood vessels that allow rapid diffusion into a patient's circulation. If inhaled or absorbed through eye or mucous membranes, death may occur in 1 to 10 minutes. With inhalation exposure, affected patients typically do not deteriorate after they have been removed from the area of vapor exposure.

Although the initial skin absorption of a lethal dose may occur within 1 to 2 minutes, it may take up to 1 to 2 hours for death to occur. With some nerve agents (particularly VX), patients may not become symptomatic for an extended time after skin exposure. Also, deterioration of the patient may continue even after the agent is removed from the surface of the skin.

If food or water contaminated with nerve agents is ingested, the patient may experience symptoms in about 30 minutes. This, of course, is dependent on the concentration, quantity, and type of nerve agent ingested.

The toxic effect of inhaled nerve agents depends on both the concentration of the nerve agent in the air and duration of exposure (C•t). The lethal dose for the most sensitive people is about 70 mg•min/m³, and it is about twice this level for the most resistant individuals. At low concentrations, the C•t does not apply, because the body is capable of limited detoxification of the agents.

Effects of Nerve Agent Exposure

Individuals poisoned by a nerve agent display similar symptoms regardless of exposure route. The intensity and sequence of the symptoms, however, are influenced by the route of absorption and by individual sensitivity. The effects of nerve agents are listed in **Table 3-1**.

Muscarinic Effects

The muscarinic effects of nerve agents include the stimulation of the endings of the parasympathetic nerves at the smooth muscle of the irises, the **ciliary bodies**, the bronchial tree, the gastrointestinal tract, the bladder, and the blood vessels.[8]

Ocular Ocular symptoms are most often caused by nerve agent inhalation or ocular exposure to nerve agent vapor. They may be early indicators of exposure to a volatile nerve agent. However, ocular symptoms are less common in patients exposed by direct skin contact. This is probably because the eye usually is not exposed directly to the agent unless it is in the form of a vapor, a splash of the agent, or contamination from rubbing the eyes.

Eye exposure to nerve agents may produce miosis, ocular pain, and dimness of vision as first effects. Miosis appears to be a consistent clinical finding with nerve agent vapor exposure.[9-11] Miosis may be absent or delayed in skin exposure to a nonvolatile agent. Miosis is often delayed in VX exposure because VX is most commonly absorbed through the skin.

Table 3-1 Effects of Nerve Agents
Rhinorrhea
Bronchial secretions
Tightness of the chest
Bronchospasm
Dimness of vision
Eye pain (in vapor or ocular exposure)
Miosis
Dyspnea
Drooling and excessive sweating
Nausea
Vomiting, cramps, and involuntary defecation and urination
Twitching, jerking, and staggering gait
Headache, confusion, coma, and convulsions
Respiratory depression and respiratory arrest

Short-range vision often deteriorates after exposure, and the patient may feel pain when he or she tries to focus on a nearby object.[12] Ciliary spasm also may cause eye pain. This is most likely from the direct effect of the agent on the eye. Attempting to focus exacerbates ciliary muscle spasm. The patient may also have conjunctival injection and lacrimation.

Respiratory Respiratory effects include rhinorrhea, wheezing, cough, increased bronchial secretions, dyspnea, and apnea. These symptoms coupled with the nicotinic (respiratory muscle paralysis) and CNS (decreased respiratory drive) effects are the primary causes of cardiac arrest in victims of nerve agent intoxication.

Patients may describe shortness of breath or chest tightness and may experience respiratory distress or gasping respirations. Bronchoconstriction and increased intrabronchial secretions may cause these sensations. These patients may develop coughing and wheezing associated with prolonged expiration as a result of the bronchoconstriction. Patients with asthma or chronic obstructive pulmonary disease may be at significant increased risk because of their diminished reserves and increased respiratory sensitivity.

Cardiovascular The patient intoxicated with a nerve agent may present with either bradycardia or tachycardia. Other cardiovascular effects include prolongation of the PR interval, and atrioventricular blocks. The cardiac rate depends on the extent of exposure. The cardiac toxicities can be divided into three phases:

1. Tachycardia and hypertension may result from the initial intense sympathetic activity.[13]
2. The patient then develops bradyarrhythmias, prolongation of the PR interval, atrioventricular blocks, and hypotension.[14-16]
3. The final phase includes QT prolongation and possible **torsade de pointes**.[17-19] (Torsade de pointes has been noted with the organophosphate insecticides, but not yet with the nerve agents.)

The bradyarrhythmias resulting from nerve agent toxicity can be lethal and should be monitored and treated accordingly. Heart blocks and premature ventricular contractions can be observed after intoxication with the nerve agents, although these are also often seen with hypoxia.

Gastrointestinal/Genitourinary Salivation, lacrimation, and involuntary defecation and urination result from the effects of the nerve agent on the gastrointestinal and genitourinary systems. The patient may develop intense crampy abdominal pain (**tenesmus**). Nausea and vomiting are common effects. The time of onset and the severity of the gastrointestinal symptoms are related to the C•t and the route of exposure.[20]

Dermal Sympathetic stimulation caused by nerve agent exposure causes flushing and sweating. Direct dermal exposure may be associated with localized sweating at the site of exposure, whereas generalized diaphoresis is associated with systemic toxicity.[21]

Mucosal Rhinorrhea is most common after a vapor exposure to a nerve agent. It can also be observed with exposure by other routes. The patient will experience increased secretions and salivation early in the exposure. These in-creased secretions may complicate airway management of the patient.

Mnemonics Two popular mnemonics for the muscarinic effects of the nerve agents are as follows:

- Military mnemonic: SLUD or SLUDGE
    - **S**alivation, sweating
    - **L**acrimation
    - **U**rination
    - **D**efecation, drooling, diarrhea
    - **G**astric upset and cramps
    - **E**mesis
- Alternative mnemonic: DUMBELS
    - **D**iarrhea
    - **U**rination
    - **M**iosis
    - **B**ronchorrhea, bronchoconstriction
    - **E**mesis
    - **L**acrimation
    - **S**alivation

Unfortunately, neither mnemonic covers all of the symptoms that nerve agents can cause. They are particularly lacking in covering the nicotinic symptoms caused by nerve agents. Both mnemonics also illustrate symptoms that may be found in the nonlethal agents that are discussed in Chapter 6.

Nicotinic Effects

Metabolic The metabolic effects of excess acetylcholine on nicotinic receptors cause metabolic abnormalities. Hyperglycemia, **ketosis**, and metabolic acidosis are common. In addition to these effects, hypoxia and respiratory depression produce a respiratory acidosis.

Pulmonary The respiratory effects of nerve agents are ultimately responsible for most deaths attributed to these chemicals. Nerve agents cause respiratory failure in three ways: increased airway resistance, weakness and paralysis of the muscles of respiration, and central depression of the respiratory drive.[22,23]

Respiratory paralysis was originally thought to be the major cause of respiratory arrest. Weakness of the diaphragm and accessory muscles of respiration does occur; however, respiratory arrest will often occur prior to a neuromuscular blockade and is not always a result of muscle paralysis.[24] The patient may develop a weakness of the muscles of the upper airway resulting in obstruction of the tongue within the oral pharynx.[25] Laryngeal muscle paralysis may cause vocal cord dysfunction and subsequent stridor.[26] With severe intoxication, the patient may rapidly develop apnea.

Cardiac As previously mentioned, the nicotinic cardiovascular effects can be seen during the early and late stages of exposure. Initially, tachyarrhythmias and hypertension occur. The final stage may produce prolongation of the QT interval and subsequent ventricular tachyarrhythmias.

Muscular The accumulation of acetylcholine at the endings of the motor nerves results in nicotinic-like signs and symptoms. For muscle, this would mean the following sequence of events would occur:

1. Spontaneous activation of **myofibrils** (**fasciculations**) as acetylcholine accumulates. Fasciculations may be described as ripples or worms moving under the skin. Localized fasciculations may be seen at the site of nerve agent skin exposure.
2. Tremors and twitching as entire muscle groups are lost
3. Progressive weakness, culminating in flaccid paralysis

A hallmark of nerve agent exposure is muscle fasciculations or twitching.[27] The fasciculation is often confined to the area of exposure early in the intoxication; it then spreads to the entire musculature. Twitching may be observed. Eventually, muscles fatigue and a flaccid paralysis ensues. This includes the muscles of respiration (the diaphragm and intercostal muscles).

When a person is exposed to a high dose of a nerve agent, the muscular symptoms are more pronounced and rapid. The victim may rapidly suffer convulsions and lose consciousness. The process of intoxication may be so rapid that the patient does not have time to develop the minor symptoms before respiratory arrest occurs.

Ocular In contrast to the miosis seen with the muscarinic signs, a patient may rarely present with **mydriasis** (dilation of the pupil). It should be noted that the majority of patients present with miosis.

Mnemonics The MTWThF (weekdays) mnemonic can be used for nicotinic effects.

- **M**etabolic (hyperglycemia, metabolic acidosis)
- **T**witching (fasciculations)
- **W**eakness
- **Th** Tachycardia/hypertension
- **F**laccid paralysis

Central Nervous System Effects

Because there are so many CNS cholinergic receptors, there are a wide variety of signs and symptoms caused by exposure to a nerve agent. The accumulation of excessive acetylcholine in the brain and spinal cord is thought to result in CNS symptoms including twitching, jerking, staggering gait, convulsions, respiratory depression, and coma. Early manifestations may include anxiety, restlessness, confusion, and ataxia. Minor exposures to the nerve agents may result in behavioral changes such as anxiety, psychomotor depression, intellectual impairment, and unusual dreams. Major exposures to the nerve agents result in rapid loss of consciousness and seizures.

Organophosphate exposure can produce both central and peripheral nervous system signs and symptoms if the patient survives the respiratory failure and other immediately lethal events. These symptoms may include impaired memory, hallucinations, fatigue, balance problems, confusion, and concentration deficits.[28-32] Signs may include both central and peripheral **neuropathies** and late seizures. Severely intoxicated patients may remain unconscious for hours or days.

Other effects and complications include hypoxia, ischemia, acidosis, hyperthermia, hypothermia, **peripheral neuropathy**, and cerebral edema. These have been seen in patients who have received convulsive doses of nerve agents.[33] It is obvious that many of the long-term effects are directly related to the problems of providing adequate ventilation to the contaminated, seizing patient who has excessive airway secretions.

Delayed Clinical Findings

Nerve gases also result in a number of delayed toxicities. The inhibition of cholinesterase enzymes is irreversible once **aging** occurs, so effects may be prolonged. Until the tissue cholinesterase enzymes are restored to normal levels, there is a period of increased susceptibility to another exposure of any nerve agent. The regeneration of enzyme levels may take as long as 2 to 3 months. During this period of regeneration, the effects of repeated exposures are cumulative.

Among the delayed effects is the sudden onset of cardiac failure in patients who have apparently recovered from the effects of organophosphate exposure.[34]

A summary of the effects of nerve agents is listed in **Table 3-2**.

Table 3-2 Effects of Nerve Agents	
Site of action	Signs and symptoms
Muscarinic Effects	
Pupils	Miosis, usually pinpoint, occasionally unequal
Ciliary body	Headache, difficulty focusing, dimness of vision, eye pain
Mucous membranes	Hyperemia, rhinorrhea, conjunctivitis, increased salivation and lacrimation
Bronchial tree	Tightness in chest, wheezing, bronchoconstriction, increased secretions, pain in chest, dyspnea, cough, pulmonary edema
Gastrointestinal	Nausea, vomiting, abdominal cramps, diarrhea, tenesmus
Sweat glands	Increased sweating
Cardiac	Tachycardia
Nicotinic Effects	
Striated muscle	Fatigue, weakness, twitching fasciculations, muscle cramps, paralysis
Sympathetic ganglia	Pallor, occasional hypertension
	Occasional bradycardia
Central Nervous System Effects	
	Tension, anxiety, restlessness, difficulty concentrating, confusion, slurred speech, ataxia, weakness, absence of reflexes
	Cheyne-Stokes respirations, apnea
	Convulsions, coma
	Depression of circulatory centers, death

Adapted from Marrs TC, Maynard RL, Sidell FR: *Chemical Warfare Agents: Toxicology and Treatment*. England, John Wiley and Sons, 1996.

INHOSPITAL INFO

Laboratory Findings

There are no laboratory tests available that would help differentiate nerve agent intoxication from other forms of cholinergic overdose.

■ G Agents: First-Generation Nerve Agents

Tabun

Tabun (GA) was the first anticholinesterase nerve agent to be developed and is the least toxic of the nerve agents. The median lethal dose is about 200 mg•min/m³ via inhalation and about 20,000 to 40,000 mg•min/m³ via dermal absorption. Tabun is a clear to brownish liquid that has a faintly fruity odor, but the dose detectable by odor is quite close to the lethal dose. Tabun produces a colorless vapor.

Tabun has a low volatility (610 mg/m³ at 25°C), but does evaporate from skin. Tabun would be expected to cause both vapor and liquid phase contamination to victims exposed to this agent.

Although tabun is considered to be outmoded and of limited use by military authorities, it is the easiest of the nerve agents to manufacture. As such, it is more likely to be used as a terrorist agent. Unfortunately, because it has not been widely explored by the US military, there is much less information available in the open-source literature about the specifics of tabun intoxication.

Tabun has a half-life in the environment of about 1 to 1.5 days. Tabun is moderately soluble in water and soluble in most organic solvents.

It is effectively detoxified on humans by bleach or soapy water. Equipment may be effectively detoxified with a dilute alkali solution, steam and ammonia, or bleach solution. Responders should be in Level A personal protection when handling grossly contaminated casualties. Level B or C is sufficient when assisting with decontamination or triage of casualties.

Sarin

Sarin (GB) is a colorless liquid that has no odor when pure. It is classified as an organophosphate anticholinesterase agent. The median lethal dose of sarin is between 70 and 100 mg•min/m³ for inhalation and about 12,000 to 15,000 mg•min/m³ for dermal absorption.

Route of Exposure

Sarin is very volatile (22,000 mg/m³ at 25°C) and is primarily absorbed by inhalation. With its high volatility, sarin is usually kept in liquid form until used **(Figure 3-2)**. As seen in the Tokyo Aum Shinrikyo incident, any container could be improvised to carry the agent. The type of dissemination that would likely create the most number of casualties is aerosolization.

The vapor pressures of sarin make it a significant inhalation hazard in any warm climate or with droplet aerosols. Indeed, sarin has a volatility that is close to that

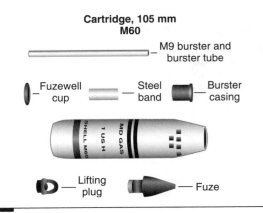

Cartridge, 105 mm M60

M9 burster and burster tube

Fuzewell cup — Steel band — Burster casing

Lifting plug — Fuze

Figure 3-2 Sarin and mustard delivery systems for a 105-mm howitzer (a unitary delivery system).

of water and is the most volatile of the nerve agents. It rapidly evaporates from the skin, thus limiting dermal exposure. The vapor is heavier than air, so it flows into low-lying areas. These volatility characteristics of sarin make it a true "nerve gas." Sarin may persist under the proper conditions for as long as 5 days, but is not considered a persistent agent.

Because sarin evaporates so quickly, it requires little cleanup. This makes it desirable for a military unit that wants to disable or kill troops and then move equipment through the resulting destruction. An act of terrorism with sarin would leave little or no property damage and minimal cleanup costs. The volatility of sarin also makes it very easy to disseminate in closed spaces through ventilation, air-conditioning, or heating ducts, thus increasing its desirability as a terrorist weapon.

Although dermal absorption requires a higher dose, this is strictly because of the low vapor pressure of sarin. If the evaporation is occluded, the median lethal dose for sarin is nearly identical to VX.

Sarin is also very soluble in water (and most other solvents), so decontamination by water irrigation is highly effective. As already noted, the evaporation of sarin and the solubility of sarin in water makes cleanup quite easy. Sarin is also effectively detoxified on humans by bleach or soapy water. Equipment may be effectively detoxified with a dilute alkali solution, steam and ammonia, or bleach solution.

The volatility of sarin creates a significant vapor hazard for the medical provider during decontamination but also makes it much less likely that the patient will spread liquid contamination. During decontamination of the patient exposed to sarin, the medical provider must have adequate respiratory protection and splash protection.[35] Level C personal protective gear with splash protection should suffice for the decontamination of most ambulatory patients. Level B protection is recommended for gross decontamination procedures. The rescuer should remember that a contaminated victim's clothing may outgas the agent for up to 30 minutes after exposure.

Table 3-3	Summary of G-Series Agents					
Name	Code name	CAS number	Appearance		Odor	Route of exposure
Tabun	GA	77-81-6	Colorless to brownish liquid, color-less vapor		Faintly fruity; odorless when pure	Inhalation, absorption
Sarin	GB	107-44-8	Colorless liquid, colorless vapor		Odorless when pure	Inhalation
Soman	GD	96-64-0	Colorless liquid, colorless vapor		Fruity, camphor	Inhalation, absorption
—	GE	1189-87-3	(unavailable)		(unavailable)	(unavailable)
Cyclohexyl sarin	GF	329-99-7	Clear liquid, colorless vapor		Odorless	Inhalation
—	GV	141102-74-1	(unavailable)		(unavailable)	(unavailable)

Soman

Soman (GD) is a colorless liquid, that has a fruity or camphor odor. Its mechanism of action is similar to sarin, and it is made by the same process, using the same equipment as sarin. Only the alcohol used is changed from isopropyl alcohol to **pinacolyl alcohol**. Whereas the United States chose sarin as their volatile agent of choice, the Russians extensively developed soman.

The median lethal dose is 50 to 70 mg•min/m³ by inhalation and only 100 mg•min/m³ by dermal absorption for a 70-kg person. The onset time of symptoms is about the same as sarin.

Soman is the second most volatile of the nerve agents, with a volatility of 3,900 mg/m³ at 25˚C. Soman is considered to be a relatively persistent agent, midway between tabun and sarin. However, soman is less stable than either tabun or sarin. The major route of action of soman is thought to be by dermal contact, not by inhalation, although there is significant vapor production, particularly at higher temperatures.

A major feature of soman is that it is difficult to treat with existing antidotes. Soman ages quite rapidly (within 2 minutes) when bound to the cholinesterase molecule. The phenomenon of aging makes treatment with 2-PAM (currently used by the US Army and discussed in the section on treatment) ineffective with soman. Because of this, soman is the most difficult of the common agents to treat with antidote therapy. The US approach to this is to initiate pre-exposure of pyridostigmine, as noted in the section on premedication. This approach is difficult to support in a civilian environment.

Considering that soman and sarin can both be produced with the same equipment and with the same process, it is theoretically possible to mix both alcohols required and make a mixture of soman and sarin. This compound would have the volatility of sarin and the difficulty of treatment of soman.

Decontamination

Soman is effectively detoxified on humans by bleach or soapy water. Equipment may be effectively detoxified with a dilute alkali solution, steam and ammonia, or bleach solution. Soman is not particularly soluble in water (2.1 g/100 g at 68˚F) and only moderately soluble in other solvents. The low solubility of soman, the persistence, and low volatility of soman make decontamination more difficult, particularly when water alone is used for decontamination.

Cyclohexyl Sarin

Cyclohexyl sarin (GF) is a nerve agent of low volatility that is produced by the same process as soman (using cyclohexyl alcohol instead of isopropyl alcohol). Cyclohexyl sarin was evaluated by the United States and was abandoned. Cyclohexyl sarin was famous as an agent cloaked in fabricated disinformation that was used by US intelligence services to deceive Russian chemical warfare experts. Open-source literature suggests that the Soviet Union and Iraq both have produced quantities of cyclohexyl sarin in unknown amounts in both unitary and binary weapons.[36]

There is very little open-source literature on this agent other than basic physical chemistry descriptions of the agent. It is absorbed through the skin or inhaled as either a gas or aerosol. Clinical signs and symptoms are simply listed as similar to sarin.

Other G Agents

Other G agents exist, but open-source data for these agents are not available. The G agents are summarized in **Table 3-3**.

■ V Agents: Second-Generation Nerve Agents

VX

The most toxic of the classic nerve agents is VX. It is an odorless, amber-colored liquid. It is more stable, less volatile, and more efficient at penetration of intact skin than the G agents.

By inhalation, VX is about twice as toxic as sarin. However, because VX is not very volatile, inhalation is not considered a major hazard with this agent. The median lethal dose by inhalation is about 30 mg•min/m³.

V agents bind to acetylcholinesterase much more potently than the organophosphate and carbamate insecticides. VX is also the slowest aging agent in common existence.

Effects

VX causes the classic nerve agent signs and symptoms. However, patients exposed to VX may not experience miosis. This is probably because the eye is often not exposed directly to the agent, unlike with the vapor of the G agents. Miosis may be a delayed sign of VX exposure and is indicative of systemic toxicity.

The ease of dermal absorption makes the median lethal dose by that route as low as 6 mg•min/m³. It is thought to be 10 times as toxic as sarin for humans by the percutaneous route. (Much of the dermal absorption of sarin is lost because of rapid evaporation.) The physiologic effects and onset times of symptoms are similar to sarin.

VX is thought to cause a delayed presentation followed by a very rapid deterioration postexposure. After receiving a lethal dose, most victims die within 15 minutes. This may well be a consequence of the amount of VX needed to penetrate the skin and circulate into the system. It may also be due to residual VX that has penetrated the skin, but has not yet affected the nervous system.

Route of Exposure

VX is an oily liquid that persists on a scene for weeks or longer. Although it is not volatile enough to pose a major inhalation hazard, it is readily absorbed through the skin. VX is considered to be a persistent nerve agent and may stay toxic for weeks. Although VX is considered to have low volatility, at temperatures greater than 100°F, vapor exposure is possible.

Other V Agents

The other agents in the V series are less known, and the information available on them is mostly classified. The other agents also have code names, including VE, VG, and VM. These V agents are approximately 10 times more poisonous than sarin.

The Soviet Union also produced several **analogues** to VX. The first was Substance 33, a compound similar to the persistent nerve gas VX, of which 15,000 tons were produced in the early 1980s. This agent is often called **V-gas** by American writers. This nerve agent is thought to be similar in persistence and effect to the V agents.

Two other similar agents were also developed: A-230, which was officially approved by the Soviet Army in 1988, and A-232 (an agent similar to A-230), which was never formally approved. The consistency of these Russian

agents is similar to oil; therefore, these agents pose less of an inhalation hazard than G agents. This consistency renders them toxic by dermal exposures. Because information on many of the agents remains classified or is otherwise unavailable in the open-source literature, this chapter discusses VX as the prototype of the series. The reader must be aware that these Russian agents may not have the same characteristics as VX.

Decontamination and Personal Protection

Most important to medical providers, VX is more difficult to decontaminate than the G agents. There are two reasons for this:

- Because VX has a low volatility, the amber-colored or clear liquid drops on the skin do not evaporate and are absorbed more readily. It is a relatively persistent agent and lasts between 2 to 6 days in soil—and may be present much longer as noted above. Any remaining agent will have an oily consistency that is difficult to remove.
- VX is only slowly hydrolyzed by water, and the **hydrolysis** products include **EA2192**, which is nearly as toxic as VX itself and longer lived. Thus, water-based decontamination schemes are not particularly effective against VX. Common bleach provides good decontamination.[37-39]

Threat

VX may be a much more attractive agent to the terrorist than sarin for several reasons. It is the most toxic of the nerve agents. When VX is dispersed, it is a persistent agent for weeks to months in the right climate. At least one of the degradation products is even longer lasting and just as toxic; this means that it is much more difficult and, hence, more expensive to clean up than the other agents. As mentioned, the Soviet Union produced large quantities of V-gas; this agent (or scientists who know how to manufacture it) may well be available to a terrorist for the right price. **Table 3-4** summarizes the V agents.

Table 3-4	Summary of V-Series Agents*				
Code name	Name	CAS number	Appearance	Odor	Route of exposure
VX	—	50782-69-9	Amber-colored or clear liquid	Odorless	Absorption, inhalation only at temperatures greater than 100°F
VE	918SN	21738-25-0	Amber-colored or clear liquid	Odorless	Absorption, inhalation only at temperatures greater than 100°F
VG	(Was sold as the pesticide Amiton)	78-53-5	Amber-colored or clear liquid Amiton oxylate is a powder.	Odorless	Absorption, inhalation only at temperatures greater than 100°F, ingestion of the powder form
V-gas	(Also designated as VR, Vx, Vsubx, RVX or Russian VX)	159939-87-4	Amber-colored or clear liquid	No odor	Absorption, inhalation only at temperatures greater than 100°F
VM	—	21770-86-5	(unavailable)	(unavailable)	(unavailable)
VS	—	73835-17-3	(unavailable)	(unavailable)	(unavailable)

*There are multiple other V agents that were investigated, but data for these agents are not available in the open-source literature.

■ Binary Agents: Third-Generation Nerve Agents

In 1948, the United States proposed production of a new variant of nerve agent—**binary munitions (Figure 3-3).** The concept is to use two chemicals that are not hazardous until mixed, transport them separately to the battlefield, then load them into the projectile just prior to use. When the projectile or bomb is fired or exploded, the two compartments rupture and the two agents combine. The final product of the resulting chemical reaction is a nerve agent.

The United States developed the **M687** binary munition in 1987. This munition was designed with two separate containers fitted into the shell **(Figure 3-4).** The second container is added just before the chemical weapon is to be fired. A disk between the two containers ruptures when the weapon is fired, and the chemicals are mixed by the rotation of the shell and react in flight. The binary munition is delivered in the usual fashion by mortar, plane, or artillery piece. The advantage is safety in transport and storage. There is no advantage in dissemination or decontamination.

Iraq used a slightly different approach. Their binary technology chemical weapon contained a single canister with one component.[40] A soldier dressed in protective gear added the second chemical into the munition just prior to delivery to the artillery unit. Needless to say, this approach can be somewhat hazardous for the soldier doing the mixing.

The Iraqi army used a mixture of pinacolyl alcohol and isopropyl alcohol to produce a mixture of sarin and soman in their binary weapon. The Russians experimented extensively with binary agents, as discussed in the next section.

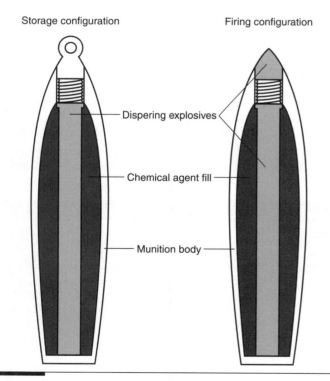

Figure 3-3 Typical chemical nerve agent shell construction of a binary munition.

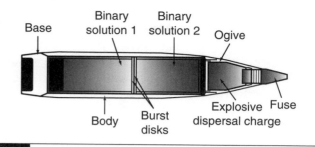

Figure 3-4 Prototype binary weapon for 155-mm artillery (M687).

■ New and Alternative Technology: Fourth-Generation Nerve Agents

Novichok

In the late 1980s and early 1990s, Russia apparently produced several new agents that were made of chemicals not controlled by the Chemical Weapons Convention. In late 1992, a Russian chemist, Vil Mirzayanov, stated that a military research institute in Moscow had developed a new binary nerve agent more potent than VX called **Novichok** (loosely translated in Russian as "newcomer"). He was subsequently arrested by the Russian Security Service for disclosing state secrets.[41] The status of this research is unknown.

The first Russian binary agent, Novichok-5, was derived from V-gas. A test batch of 5 to 10 metric tons was produced at a pilot-scale plant in Volgograd and field-tested at the chemical warfare testing ground at Nukus.

The Russian Federation Science Center State Research Institute of Organic Chemistry and Technology (**GosNIIOKhT**) developed a second binary form of Substance 33 that has no established name, but which Mirzayanov called Novichok-#. It also was tested at Nukus and adopted as a chemical warfare agent in 1990. Mirzayanov stated that the organization developed a third binary agent called Novichok-7, which has a similar volatility to soman but is about 10 times as effective. It was produced in experimental quantities (tens of tons) in Shikhany, as well as Volgograd. Two additional binary nerve agents, Novichok-8 and Novichok-9, were under development but were never produced.

The program that developed the Novichok agents was called **Foliant** by the Russians. Some open-source data about Novichok agents reveal the following:

■ These agents, referenced by a variety of code names including Substance 33, A-230, A-232, A-234, Novichok-5, and Novichok-7, are designed to be deployed as binary munitions.

■ These chemicals are at least as toxic and persistent as the most lethal nerve agent, VX, and some are reported to be 10 times as toxic.

- The Novichok agents apparently do not owe their toxicity to being an acetylcholinesterase inhibitor, at least according to Mirzayanov. They may inhibit acetylcholinesterase, but this may be only a minor or secondary effect. (This means that our conventional antidotes may be ineffective.)
- The Novichok agents are thought to be far more difficult to detect during manufacturing and far easier to manufacture covertly, because they can be made with common chemicals in relatively simple pesticide factories. In the words of Vil Mirzayanov regarding the agent, "The weapon's originality lies in the simplicity of its components, which are used in civilian industry and which cannot, therefore, be regulated by international experts."
- The Novichok agents may have been given to Iraq by Russian sources. The agent may have accounted for strange readings on US chemical weapons detectors that were labeled as spurious or bogus readings. This may indicate that current detection equipment may not be able to reliably detect the Novichok agents.
- The disabling effects of the Novichok agents, as described by Russian scientists, may include permanent neuropathy.
- Finally, unlike VX, which can be defeated quickly with injectable antidotes, the Novichok agents are at least as resistant to treatment as soman.

With the breakup of the Soviet Union, as with V-gas, the Novichok agents (or scientists who know how to manufacture them) may well be available to a terrorist at the right price. Considering that detection and treatment of these agents are not well established, the Novichok agents would prove to be quite problematic if used as a weapon of terrorism. The ability to manufacture them free of controls makes them quite appealing to terrorists. **Table 3-5** lists known open-source information regarding these agents.

Carbamates

Carbamates are a class of toxic pesticides that resemble the organophosphorus nerve agents in action. Carbamates are used in industry, agriculture, and households.

Like the organophosphates, they are well absorbed through all routes including the skin. Inhalation effects of the agent are uncommon, because carbamates are solid at room temperature, but it is not difficult to foresee a dispersal of a fine carbamate powder and the development of subsequent inhalation effects. To date, carbamates are not considered chemical warfare agents, because they have a number of operational drawbacks. However, if massive numbers of casualties resulted from a terrorist attack with this agent, medical treatment facilities would still be overwhelmed despite the availability of an antidote. Carbamates may be the basis of some of the Novichok agents.

Clinical Picture

The clinical picture of the patient with carbamate poisoning is just like the patient with organophosphate toxicity. The SLUDGE syndrome should be obvious and should point the examiner to cholinergic crisis.

The clinical syndrome of carbamate intoxication is shorter and milder than that caused by organophosphates. The carbamates do not penetrate into the CNS well, and cause less CNS effects. Convulsions are thought to be quite uncommon with carbamate intoxication.

Serum and red cell cholinesterase levels are unreliable predictors of carbamate toxicity. The enzyme activity reverts to normal within a few hours and does not correlate well with the patient's symptoms.

Thickened and Dusty Agents
Thickened Agents

Military researchers have investigated ways to change the physical characteristics of a chemical warfare agent in order to facilitate the agent's delivery. The researchers adjust the surface tension, density, storage parameters, and the droplet-forming shear rate using polymers and other chemical additives. These new formulations can also make decontamination more difficult.

A number of compounds have also been used to make some agents thicker and thus more persistent. These ad-

Table 3-5 Novichok Agents					
Name/symbol	Means of exposure	Lethal dosage	Rate of action	Effects	Antidotes/methods of treatment
Novichok agents*	Thought to be both liquid and vapor	*Novichok-5*: Estimated to exceed effectiveness of VX by 5 to 8 times *Novichok-7*: Estimated to exceed effectiveness of soman by 10 times	Very rapid	Assumed to be similar to the effects of other nerve agents. (This assumption has not been validated.)	Assumed to be similar to treatment methods for other nerve agents. (This assumption has not been validated.)

*For more information regarding Novichok agents, refer to Mirzayanov V: Dismantling the Soviet/Russian chemical weapons complex: An insider's view, in [Editors (eds):] *Chemical Weapons Disarmament in Russia: Problems and Prospects.* Washington, DC, Henry L. Stimson Center, 1995.

ditives make the agents cling to people and material without evaporating and also make the agents less susceptible to decontamination.

In 1969, the US military applied for a patent to thicken a number of chemical warfare agents, including lewisite, mustard, tabun, sarin, soman, and VX. Such a preparation was designed "to adhere to and prolong the level of contamination in the treated area."[42] The Russians also thickened soman, their version of VX, and lewisite.

Dusty

Dusty agents use a solid material that enhances aerosol formation. The term dusty refers to the use of a carrier particle, such as talc or **diatomaceous earth,** in order to form a particulate aerosol from the liquid agent.[43] Dusty agents increase the effectiveness of the base chemical warfare agent in three ways: increased coverage area, increased inhalation injury, and increased penetration of chemical warfare protective garments.

Use of a dusty agent enables the terrorist or chemical warfare specialist to increase the area of coverage with the base agent. The agent disperses in a large, concentrated cloud, making it possible for many more particles to reach soldiers or civilians and contaminate them, their clothing, and their equipment.

Dusty agent formulation increases the ability of VX to cause symptoms from inhalation. The fine particles containing VX are much more easily inhaled than the poorly vaporizing VX.

In addition to increasing the amount of agent that can be spread across an area, dusty agents also frustrate and defeat chemical protection measures. The very fine particles exploit weaknesses in chemical defensive gear by making their way into gaps and spaces of clothing, no matter how well they are fitted. Potentially, this includes full-body protective gear (Level A protection). Considering the persistence of VX along with the ability of VX to cause symptoms with skin exposure, this fine dust represents a significant chemical threat.[44]

The US military advocates using a poncho over **mission oriented protective posture (MOPP)** gear when the soldier is exposed to dusty agents:

WHILE EMPHASIZING THAT THERE IS NO EVIDENCE THAT IRAQ HAS DEVELOPED A DUSTY V-AGENT, FATALITIES RANGING FROM 3 TO 38 PERCENT ARE PROJECTED FOR THE SAME CONCENTRATIONS CITED ABOVE FOR TROOPS IN FULL MOPP IF SUCH AN AGENT WERE USED. USE OF THE PONCHO OVER THE MOPP GEAR IS EXPECTED TO REDUCE THESE PROJECTED CASUALTIES TO NEAR ZERO EVEN FOR A DUSTY NERVE AGENT.[45]

One senses that this recommendation was given in the face of few other options, considering that the open poncho could not possibly stop the very small particles of the dusty agent. A better protection (SERPACWA) was urgently developed and is discussed subsequently.

■ General Treatment of Nerve Agents

Nerve agents have an extremely rapid effect—particularly when inhaled. Treatment must be started rapidly after initial symptoms, or life support will be needed as respiratory arrest occurs. If multiple people have severe exposure to a nerve agent, it is quite likely that some of them will die. The cardinal principles of treatment for nerve agent intoxication are listed in **Table 3-6**.

Triage of the patient should be based on the available resources, the type of exposure (liquid or vapor), and the need for decontamination before therapy is attempted (**Table 3-7**). Based on the experience in Japan, those patients who have had exposure to nerve agent vapor and are still awake are not likely to get worse after arrival at the hospital.[46] Minimal decontamination should consist of the removal of all clothing and the washing of hair to remove residual vapor.[47]

This is not true if the patient has liquid nerve agent exposure. Following exposure to a nerve agent liquid, formal decontamination is a priority. Any residual nerve agent poses a continuing threat to the patient and to the medical staff caring for him or her.

Formal decontamination begins with removal of all clothing and irrigation with water. The patient's hair should be scissor trimmed close to the scalp and the scalp washed with soap and water. Do not use shears or razors, as this may cause scratches and ease the entry of residual nerve agent. After the irrigation and trim, the patient should be washed with soap and water or with bleach. The provider should avoid razors, stiff brushes, hot water, or scrubbing, as all of these can abrade skin and enhance the absorption of the nerve agent.[48,49] Antidotes are not needed for asymptomatic patients.

Table 3-6 Principles of Treatment for Nerve Agent Intoxication

1. Protect yourself.
   - The medical provider should wear full protective gear.
   - If possible, he or she should be pretreated with **pyridostigmine bromide**.
2. Terminate exposure by removing the individual from the contaminated area.
3. Assist ventilation (do NOT perform mouth-to-mouth resuscitation).
4. Administer atropine. The dose depends on the symptoms. Initial therapy of mild to moderate symptoms will require at least 2 mg IM or IV and may well require up to several milligrams over a period of time.
5. Decontaminate the patient.
6. Reactivate enzymes with an oxime. Administer 2-PAM in an initial dose of 500-1,000 mg intravenously. This is repeated every 4-6 hours as needed.
7. Confirm the diagnosis by assaying red blood acetylcholinesterase and/or plasma acetylcholinesterase.

Table 3-7 Triage for Individuals Exposed to Nerve Agents

Category	Definition	Description
IMMEDIATE	• Victim requires immediate lifesaving care when that care is available and of short duration.	• Circulation intact, talking, unable to walk. • Circulation intact, unable to talk or walk. • Circulation not intact, unable to talk or walk. Classification of these patients depends on the facilities available. If adequate facilities for all patients are unavailable, classify these patients as **expectant**.
DELAYED	• Victim requires major prolonged care, but a delay of care will not adversely affect the outcome of the injury.	• Has been given or used antidotes (eg, autoinjector); is showing signs of recovery.
MINIMAL	• Victim has relatively minor injuries that can be cared for by nonphysicians.	• Capable of walking, capable of talking, capable of self-care.
EXPECTANT	• Victim has severe injuries that will not be survivable even if given optimal care with available resources.	• Not talking, circulation failed. (These patients may be classified as immediate if treatment resources are adequate for all patients involved in the incident.)

NOTE: The categories above are based on military triage categories in the *Textbook of Military Medicine*, Part 1, Medical Aspects of Chemical and Biological Warfare. Office of the Surgeon General, Department of the Army, 1997.

Atropine

For over 40 years, the standard therapy for emergency treatment of anticholinesterase agents has been **atropine sulfate**. Atropine relieves the symptoms but does not attack the cause of the toxicity.

Atropine only works in certain parts of the cholinergic nervous system. Atropine reverses the muscarinic effects of nerve agent poisoning, such as bronchospasm, excessive respiratory secretions, and intestinal **hypermotility**. Atropine provides no protection from the effects of the organophosphates on the nicotinic receptors at the muscular junctions.

Large doses of atropine may be required for the reversal of the muscarinic effects of nerve agents. Although the military issues three autoinjectors with 2 mg of atropine each, this may be an inadequate dose for field treatment. Well-documented exposures requiring 20 to 40 mg of atropine are not unusual with exposure to nerve agents. Doses of more than 2000 mg/day have been required in organophosphate pesticide poisonings.[50]

In the sarin release in the Tokyo subway, one report noted less use of atropine than was expected.[51] It has been suggested that most patients from the Tokyo subway had only limited exposure because of the ineffectiveness of the delivery system of the sarin. It has been further pointed out that 82% of these patients had only minimal aerosol exposure to the agent and that the decreased use of atropine was therefore a result of the decreased exposure.

Few ambulances are equipped with more than a total of 10 to 15 mg of atropine in all of the drug boxes and resupplies carried on the ambulance. Likewise, few emergency departments have access to enough atropine to treat substantial numbers of severely affected victims. The ideal solution is rapid movement to the site of prepositioned supplies of atropine, but this may not be available or practical. Additional sources of atropine include the operating rooms where atropine may be stored. Field-expedient atropine sources include ophthalmic atropine and veterinary atropine.[52]

Pralidoxime

In 1951, oximes (of which pralidoxime chloride [2-PAM] is the most relevant to this discussion) were first proposed as a treatment of poisoning by nerve agents (**Figure 3-5**). These drugs are used to reactivate acetylcholinesterase bound by the nerve agent (**Figure 3-6**). The efficiency of the oxime depends on the enzyme, the oxime used, and the nerve agent that is in action. There is no single oxime available that is effective for all nerve agents. The US Army uses 2-PAM to treat nerve agent exposure. One other oxime, obidoxime (Toxogonin), has been tested successfully for sarin and tabun intoxication. Atropine and the oximes should be considered to complement each other, and the two antidotes appear to have a synergistic effect.

After the aging period, cholinesterase cannot be reactivated with conventional oximes. Aging takes place in hours

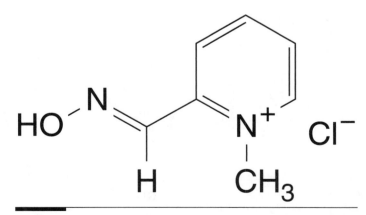

Figure 3-5 Pralidoxime chloride (2-PAM) molecular structure. Copyright © 1996–2002 Mitretek Systems, used with permission.

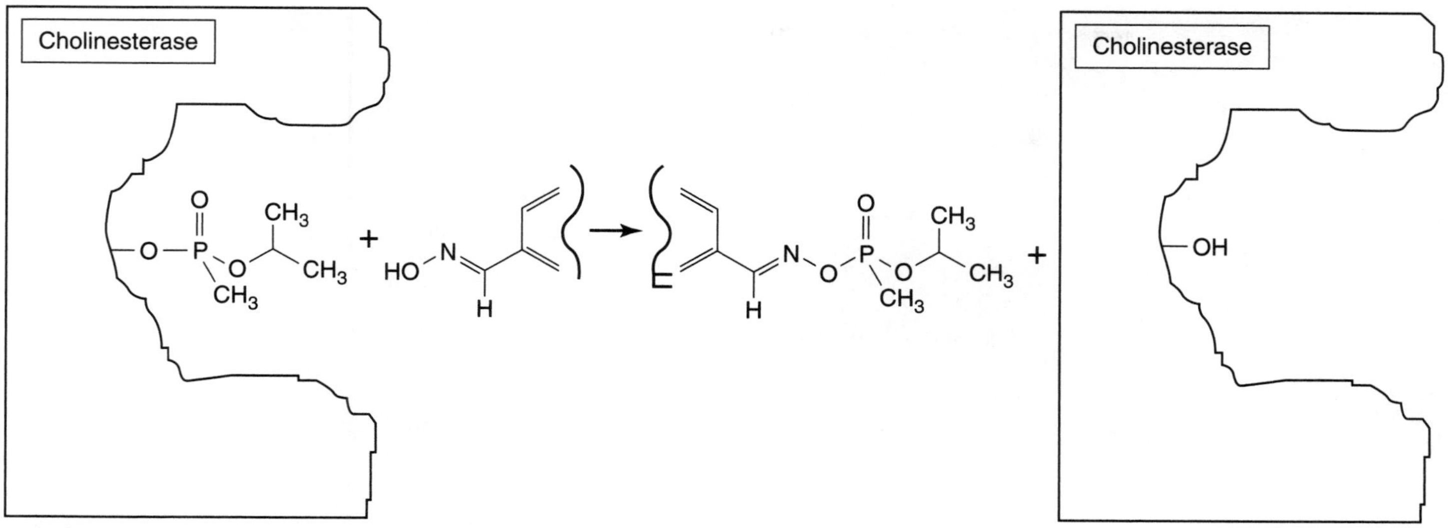

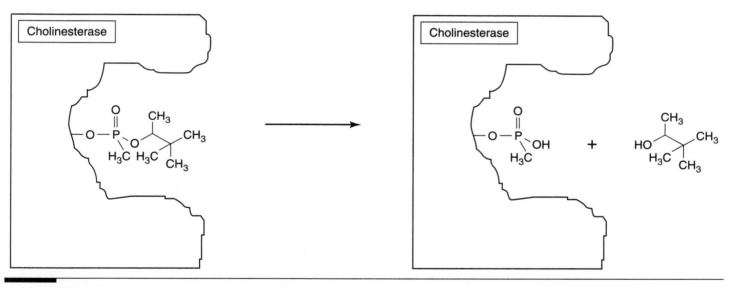

Figure 3-6 Regeneration of cholinesterase by 2-PAM. Copyright © 1996–2002 Mitretek Systems, used with permission.

Figure 3-7 Aging of cholinesterase associated with soman.

for sarin and VX, but occurs in about 2 minutes for soman; this makes soman exposure particularly difficult to treat with oximes **(Figure 3-7)**. For this reason, VX and sarin are the easiest of the nerve agents to treat, and all oximes increase the chances of survival with these agents. For commercial organophosphates, aging occurs after 24 to 48 hours.

H Oximes

A subset of conventional oximes is the **H oximes**. These include agents such as **HI-6**, **HGG-12**, and **HGG-42**. These oximes have been studied in the military setting but are not available for use in the United States. HI-6 **(Figure 3-8)** is approved for use in other countries **(Figure 3-9)**.

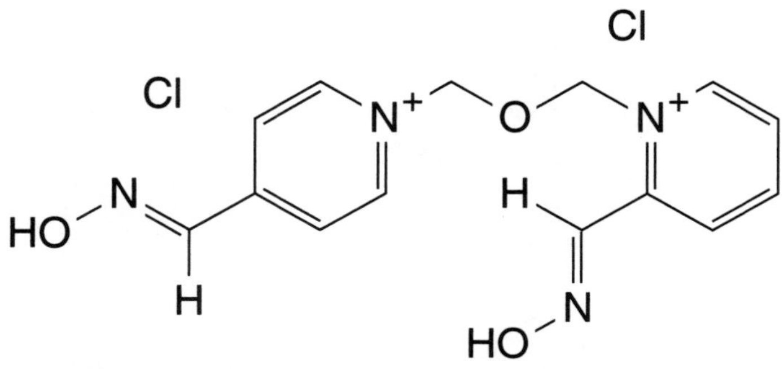

Figure 3-8 HI-6 molecular structure.

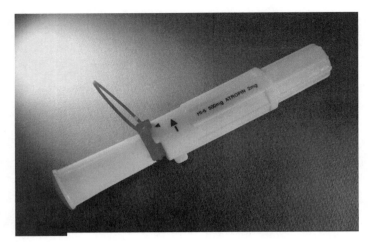

Figure 3-9 Swedish autoinjector with HI-6.

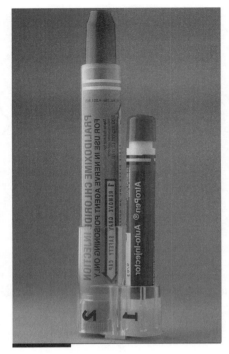

Figure 3-10 US Mark I Nerve Agent Antidote Kit (NAAK).

H oximes have shown promise in reactivating aged enzyme after soman exposure.[53] HI-6 appears to be the most effective antidote against tabun poisoning. It is possible that HI-6 has some positive antidotal effects in addition to reactivation of the aged enzyme.[54]

Use of Pralidoxime

Endpoints for therapy are the elimination of **bronchorrhea** (via atropine) and improvement of muscle strength (via oximes). Currently the US Army uses pralidoxime chloride (2-PAM) to reactivate cholinesterase. As stated, it is not completely effective, and it is least effective against soman. VX, on the other hand, has an aging period of several hours, and the use of 2-PAM is helpful in the treatment of this agent.

The US military NAAK (Nerve Agent Antidote Kit) **Mark I (Figure 3-10)** contains 2 IM autoinjectors, 1 with 2 mg of atropine and the other with 600 mg of pralidoxime, to be administered simultaneously in the event of nerve gas exposure. US soldiers carry three Mark I kits. They are trained to administer one combination injector through protective clothing and undergarments if any symptoms of exposure occur **(Figure 3-11)**. The recommended number of Mark I kits to be administered to a victim depends on the route of exposure, severity of clinical effects, and elapsed time after exposure.

Recently, a single-needle autoinjector combining both 2-PAM and atropine has been developed, called Advanced Treatment Nerve Agent Antidote or ATNAA **(Figure 3-12).**

INHOSPITAL INFO

Continuous intravenous infusion of 2-PAM for insecticidal organophosphate poisoning has been shown to be safe and effective. Current therapeutic guidelines suggest administration of 1 g of 2-PAM every 4 to 6 hours for organophosphate intoxication. Infusion (0.5 g/hr) provides serum levels of about 15 μg/mL in steady-state simulation in adults and may provide better therapy in patients with organophosphate intoxication.[55]

In available case reports of nerve agent intoxication, severe toxic effects often last only a few hours if the patient is thoroughly decontaminated and treatment with both atropine and 2-PAM is administered early. In contrast to organophosphate insecticides, repeated pralidoxime dosing may not be necessary for nerve agent poisoning.

Pralidoxime is rapidly excreted in the urine, and the patient should have adequate hydration during therapy. Patients with renal failure will require lower doses for continued therapy.

If intravenous access is difficult, a solution for intramuscular use can be made by mixing the contents of a 1-g

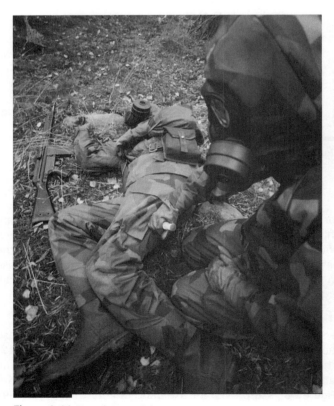

Figure 3-11 Use of an autoinjector.

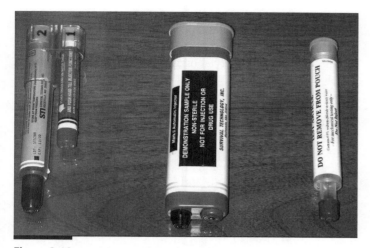

Figure 3-12 Autoinjectors (shown from left to right): NAAK Mark I, ATTNA, and CANA.

vial with 3 mL of sterile saline. Intramuscular administration to a patient with an adequate blood pressure produces plasma concentration of 4 mg/L within 10 minutes.[56]

In cases where the medical provider does not know the nature of the agent, use of 2-PAM will cause no harm to the patient and will protect the patient from organophosphate poisoning.

Carbamate Poisoning Treatment

The drug of choice for carbamate intoxication is atropine. The initial dose is 0.5 to 2 mg intravenously. This can be repeated every 15 to 30 minutes. Massive doses of atropine are not usually required for patients with carbamate intoxication. The rationale for atropine use is exactly the same for carbamate intoxication as for organophosphate intoxication, described previously.

Pralidoxime is not indicated for carbamate intoxication, because the acetylcholine complex is reversible. Pralidoxime may be used for patients in whom the diagnosis is in doubt or when the patient has ingested both types of acetylcholinesterase inhibitors. There is some controversy about whether the patient who is given pralidoxime for carbamate toxicity improves or worsens as a result. This controversy appears to be resolving in favor of administering pralidoxime.

Recovery is usually without event in patients who survive.

Diazepam and Other Benzodiazepines

If the patient presents with seizures or signs of severe intoxication, then diazepam should be administered in usual anticonvulsive doses. The addition of diazepam to the treatment protocol is recommended, because diazepam helps protect against seizures commonly found in nerve agent poisoning. Rapid treatment of seizures is essential to protect neurons.

In addition, diazepam has improved morbidity and mortality of soman poisoning.[57] Diazepam appears to provide some protection against permanent damage that may result from heavy exposure to nerve agents.[58] It is expected that all of the other benzodiazepines employed as usual antiseizure medications (such as lorazepam and midazolam) would be equally

useful in this regard in the context of nerve agent therapy. The US military issues diazepam as an autoinjector labeled CANA (**C**onvulsant **A**ntidote, **N**erve **A**gent).

Diazepam is an FDA Category D agent and may potentially damage the fetus, but the provider should realize that seizure associated with nerve agent intoxication is a potentially life-threatening disorder for the patient and proceed accordingly. Ativan is not associated with birth defects and would represent a better choice for the pregnant patient, if it is available.

Pediatric Antidote Doses

For all children less than 32 kg, the Mark I nerve agent antidote kit represents a serious overdose of atropine and 2-PAM. Risks versus benefits should be considered quite carefully before it is used. Endpoints for therapy are the same as for adults: elimination of bronchorrhea (via atropine) and improvement of muscle strength (via oximes).

Pediatric Atropine Suggested Doses

There is no available evidence regarding the use of atropine for treatment of nerve agent poisoning in the pediatric population. There is abundant literature about the use of atropine and similar agents as preoperative medications for the treatment of pediatric patients. There is also some experience with pediatric overdoses on commercial organophosphates, but how this experience relates to nerve agent exposure is unknown. Doses have been extrapolated for pediatric populations based on weight, but there are no experimental or even good anecdotal data that validate these extrapolations. These extrapolations are given in **Table 3-8**. The minimum dose used should be 0.1 mg.

Pediatric 2-PAM Suggested Doses

Table 3-9 shows suggested pediatric doses of 2-PAM. Larger doses may be needed in severe intoxications. There is limited experience with the use of oximes to treat organophosphate intoxication with commercial organophosphates in children. There is no practical experience with

Table 3-8	Pediatric Atropine Suggested Doses: 0.02 mg/kg Dose (2 mg/mL Concentration)			
Estimated age	Estimated weight	Dose in mL (route: IM) Exposure severity		
		Mild	Moderate	Severe
3 months	5 kg (11 lb)	0.1	0.1	0.2
12 months	10 kg (22 lb)	0.1	0.2	0.3
3 years	15 kg (33 lb)	0.2	0.3	0.5
6 years	20 kg (44 lb)	0.2	0.4	0.6
8 years	25 kg (55 lb)	0.3	0.5	0.8
10 years	30 kg (66 lb)	0.3	0.6	0.9
11 years	35 kg (77 lb)	0.4	0.7	1.1
12 years	40 kg (88 lb)	0.4	0.8	1.1
13 years	45 kg (99 lb)	0.5	0.9	1.4
14 years to adult	50+ kg (110+ lb)	1.0	2.0	3.0

Adapted from: Holstege CP, Kirk T, Sidell FR: Chemical warfare: Nerve agent poisoning. *Crit Care Med* 1997:13:923.

Table 3-9 Pediatric 2-PAM Chloride Suggested Doses: 10 to 25 mg/kg Dose (300 mg/mL Concentration)

Estimated age	Estimated weight	Dose in mL (route: IM) Exposure severity		
		Mild	Moderate	Severe
3 months	5 kg (11 lb)	0.5	1.0	1.25
12 months	10 kg (22 lb)	1.0	2.0	2.5
2 to 5 years	15 to 20 kg (33 to 44 lb)	1.5	3.0	3.75
6 years to adult	20 to 50+ kg (44 to 110+ lb)	2.0	4.0	4.5

Adapted from: Holstege CP, Kirk T, Sidell FR: Chemical warfare: Nerve agent poisoning. Crit Care Med 1997:13:923.

the use of this drug in the pediatric population for nerve agent exposure.

Pediatric Diazepam Suggested Doses

There is abundant literature about the use of diazepam and similar agents in the treatment of pediatric patients with seizures **(Table 3-10)**. There is limited experience with the use of diazepam and similar agents to treat seizures resulting from organophosphate intoxication with commercial organophosphates. There is no practical experience with the use of diazepam in the pediatric patient for nerve agent intoxication.

Geriatric Antidote Doses

As with pediatric patients, there is no evidence that supports (or refutes) a different dose of atropine for the geriatric population. However, note that any contraindication to atropine is relative in the face of a surely lethal exposure to a nerve agent.

Pregnancy

The doses for each of the agents mentioned above are the same for the adult pregnant patient as for nonpregnant adults. Although 2-PAM is a class C drug (use with caution—effects

Table 3-10 Pediatric Diazepam Suggested Doses: 0.2 mg/kg Dose (5 mg/mL Concentration)

Estimated age	Estimated weight	Dose in mL (route: IM)
3 months	5 kg (11 lb)	0.2
12 months	10 kg (22 lb)	0.4
3 years	15 kg (33 lb)	0.6
6 years	20 kg (44 lb)	0.8
8 years	25 kg (55 lb)	1.0
10 years	30 kg (66 lb)	1.2
11 years	35 kg (77 lb)	1.4
12 years	40 kg (88 lb)	1.6
13 years	45 kg (99 lb)	1.8
14 years to adult	50+ kg (110+ lb)	2.0

Adapted from: Holstege CP, Kirk T, Sidell FR: Chemical warfare: Nerve agent poisoning. Crit Care Med 1997:13:923.

unknown in pregnancy), there is simply no question that the choice between antidotes and death would lean heavily towards the use of 2-PAM. Pregnant women have been successfully treated for commercial organophosphate poisoning with atropine and pralidoxime in the second and third trimesters of pregnancy and have delivered healthy newborns.

Pretreatment

Because atropine/oxime antidote therapy has limitations, another approach is to competitively inhibit the nerve agent with a pretreatment drug. This drug must be relatively nontoxic and easily tolerated, and it must compete with nerve agents for acetylcholinesterase.

A high dose of nerve agent may permanently inactivate all remaining acetylcholinesterase and cause death. A lower, but otherwise lethal, dose may be inhibited by the reversible carbamate-bound acetylcholinesterase. The current carbamate of choice is **pyridostigmine**. It has a wide therapeutic margin of safety and appears to have no long-term toxicity to humans. Pyridostigmine has been used in the United States for years as a therapy for myasthenia gravis and is readily available in 30-mg tablets. The usual pretreatment dose is 30 mg orally every 8 hours, starting 6 to 8 hours prior to exposure.[59]

Data show that the use of atropine and 2-PAM will protect an animal for about 1.6 times the median lethal dose. With the addition of pretreatment, the protective ratio was increased to well over 20 times the median lethal dose. A human who survives a multiple exposure with the use of this combination therapy may require weeks to recover full functionality, however.

Pretreatment with cholinesterase inhibitors may improve survival when administered prior to exposure to tabun, soman, and cyclohexyl sarin. No evidence demonstrates that pretreatment before exposure to sarin or VX is effective.

The major problem with pretreatment is that it does not protect the individual against nerve agent–induced convulsions. Again, one expects multiple casualties from the combinations of convulsions, copious secretions, and decreased respiratory effort. Benzodiazepine will help protect against these convulsions, but it cannot be effectively administered as a pretreatment.

Barrier Creams

The US Army has developed a barrier cream, which is to be applied before entry into areas contaminated with dusty mustard and other chemical agents.[60] This cream is called **SERPACWA,** which stands for Skin Exposure Reduction Paste Against Chemical Warfare Agents **(Color plate 3-2).**[61] This cream has been tested against dusty mustard and chemical agents in animals. It has not been tested as chemical agent protection for humans. It appears to be effective against dusty mustard, but the protective effect of SERPACWA against dusty VX is unknown. The FDA made final approval of this cream in February 2000.[62] SERPACWA has only been tested in humans against nondangerous substitutes for chemical warfare agents (such as **urishiol**).[63]

This formulation appears to provide a prolonged protection for both mustard and exposure to organophosphates (about 4 hours' duration). This protective agent could be used for protection of the troops against chemical warfare agents. It is available in 84-g camouflaged plastic, single-use containers. This barrier cream has been approved for EMS and law enforcement agency purchase.

Fumes from SERPACWA are harmful and can cause **polymer-fume fever**. The fumes are released during burning. Clothing or other products that have been exposed to SERPACWA should not be destroyed by burning. Cigarettes that have been contaminated with SERPACWA can release these fumes, so smoking while using this cream is dangerous.

SERPACWA is designed to augment the protection afforded by MOPP gear. It was not designed to be used alone. SERPACWA's ability to reduce or delay absorption of chemical warfare agents after 5 hours from its application is unknown. **DEET** and some camouflage paints are known to reduce the effectiveness of SERPACWA. It should be presumed that some cosmetics would likewise reduce the effects of SERPACWA.

A second-generation SERPACWA known as **active Topical Skin Protectant** (aTSP) is in development. The active ingredient is designed to inactivate chemical warfare agents before they can penetrate the barrier cream. A **chloroamide** (S-330) has been shown to provide further protection from mustard when added to the barrier cream.[64] This product increases the effectiveness of SERPACWA by adding a component that neutralizes any chemical warfare agent that penetrates into the base cream. The availability of the improved formula is unknown.

The US Army is also working on another skin protective cream that will neutralize any chemical weapon agent and protect the wearer against the effects of the agent (**decontaminating protective skin cream**). These protective barrier creams would augment the protection afforded by protective garments or decrease the need for these garments in cases of lesser exposure. These creams have been described in military dermatology articles, but details are not available.

Decontamination

Self-protection is paramount in the care of these victims. As the Tokyo experience clearly demonstrated, large numbers of casualties will overwhelm emergency systems.[65] Contaminated patients may render an emergency department or even large parts of a hospital unusable.

Furthermore, the medical provider must not assume that the fire department or hazardous materials crew will contain the scene and decontaminate all patients before they are transported for care in the emergency department. It is likely that well-meaning police, passersby, friends, or family will bring some casualties directly to the emergency department. These casualties may have both vapor and liquid contamination of skin, hair, and clothing that can cause casualties among emergency providers.

All health care providers must wear full protective gear at all times during care for the patient until an environmental health specialist who is trained to detect these agents clears the patient. Because these are lethal agents, decontamination should be accomplished in complete protective gear with self-contained breathing apparatus if available. Although this should be a standard, most hospitals simply don't have a large enough budget to afford self-contained breathing apparatus and protective ensemble for most of the emergency staff.

In addition, the emergency provider must not depend on state or federal help for these incidents. Vast numbers of casualties will be seen, triaged, and either cared for or lost by the time additional federal or state help can be summoned, briefed, and clad in protective gear. This help may be assembled in a more timely fashion when terrorists strike at a popular event with preplanning, such as the Olympics. For most events, the provider must assume that no significant help will be available for a minimum of 2 to 4 hours after the incident has occurred.

A minimum for decontamination of the nerve gas intoxicated patient is Level C protection consisting of overgarments and a properly fitted canister-filter respirator (gas mask). Multipurpose inserts for protective masks have only a limited life span and should be carefully checked and replaced promptly. **Tyvek** and double layers of latex gloves provide little protection from nerve agents and should not be used, even in training. Nitrile or **butyl** rubber gloves and overgarments provide the best protection from dermal exposure.

The need for decontamination of patients presenting to the emergency department depends partly upon the nature of exposure. If the patient has only vapor exposure, contamination of clinical workers will be minimal.[66] Decontamination may consist of removal of the patient's clothing and washing with plain water.

Liquid contamination presents both vapor and dermal hazards to the staff. Local decontamination of the G agents may be accomplished with soap and water. As noted earlier, VX does not decompose with water and should be treated with bleach.

■ Threat of the Nerve Agents

Chemical warfare agents are not difficult to synthesize, and the synthesis procedures are readily available in scientific literature. The nerve agents can be manufactured by using fairly simple chemical techniques. The raw materials are inexpensive and available through common sources. Great caution is required, but a knowledgeable user can handle the agent.

As noted, one terrorist group, Aum Shinrikyo, has already produced and deployed a nerve agent as a terror weapon. With the great psychological effects that these agents cause when used in a terror campaign and the increasing threats against US civilians, there can be no doubt that emergency providers in the United States will see these agents employed.

The technologies required for the production of nerve agents have been known for over 40 years and are easily within the capabilities of anyone with a master's degree in chemistry or the equivalent. In addition, chemical weapons can be made with commercial equipment that is generally available in any country.

The most common nerve agents can be clustered into three production process groups: tabun, sarin/soman, and VX. There are a wide variety of alternative production techniques within each group. These production techniques have been published in a wide variety of open-source chemical literature and include data on reaction kinetics, catalysts, and operating parameters. At the same time, thousands of applied organic chemists and chemical engineers from developing countries have been trained in related chemical production techniques at universities in the United States, Europe, and the former Soviet Union.

The technical hurdles associated with the production of small quantities of nerve agents are not fundamentally different from those associated with commercial products, such as organophosphate pesticides. These hurdles are well described in the open-source literature.

Production hurdles for nerve agents include the following:

■ The cyanation reaction for tabun, which involves the containment of a highly toxic gas
■ The alkylation step for sarin, soman, and VX, which requires the use of high temperatures and the processing of corrosive and dangerous reactants, such as hot hydrochloric acid or hydrogen fluoride
■ The careful control of temperature, including the cooling of the reactor vessel during exothermic reactions.
■ The safe handling of intermediates that can react explosively with water
■ The distillation step, if high purity agents are required (unnecessary for terrorism)

Although some of the steps in the production of nerve agents are difficult and hazardous, they represent a nuisance more than an obstacle to a determined terrorist group. This has already been demonstrated by the production of nerve agents by Aum Shinrikyo. Germany produced tons of tabun very effectively with 1940s technology and without the stringent safety and environmental standards that would be invoked today. In an attempt to conceal the production of nerve agents, a terrorist organization may well resort to production processes that have been discarded by the military because they cost too much, were inefficient, or needed an unusual catalyst or precursor.

Tabun was the first militarized nerve agent and is the simplest to produce. Tabun is made from four precursor chemicals: phosphorus oxychloride ($POCl_3$), sodium cyanide, dimethylamine, and ethyl alcohol. Two of these chemicals (dimethylamine and phosphorus oxychloride) are restricted chemicals, but they are still available in small quantities and are produced in several countries for commercial applications in the production of pharmaceuticals, pesticides, and gasoline additives.

The basic batch process for tabun was developed by Germany during World War II and was employed by Saddam Hussein's Iraq. Synthesis of tabun does not require the use of corrosives and does not produce reactive intermediates. It is a two-step process that requires that the chemicals be added in the correct order and kept from heating, and it does not require further distillation of the toxic products. The Iraqis produced 40% tabun in large quantities with this process. There is simply no reason why small quantities for use in terrorist operations could not be produced in a small laboratory with appropriate apparatus and protective gear.

Sarin and soman are both made in a batch process with the same reaction steps and apparatus. As noted previously, they differ only in the alcohol used in the reaction: isopropyl alcohol is used for sarin and pinacolyl alcohol is used for soman. Phosphorus trichloride (PCl_3) is the basic starting material for synthesis of both agents. Depending on which of several alternative pathways are chosen for the synthesis, from two to five steps are required to produce the nerve agent.

There are three major obstacles specific to small-batch synthesis of G agents by terrorists:

1. The synthesis of G agents requires the use of hot hydrochloric acid and hydrogen fluoride, both of which are extremely corrosive. If corrosion-resistant reactors and pipes are not used, the chance of major leaks with resultant danger to the manufacturer is significantly increased.
2. G agent manufacture also requires an alkylation reaction, which is not used in the production of commercial pesticides and is technically difficult.
3. Distillation of the final product may be necessary, which is an extremely hazardous operation. When an agent is not distilled, the quality is poor and the agent deteriorates rapidly. If the terrorist organization were to make G agents without this process, the sarin or soman would have to be refrigerated and used within a short time.

There are at least three practical synthesis routes for V agents that could be used by a terrorist. As with G agents, production of VX involves an alkylation reaction that is technically difficult. However, because there is no fluorine involved in the synthesis, corrosion-resistant plumbing and vessels are not required. After the alkylation step is completed, the remainder of the synthesis is relatively simple.

Aside from proliferation, effective dissemination poses a quandary for nonmilitarized would-be purveyors of chemical weapons. The major problem with deployment of the agents is delivery and dispersal. Traditionally, military planners have used munitions, mines, and aerial sprays for these agents. These military planners point out that design of these munitions for effective dispersal requires significant knowledge. However, a significant consideration is that *effective* is a very relative term. As the Tokyo experience with sarin showed, the number of casualties produced by a terrorist attack would be out of proportion to the amount of agent employed as a result of the fear and panic that followed the first few casualties.[67] This is not necessarily true of trained and properly equipped soldiers.

What might be a terrorist target for a nerve agent? The agent would be most effective in an enclosed area, such as a stadium, subway, airport, shopping mall, or commercial building. Sidell points out with simple arithmetic that, for a building that is 100 m on a side by 50 m high (a large office building, typical sports arena, auditorium, or convention hall), a concentration of 10 mg/m³ can be produced with about 5 kg of agent or about 7.5 L.[68] If this amount of agent were dispersed evenly, most of the people within the building would be severely poisoned. Because sarin evaporates rapidly, this dispersal could be accomplished through the ventilation or air-conditioning system. The use of simple explosives to seal doors would markedly increase both the psychological and lethal effects.

If the agent were used out of doors, a substantially larger quantity would be required. In this setting, the volatility of sarin may work against the terrorist and a persistent agent such as VX may be more suitable. The agent would vaporize and the vapor would be susceptible to wind currents. A crop sprayer or other aerosol-producing equipment could be used to form a dense fog of nerve agent over a large crowd such as at a sporting event. Although airplane spraying is one consideration, such a means of dissemination is not necessary. As recent events have shown, the terrorists may not expect their survival to be a necessary condition for the terrorism, which makes their planning much simpler.

■ References

1. Pittaway AR: *The Difficulty of Converting Pesticide Plants to CW Nerve Agent Manufacture.* Task IV, Technical Report No. 7, Kansas City, MO, Midwest Research Institute, February 20, 1970.

2. Paxman J, Harris R: *A Higher Form of Killing: The Secret Story of Chemical and Biological Warfare.* New York, NY, Hill and Wang, 1982, pp 53-67, 138-139.

3. Compton JAF: *Military Chemical and Biological Agents.* Caldwell, NJ, Teleford Press, 1987, p 135.

4. Pine A: Pentagon Reports 15,000 Troops Possibly Exposed to Iraqi Toxins. *Los Angeles Times,* October 2, 1996, on page 2. Found at http://www-tech.mit.edu/V116/N47/pentagon.47w. html (accessed March 22, 2004).

5. Harris LW, Heyl WC, Stitcher DL, et al: Effects of 1.1' -oxydimethylene bis-(4-tertbutylpyridinium chloride) (SAD-128) and decamethonium on reactivation of soman and sarin-inhibited cholinesterase by oximes. *Biochem Pharmacol* 1978;27:757-761.

6. Brown JH, Taylor P: Muscarinic receptor agonists and antagonists, in Hardman JG, Kimberd LE (eds): *Goodman and Gilman's The Pharmacologic Basis of Therapeutics.* New York, NY, McGraw-Hill, 1996, vol 9, p 141.

7. Taylor P, Brown JH: Acetylcholine, in Seigel GJ, Agranoff BW, Albers RW, et al (eds): *Basic Neurochemistry.* New York, NY, Raven Press, 1994, vol 5, p 231.

8. Rengstroff RH: Accidental exposure to sarin: Vision effects. *Arch Toxicol* 1985;56:201-203.

9. Kato T, Hamanaka T: Ocular signs and symptoms caused by exposure to sarin gas. *Am J Ophthalmol* 1996;121:209.

10. Morito H, Yanagisawa N, Nakajima T, et al: Sarin poisoning in Matsumoto, Japan. *Lancet* 1995;346:290.

11. Yokoyoma K, Yamada A, Mimura N: Clinical profiles with sarin poisoning after the Tokyo subway attack. *Am J Med* 1996;100:586.

12. Anonymous: Nerve agents: A FOA briefing book on chemical weapons. FOA, S-172 90 Stockholm, Sweden http://www.opcw.nl/chemhaz/nerve.htm (accessed October 29, 2001).

13. Ludomirsky A, Klein HO, Sarelli P, et al: Q-T prolongation and polymorphous ("torsades de pointes") ventricular arrhythmias associated with organophosphorus insecticide poisoning. *Am J Cardiol* 1982;49:1654.

14. Anzueto A, Berdine G, Moore G, et al: Pathophysiology of soman intoxication in primates. *Toxicol Applied Pharmacol* 1986;86:56.

15. Ludomirsky A, Klein HO, Sarelli P, et al: Q-T prolongation and polymorphous ("torsades de pointes") ventricular arrhythmias associated with organophosphorus insecticide poisoning. *Am J Cardiol* 1982;49:1654.

16. Robineau P, Guittin P: Effects of an organophosphorus compound on cardiac rhythm and haemodynamics in anaesthetized and conscious beagle dogs. *Toxicol Lett* 1987;37:95.

17. Ludomirsky A, Klein HO, Sarelli P, et al: Q-T prolongation and polymorphous ("torsades de pointes") ventricular arrhythmias associated with organophosphorus insecticide poisoning. *Am J Cardiol* 1982;49:1654.

18. Kiss Z, Fazekas T: Arrhythmias in organophosphate poisonings. *Acta Cardiol* 1979;34:323.

19. Robineau P, Guittin P: Effects of an organophosphorus compound on cardiac rhythm and haemodynamics in anaesthetized and conscious beagle dogs. *Toxicol Lett* 1987;37:95.

20. Grob D: The manifestations and treatment of poisoning due to nerve gas and other organic phosphate anticholinesterase compounds. *Arch Intern Med* 1956;98:221.

21. Grob D, Harvey JC: Effects in man of the anticholinesterase compound sarin (isopropyl methyl phosphonofluoridate). *J Clin Invest* 1958;37:358.

22. Johnson RP, Gold AJ, Freeman G: Comparative lung-airway resistance and cardiovascular effects in dogs and monkeys following parathion and sarin intoxication. *Am J Physiol* 1958;192:581.

23. Wright PG: Analysis of the central and peripheral components of respiratory failure produced by anticholinesterase poisoning in the rabbit. *J Physiol* 1954;126:52.

24. Holstege CP, Kirk M, Sidell FR: Chemical warfare: Nerve agent poisoning. *Crit Care Clin* 1997;13:923.

25. Grob D: The manifestations and treatment of poisoning due to nerve gas and other organic phosphate anticholinesterase compounds. *Arch Intern Med* 1956;98:221.

26. Anzueto A, Berdine G, Moor G, et al: Pathophysiology of soman intoxication in primates. *Toxicol Applied Pharmacol* 1986;86:56.

27. Grob D, Harvey JC: Effects in man of the anticholinesterase compound sarin (isopropyl methyl phosphonofluoridate). *J Clin Invest* 1958;37:358.

28. Abou-Donia M: Organophosphorus ester-induced delayed neurotoxicity. *Ann Rev Pharmacol Toxicol* 1981;21:511-548.

29. Laskowski MB, Olson WH, Dettbarn WD: Ultrastructural changes at the motor end-plate produced by an irreversible cholinesterase inhibitor. *Exp Neurol* 1976;47:290-306.

30. Nishiwaki Y, Maekawa K, Ogawa Y, et al: Effects of sarin on the nervous system in rescue team staff members and police officers 3 years after the Tokyo subway sarin attack. *Environ Health Persp* 2001;109:A542.

31. Yokoyama K, Araki S, Murata K, et al: A preliminary study on delayed vestibulo-cerebellar effects of Tokyo

subway sarin poisoning in relation to gender difference: Frequency analysis of postural sway. *J Occ Environ Med* 1998;40:17.

32. Nakajima T: Sequelae of sarin toxicity at one and three years after exposure in Matsumoto, Japan. *J Epidemiol* 1999;9:337-343.

33. McLeod CG: Pathology of nerve agents: Perspective on medical management. *Fund Appl Toxicol* 1985;5:S10-S16.

34. Ludomirsky A, Hlein HO, Sarelli P, et al: Q-T prolongation and polymorphous ("torsade de pointes") ventricular arrhythmias associated with organophorus insecticide poisoning. *Am J Cardiol* 1982;49:1654-1658.

35. Okumura T, Takasu N, Ishimatsu S, et al: Report on 640 victims of the Tokyo subway sarin attack. *Ann Emerg Med* 1996;28:129-135.

36. Anonymous: FAS nerve agents briefing. http://www.fas.org/irp/gulf/oia/970825/970613_dim37_91d_txt_0001.html (accessed April 19, 2003).

37. Yang YC, Baker JA, Ward JR: Decontamination of chemical warfare agents. *Chem Rev* 1992;92:1729-1743.

38. Yang YC, Szfraniec LL, Beaudry WT, Rohrbaugh DK: Oxidative detoxification of phosphonothiolates. *Am Chem Soc* 1990;112(18):6621-6627.

39. Anonymous: Chemistry of VX. Mitretek, http://www.mitretek.org/offcr/energylcw_page/vx.htm (accessed January 3, 1999).

40. Anonymous: Nerve agents: FOA briefing book on chemical weapons. FOA, S-172 90 Stockholm, Sweden. http://www.opcw.nl/chemhaz/nerve.htm (accessed March 22, 2002).

41. Englund W: Ex-Soviet scientist says Gorbachev's regime created new nerve gas in '91. *Baltimore Sun*, September 16, 1992:3.

42. The United States of America as represented by the secretary of the Army. US patent application number 855078, September 2, 1969.

43. Hassall, KA: *The Chemistry of Pesticides*. Deerfield Beach, FL, Verlag Chemie, 1982, p 31.

44. Iraq-Kuwait: Chemical warfare dusty agent threat. US Defense Intelligence Agency (Filename:73349033), October 10, 1990, http://www.desert-storm.com/Gulflink/950719dl.txt (accessed December 10, 2002).

45. Iraq-Kuwait: Chemical warfare dusty agent threat. US Defense Intelligence Agency (Filename:73349033), October 10, 1990, http://www.desert-storm.com/Gulflink/950719dl.txt (accessed December 10, 2002).

46. Okumura T, Takasu N, Ishimatsu S, et al: Report on 640 victims of the Tokyo subway sarin attack. *Ann Emerg Med* 1996;28:129-135.

47. Holstege CP, Kirk T, Sidell FR: Chemical warfare: Nerve agent poisoning. *Crit Care Med* 1997:13:923.

48. Weber LW, Zesch A, Rozman K: Decontamination of human skin exposed to 2,3,7,8-tetrachlorodibenzo-p-dioxin (TCDD) in vitro. *Arch Environ Health* 1992;47:302.

49. Wester RC, Maibach HI: In vivo percutaneous absorption and decontamination of pesticides in humans. *J Toxicol Environ Health* 1985;16:25.

50. DuToit P, Muller F, Van Tonder W, et al: Experience with the intensive care management of organophosphate insecticide poisoning. *S African Med J* 1981;60:227-229.

51. Okumura T, Takasu N, Ishimatsu S, et al: Report on 640 victims of the Tokyo subway sarin attack. *Ann Emerg Med* 1996;28:129-135.

52. Holstege CP, Kirk T, Sidell FR: Chemical warfare: Nerve agent poisoning. *Crit Care Med* 1997:13:923.

53. Exner 0, Benn MH, Willis F: *Can J Chem* 1968;46:1873.

54. Anonymous: Nerve agents: FOA briefing book on chemical weapons. FOA, S-172 90 Stockholm, Sweden, http://opcw.nl/chemhaz/nerve.htm (accessed March 22, 2002).

55. Hoidal CR, Hall Kulig KW, et al: Pralidoxime chloride continuous infusions. Letter. *Ann Emerg Med* 1987;16:831.

56. Holstege CP, Kirk T, Sidell FR: Chemical warfare: Nerve agent poisoning. *Crit Care Med* 1997:13:923.

57. Kusic R, Jovanovic D, Randjeovic D, et al: HI-6 in man: Efficacy of oxime in poisoning by organophosphorus insecticides. *Hum Exp Toxicol* 1991;10:113-118.

58. Anonymous: Nerve agents: FOA briefing book on chemical weapons. FOA, S-172 90 Stockholm, Sweden, http://opcw.nl/chemhaz/nerve.htm (accessed March 22, 2002).

59. *Pyridostigmine Pretreatment for Nerve Agents.* US Army Academy of Health Sciences (Field Circular No 8-48), March 26, 1987.

60. Smith KJ, Hurst CG, Moeller RB, et al: Sulfur mustard: Its continuing threat as a chemical warfare agent, the cutaneous lesions induced, progress in understanding its mechanism of action, its long term health effects, and new developments for protection and therapy. *J Am Acad Derm* 1995;32:765-776.

61. Smith KJ, Hurst CG, Moeller RB, et al: Sulfur mustard: Its continuing threat as a chemical warfare agent, the cutaneous lesions induced, progress in understanding its mechanism of action, its long term health effects, and new developments for protection and therapy. *J Am Acad Derm* 1995;32:765-776.

62. Drugs approved by the FDA: Drug name: Skin exposure reduction paste against chemical warfare agents (SERPACWA). Centerwatch, http://www.centerwatch.com/patient/drugs/dru606.html (accessed April 20, 2002).

63. Liu DK: Efficacy of the topical skin protectant in advanced development. *J Appl Toxicol* December 1,1999;19(suppl 1): S40-S45.

64. Braue EH Jr: Development of a reactive topical skin protectant. *J Appl Toxicol* December 1, 1999;19(suppl 1):S47-S53.

65. Okumura T, Takasu N, Ishimatsu S, et al: Report on 640 victims of the Tokyo subway sarin attack. *Ann Emerg Med* 1996;28:129-135.

66. Okumura T, Takasu N, Ishimatsu S, et al: Report on 640 victims of the Tokyo subway sarin attack. *Ann Emerg Med* 1996;28:129-135.

67. Romano JA Jr: Psychological casualties resulting from chemical and biological weapons. *Mil Med* 2001;166 (suppl 12):21-22.

68. Sidell FR: Chemical agent terrorism. *Ann Emerg Med* 1996;28:223-224.

Pulmonary Agents

■ Introduction

Chemical agents that attack lung tissue are classified as lung-damaging agents. These choking or pulmonary agents are characterized by pronounced irritation of the upper and lower respiratory tract. The military list of pulmonary agents includes phosgene, **diphosgene**, **chlorine**, **perfluoroisobutylene** (PFIB), and **chloropicrin**. Inhalation of organohalides, oxides of nitrogen, and many other compounds can cause the same pulmonary irritation as chlorine and phosgene. PFIB is a toxic combustion product of Teflon non-stick coating and other polymers encountered in civilian and military construction. The oxides of nitrogen are used in industry and in components of blast weapons, and they can be products of toxic decomposition. Smoke-producing devices may contain toxic compounds that cause the same effects as phosgene. The medical management of phosgene and chlorine exposure also applies to casualties of compounds such as PFIB or nitrogen oxides.

The effects of the pulmonary agents can be particularly difficult to diagnose and treat because they often have a latent period of several hours following exposure. Chemically induced acute lung injury by these agents involves a permeability defect in the blood-air interface (the alveolar-capillary membrane). After exposure, a victim's symptoms of dyspnea and mild chest discomfort may progress in severity over a few hours.

■ Chlorine

Chlorine (CL) is a slightly water-soluble, yellowish gas that is about 2.5 times heavier than air. The use of 498 tons of chlorine released from 20,730 cylinders on April 22, 1915, was the cause of more than 7,000 casualties at Ypres, Belgium **(Figure 4-1).** This agent has fallen into military disfavor because it is quite easy to detect and protect against. However, it is readily available as an improvisational weapon for those seeking unconventional weapons. Millions of tons of chlorine are used in bleaching, water purification (including water for swimming pools), and chemical processes. Chlorine is one of the greatest causes of accidental industrial toxic exposure.[1]

Adding chlorine bleach to an acidic cleaning agent will produce free chlorine gas. The extent of the resulting injury depends on the concentration and duration of the exposure. Symptoms begin within moments of exposure; no delayed symptoms are noted.

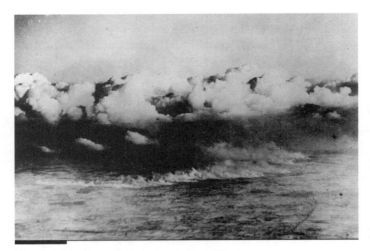

Figure 4-1 Release of chlorine gas in World War I.

When chlorine is dissolved in water, it forms hypochlorous acid and hydrochloric acid.

$$HOH + Cl_2 5 \Rightarrow HOCl + HCL$$

Threat

Use of chlorine gas in an unconfined area would require massive amounts of chlorine to be released in a short period of time. This would be a daunting undertaking for the terrorist wishing to deploy chlorine as a weapon. Chlorine could well be effective within a closed environment such as subway or auditorium. However, because other, more effective agents are readily available, chlorine is an unlikely terrorist weapon. Because accidental exposures to chlorine are quite common, the emergency provider needs to be well aware of the toxicity of chlorine and the treatment for its effects.

Delivery

Chlorine gas is heavier than air and can be delivered by bomb, artillery, or mortar round, or it can simply be released from a canister. It will follow the curves of hills and will flow into caves, trenches, and hollows. Chlorine has a strong and distinctive odor. Because the odor threshold of chlorine is 0.08 ppm and is well below the threshold of toxicity, the sense of smell usually provides appropriate warning that chlorine is present.

Effects

Chlorine readily dissolves in the moist mucosa of the upper respiratory tract. The resulting reaction with water causes rhinorrhea, hypersalivation, and may cause **laryngeal edema**. In the lower respiratory tract, the reaction causes coughing, wheezing, and may cause rales and pulmonary edema. High concentrations of chlorine gas will produce chemical skin burns. **Table 4-1** lists the effects of various concentrations of chlorine gas.

Chlorine effects are usually related to the extent of the pulmonary damage. The typical pulmonary pattern of those exposed to a moderate concentration of chlorine gas is increased airway resistance. Pulmonary function will return to normal in most patients within months.[2] As might be expected, patients with worse subjective complaints tended to have slower resolution than those with simpler complaints such as cough.[3]

Treatment

There is no specific antidote for the inhalation of chlorine. Treatment is entirely supportive and includes supplemental oxygen and early intubation for patients with pulmonary edema.

Eye injuries should be evaluated with **fluorescein staining** (preferably with a slit lamp). For eye irritation, irrigate the eye promptly with copious amounts of water. If available, monitor the irrigation of the eye with a pH reagent strip.

Most victims exposed to chlorine gas will recover without problems. Only if the patient has exposure to high concentrations of chlorine would significant aftereffects be found. Prolonged pulmonary disease after exposure to chlorine is uncommon.

Table 4-1	Effects of Various Concentrations of Chlorine Gas	
Exposure level	Concentration (ppm)	Effects
Mild	0.002	Odor detection threshold.
	1	US TLV-TWA limit.*
	1–3	Mild mucous membrane irritation. U.S. short-term exposure is limited to 1 ppm.
Moderate	5–15	Moderate mucous membrane and upper respiratory tract irritation. Lacrimation, conjunctival irritation, and rhinorrhea.
Severe	30	Chest pain, dyspnea, cough, severe upper respiratory tract irritation, headache, and vomiting. Laryngeal edema may produce hoarseness.
	40–60	Pulmonary damage—ulcerative tracheobronchitis, laryngeal edema, pneumonitis, and pulmonary edema. Corneal abrasions and burns. Cutaneous burns may be present in moist areas.
Lethal	430	Potentially lethal for exposure of about 30 minutes.
	1000	Fatal within minutes.

*TLV (threshold limit value) The permissible exposure that a worker can tolerate without fear of damage. TWA (time weighted average) An average exposure over a specified time—usually 8 hours.

Oxygen

Measure the oxygen saturation in all symptomatic patients, because hypoxia is common. These patients frequently need oxygen supplementation. Humidified oxygen treatment should be continued until symptoms abate.

Early administration of **Intermittent Positive Pressure Breathing (IPPB)**, **Positive End Expiratory Pressure (PEEP)**, or Bi-level Positive Airway Pressure (BiPAP) may be quite helpful in minimizing the pulmonary edema and reducing the degree of hypoxia.[4] Intubation with or without a ventilator may be appropriate.

Nebulizer Treatments

Patients with hyperactive airways may benefit from aerosolized bronchodilators such as albuterol or terbutaline.[5] **Beta-adrenergic agonists** relax airway smooth muscle and reduce hyperactivity and resultant airway narrowing in patients with chlorine inhalation. Aminophylline or theophylline may be considered for these patients.[6]

Corticosteroids

Administration of corticosteroids has been recommended, but there is no solid proof of their beneficial effects in the treatment of pulmonary edema resulting from chlorine inhalation. When corticosteroids are used, they should be given in high doses by inhalation or intravenously. There are two regimens in use: one uses dexamethasone and the other uses beclomethasone. The doses of corticosteroids used for chlorine-induced pulmonary edema are much higher than those used for asthma.

Antibiotics

Antimicrobial therapy should be reserved for a proven bacterial bronchitis or pneumonia. Bacterial **superinfection** resulting in bronchitis or pneumonia may develop 3 to 5 days after exposure to chlorine. The medical provider should search for this infection if the patient does not improve within 3 to 4 days after exposure to chlorine. Prophylactic antibiotic therapy is inappropriate.

Rest

It is important that a patient exposed to chlorine be kept at rest until the danger of pulmonary edema is past. This may not be possible in some situations, however. If the patient has significant respiratory involvement, litter evacuation is necessary.

Diuretics

The pulmonary edema associated with chlorine is noncardiac. Treatment of the chlorine-induced noncardiac pulmonary edema is supportive. Diuretics such as furosemide have only a very limited utility in these patients and should generally not be used.

Decontamination

Decontamination of the victim should begin with extensive irrigation of irritated areas. Chlorine is quite soluble in water and is easily dispersed. The patient's clothing should be removed if it is contaminated with liquid chlorine. Following irrigation of the patient and removal of the patient's clothing, the medical provider needs no special contamination protection for pure chlorine exposure. Chlorine gas exposure represents little risk for the medical care provider. A chemical protective mask will suffice, after chlorine is confirmed as the responsible agent.

If chlorine exposure of the skin is significant, thoroughly flush the skin with water. If there is eye irritation, then the eye should also be irrigated with copious amounts of water.

If available, a pH reagent strip can be used to monitor irrigation of the eye.

Personal Protection

Operations teams are advised to don Level B or A protection when handling casualties until chlorine is confirmed as the responsible agent. Filter-type protective masks are effective for chlorine, so Level C protection is sufficient when contamination with chlorine is confirmed.

■ Phosgene

Phosgene (CG) is a chemical agent used to cause pulmonary damage and asphyxia. During World War I, liquid-filled explosive shells were used to deliver this agent. Although phosgene is a liquid, it rapidly vaporizes into a colorless, low-lying gas that is three times as dense as air. It does not cause immediate damage and thus often permits a lengthy and profound exposure as the victim continues to breathe.

It is one of the most deadly of the chemical war munitions. The average lethal dose of phosgene is 500 to 800 ppm/min. This means that a 10-minute exposure to only 50 to 80 ppm would likely be lethal. The military defines a 2-ppm concentration of phosgene as being immediately dangerous to life and health.[7] Mild symptoms occur at 3 to 5 ppm (eye, nose, and throat irritation). Pulmonary edema occurs at doses exceeding 600 mg•min/m^3.[8] Though phosgene is less potent than almost all of the subsequently developed chemical warfare agents, its danger should not be underestimated; deaths have occurred after only a few breaths of this gas.

Phosgene is variously described as smelling like decaying fruit, freshly cut grass or hay, and moldy hay. The odor threshold is about 1.5 ppm, but trained workers can detect it at concentrations below 1 ppm. Sense of smell is a poor guide to concentration of phosgene. At higher concentrations, olfactory fatigue rapidly sets in, and the victim loses his or her sense of smell as well as the ability to assess danger. The sense of smell is not a sufficient warning to prevent toxicity.

Threat

Phosgene is a commercial precursor to plastics manufacture. The United States produces over a billion pounds (about 500 million kilograms) of phosgene per year for industrial uses. It is shipped in large containers in public commerce, making it vulnerable to illegal procurement. It has a proven track record as a significant war agent in World War I. As such, it is an attractive improvisational agent for the terrorist.

Mechanism of Action

The mechanism of action of phosgene is not fully understood. Theories for its action include the dissolution of phosgene within the alveolus to hydrochloric acid, resulting in subsequent alveolar damage, inhibition of enzymes, and a direct reaction at the alveolar and capillary wall interface. Once phosgene dissolves, it rapidly hydrolyzes to form carbon dioxide and hydrochloric acid. The early effects of this are onset of ocular, nasal, pharyngeal, and central airway irritation.

Whatever the mechanism of action, phosgene increases the permeability of the alveolar capillary, allowing plasma to flood the alveolus. This leakage increases over 24 hours, leading to pulmonary edema. The effects reach a maximum at about 12 to 24 hours after exposure. The greater the exposure, the more quickly the effects occur.

Effects

Initial exposure to a low concentration of phosgene can cause burning and watering of the eyes, pharyngitis, dry cough, chest tightness, and dyspnea. Nausea and headache may also be present. These symptoms occur during and immediately after the exposure but clear within a short time. The presence or absence of these symptoms may be of little value in the ultimate prognosis.[9]

At exposures exceeding 120 mg•min/m^3 (30 ppm/min) the initial respiratory symptoms are followed by a latent phase lasting 2–48 hours.[10] Duration of this latent phase is inversely proportional to the inhaled dose. A small dose may have a latent phase of 24 to 48 hours or may have no further symptoms. A large inhalation dose may be followed by additional symptoms within 1 to 4 hours after exposure.

The most significant feature of phosgene intoxication is massive pulmonary edema. After a latent period of about 2 to 24 hours, pulmonary edema develops with the production of large amounts of frothy sputum.[11] The patient may have an initial cough, followed by dyspnea, rapid, shallow breathing, and cyanosis. As the edema progresses, discomfort, apprehension, dyspnea, and cyanosis increase. The patient may have rales and rhonchi or have diminished breath sounds. Extensive fluid loss into the lungs may cause hypovolemic shock. Although the major determinant of the pulmonary damage is the inhaled dose of phosgene, increased physical activity will shorten the latent period and increase the respiratory distress. Very large inhalation doses of phosgene can also cause laryngeal irritation, laryngeal spasm, and death.

A prominent symptom occurring after the latent period is dyspnea. This may be accompanied by chest tightness. Dyspnea reflects the increasing accumulation of pulmonary fluid, decreased lung compliance, and increased ventilatory drive. The provider may hear fine crackles and rales, first in the bases, then in the entire lung. Severe mucous membrane irritation is also associated with phosgene exposure; it occurs after a high-level exposure and indicates serious toxicity.

If the patient develops pulmonary edema within 4 hours of exposure, the patient has a poor prognosis. Unless there is intensive medical care immediately available, these patients are at very high risk of death. The terminal clinical phase of lethal phosgene poisoning is described as extreme distress with intolerable dyspnea until the respiration ceases. If the provider is confronted with multiple casualties and limited resources, these patients may need to be classified as expectant.

In most cases, the pulmonary edema reaches a maximum in 24 hours. If the patient survives for 48 hours, there is a very good prognosis and, in the absence of complicating infections, the patient may have little or no long-term damage. Residual bronchitis, however, may last for several days.

At very high concentrations, phosgene will pass through the alveolar-capillary membrane and cause hemolysis in the pulmonary capillaries. The red cell fragments may block the capillary circulation. Death occurs in these patients within a few minutes of acute cor pulmonale.

Symptomatic patients should have a chest radiograph taken to assess the possibility of noncardiogenic pulmonary edema. Common radiologic abnormalities include **diffuse interstitial infiltrates, normal cardiac shadow**, and possibly a **bilateral perihilar fluffy infiltrate**. These radiologic changes frequently lag behind the clinical presentation with phosgene inhalation. If the patient becomes worse, then a repeat radiograph is appropriate.

Another result of phosgene exposure is hypoxia. Hypoxia may be accompanied by hypotension, as vast quantities of fluid are coughed up from the lungs. Death can result from respiratory failure, hypoxia, hypovolemia, or a combination of these. Rapid progression of hypoxia and hypotension suggest a poor prognosis.

Most survivors of acute exposure to phosgene will have a good long-term prognosis. Shortness of breath and reduced tolerance for physical activity may persist in some patients. Smoking appears to worsen the chances of full recovery. Preexisting lung disease, such as emphysema, will exacerbate the effects of phosgene exposure.[12] Late complications include infections and slow respiratory failure. **Table 4-2** lists the effects of various concentrations of phosgene gas.

Decontamination

Phosgene will not remain in liquid form unless the temperature is nearly freezing. Indeed, exposure to liquid phosgene can cause cold injury or frostbite. Decontamination stations should be well ventilated, because much of the decontamination is accomplished by simple aeration. No further decontamination is required unless phosgene has been used in a very cold climate.

Phosgene decomposes to carbon monoxide and hydrochloric acid in the presence of moisture. Therefore, decontamination with copious amounts of water will sufficiently decompose any residual of this agent.

Phosgene and similar pulmonary agents are absorbed by inhalation and do not cause significant skin damage. Removal of clothing will prevent outgassing. The activated charcoal in the canister of a military chemical protective mask adsorbs phosgene, and the military mask provides full protection from this gas for a variable time period, depend-

Table 4-2 Effects of Various Concentrations of Phosgene Gas

Exposure level	Concentration (ppm)	Effects
Mild	1	U.S. TLV-TWA limit.*
	1.5	Odor detection threshold.
Moderate	3–5	Mild mucous membrane irritation. U.S. short-term exposure is limited to 3 ppm.
	5–15	Moderate mucous membrane and upper respiratory tract irritation. May develop mild pulmonary edema after a latent period of 4–6 hours.
Severe	15+	Lacrimation, conjunctival irritation, and rhinorrhea. Massive pulmonary edema (within 4 hours) often with hypovolemic shock.
Lethal	50–80	Lethal with a 10-minute exposure.
	500–800 ppm/min	Average lethal dose.

*TLV (threshold limit value) The permissible exposure that a worker can tolerate without fear of damage. TWA (time weighted average) An average exposure over a specified time—usually 8 hours.

ing on concentration. Various civilian protective masks may or may not provide protection. Medical providers in decontamination stations should be protected at a minimum with phosgene-rated charcoal filter respirators.

Treatment

There is no specific antidote for the inhalation of phosgene. Treatment should be focused on supportive care, with special attention to ventilatory support and fluid replacement as needed.

Because there is a distinct latent period associated with inhalation of phosgene, it is important to observe these patients for a minimum of 6 hours after exposure. Onset of pulmonary edema before 6 hours is indicative of severe inhalation injury.

Oxygen and Similar Therapy

Measure the oxygen saturation in all symptomatic patients, because hypoxia is a common effect of phosgene inhalation. These patients frequently need oxygen supplementation. Early administration of intermittent positive pressure breathing (IPPB), positive end expiratory pressure (PEEP), or bi-level positive airway pressure (BiPAP) may be quite helpful in minimizing the pulmonary edema and reducing the degree of hypoxia. Intubation with or without a ventilator may be appropriate.[13-15]

Patients with bronchospasm may benefit from aerosolized bronchodilators such as albuterol and terbutaline.[16] Beta-adrenergic agonists relax airway smooth muscle and reduce hyperactivity and resultant airway narrowing in patients with phosgene inhalation. Aminophylline or theophylline may be considered for these patients.[17]

Antibiotics

Antimicrobial therapy should be reserved for a proven bacterial bronchitis or pneumonia. Prophylactic therapy is inappropriate.

Rest

It is important that patients exposed to phosgene be kept at rest until the danger of pulmonary edema has passed. This may not be possible in some situations, however. If the patient has significant respiratory involvement, litter evacuation is necessary.

Diuretics

Pulmonary edema associated with phosgene is noncardiac. Therefore, diuretics such as furosemide have only a very limited utility in these patients and should generally not be used. Because the pulmonary edema is of such scope as to cause hypovolemia, EMS providers should be aware that use of diuretics may not only be ineffective, but may cause hypotension.

Detection and Laboratory Aids

Chest radiographs may show hyperinflation early, followed by pulmonary edema without **cardiomegaly**. Early pulmonary edema can be detected by a chest radiograph using 50 to 80 KV exposure. The use of 100 to 120 KV exposure may not capture these early signs.[18]

Peak expiratory flow may decrease early after a massive phosgene exposure. Peak expiratory flow may indicate the degree of airway damage and indicate how much of the bronchoconstriction is reversible with bronchodilators. Pulmonary function testing will show increased work of breathing, increased airway resistance, decreased lung compliance, and decreased flow rates in the presence of a pulmonary injury. The presence of normal **spirometry** values probably excludes a significant injury to the lower respiratory tract.[19] However, pulmonary function tests are often not obtainable if the patient is a young child, unconscious, or uncooperative.

With phosgene exposures, arterial blood gasses will show nonspecific hypoxia. The hematocrit may increase as fluid is lost within the lung.

Decontamination and Personal Protection

Decontamination of casualties with soap and water is recommended. Operations teams are advised to don Level B or A protection when handling casualties, at least until phosgene has been confirmed as the toxic agent. Filter-type protective masks are effective for phosgene, so Level C protection is sufficient when contamination with phosgene is confirmed.

INHOSPITAL INFO

■ Diphosgene

Diphosgene (DP) is produced by combining phosgene with chloroform, which creates an unstable compound that breaks down easily into its components. Diphosgene was used in World War I, because the chloroform would destroy the chemical filters within the gas masks of the era. Diphosgene is liquid at room temperature, but rapidly vaporizes into a colorless gas.

Threat

Diphosgene is commercially available and is therefore a credible threat as a terrorist weapon. When its ability to penetrate a carbon-based protective mask is considered, it becomes even more attractive to the terrorist.

Effects

Clinically, diphosgene behaves like phosgene. Like phosgene, the outstanding attribute of diphosgene as a chemical weapon is its ability to cause delayed pulmonary edema. The mechanism of this pulmonary edema is thought to be the same as for phosgene, because diphosgene rapidly decomposes into phosgene and chloroform. The chloroform that is formed does not reach sufficient levels to cause toxicity.

Respiratory effects start to occur at 1 to 10 ppm (4 to 40 mg•min/m³). A dose of more than 25 ppm for a few minutes can be rapidly fatal. As with all of the inhalation agents, the toxicity varies with the concentration and duration of exposure to the vapor.

Decontamination

Decontamination of casualties with soap and water is recommended. Operations teams are advised to don Level B or A protection when handling casualties. Filter-type protective masks may be rendered useless because of the chloroform and are not recommended.

Treatment

Exposure to diphosgene should be treated in the same manner as exposure to phosgene. Pulmonary edema can be precipitated by exertion, so litter evacuation is recommended.

■ Chloropicrin

Chloropicrin (PS) was one of the first agents used in World War I and is quite easy to produce. It was first synthesized from picric acid (2,4,6-trinitrophenol) and calcium hypochlorite (chloride of lime) in 1848. Chloropicrin was manufactured by both sides during World War I for use as both an irritant and a lethal chemical. Although its toxicity makes chloropicrin a poor riot control agent, it is still used as a soil sterilant, a grain disinfectant, and an intermediate in chemical synthesis. It is also used as an odor maker in pesticide formulations.

Effects

The odor threshold of chloropicrin is 1.1 ppm, which is above the level that will cause eye irritation. Concentrations of 1 to 3 ppm will cause lacrimation and a 1-minute expo-

sure to 15 ppm will result in pulmonary injury.[20] Exposure to 4 ppm for even a few seconds renders an individual unfit for activity.

Chloropicrin has been used as a homicidal agent and would serve as an easy weapon for a terrorist to acquire and deploy.[21] None of the chemicals used to make chloropicrin are particularly difficult to acquire.

Decontamination and Personal Protection

If the concentration of chloropicrin exceeds 4 ppm, an air-supplying respirator or SCBA is required. Chemical-resistant clothing is necessary when handling this agent. Operations teams are advised to don Level B or A protection when handling casualties. Filter-type protective masks may be rendered useless against chloropicrin and are not recommended. Organic vapor mask filters are ineffective against chloropicrin.

Chloropicrin has a dual classification as both a lacrimator agent and a choking agent. Chloropicrin is covered fully in Chapter 6 as a lacrimator. Because there is considerable bulk production of chloropicrin, it is conceivable that an improvisational chemical weapon could be made from this agent.

■ PFIB

PFIB is an extremely toxic product of Teflon non-stick coating and other polymers encountered in civilian and military construction.[22] PFIB is 10 times more lethal than phosgene. Although PFIB was once used as an industrial chemical, it fell into disuse decades ago because it was so hazardous. It was prepared by the former Soviet Union as a chemical warfare agent.[23]

Threat

This agent is an attractive potential terrorist weapon. A protective mask containing charcoal filters would be ineffective against any substantial concentration of this agent. PFIB is not readily available, but Teflon (a key ingredient) is. This agent could be easily produced by heating Teflon to above 400°F and collecting the gas.

Fortunately, making this compound in miniscule quantities is not the same as collecting a sufficient quantity at a sufficient concentration and deploying it in an improvisational munition. This task would be significantly more difficult. However, considering that the former Soviet Union investigated this agent extensively because of its ability to penetrate a charcoal mask, there may be quantities of it for sale on the black markets.

Effects

Inhalation exposure may cause symptoms of pulmonary edema with wheezing, difficulty breathing, production of sputum, and cyanosis. The patient may experience initial coughing and chest pain, followed by a latent period of several hours; the patient will then rapidly decompensate.

High concentrations may produce irritation of the eyes, nose, and throat, but the major target organ of this agent is the lungs. Systemic effects seen in animal studies only occur after there is substantial injury to the lungs. Hypoxia is considered a major contributing factor.

There are few data on the exposures that cause symptoms in human beings. In rodents, exposures of 150 to 180 ppm/min (1,250 to 1,500 mg•min/m³) will kill 50% of the test population. A comparable dose of phosgene is 750 ppm/min.[24,25] High concentrations of PFIB have caused sudden death in animals. There is no such reported death in human beings, although reported experience is scanty.

A comparable syndrome known as polymer fume fever has been described following the inhalation of the products of combustion of Teflon coating.[26-29] These inhalation injuries have resulted from fires, smoking cigarettes contaminated with Teflon coating or similar products, and welding around Teflon coating.

A few hours after exposure, the patient experiences a gradual increase in temperature (hence the moniker polymer fume fever), pulse, and respiratory rate. Shivering and sweating usually follow. Auscultation of the lungs may reveal moist, diffuse rales in the most severe cases. Toxic pulmonary edema may be more severe and appear earlier if the patient exercises after exposure.

Decontamination and Personal Protection

Air purifying respirators are inadequate protection against this agent. PFIB is not well adsorbed by activated charcoal. If PFIB exposure is suspected, providers should wear a positive pressure supplied air respirator.

When dissolved in water, PFIB decomposes rapidly to various reactive intermediates and fluorophosgene, which in turn decomposes to carbon dioxide, a radical anion, and hydrogen fluoride. Because a reactive product is hydrogen fluoride, use of water for decontamination of this agent cannot be recommended. Fortunately, this agent is extremely volatile, and ventilation with air should provide adequate decontamination.

Specific Treatment

There is no prophylaxis or antidote for the inhalation of PFIB.

Because there is a distinct latent period associated with the inhalation of PFIB, it is important to observe these patients for a minimum of 6 hours after exposure. Onset of pulmonary edema before 6 hours is indicative of severe inhalation injury.

Oxygen

Measure the oxygen saturation in all symptomatic patients, because hypoxia is common. These patients frequently need oxygen supplementation. Early administration of IPPB, PEEP, Continuous Positive Airway Pressure (CPAP), or BiPAP may be quite helpful in minimizing the pulmonary edema and reducing the degree of hypoxia. Intubation with or without a ventilator may be appropriate. Patients with bronchospasm may benefit from aerosolized bronchodilators such as albuterol.

Antibiotics

Antimicrobial therapy should be reserved for a proven bacterial bronchial pneumonia. Prophylactic therapy is inappropriate. Bacterial superinfection is sufficiently common to warrant a careful watch.

Rest

It is important that a patient exposed to PFIB be kept at rest until the danger of pulmonary edema is past. This may not be possible in some situations, however. If the patient has significant respiratory involvement, litter evacuation is necessary. As noted, pulmonary edema may be more severe and appear earlier if the patient exercises after exposure.

Diuretics

The pulmonary edema associated with PFIB is noncardiac. Therefore, diuretics such as furosemide have only a very limited utility in these patients and should generally not be used. Because the pulmonary edema is of such scope as to cause hypovolemia, providers should be aware that use of diuretics may not only be ineffective, but may cause hypotension. Fluid replacement is mandatory if the patient becomes hypotensive. Combined hypotension and hypoxia may cause multi-organ failure.

A summary of the pulmonary agents is provided in **Table 4-3**.

Table 4-3 Summary of Pulmonary Agents					
Name	Code name	CAS number	Appearance	Odor	Route of exposure
Chlorine	CL	7782-50-5	Yellowish gas	Strong, distinctive odor	Inhalation
Phosgene	CG	75-44-5	Liquid Colorless, low-lying, dense gas	Decaying fruit, freshly cut grass or hay, moldy hay	Inhalation
Diphosgene	DP	503-38-8	Liquid at room temperature Colorless gas	Vapor has odor of phosgene	Inhalation
Chloropicrin	PS	76-06-2	Heavy, colorless liquid	Sharp odor	Inhalation
Perfluoroisobutylene	PFIB	382-21-8	Colorless gas	Odorless	Inhalation

■ General Management of Toxic Inhaled Agents

The basic treatment of inhalation agents is supportive. There is no antidote for these chemicals. The victim of pulmonary agent poisoning should be treated as if the victim suffers from severe smoke inhalation.

Terminate Exposure

Remove the patient from the contaminated environment. Remove the patient's clothing to prevent outgassing and continued exposure. Provide a mask for the patient if available. Decontaminate the patient with copious amounts of water. (With the exception of PFIB, all of the inhalation agents discussed in this chapter can be decontaminated with water.)

Manage ABCs

The patient should be carefully evaluated for potential airway obstruction. Intubation may be lifesaving and may allow the clearance of secretions when they occur. Because these patients may develop hypoxia or hypotension rapidly, they must be monitored carefully. High-flow humidified oxygen should be immediately instituted.

Treat Hypoxia

Supplemental oxygen is indicated. Intubation with or without ventilatory assistance may be required. Management of patients with inhalation injuries often requires aggressive pulmonary toilet. Frequent postural drainage, coughing, and encouragement of deep breathing all aid in clearing the airway of debris and secretions. Frequent airway suctioning is often needed to help remove this material.

Treat Bronchospasm

If the patient has bronchospasm or wheezing, a trial of nebulized aerosol bronchodilators such as albuterol or terbutaline is indicated. There is no evidence that there is any benefit from the use of corticosteroids in the specific treatment of phosgene inhalation, but there have been only a few reported cases of phosgene inhalation since the 1950s and the availability of corticosteroids. Corticosteroids have been advocated for patients with the inhalation of ammonia and chlorine. Considering that there is good evidence that the use of corticosteroids will decrease the inflammatory component of bronchospasm in asthma and that there is little risk from a short dose of corticosteroids, this may be an appropriate option for all patients with inhalation injury.

Symptomatic treatment can include the inhalation of a nebulized mixture of 2 mL 8.4% $NaHCO_3$ with 2 mL normal saline. This has been shown to be effective for chlorine inhalation, and may well be effective in cases of phosgene inhalation.

Manage Airway Secretions

Watery secretions may serve as a marker of the degree of pulmonary edema present. They should be suctioned as frequently as needed.

Treat Pulmonary Edema

As noted, the pulmonary edema associated with phosgene toxicity is attributed to capillary-alveolar membrane damage. Pulmonary edema from toxic gas exposure does not resolve with diuretics. Positive pressure breathing such as positive end expiratory pressure and intubation are often required. Positive airway pressure can decrease some of the effects of phosgene-induced pulmonary edema. High peak inspiratory pressures should be avoided, because they can be associated with barotrauma. Unfortunately, this positive airway pressure can also exacerbate hypotension. This may put the provider in the unenviable position of pushing fluids on a patient with pulmonary edema.

Treat Hypotension

The pulmonary edema of phosgene gas exposure has been associated with massive fluid loss from the lungs and may require fluid replacement.[30] Urgent intravenous administration of either colloid or crystalloid may be needed for treatment of fluid-loss induced hypotension. The use of vasopressors may be considered until fluids can be replaced.

Treat Mucous Membrane Irritation

Treatment is symptomatic for limited exposures. Eyes should be well irrigated and checked for corneal burns. Humidification of the air or oxygen will help for cough and sore throat. Cutaneous burns should be treated as all caustic acid injuries, with excessive irrigation with high-flow, low-pressure tap water.

Enforce Rest

Even modest exercise may decrease the latent period and increase the severity of the symptoms. Physical exertion in a symptomatic patient may precipitate respiratory failure and death. These patients should be placed on strict bed rest.

■ References

1. Jones FL: Chlorine poisoning from mixing household cleaners. *JAMA* 1972;222:1312.
2. Kaufman J, Burleons D: Clinical roentgenologic and physiologic effects of acute chlorine exposure. *Arch Environ Health* 1971;23:39–44.
3. Hasan FM, Gehshan A, Fuleihan FJD: Resolution of pulmonary dysfunction following acute chlorine exposure. *Arch Environ Health* 1983;38:76–80.
4. Hedges JR, Morrisey WL: Acute chlorine gas exposure. *JACEP* 1979;8:59–63.
5. Sexton JD, Pronchik DJ: Chlorine inhalation: the big picture. *J Toxicol Clin Toxicol* 1998;36:87–93.
6. Sciuto AM. Postexposure treatment with aminophylline protects against phosgene-induced acute lung injury. *Exp Lung Res* 1997;23:317–332.
7. [Author: anonymous] Pulmonary agents. http://ccc.apgea.army.mil/Documents/RedHandbook/003PulmonarAgents.htm (accessed October 31, 2001).
8. Wells BA: Phosgene: A practitioner's viewpoint. *Toxicol Ind Health* 1985;1(2):81–92.
9. Diller WF: Early diagnosis of phosgene overexposure. *Toxicol Ind Health* 1985;1(2):73–79.
10. [Author: anonymous] *Phosgene.* Geneva, Switzerland, World Health Organization, International Programme of Chemical Safety, 1997.
11. Diller WF: Medical phosgene problems and their possible solutions. *J Occup Med* 1975;32:271–277.
12. Diller WF: Early diagnosis of phosgene overexposure. *Toxicol Ind Health* 1985;1(2):129–136.
13. Diller WF: Early diagnosis of phosgene overexposure. *Toxicol Ind Health* 1985;1(2):73–79.
14. Wells BA: Phosgene: A practitioner's viewpoint. *Toxicol Ind Health* 1985;1(2):81–92.
15. Regan RA: Review of clinical experience in handling phosgene exposure cases. *Toxicol Ind Health* 1985;1(2):69–80.
16. Sexton JD, Pronchik DJ: Chlorine inhalation: the big picture. *J Toxicol Clin Toxicol* 1998;36:87–93.
17. Sciuto AM. Postexposure treatment with aminophylline protects against phosgene-induced acute lung injury. *Exp Lung Res* 1997;23:317–332.
18. Diller WF: Early diagnosis of phosgene overexposure. *Toxicol Ind Health* 1985;1(2):73–79.
19. Whitener DR, Whitener LM, Robertons KJ, et al: Pulmonary function measurements in patients with thermal injury and smoke inhalation. *Am Rev Resp Disease* 1980;122:731.
20. *Chloropicrin.* Hamilton, ON, Canadian Centre for Occupational Health and Safety (CHEMINFO No. 2000-2003); available at http://www.ccohs.ca/products/databases/cheminfo.html (accessed June 6, 2005).
21. Gonomori K, Muto H, Yamamoto T, et al: A case of homicidal intoxication by chloropicrin. *Am J Forensic Med Pathol* 1987;8:135-138.
22. Lee CH, Guo YL, Tsai PJ, et al: Fatal acute pulmonary oedema after inhalation of fumes from polytetrafluoro-ethylene (PTFE). *Euro Respir J* 1997;10:1408–1411.
23. Stamgaugh JJ: Deadly toxin missing. *KnoxNews.com,* June 10, 2000, http://www.knoxnews.com/news/10242.shmtl (accessed October 31, 2001).
24. Urbanetti JS: Toxic inhalation injury, in Sidell F, Takafuji ET, Franz DR (eds): *Medical Aspects of Chemical and Biological Warfare.* Washington, DC, Walter Reed Army Medical Center, 1997.
25. Maidment MP, Rice P, Upshall DG: Retention of inhaled hexaflurocyclobutene in the rat. *J Appl Toxicol* 1994;14:395-400.
26. Harris DK: Polymer fume fever. *Lancet* 1951;2;1008-1011.
27. Robbins JJ, Ware RL: Pulmonary edema from Teflon fumes. *NEJM* 1964;271:360–361.
28. Lewis CE, Kerby GR: An epidemic of polymer-fume fever. *JAMA* 1965:191:103–106.
29. Shusterman DJ: Polymer fume fever and other fluorocarbon pyrolysis related syndromes. *Occ Med* 1993;8:519–531.
30. Everett ED, Overholt EL: Phosgene poisoning. *JAMA* 1968;205:103–105.

5 Vesicant Agents

■ Introduction

A vesicant is a chemical that produces blisters or **vesicles** on exposed tissues. These chemicals are toxic to skin, lungs, eyes, and mucous membranes. If a significant amount of any of these chemicals is absorbed, a systemic illness may result. With many of these agents, the effect will be delayed **(Table 5-1).** Even though these contact poisons can cause serious skin and ocular lesions, pulmonary involvement is the most common cause of death.[1,2]

There are three subclasses of vesicants: mustards, arsenicals, and halogenated oximes. The effects and properties of the halogenated oximes are quite different from those of the other vesicants.

These chemicals are far less lethal than nerve agents under comparable conditions of exposure. Although vesicants have a relatively low lethality, they are quite effective in causing injury. Vesicant agents inflict painful burns and blisters that require medical attention even at low doses.

Vesicant agents are ideal terrorism agents, because they are easy to produce, available in industrial quantities, and can inflict substantial injuries on an unprotected populace. Blister agents force police and emergency response workers to wear full protective equipment, which degrades performance and efficiency. Vesicant agents could easily be added as secondary or tertiary effect agents to endanger emergency response workers after an initial attack.

■ Mustard and Similar Agents

The **mustard agents** are a family of sulfur-, nitrogen-, and oxygen-based compounds with similar chemical and biological effects. The military prototype of this class of chemicals is sulfur mustard, also called Levinstein mustard, named after the inventor of a major manufacturing process for sulfur mustard. There are two types of sulfur mustard: distilled sulfur mustard (HD) and impure mustard (H). Other similar agents include **Agent Q**, **Agent T**, and nitrogen mustards.

History

The most dangerous chemical warfare agent of World War I was sulfur mustard. Sulfur mustard was first synthesized by Dr. Guthrie in 1859. Mustard gas was used for the first time in

Table 5-1 Vesicant Agents and Onset of Symptoms

Agent	Code	Onset of Symptoms
Mustard (sulfur and nitrogen mustard agents)	HD, HN, T, HT, Q, dusty mustard	Delayed
Lewisite	L	Immediate
Phosgene oxime	CX	Immediate, also causes nausea

Ypres, Belgium, in 1917 during World War I. The Germans chose the same battlefield where chlorine was released 2 years earlier to debut this new agent. Mustard is still considered a major chemical warfare threat.

Although mustard was introduced late in World War I, it caused more chemical casualties than all other agents combined. Although the agent has a low lethality, casualties are common and numerous. Sulfur mustard is often called the king of chemical agents, because it is easily produced, inexpensive, persistent, has predictable properties, and causes resource-devouring casualties rather than fatalities.[3]

Sulfur mustard is still considered by the military to be a modern chemical warfare agent because of its powerful penetrating potency, persistence, and difficult detection. Mustard penetrates ordinary clothing, leather, and most common plastics without burning them and attacks only living tissue.[4] Moreover, those exposed are often asymptomatic for quite some time (usually hours). This combination makes personal protection very difficult.

Mustard on the skin causes no immediate sensation, and symptoms do not normally appear until several hours after exposure. At incapacitating levels of mustard, symptoms may not be evident for as long as 12 hours. Not only is the air poisonous after a mustard attack, but everything that the mustard agent touches is potentially toxic.

Physical Characteristics

Sulfur mustard (H) is a clear, yellow, or amber-colored oily liquid with a faint, sweet odor of mustard or garlic. Mustard vaporizes slowly at temperate climates and may be aerosolized by spray or by explosive blasts. The vapor is heavier than air and settles slowly into low areas.

Because of its low volatility at lower temperatures, mustard is considered to be a persistent agent at temperate climates, and it remains for up to a week after dispersal. It is only slightly soluble in water, but it is highly soluble in organic solvents and in skin oils. Mustard is slowly hydrolyzed in water to form hydrochloric acid.

Mustard freezes at 13.9°C (57°F), so it is difficult to use in winter or to deliver by air in cool climates. Mustard's high freezing point makes it quite dangerous during the times of year when temperatures fall at night to below 10°C. The mustard will freeze in low-lying parts of the ground at night and then thaw by the sun during the day and evaporate, creating a "second attack" several hours after daybreak.

Dissemination

Mustard agents may be delivered by bomb, artillery, or mortar round, or by release from canisters. Missiles are readily adapted to deliver this agent in large quantities. It is possible to disseminate mustards that have been adsorbed to small particles (dusty mustard). This preparation of mustard is discussed in detail later in the chapter. Mustard is a chemical agent that is likely to be used on the modern battlefield; it has been used by Iraq in recent times. Mustard is easy to produce from commonly available materials using processes that are well described in the open-source literature.

Mustard is strategically attractive for use as a weapon of mass casualties for the following reasons:
- It is potent.
  - It inflicts casualties despite the appropriate use of respiratory protective devices.
  - It causes prolonged disability.
  - It produces delayed effects.
  - It is rapidly effective, despite the delayed presentation.
- It is not easy to detect.
- It is easy and inexpensive to produce.
- It is difficult to decontaminate.
  - It is persistent.
  - It penetrates many types of protective garments.
- It is easily deployed in explosive devices.
- It is effective in gas (vapor), liquid, and aerosol forms.

Mechanism of Action on Tissues

Mustard is a primary tissue irritant. Mustard penetrates intact skin rapidly. It has been estimated that between 12% and 50% of mustard that is absorbed will react with the skin and skin components.

The molecular mechanisms that cause toxicity from mustard are far from clear.[5] Sulfur mustard **alkylation reactions** are rapid and irreversible. Mustard's most important metabolic effect, at least for acute toxicity, is the inhibition of cellular glycolysis. Disruption of that metabolic pathway is found after exposure to nearly all vesicant chemicals.[6] Mustard gas binds to DNA, forming cross-links that prevent further replication of cells. The process takes about an hour and leads to the inhibition of glycolysis, the release of tissue proteases, and cellular death.

Mustard also damages RNA and proteins. Although mustard can react with a large variety of molecules, the dose of mustard encountered by most victims will not inhibit the cell's energy metabolism, protein synthesis, RNA synthesis, or other enzymatically mediated activities to any significant degree. In mammalian cells there are multiple pathways for DNA repair that may minimize permanent damage from mustard.

Mustard is **mutagenic**, **carcinogenic**, and **teratogenic**. Dividing cells are the most sensitive, but mustard at a significant concentration will kill any cells. Cells with high cell turnover such as bone marrow, intestinal mucosal cells, and skin elements are especially sensitive to mustard.

The effects of mustard exposure are cumulative if exposures occur within 12 hours.[7] At more prolonged intervals between exposures, the effects are probably less cumulative.[8]

Effects

Mustard readily penetrates skin and mucous membranes. Moist body parts, such as the eyes, mouth, respiratory tract, scrotum, and anus, are most affected by all of the mustard agents **(Table 5-2)**.

The effects of mustard depend on the duration of exposure and the concentration of the agent **(Table 5-3)**. There is a characteristic latent period of 4 to 12 hours before the onset of symptoms after exposure. The rate of onset is related to the dose of agent absorbed. Higher concentrations and longer exposures cause symptoms to develop more rapidly. There is also a significant variation in sensitivity to mustard among individuals.

Battlefield concentrations during World War I mustard gas attacks were estimated to be in the range of 19 to 33 mg/m³.[9] At these concentrations, exposure for several minutes causes skin and eye damage, and exposure for 30 to 60 minutes causes severe respiratory injury, systemic poisoning, and probable death.

Victims of mustard toxicity generally have lesions in multiple sites. In most patients, lesions are primarily **cutaneous**, but respiratory, ocular, and gastrointestinal injuries are common. If the patient was wearing a protective mask at the time of exposure, only cutaneous manifestations are likely.

Dermal

Mustard does not produce uniform skin injuries. As noted earlier, the face, scrotum, and anal areas are frequently involved, while the thicker skin on the hands may be spared. Moist or wet skin, such as that of the groin and axilla, is especially prone to damage.[10] There are no available data about perineal and vulvar involvement in females, but these injuries would be expected to parallel those of males. If the skin is directly exposed to mustard liquid, ulcerations and skin necrosis develops after only a very short latent period **(Color plate 5-1)**. Skin toxicity increases as ambient temperature increases.[11]

There are large differences in reactivity to sulfur mustard among individuals. As much as 100 times the agent needed to cause a lesion in a sensitive person may be required to cause similar lesions in a resistant person.[12]

After a latent period of 4 to 12 hours, patients may develop diffuse **erythema** that progresses to blister formation and widespread **bullae**.[13] The affected areas may turn black. Mild exposures may only produce erythema similar to a sunburn. Serious mustard exposures are likely to produce systemic effects. The most severely exposed patients may experience marked fluid losses, hypovolemia, and renal failure.

Skin lesions in children appear to be more severe than in adults. The time of onset of symptoms is shorter for children when compared with adults. Both phenomena could be attributed to the thinner, more delicate skin of the young patients.[14]

Skin injuries take the form of a chemical burn that heals in about 4 to 6 weeks unless there is an infection. After the inflammation subsides, there is often a distinctive residual black to brown **punctate perifollicular pigmentation**.[15]

Skin lesions caused by mustard can recur at sites of prior injury. Exposed German and Japanese mustard workers developed multiple skin tumors such as basal cell carcinoma, Bowen's carcinoma, and squamous cell skin cancer.[16] These lesions developed only after repeated exposure.

Ocular

In World War I, American physicians noted that the eye was the most commonly damaged organ in a mustard attack.[17] This was reconfirmed by data on the Iranian victims of mustard.[18] The eye is affected at lower vapor concentrations than any other organ, and the latent period is shortest for ocular injuries. Increased doses of mustard cause progressively more severe conjunctivitis, intolerance to light (**photophobia**), spasm of the eyelids (**blepharospasm**), pain, and corneal damage.

Severe conjunctivitis, blepharospasm, lid edema, and conjunctival edema may be noted in patients and may take 2 to 5 weeks to resolve. Moderate corneal involvement may be noted as corneal erosion that stains with fluorescein. This may be followed by superficial corneal scarring, **vascularization**, and **iritis**. These injuries may take as long as 2 to 3 months to resolve.

If severe corneal involvement is noted, the patient may have dense corneal **opacification** and deep ulcer formation. These patients will require ophthalmologic intervention and may require hospitalization. Some of these

Table 5-3 Effects of Mustard on Humans

Concentration (parts per million)	Duration (minutes)	Effects
0.1	10	Eye and skin damage
1.0	60	Serious lung damage
10.0	60	Dangerous to life
100.0	10	Lethal (within a few hours)

Adapted from: Eisenmenger W, Drasch G, von Clarmann M, Kretschmer E, Roider G: Clinical and morphological findings on mustard gas [bis(2-chloroethyl)sulfide] poisoning. *J Forensic Sci* 1991;36:1688-1698.

Table 5-2 Body Parts Most Affected by Mustard

Body part	Exposed patients
Eyes	86%
Respiratory tract	75%
Scrotum	42%
Face	27%
Anus	24%

Note: Percentages add to greater than 100% because multiple sites of injury were common.

Adapted from: Requena L, Requena C, Sanches M, et al: Chemical warfare: Cutaneous lesions from mustard gas. *J Am Acad Dermatol* 1988;19:529-536.

INHOSPITAL INFO

INHOSPITAL INFO

patients will develop blindness as a result of the ocular damage. Recurrent corneal ulcers may occur for years after severe exposure. Patients may also have chronic conjunctivitis after severe exposure to mustard.

Respiratory

Inhalation of mustard aerosol or vapor produces a serious upper respiratory tract irritation and can lead to respiratory failure and death. In World War I, the mortality rate of mustard gas casualties was about 2.5% and nearly all of the deaths were from inhalation of the agent. The respiratory injuries that develop after inhalation of mustard vapor (and presumably dusty mustard) primarily affect the **laryngeal** and **tracheal-bronchial mucosa**.

After a delay of several hours, victims suffer **tracheobronchitis** with symptoms such as chest pressure, hacking cough, sore throat, and hoarseness. Sinusitis, sinus pain, increasing cough, and tachypnea develop as symptoms progress over the next 12 hours. The severe cough responds poorly to cough suppressants, steam, bronchodilators, and corticosteroids.

Over several days, the damage to the pulmonary tree develops with marked inflammation of the pulmonary mucosa and airway. This may be followed later by necrosis of the mucosa and airway musculature. The tracheal and bronchial mucosa may slough and obstruct the bronchi. Pulmonary edema appears to be less common with mustard gas than with the choking agents. However, severe mustard exposures do lead to hemorrhagic pulmonary edema, secondary pneumonia, and respiratory failure after 24 to 48 hours. Bronchopneumonia is a common complication in inhalation injuries resulting from mustard and lewisite. Radiographs may be consistent with adult respiratory distress syndrome. Lesions may take many weeks to heal and may lead to chronic airway problems.

Gastrointestinal

Gastrointestinal injury can result from systemic toxicity that occurs following massive exposures (more than 1,000 mg•min/m^3) or the swallowing of contaminated food, water, or saliva. Nausea and vomiting are common after exposure, though diarrhea and gastrointestinal bleeding are uncommon.[19] Both the liquid and vapor forms can contaminate food, causing gastrointestinal disease.

When gastrointestinal symptoms occur within hours after exposure, they have little prognostic significance. It is the gastrointestinal symptoms that occur 4 to 5 days after exposure that are indicative of a systemic effect of mustard and a poor prognosis.

Hematologic

High-dose exposures (more than 1,000 mg•min/m^3) that produce systemic toxicity may cause bone marrow suppression. The patient may develop an initial **leukocytosis** that lasts several days. This is followed by **leukopenia**, which develops within 3 to 5 days after exposure. The lowest white blood cell count is reached at about 10 days after exposure.[20] At this time, the patient is at great risk

of sepsis, often from a pulmonary focus. **Thrombocytopenia** may accompany the leukopenia. Anemia is seen less common, although all elements of the marrow are suppressed.

Cardiovascular

Large exposures to mustard can cause cardiovascular collapse, shock, and death. A patient's declining condition may be unresponsive to fluid replacement. Patients with large skin burns experience hypovolemia, hemoconcentration, peripheral edema, and bradycardia followed by tachycardia.

Immune System

Seven to 10 days after exposure, sulfur mustard can also cause the impairment of immune functions. This can increase vulnerability to bacterial infection and multiple septic complications.

Lethality

Mortality rates after battlefield exposure to mustard are between 1% and 3%. The cause of death may be burns, respiratory tract damage, bone marrow depression, or infection.[21] The development of mustard-induced **hematological effects** is an especially poor prognostic sign but is a late finding.

Marked increases in the lethality of a mustard attack will occur if victims continue to wear mustard-soaked clothing and inhale the emanating fumes. Because of the rapid effects combined with the long latent period of mustard, patients with a surely lethal exposure to mustard may still be ambulatory shortly after exposure. These patients may be quite contaminated and dangerous to others.

Dusty Mustard

As discussed in Chapter 3, dusty agents are created using a solid material that enhances aerosol formation. Dusty mustard may decrease the latent period before mustard causes visible skin damage.

Dusty mustard is easy to disperse as an aerosol in a large, concentrated cloud. This aerosolization increases the area of coverage with the chemical agent. Contamination of clothing and equipment by the agent will be markedly increased from the usual patterns associated with blast or vapor aerosols. Dusty agent formulation also appears to increase inhalation symptoms from mustard. The fine particles containing mustard are apparently much more easily inhaled than the merely vaporized mustard.

In addition to increasing the amount of agent that can be spread across an area, dusty agents also frustrate and defeat chemical protection measures. The very fine particles exploit weaknesses in chemical defensive gear by making their way into gaps and spaces of clothing, no matter how well the clothing is fitted. Considering the ability of mustard to cause symptoms with skin exposure, this fine dust represents a significant chemical threat.[22]

As with other dusty agents, the US military advocates using a poncho over MOPP gear to protect from this agent. However, SERPACWA and aTSP protective creams may lend better protection. It is unknown how effective detec-

INHOSPITAL INFO

tion or decontamination of this agent would be, as implied in the following statement from the US Defense Intelligence Agency.

> THE PROTECTIVE MASK PROVIDES FULL PROTECTION AGAINST ALL THREATENED CHEMICAL HAZARDS, INCLUDING DUSTY AGENTS. HOWEVER, DETECTION OF DUSTY MUSTARD WITH CURRENT SYSTEMS IS PARTICULARLY DIFFICULT, AND CONFIRMATION OF USE OF DUSTY MUSTARD MAY ALSO BE DIFFICULT AND TIME CONSUMING. FIRST BATTLEFIELD USE WILL MOST LIKELY BE DETECTED BY THE ONSET OF SYMPTOMS AMONG EXPOSED PERSONNEL. ONSET OF SYMPTOMS ON THE SKIN CAN BE EXPECTED APPROXIMATELY 15–90 MINUTES AFTER EXPOSURE. EFFECTS FROM INHALATION OF DUSTY MUSTARD CAN BE MUCH MORE RAPID.[23]

Similar Agents
Agents T and Q
Agent T is a by-product of one manufacturing process for making mustard gas. Very little information is available on the long-term toxicity of Agent T, which has a much lower volatility than mustard. Agent T is thought to be a more potent vesicant than sulfur mustard. Agent T is also more stable than sulfur mustard and has a lower freezing point.

However, Agent T has a lower vapor pressure than sulfur mustard, which makes it inefficient as a respiratory agent. Agent T may be mixed with mustard to increase the potential for inhalation injury over Agent T alone (this may be referred to as Agent HT). Agent T adds stability to the mixture so that it is more persistent. This combination is thought to be two to three times as toxic as sulfur mustard.[24] The mixture is a clear, yellowish liquid with an odor similar to that of distilled sulfur mustard. It has a strong blistering effect and a longer duration of effectiveness.

Agent Q is a potent vesicant agent and pulmonary agent. It is considered to be significantly more toxic than sulfur mustard. It has a very low vapor pressure, so it does not present a significant respiratory threat unless it is aerosolized.

The overall effects of both Agent Q and Agent T are quite similar to mustard and require the same protection for the provider. Treatment and decontamination should proceed as if the patient has been exposed to mustard.

Nitrogen Mustard
Nitrogen mustard (HN) is an oily, pale yellow or colorless liquid that is freely soluble in organic solvents but insoluble in water. There are three variants of nitrogen mustard: HN-1, HN-2, and HN-3. All three variants may be formed during the manufacture of the agent.

Nitrogen mustard has never been used in chemical warfare, so there is not a large body of literature on the effects of this agent. The US military produced substantial quantities of nitrogen mustard towards the end of World War II, but this was apparently disposed of in the sea.

A terrorist would likely find nitrogen mustard just as attractive as sulfur mustard, because they share many properties, and neither has an antidote. The lethal dose for inhalation of HN-1 is substantially smaller than that of sulfur mustard, so more deaths could be expected if this agent is ever used.

Effects
Ocular In mild exposures to nitrogen mustard, there is significantly more eye damage than skin or respiratory damage. This irritation appears sooner than that of sulfur mustard. Mild exposure produces edema and erythema of the conjunctiva and haziness of the cornea. The patient may experience eye pain, miosis, photophobia, and profuse **lacrimation**. After more severe exposure, the patient may have hemorrhagic discolorations of the iris. Local necrosis of the cornea may lead to rupture of the globe.

Dermal In mild exposures to nitrogen mustard, the patient may be free of skin lesions. Skin lesions that do occur are similar to those caused by sulfur mustard. When the exposure is severe, the patient's symptoms may appear earlier than with sulfur mustard exposure. The rate of absorption of nitrogen mustard is slower than that of sulfur mustard.

Respiratory The effects of nitrogen mustard are similar to those caused by sulfur mustard.

Systemic The most specific effects of nitrogen mustard appear to be on the **hematopoietic** and **lymphoid tissues**. The degenerative changes within the bone marrow can be detected within 12 hours after significant exposure. The patient may develop **aplasia**. This is detected as a transient leukocytosis followed by a severe **lymphopenia**. The various forms of nitrogen mustard differ in their ability to produce these changes.

Severe leukopenia, thrombocytopenia, and hemorrhage are quite ominous. The probability of severe infections with this leukopenia is significant, and any infection found should be treated rapidly.

Decontamination
Responders should wear Level A protection when conducting containment operations or gross decontamination of patients exposed to any form of mustard gas. Level B protection with butyl rubber or nitrile gloves and apron should be used when in contact with contaminated casualties. Because of the splash and vapor hazards of this agent, lower levels of protection are not recommended at any time. (Remember that a patient may have a surely lethal skin and systemic exposure and still be able to ambulate because of the delayed effects of mustard.)

Decontamination within 1 to 2 minutes after exposure is the only known effective means of preventing or decreasing tissue damage from mustard exposure. If decontamination is performed when symptoms appear, it is of only limited usefulness to the patient. However, decontamination may protect medical staff and others from contamination and may prevent the spread of contamination to other parts of the patient's body. Decontamination of every patient potentially exposed to mustard should be completed BEFORE they are allowed into a medical treatment facility. Contaminated litters, blankets, and equipment should be left outdoors so that vapor does not accumulate indoors. These items will not be able to be decontaminated and must be safely destroyed.

Symptoms should NOT guide decontamination efforts. Mustard on the skin causes no immediate symptoms, and symptoms may not be present for several hours after exposure. Every patient (as well as EMS, fire, and law enforcement personnel) should be checked for mustard and decontaminated if it is found.

Droplets of the oily agent on the skin should be removed by blotting and then cleansing with soap and water or a decontamination solution. Washing with 0.5% hypochlorite (household bleach diluted 1:10) is the decontamination technique most often recommended.[25] This solution not only removes the mustard from the skin, but also destroys it.

All clothing, jewelry, and leather should be removed, and the underlying skin must be washed. Washing should include the groin, axillae, and perianal areas, because these areas are quite frequently involved. Scrubbing and hot water should be avoided, as both enhance the absorption of the agent.

Chloramine solution wash has been recommended by some authors, but it is not generally available. Currently, the US military uses M258A1 kits for skin decontamination from mustard, which contain three sets of two paper towels each, one towel containing phenol and hydroxide and the other containing chloramine.

If water supplies are limited, a limited skin decontamination can be performed with adsorbent powders, such as flour or talcum powder.[26] The powder should be liberally dusted onto the contaminated exposed skin, allowed to adsorb mustard from the skin, and then wiped off with a moist paper or towel. This procedure will markedly decrease contamination and subsequent exposure to the patient and provider.

Mustard agent penetrates rapidly through or into porous materials such as wood, fabrics, and rubber. This makes decontamination of these materials quite difficult and these materials must generally be discarded. Only nonporous items can be safely decontaminated. All contaminated clothing and nonmetallic personal effects must be destroyed in a safe manner.

Hard, nonporous surfaces are not as difficult to decontaminate as they do not absorb mustard. Possible methods of decontamination include high-pressure steam, hot water spray, or DS2 (DS2 is a mixture of 70% diethylenetriamine, 2% sodium hydroxide, and 28% ethylene glycol monomethyl ether). DS2 is corrosive to eyes and skin and is harmful to breathe. It should never be used to decontaminate patients.

Treatment

After over 75 years of exposure to this agent, there is not yet an effective antidote for mustard. Treatment is supportive, and most patients exposed to mustard gas will recover completely.[27] Some typical treatment modalities are described in **Table 5-4**. At the beginning of the last large use of mustard (the Iran–Iraq War), the treatment varied considerably. Europeans were consulted about these casualties, and eventually a relatively standardized protocol evolved. This protocol included ocular treatment, skin decontamination, pulmonary treatment, bone marrow suppression treatment for patients with massive intoxication, and general measures for the comfort of the patient.

The primary effects of an attack with sulfur mustard are painful skin and eye irritations and pulmonary injuries. Mustard injuries are slow to heal and often take over 6 weeks of **convalescence**. Only a small proportion of patients will have long-term eye or lung damage. Unfortunately, there are no studies about the incidence of cancer or birth defects following exposure to mustard.

Patients who have been exposed to mustard gas can be classified into three categories: severe (those whose injuries are life threatening), moderate (those who will require ongoing hospital care), and minimal. There will be many patients with minimal injuries, and the majority will require hospitalization. Only a very small percentage will have life-

Table 5-4 Emergency Treatment of Mustard Vesicant Injuries		
Symptom	Standard treatment	Advanced treatment
All symptoms—immediate treatment	Irrigation and decontamination	Consider the use of 2% sodium thiosulfate solution irrigation within 3 hr of exposure.
Mild skin irritation	Protection of the skin from further trauma	Ensure that there is no further trauma or exposure to this area.
Severe skin lesions, blisters	Careful cleansing	Apply a silver sulfadiazine dressing. Consider the use of 2% sodium thiosulfate solution and 20 g of IV sodium thiosulfate. Intravenous fluids may be necessary.
Eye lesions	Copious irrigation, eye patch	Consider corticosteroids and antibiotics.
Severe pain	Morphine IV	Administer morphine intravenously.
Respiratory distress	Oxygen	Consider intubation. Consider bronchodilators. Consider antibiotics.

threatening injuries. The provider should remember that there is no antidote for mustard.

Severe: Patients who become critically ill from exposure to mustard present with large areas of burns, major pulmonary damage, and subsequent immunosuppression. Patients who present with the early onset of moderate-to-severe respiratory symptoms or large surface area burns caused by liquid mustard probably have life-threatening injuries. Dyspnea that occurs within 4 to 6 hours after inhalation of mustard suggests that the patient has inhaled a lethal amount of the agent. In the Iran–Iraq War, many fatalities occurred because Iranian soldiers continued to wear mustard-soaked clothing and inhaled the emanating fumes. The cause of death from mustard exposure may be burns, respiratory tract damage, bone marrow depression, or infection.[28]

Moderate: Patients with a large area of blisters or erythema will require hospitalization. Those who have eye injuries that obscure vision or are very painful will also require hospital care. Patients with respiratory symptoms, including dyspnea or a productive cough, will likely require inpatient respiratory care. Some of these patients may later progress to life-threatening symptoms. Moderately exposed casualties constitute the largest group of patients, and include those who will benefit most by medical care.

Minimal: Patients with only a small area of blister or erythema and patients with late-onset mild upper respiratory symptoms will not require hospitalization.

General

Patients who have been exposed to mustard will often require significant pain medication for relief. Providers must pay strict attention to fluid and electrolyte replacement. The patient will likely need intravenous therapy for hydration.

For some patients, intravenous **hyperalimentation** will be required to treat the persistent nausea, vomiting, and diarrhea seen with exposure to large amounts of mustard. Patients with extensive genital lesions may require a urinary catheter.

Systemic

Systemic symptoms are uncommon in military exposure to sulfur mustard. Physicians familiar with the effects of other alkylating agents used in clinical medicine deal mainly with the agents' systemic toxicity to cells of the bone marrow, lymphoid tissue, and gut mucosa. Exposure to sulfur mustard in situations of war and terrorism involves external epithelial surfaces rather than primary systemic absorption. This probably accounts for the paucity of systemic effects seen in World War I.

Systemic symptoms have been treated with high doses of sodium thiosulfate and vitamin E. Intravenous n-acetylcysteine has been used in some patients with systemic symptoms and may have some internal decontamination effect.[29] Intravenous cysteine 0.5%, 10 mg four times daily was used in 10 Iraqi patients in one study.[30] In that same study, charcoal hemoperfusion was used for patients with the most severe exposures.

Respiratory

Death from exposure to mustard usually results from pulmonary complications, such as **acute chemical pneumonitis** or pneumonia.[31] Appropriate respiratory care is a major contributor to survival.

The therapeutic goal in treating a patient exposed to mustard with skin burns and mild respiratory symptoms is pain management. Patients with mild upper airway lesions may benefit from cough suppressive drugs and increased humidity of the inhaled air. Bronchodilator therapy and supplemental oxygenation are needed in all but the mildest exposures. Steroids should be considered for patients with underlying asthma, chronic obstructive pulmonary disease, or hyperreactive airways disease.

Patients with severe respiratory exposure must have respiratory support. If the large lower tract airways are involved, the patient may develop fever and leukocytosis, and an **infiltrate** may appear on the chest radiograph during the first 2 days after exposure. This is almost always a chemical pneumonitis and not pneumonia, so antibiotics should be withheld. The patient may subsequently develop purulent sputum. This should be examined before the patient is started on antibiotics. Pulmonary function tests may show obstruction to airflow and hyperinflation, as well as **restrictive phenomena** and progressive impairment of gas exchange.[32]

A patient with severe respiratory signs should have early intubation. Subsequent laryngeal spasm may make later intubation problematic. **Bronchoscopy** may be needed to remove secretions and plugs. Early use of positive end expiratory pressure or constant end expiratory pressure is beneficial. A requirement for ventilation support is ominous. Over 80% of Iranian casualties treated in Western European hospitals who required assisted ventilation died.[33]

Ocular

Rapid decontamination is essential, as eye injury occurs within moments of mustard gas exposure. Eye exposures may be treated with copious irrigation with 2.5% sodium thiosulfate. Minor eye lesions may be treated with soothing eye solutions, such as eye drops available over the counter. More severe eye injuries should be treated with topical antibiotics and atropine or other topical **cycloplegic** drugs. The patient should be treated with frequent irrigation to remove inflammatory and necrotic debris. **Topical ophthalmologic corticosteroids** may be used for the first few days, but there are few data to support continued use. Topical anesthetics should be used only for examinations to prevent self-injury of the intensely inflamed eyes. Lid edge inflammation should be covered with petrolatum to ensure that lids do not adhere to each other. Dark glasses and reassurance are very important, as the eye lesions will produce severe photophobia and possibly subsequent blindness.[34] To prevent complications, the patient should be treated by an ophthalmologist as soon as possible.

Dermal

Chemical burns resulting from mustard are deceptively superficial on initial presentation. A potential lethal exposure is approximately 100 mg/kg or 5 to 7 mL of distilled mustard, the amount of mustard that will lightly cover about 25% of the body surface area. Patients who have sustained a potentially lethal dose of sulfur mustard may present initially with what appears to be a large first- or second-degree burn **(Color plates 5-2 and 5-3)**.

The blister fluid is described as nontoxic, but skin may well have residual agent present. Bullae and surrounding skin should be carefully decontaminated to remove residual agent.[35]

A major goal of skin therapy is to prevent infection. This may be accomplished by frequent irrigation of the burned areas and liberal use of topical measures, including cleansing with povidone-iodine solution and application of 1% silver sulfadiazine cream. The injured areas should be bathed daily with tap water and rinsed with physiological saline solutions.

Large areas of denuded skin (skin which is stripped of the protective outer layer) require the same treatment as needed for the care of other serious burns. Even under the best conditions, injuries from mustard exposure heal slowly, with repeated vesicles and ulcers. Systemic toxicity from mustard may contribute to the high incidence of secondary infection. Like other major burns, mustard lesions require months of medical care.

Protection

Skin Barriers and Reactive Skin Protectant

Because mustard is absorbed and reacts with the skin within minutes after exposure, the development of any protective ointment or lotion has been extremely difficult. Protective masks and clothing have been developed, but they markedly limit agility and endurance, thus compromising patient care and evaluation. More importantly to EMS, they simply may not be available when urgently needed. SERPACWA, discussed in Chapter 3, appears to provide prolonged protection from exposure to both mustard and organophosphates.

■ Lewisite and Similar Arsenical Agents

History

Lewisite (L) was developed near the end of World War I by a team of Americans headed by Captain W. Lee Lewis.[36,37] Lewisite was never used in World War I because hostilities ceased before the agent was deployed. The United States, Great Britain, France, Italy, the Soviet Union, and Japan produced large quantities of lewisite in the immediate post–World War I years.

Following World War II, lewisite was abandoned by the militaries of most countries. The development of British anti-lewisite (BAL), which is an inexpensive and effective antidote to lewisite exposure, caused these forces to consider lewisite to be obsolete. However, lewisite is easy and inexpensive to produce, making it attractive for terrorist activities. Lewisite and similar arsenicals are much more dangerous as liquids than as vapors.

Description

Lewisite is an oily, colorless liquid when pure. Impure lewisite is amber or dark brown in color. It is described as having an odor of geraniums. Lewisite is much more volatile than mustard, and it is more persistent in colder climates. It degrades rapidly under humid conditions.

Lewisite is easily mixed with other chemical agents to augment certain toxic effects. Lewisite can be mixed with mustard to form mustard-lewisite mix (HL). The resulting mixture has a lower freezing point than mustard alone, so it is less likely to freeze when dropped from high attitudes. Lewisite can be quite effective when mixed with nerve agents. Because lewisite can induce vomiting, it makes the use of protective masks less practicable. The resultant skin burns from lewisite allow rapid absorption of nerve agents.

When lewisite is manufactured, a complex mixture of several compounds is formed, forming substances L-1, L-2, and L-3. When lewisite is produced for chemical weapons, L-1 generally predominates as the major toxic substance. L-1 is a vesicant chemical warfare agent. L-1 forms initially, but it will react during production with additional acetylene to form L-2, which will in turn react to form L-3. Substances L-2 and L-3 are also toxic, but considerably less so than L-1.

Mechanism of Action

Like mustard, the complete mechanism of toxicity of lewisite on the body's cells is not completely known. As with the other arsenical compounds, lewisite inhibits many enzymes. In particular, lewisite affects cellular enzyme systems and damages the mucous membranes, liver, gallbladder, kidneys, and skin. Lewisite is widely distributed throughout the body, with high concentrations in the liver, lungs, and kidneys. Lewisite and metabolites are excreted through the kidneys and, to a lesser extent, the biliary tract.

Effects

Like sulfur mustard, lewisite causes damage to the skin, eyes, and airways, with direct-contact toxicity **(Color plate 5-4)**. It also causes systemic effects.

Dermal

Like mustard, arsenical vesicants are designed to irritate the skin. Lewisite and mustard are about equal in inhalation toxicity, but lewisite is faster acting and more toxic to the skin. Lewisite produces pain or irritation within minutes to seconds after contact with the skin.

Although erythema, burning, and pain occur immediately after exposure, blister formation takes 2 to 4 hours. A skin contact of only 5 minutes will cause a chemical burn resulting in a deep ulceration. This worsens over 3 to 4 days with the enlargement of the painful vesicles. Pain often decreases after blisters form. Gradually, the vesicles dry out, and a crust forms **(Color plate 5-5)**. The affected skin will show degenerative necrotic changes, including hemorrhage, edema, and generalized inflammation. Like mustard, the scrotum, axillae, and neck are especially sensitive to arsenical agents.

Lewisite blisters are thought to begin in the center of an exposed area and expand to include the entire lesion. Mustard blisters begin as a "string of pearls" on the edges of the exposed area and then grow to merge.[38] Lewisite skin lesions heal faster than lesions caused by mustard. Secondary infection within these lesions is much less likely, because lewisite does not suppress the immune functions. Loss of pigmentation within the healed lesions is also thought to be less common than with mustard.

Ocular

If moderate ocular exposure occurs, lewisite causes immediate pain, blepharospasm, and rapid formation of **eyelid edema**. Within 1 hour after exposure, the patient's lids will be swollen shut, and the patient will experience photophobia (presumed to be from ciliary spasm) and headache. After a few hours, the swelling will subside, but the patient may have areas of clouding in the cornea (cataract formation) and inflammation of the iris (iritis). This is quite similar to an acid burn of the eyes.

With mild exposure to very low levels of lewisite, the victim may only sustain conjunctivitis. Severe exposures may produce necrosis of the iris, with depigmentation and the formation of pus in the anterior chamber of the eye (**hypopyon**).

A relapsing syndrome has not been described for lewisite. Unlike mustard, there is no latent period for the eye damage. Because lewisite has an immediate onset, ocular irrigation must be equally rapid in order to prevent damage to the eyes. Since the patient has immediate pain, treatment is more likely than with mustard.

Respiratory

When inhaled, lewisite vapors cause sneezing and produce irritation of the upper respiratory tract. Mild respiratory exposure may resemble upper respiratory illness, with cough, inflammation of the mucous membrane of the nose (**rhinitis**), and mucous membrane erythema. There is abundant mucus and sputum. Some victims may complain of **retrosternal** pain. The examiner may hear crackles and rales over the lung fields. Concentrations of vapor in the lung fields are unlikely to cause more significant respiratory injury. Lewisite may cause more nasal irritation than mustard.

Chronic cough can be expected from exposure to lewisite. Reactive airway disease after severe exposure to lewisite has been noted.

Systemic

Systemic effects of the arsenicals include an increased capillary permeability. This phenomenon may cause extensive **interstitial fluid losses** and allow sufficient fluid to exude from the bloodstream (third-space shift) to cause **hemoconcentration**, shock, and even death. This effect is called **lewisite shock** and is noted with higher dose exposures. If the patient is hypotensive, hypovolemia should be presumed and corrected before the use of **sympathomimetics**.

Acute systemic toxicity of the arsenical vesicants may result from absorption through large skin burns. In animals, this caused pulmonary edema, diarrhea, and hypovolemic shock. Burns large enough to cause systemic poisoning in humans should be presumed to be life threatening.

Experience with ingestion of lewisite has not been documented. Nausea and vomiting occur with respiratory or significant skin exposure. (This effect is so pronounced that a Chinese chemical warfare analyst has classified lewisite as a vomiting agent.[39])

Lethality and Toxicity

Lewisite is faster acting and more toxic to the skin than mustard gas. A 2-mL dose of lewisite (about 30 mg/kg) applied to the skin is fatal to an adult. Lethal exposures for lewisite are listed in **Table 5-5**. Blisters will be caused by about 15 mg of lewisite applied to the skin. A very small amount of liquid in the eye (0.1 mL) blinded rabbits.

Intravascular hemolysis and subsequent hemolytic anemia may complicate the clinical picture. In extreme cases, these hemolytic manifestations may cause renal failure.

Similar Agents

Mustard-lewisite mix is a combination of both mustard and lewisite, which comprises the rapid effects of lewisite and the delayed effects of mustard. It has a garlic odor because of the mustard component. As previously noted, this mixture has a lower freezing point than mustard alone. This mixture does not produce more severe lesions than either agent alone, but it may confuse the diagnosis, making treatment more difficult for the medical provider.

From a battlefield perspective, mustard does not produce rapid casualties. In order to increase the number of early casualties, many countries that stocked chemical agents developed a mixture of mustard and lewisite. Much of the vesicant stocks of the former Soviet Union were mixtures of lewisite and sulfur mustard.

Decontamination and detection are similar to mustard. Medical providers require protective masks and full protective clothing ensemble for casualty management, although Level A or B protection is more appropriate.

PD

Phenyldichloroarsine (PD) is a variant of lewisite that is very irritating to eyes and mucous membranes. It causes rapid blister formation on exposed skin (0.5 to 1 hour). Exposure to this agent can also cause nausea and vomiting. (This would cause the affected victim to remove the protective mask and possibly expose the victim to other agents.)

Casualty management requires the use of a protective mask with charcoal inserts and protective clothing at a minimum, although Level A or B protection is much more appropriate. Decontamination of closed areas and personnel may be accomplished with bleach or bicarbonate solutions. Decontamination of open areas is unnecessary.

Table 5-5 Lethal Exposures of Lewisite by Route	
Route	Lethal exposure (mg•min/m³)
Eye	150
Inhalation	500
Dermal	1,500

ED

Ethyldichloroarsine (ED) is an arsenical agent that produces a vapor that is harmful only after a long exposure. The liquid form causes blisters after exposures of less than 1 minute. Immediate irritation occurs with delayed formation of bullae. If liquid droplets are inhaled, pulmonary edema and respiratory damage may occur. Eye injury may occur as a result of exposure to either vapor or liquid; however, the liquid form causes injury more rapidly than the vapor form, and the damage from liquid exposure is much more severe.

Medical providers should wear both supplied air protective masks and impermeable overgarments (Level A or B protection). Decontamination of closed areas may be accomplished with bleach. Decontamination of open areas is unnecessary, as the substance decomposes rapidly.

MD

Methyldichloroarsine (MD) is another rapidly acting arsenical blister agent, with effects and decontamination requirements that are similar to ED and lewisite. It also requires Level A or B protection for the medical provider.

Decontamination

Responders should don Level A protection when conducting containment operations or gross decontamination of incapacitated casualties. Level B protection with butyl rubber or nitrile gloves and apron is the minimal protection for those in close contact with contaminated patients. Because of the splash and vapor hazards of this agent, lower levels of protection are not recommended.

Exposed skin may be decontaminated by flushing with cool water, although this is controversial and bleach is more rapid and effective. Water will decompose lewisite to hydrochloric acid and chlorovinyl-arsenious oxide. The latter is a nonvolatile blister-forming solid that is not readily washed away by water. This substance may be deactivated with 0.5% bleach. Bleach will rapidly destroy the vesicant properties of lewisite. Avoid scrubbing and hot water, because they enhance absorption and toxicity. Blisters should be opened and drained of fluid. Although the blister fluid does not contain lewisite, it will contain arsenicals.

Treatment

Emergency care for casualties exposed to lewisite should focus on supportive care (Table 5-6). Once properly decontaminated, the patient's airway, breathing, and circulation should be continuously evaluated and supported as needed. As with the other vesicants, early interventions (other than decontamination) are usually unnecessary because of the delayed presentation of symptoms.

British Anti-Lewisite (BAL)

The British developed an effective antidote, BAL, that reverses the toxic symptoms of lewisite. BAL is available as an injectable agent or as a protective ointment applied to the skin. It chelates unbound lewisite and reactivates metabolically critical enzymes that have been inactivated by lewisite (Figure 5-1).[40] BAL reacts with lewisite to form a stable nontoxic product.

Table 5-6 Emergency Treatment of Lewisite Vesicant Injuries

Symptom	Standard treatment	Advanced treatment
All symptoms—immediate treatment	Copious irrigation and decontamination with bleach	
Mild skin irritation	Careful cleansing	Protect the skin from further trauma. Consider the use of BAL cream.
Severe skin lesions, blisters	Careful cleansing	Cover with a liberal application of BAL cream.
Severe eye lesions	Copious irrigation, eye patch	Consider corticosteroids and antibiotics. BAL may be used in the eye, but it can cause irritation.
Severe pain	Morphine IV	Administer morphine intravenously.
Respiratory distress	Oxygen	Consider intubation. Consider bronchodilators.

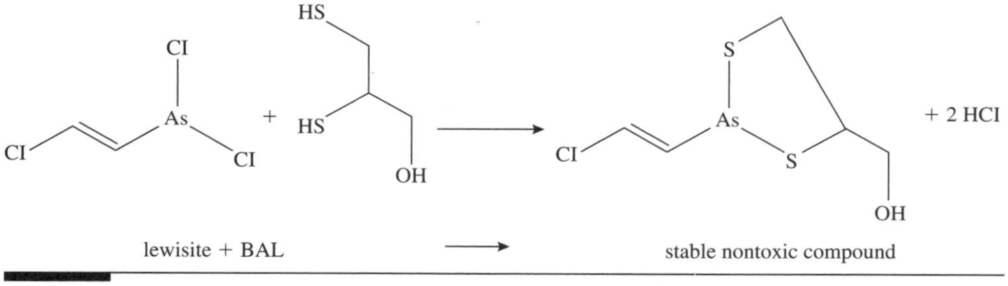

Figure 5-1 BAL chemical reaction with lewisite to form a nontoxic product.

There are two basic methods of treatment with BAL for lewisite toxicity:

- Local neutralization and use of BAL ointment
- Intramuscular administration of BAL

Local neutralization provides some limited protection against the effects of lewisite and is most useful for the patient with small lesions. The affected skin is thoroughly decontaminated and then covered with a liberal layer of BAL ointment. Any other protective ointment should be removed prior to treatment with BAL. BAL can be used in the eye, but greater than 20% concentration will cause the patient to develop conjunctivitis.

The intramuscular administration of BAL provides relief from exposure to larger doses of lewisite and the resulting systemic symptoms. Because the agent continues to burn until removed or detoxified, the first dose should be given as soon as possible, simultaneously with detoxification.

Dosage must be adjusted to the estimated weight of the patient (0.5 mL of 10% BAL in oil per 11.25 kg up to a maximum of 4.0 mL).[41] The dose should be repeated at different sites in the buttocks at 4, 8, and 12 hours after the initial injection for a total of four doses. An alternative dose of BAL is 4 mg/kg IM every 4 hours for 3 to 4 days.

Systemic signs requiring BAL treatment are as follows:[42]

- Signs of pulmonary edema
- Hypotension
- Any skin burn greater than 1% of total body surface area (greater than one palm size of the patient's hand) which was not decontaminated in the first 15 minutes
- Skin contamination greater than 5% of total body surface area with erythema or immediate skin damage

If the patient has pulmonary symptoms or signs of severe arsenical poisoning, then the interval between the first and second dose may be shortened to 2 hours. In these severe cases, additional doses of 0.25 mL per 25 lb (11.25 kg) may be given daily for 3 to 4 more days.

BAL ointment can cause stinging, itching, and urticarial wheals at the site of application. The skin lesions caused by BAL usually subside after about an hour and should not be treated. Mild dermatitis can occur if BAL ointment is used frequently. BAL ointment is not suitable for a protective barrier because of this dermatitis.

BAL is not innocuous. The preparation is in peanut oil, and patients who have severe allergies to peanut products will have reactions to this product. Side effects are relatively frequent, but, at the therapeutic dosage employed, they are seldom severe enough to warrant cessation of treatment and are almost invariably reversible.

BAL in oil has been shown to cause the following symptoms:

- A feeling of constriction in the throat and a sense of pressure in the chest
- Sweating of the forehead and hands
- Apprehension, restlessness, and nervousness
- Burning of the lips and dryness of the mouth and throat
- Lacrimation and reddening of the eyes
- Generalized muscular aches and spasms
- Nausea, vomiting, and abdominal pain

- Moderate tenderness at the injection site
- Hypertension (transient) accompanied by tachycardia
- Local pain (This may occur at the site of injection, and gluteal abscess has occasionally been encountered.)
- Fever (This is apparently particular to children, and it develops after the second or third injection and persists until treatment is terminated.)
- Acute renal insufficiency (BAL should be used with care in patients with hypertension or impaired renal function. It should be discontinued or continued with extreme caution if acute renal insufficiency develops during therapy. BAL may not be as effective in cases of **concomitant** renal failure.)

There is some evidence to indicate that 30 to 60 mg of ephedrine sulfate by mouth, given 0.5 hour before each injection of BAL, will reduce these reactions. Also, a minimum interval of hours between doses appears to reduce side effects.

The use of SERPACWA as a protection for lewisite exposure was researched by the United States, but the results are not available in the open-source literature. It can be presumed that SERPACWA offers some protection from lewisite as well as from mustard.

■ Halogenated Oximes: Phosgene Oxime

Phosgene oxime (CX) is an example of the class of chemical agents called urticariants or nettle gases. These agents produce an immediate sense of pain that may vary from a mild prickling to an intense pain. Phosgene oxime produces erythema, wheals, and urticaria. The lesions have been compared to those caused by the stinging nettle.

Phosgene oxime is a white crystalline powder that melts between 39° to 40°C and boils at 129°C (but it decomposes rapidly at this temperature). It is fairly soluble in water and in organic solvents. It has a high vapor pressure, and its odor is very unpleasant and irritating. Even as a dry solid, phosgene oxime decomposes spontaneously and has to be stored at low temperatures. By adding other chemicals, it is possible to liquefy phosgene oxime at room temperature. The liquid form is much more readily dispersed.

Phosgene oxime is unique, because it penetrates garments and rubber much more quickly than other chemical agents do. It is also a very rapidly acting agent on the skin. It can be mixed with other chemical agents (such as VX) so that the skin damage caused by phosgene oxime will allow a second agent to more easily penetrate the skin. Fortunately, a relatively high concentration of phosgene oxime is required for toxic effects.

Mechanism of Action

The mechanism of action of phosgene oxime is unknown. The agent seems to cause the greatest systemic effects in the first capillary bed that is encountered. Cutaneous application or intravenous injection of phosgene oxime causes pulmonary edema. Injection into the portal vein causes hepatic necrosis, but does not cause pulmonary edema.[43]

Phosgene oxime causes more severe tissue damage at a given concentration than other vesicant agents. The lethal dose in humans is unknown, but it is estimated to be about 30 mg/kg or a LC•t$_{50}$ of about 3,200. The skin irritation is manifest at 1 to 3 mg/m^3. The minimum effective respiratory dose is thought to be 300 mg/m^3.

Effects

Phosgene oxime is a powerful irritant that produces immediate effects, varying from a mild irritation to severe local pain. Phosgene oxime affects the skin, the eyes, and the lungs. Pain occurs immediately on contact with either the liquid or the solid form of phosgene oxime.

A diagnostic characteristic of phosgene oxime is this rapid onset of pain and irritation. Few other chemical agents produce such an immediate pain followed by rapid tissue necrosis.

Dermal

When phosgene oxime contacts the skin, the site of contact becomes blanched within 30 seconds. The blanched area is surrounded by erythema. The patient may then develop severe itching, hives, and painful blisters that resemble nettle stings. A wheal forms in about 30 minutes, and the blanched area turns brown in about 24 hours. A dark **eschar** forms over the next week. The eschar generally falls off in about 3 weeks, but healing may be incomplete for as long as 4 to 6 months after exposure. Itching may be present throughout the healing process.

The lesions of phosgene oxime extend into the subcutaneous tissue, fat, and muscle. Congestion and hemorrhage are found with thrombosis in both small arteries and veins.

Ocular

The lesions caused by phosgene oxime are similar to those caused by lewisite. Victims experience immediate pain and conjunctivitis.

Respiratory

Inhaled phosgene oxime causes rapid pulmonary edema. The pulmonary edema may be accompanied by a necrotizing bronchiolitis and thrombosis of the pulmonary vessels. Pulmonary edema also follows systemic absorption of large amounts of phosgene oxime from the skin. There are no known long-term respiratory injury data.

Treatment

There is no antidote for phosgene oxime. There are no medications that are specific to the treatment of phosgene oxime exposure. Analgesics are appropriate because of the intense pain caused by this agent.

Treatment of the skin lesions is the same as for other causes of skin necrosis, including diligent attention to cleanliness and avoidance of secondary infection. The eye lesions should be treated as any other eye injury resulting from a corrosive substance. Other treatment regimens are listed in **Table 5-7**.

Decontamination

Because phosgene oxime penetrates garments and rubber much more rapidly than other chemical agents, responders should use Level A protection when conducting containment operations or gross decontamination of incapacitated patients. Responders who are in close contact with contaminated patients may use Level B protection with butyl rubber or nitrile gloves and aprons.

Decontamination must be accomplished within seconds after contact to be effective. The U.S. military recommends use of the M291 decontamination kit with impregnated towelettes. The U.S. military also recommends flushing the skin with large amounts of water as rapidly as possible to remove any phosgene oxime that has not yet reacted with tissue. Phosgene oxime is readily soluble in water and is very soluble in organic solvents.

Phosgene oxime is considered to be a highly reactive agent and does not persist in the environment. The M256A1 detector can detect phosgene oxime and responds to levels within 3 to 5 mg/m^3. It is also possible to program the MM1 detector in the military "Fox" chemical detection vehicle to detect phosgene oxime. (Both of these are military detection devices, some of which are available to civilians.)

■ Threat Analysis

Mustard is a chemical agent that is likely to be used on the modern battlefield. As mentioned, mustard is easy to produce from commonly available materials with processes that are well described in the open-source literature. It should be presumed that terrorists may have access to mustard gas in

Table 5-7 Emergency Treatment of Phosgene Oxime Vesicant Injuries		
Symptom	Standard treatment	Advanced treatment
All symptoms—immediate treatment	Copious irrigation and decontamination	Administer pain medication.
Mild skin irritation	Protection of the skin from further trauma	Ensure that there is no further trauma or exposure to this area.
Severe skin lesions, blisters	Careful cleansing	Apply a silver sulfadiazine dressing.
Severe eye lesions	Copious irrigation, eye patch	Consider corticosteroids and antibiotics.
Severe pain	Morphine IV	Administer morphine intravenously or alternative pain medications.
Respiratory distress	Oxygen	Consider intubation. Consider bronchodilators.

small quantities and could employ it in confined spaces or at events with large attendances.

The need for protective measures for handling and dispersing this agent is the major drawback for a terrorist's use of mustard and analogues. The terrorist organization must accept casualties in the delivery team, use delayed fused munitions, or deliver the agent while dressed out in protective gear. However, if the person delivering the munition is expendable, the potential delivery scenarios are mind-boggling.

Covert Production

Almost all producers of chemical weapons since World War I have manufactured the vesicant agents, principally sulfur mustard. The chemical processes used to produce these agents are well documented in chemical literature and readily available from open sources. Indeed, the open-source literature includes data on reaction kinetics, necessary catalysts, and appropriate operating parameters of the reactions. These chemicals can be made with primitive equipment if the producers are not overly concerned with worker health and safety or environmental impact.

There are at least nine separate chemical routes to manufacture mustard, none of which require sophisticated technology or special materials. At least three of these methods could be used by terrorists to produce small quantities of mustard gas. (Small quantities of sulfur mustard can be easily prepared by bubbling ethylene through sulfur chloride or by utilizing hydrogen chloride and thiodiglycol.)

During World War I, thousands of tons of mustard gas were produced from alcohol, bleaching powder, and sodium sulfite. These are commonly available chemicals. The most common mustard production technique used in World War II was the Levinstein process, which consists of bubbling dry ethylene through sulfur monochloride. Only two chemicals are required in bulk and both of these are common industrial chemicals.

More recent production involves chlorination of thiodiglycol, a common material with dual use as an ingredient in some plastics and ballpoint pen inks. Known as the Victor Meyer-Clarke process, the chlorination of thiodiglycol was developed by Germany during World War I and used extensively by Iraq in the 1980s. Drums of thiodiglycol, produced in the United States and diverted from the intended recipients, were found by international inspectors in Iraq after the first Gulf War. Creation of mustard by this method is a one-step process and could be performed in a basement laboratory.

Processes for production of lewisite and nitrogen mustards are equally simple. The major problem for the terrorist who engages in covert production of mustard and similar agents is the potential casualties from accidental exposure to the agent. If the junior members of the production team are considered expendable, this is an insignificant problem.

■ References

1. Prakash UBS: Chemical warfare and bronchoscopy. *Chest* 1991;100:1486-1487.
2. Frietag L, Firusian N, Stamatis G, Greshuchna D: The role of bronchoscopy in pulmonary complications due to mustard gas inhalation. *Chest* 1991;100:1436-1441.
3. Borak J, Sidell FR: Agents of chemical warfare: Sulfur mustard. *Ann Emerg Med* 1992;21:303-308.
4. Heully F, Gruninger M, et al: Collective intoxication caused by the explosion of a mustard gas shell. (Trans US Army) *Annales d Medicine Legale* 1956;36:195-204.
5. Papirmeister B, Gross CL, Meier HL, Petrali JP, Johnson JB: Molecular basis for mustard-induced vesication. *Fund Appl Toxicol* 1985;5:S134-S149.
6. Borak J, Sidell FR: Agents of chemical warfare: Sulfur mustard. *Ann Emerg Med* 1992;21:303-308.
7. Papirmeister B, Feister AJ, Robinson SI, et al: *Medical Defense Against Mustard Gas: Toxic Mechanisms and Pharmacological Implications*. Boca Raton, FL, CRC Press, 1991.
8. Papirmeister B, Feister AJ, Robinson SI, et al: *Medical Defense Against Mustard Gas: Toxic Mechanisms and Pharmacological Implications*. Boca Raton, FL, CRC Press, 1991.
9. Borak J, Sidell FR: Agents of chemical warfare: Sulfur mustard. *Ann Emerg Med* 1992;21:303-308.
10. Haber L: *The Poisonous Cloud*. Oxford, England, Clarendon Press, 1986.
11. Ruhl CM, Park SH, Danisa O, et al: A serious skin sulfur mustard burn from an artillery shell. *J Emerg Med* 1994; 12(2) 159-166.
12. Watson AP, Griffin GD: Toxicity of vesicant agents scheduled for destruction by the chemical stockpile disposal program. *Environ Health Persp* 1992;98:259-280.
13. Requena L, Requena C, Sanches M, et al: Chemical warfare: Cutaneous lesions from mustard gas. *J Am Acad Dermatol* 1988;19:529-536.
14. Momeni AZ, Aminjavaheri M: Skin manifestations of mustard gas in a group of 14 children and teenagers: A clinical study. *Int J Dermatol* 1994;33(3):184-187.
15. Barranco V: Mustard gas and the dermatologist. *Int J Dermatol* 1991;30:684.
16. Augerson, WS.: Rand report on war gas exposure in the Gulf War. http://www.rand.org/publications/MR/MR1018.5/MR1018.5.chap3.html (accessed November 11, 2001).
17. Eisenmenger W, Drasch G, von Clarmann M, Kretschmer E, Roider G: Clinical and morphological findings on mustard gas [bis(2-chloroethyl)sulfide] poisoning. *J Forensic Sci* 1991;36:1688-1698.
18. Momeni AZ, Enshaeih S, Meghdadi M, Aminjavaheri M: Skin manifestations of mustard gas: A clinical study of 535 patients exposed to mustard gas. *Arch Dermatol* 1992:128:775-780.
19. Willems JL: Clinical management of mustard gas casualties. *Ann Med Milit Belg* 1989;3S:1-61.
20. Willems JL: Clinical management of mustard gas casualties. *Ann Med Milit Belg* 1989;3S:1-61.
21. Murray VSG, Volans GN: Management of injuries due to chemical weapons. *BMJ* 1991;302:129-130.
22. Anonymous: Iraq–Kuwait: Chemical warfare dusty agent threat. US Defense Intelligence Agency (Filename:73349033), October 10, 1990, http://www.desert-storm.com/Gulflink/950719dl.txt (accessed December 10, 2002).
23. Anonymous: Iraq-Kuwait: Chemical warfare dusty agent threat. US Defense Intelligence Agency (Filename:73349033), October 10, 1990, http://www.desert-storm.com/Gulflink/950719dl.txt (accessed December 10, 2002).
24. Augerson, WS.: Rand report on war gas exposure in the Gulf War. http://www.rand.org/publications/MR/MR1018.5/MR1018.5.chap3.html (accessed November 12, 2001).

25. Smith KJ, Hurst CG, Moeller RB, et al: Sulfur mustard: Its continuing threat as a chemical warfare agent, the cutaneous lesions induced, progress in understanding its mechanism of action, its long term health effects, and new developments for protection and therapy. *J Am Acad Derm* 1995;32:765-776.

26. van Hooidonk C: CW agents and the skin: Penetration and decomposition, in: *Proceedings of the International Symposium on Protection Against Chemical Warfare Agents Stockholm*. Stockholm, Sweden. National Defense Research Institute. 1983, pp 153-160.

27. Murray VSG, Volans GN: Management of injuries due to chemical weapons. *BMJ* 1991;302:129-130.

28. Murray VSG, Volans GN: Management of injuries due to chemical weapons. *BMJ* 1991;302:129-130.

29. Leonard RB, Teitelman U: Manmade disasters. *Crit Care Clin* 1991;7:293-320.

30. Murray VSG, Volans GN: Management of injuries due to chemical weapons. *BMJ* 1991;302:129-130.

31. Davis KG, Aspera G: Exposure to liquid sulfur mustard. *Ann Emerg Med* 2001;37:653-656.

32. Freitag L, Firusian N, Stamatis G, Greschuchna D: The role of bronchoscopy in pulmonary complications due to mustard gas inhalation. *Chest* 1991;100:1436.

33. Willems JL: Clinical management of mustard gas casualties. *Ann Med Milit Belg* 1989;3S:1-61.

34. Murray VSG, Volens GN: Management of injuries due to chemical weapons. *BMJ* 1991;302:129-130.

35. Momeni AZ, Enshaeih S, Meghdadi M, Aminjavaheri M: Skin manifestations of mustard gas. *Arch Dermatol* 1992;128:775-780.

36. Paxman J, Harris R: *A Higher Form of Killing: The Secret Story of Chemical and Biological Warfare*. New York, NY, Hill and Wang, 1982, p 32.

37. Stockholm International Peace Research Institute: *The Problem of Chemical and Biological Warfare: A Study of the Historical, Technical, Military, Legal, and Political Aspects of CBW and Possible Disarmament Measures*. New York, NY, Humanities Press, 1971, vol 1, pp 50, 62.

38. Sidell FR, Urbanetti JS, Smith WJ, Hurst CG: Vesicants in medical aspects of chemical and biological warfare.

39. Rand report on war gas exposure in the Gulf War. http://www.rand.org/publications/MR/MR1018.5/MR1018.5.chap3.html (accessed November 12, 2001).

40. Goldman M, Dacre JC: Lewisite: Its chemistry, toxicology, and toxicologic effects. *Ref Environ Contam Toxicol* 1989;110:75-115.

41. *NATO Manual FM8-285*. North Atlantic Treaty Organization.

42. *NATO Manual FM8-285*. North Atlantic Treaty Organization.

43. McAdams AJ Jr, Joffe MH: *A Toxico-Pathologic Study of Phosgene Oxime*. MD, Army Chemical Center (Medical Laboratories Research Report No 381), 1955.

CHAPTER

6 Nonlethal Agents

■ Introduction

Nonlethal chemical agents are chemicals that cause the temporary incapacitation of the victim. Nonlethal agents can be grouped into four general categories: **lacrimators**, which cause tearing of the eye and eye irritation; **sternutators**, which primarily cause sneezing and irritation of the upper respiratory tract; **vomiting agents**, which cause upper respiratory irritation and intense vomiting; and **incapacitating agents**, which render the victim mentally incapacitated and unable to resist. Of these four general categories, the first three are often lumped together as the riot control agents, because they have many common characteristics. These agents often act by irritation of the eyes, irritation of the upper respiratory tract, and vomiting **(Table 6-1)**. The public usually describes them as tear gases, but nonlethal agents may also be called riot control agents, irritant agents, or harassing agents.

In general, the acute toxicity of these agents is low, with a wide margin between the concentration that causes injury. If very high concentrations are used within an enclosed area or in very large amounts, then injury may result. The weapons used to disperse these agents may cause death or serious injury if not used as directed.

The use of nonlethal agents began before the use of lethal chemical warfare agents. Modern use of nonlethal gases began just before World War I in France with the use of ethylbromoacetate against criminals by the French police. When World War I started, many of these French policemen were recruited into the army and brought their skills with them. Ethyl bromoacetate, chloroacetone, and mixtures of xylyl bromide, xylylene bromide, and benzyl bromide were all used in World War I. CA was used by both the French and Americans towards the end of World War I. All these compounds are extreme irritants, capable of severely limiting the effectiveness of unprotected troops.

As noted in Chapter 4, chloropicrin was first synthesized from picric acid (2,4,6-trinitrophenol) and calcium hypochlorite (chloride of lime) in 1848. Chloropicrin was manufactured by both sides during World War I and used both as an irritant and a lethal chemical during that conflict. Although its toxicity makes chloropicrin a poor riot control agent, it is still used as a soil sterilant, a grain disinfectant, and an intermediate in chemical synthesis.

Table 6-1 Effects Common to All Riot Control Agents

Eye	Blepharospasm Burning, irritation Conjunctival injection Photophobia Tearing
Skin	Burning Erythema Bullous lesions in high concentration or long exposure
Gastrointestinal tract	Gagging Retching Vomiting
Respiratory tract	Burning pain Chest tightness Coughing Bronchospasm Irritation Rhinorrhea Secretions Sneezing
Mouth	Burning of mucous membranes Increased salivation

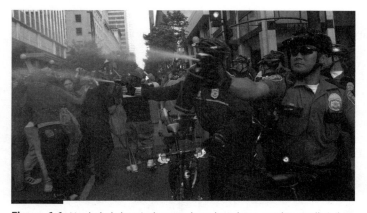

Figure 6-1 Nonlethal chemical agents have long been used to quell civil disturbances.

Nonlethal chemical agents have been used to quell civil disturbances in many countries for many years **(Figure 6-1)**. These agents have been used to stop prison riots, to roust hiding criminals, and to incapacitate belligerent forces, and they have even been used by civilians to foil rape and assault.

Although these agents may not be the ideal terrorist agents because they do not normally cause death, they may be quite useful in a terrorist's hands. Imagine, for example, the chaos that would be caused by the release of one of these agents in a crowded subway system. Lethality is not necessary to strike terror into the public's mind.

INCIDENTS INVOLVING Chemicals

E2 Nightclub Riot

In February, 2003, 21 people were killed in a panic sparked by a riot control agent that was sprayed in a confined area in a Chicago nightclub known as E2. Although the agent used (OC) was supposed to be nonlethal, the panic that ensued caused 21 deaths, mainly from crush injuries. Dozens of others were seriously injured.

■ Lacrimator Agents

Perhaps the most information on chemical agents available to the public exists about the lacrimator agents. This is simply because they are in current use by many law enforcement agencies in the United States and other countries. Most of these agents are entirely unclassified, and access to data about them is easily obtained. At least three of these agents are available to the public in small quantities. Although they have been marketed for self-defense, they are certainly able (and have been used) to incapacitate a victim during a crime.

The agents are not gases. Rather, they are highly refined, submicron-sized crystals or particles of chemical compounds that are highly irritating to the skin, upper respiratory system, and the **lacrimal glands**. They may also be carried in a carrier solution that evaporates quickly and leaves the crystals behind.

The acute toxicity of the lacrimator agents is very low, meaning that the margin between the concentration that causes an intolerable effect and that which causes injury is large. Only very high concentrations can cause serious or lethal injuries. In practice, this requires exposure in closed spaces. Common lacrimator agents are listed in **Table 6-2**.

■ Lacrimator Dispersement Methods

Blast Dispersion

Lacrimator agents can be dispersed from a container with an explosive charge. The charge expels the agent with great force when the explosive is detonated. This form of dispersal is used solely by the military, because the explosive and shrapnel can cause as many injuries as standard explosive devices.

Smaller alternative devices include liquid-filled grenades that use the force of an explosive charge to activate an aerosol unit or to provide compressed air to expel powder **(Figure 6-2)**. These may be used by law enforcement agencies.

Thermal Dispersion

Thermal dispersion is the most commonly used technique for the dispersion of lacrimator agents in a riot. With this method, the agent is vaporized by a heat source, and the

Table 6-2 Lacrimator Agents

Code name	Chemical name	Comments
CA	Bromobenzylcyanide	Outdated and not stocked
CN	2 Chloroacetophenone	Riot agent and Mace tear gas
CNC	Chloroacetophenone in chloroform	Similar to CN, but chloroform penetrates clothes easily
CNS	Chloroacetophenone and chloropicrin in chloroform	Actions are the same as CN, but chloropicrin can also cause intense nausea and pulmonary injury
CR	Dibenzoxazepine	Available in Britain
CS	Ortho-chlorobenzylidenemalononitrile	Current riot agent of choice, available to police and military
DM	Adamsite, vomit gas, diphenylaminochloroarsine	Not used or stockpiled in the United States
OC	Oleoresin capsicum	Widely available in the United States—component of most self-defense sprays, and current police agent of choice
PS	Chloropicrin	Chloropicrin causes nausea, lacrimation, and pulmonary irritation. It is also discussed as a pulmonary agent.

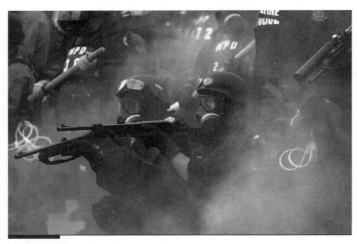

Figure 6-2 A blast dispersion of a powdered lacrimator agent.

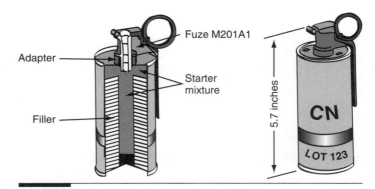

Figure 6-3 Cross-sectional diagram of a CN thermal gas grenade. (Note that this device does not deliver a gas and is not an explosive grenade.)

resulting vapors are spread into the area desired. Included in this method of dispersion are thermal fogger systems that heat the agent and a carrier that vaporizes the agent and blows the vapors into the desired area. Once aerosolized in this manner, prevailing atmospheric conditions determine the path of the agent. This dependence on airflow may lead to substantial toxicity in enclosed areas. The application of this technique ranges from the older military training capsules heating CN in an enclosed tent to modern pyrotechnic grenades and projectiles.

Handheld "gas grenades" are usually pyrolytic smoke generators, and not bursting devices (**Figure 6-3**). The pyrotechnic devices release the agent by a chemical reaction that boils off the chemical agent. When it hits the cooler ambient air, a cloud of small particles is formed. Because the projectile or grenade is literally a fire, victims may suffer burns.

The pyrolytic devices have been implicated in many fires, including the fire that destroyed the Branch Davidian compound in Waco, Texas in 1993 (**Figure 6-4**).

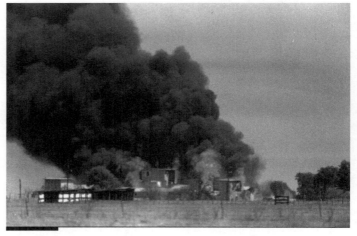

Figure 6-4 The fire that destroyed the Branch Davidian compound in Waco, Texas was attributed to pyrolytic devices.

Projectiles from kinetic or explosive effects may also cause serious or even lethal injury if they strike a victim. The shrapnel fragments are contaminated with the agent used in the device, further complicating care. Smaller dispersion

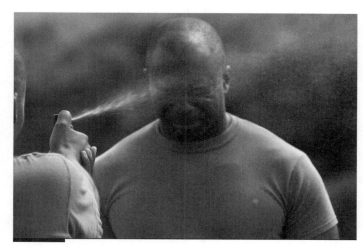

Figure 6-5 Small nonblast dispersion device.

devices may be aimed at the face, and both ocular and facial trauma may result.

Nonblast Dispersion

Powders and liquids can also be dispersed with a high-velocity air or water stream that carries the powder into the desired area. These dispersion devices range from water cannons to handheld aerosol streamers, mists, and foggers **(Figure 6-5)**.

■ Specific Lacrimator Agents

CS

CS is the standard riot control agent used by the US armed forces. The compound was first synthesized by Corson and Stoughton, hence the code name *CS*. It was adopted by most US law enforcement agencies and the military during the late 1950s.

CS exists as a family of three forms: CS, CS1, and CS2. CS is the white crystalline form. CS is insoluble in water, and minimally soluble in alcohol, ether, and carbon disulfide. This means that it is quite difficult to decontaminate buildings, furniture, and other material after the use of CS.

CS is available in a variety of munitions designed for both small and large area dispersion. It is effective in the form of aerosolized particles generated by pyrolytic generators. An aerosolized spray may also be generated using Freon or similar propellants (Paralyzer or Mace tear gases). CS1 is a mixture consisting of 95% crystalline CS blended with 5% silica aerogel to reduce **agglomeration**. This mixture is micropulverized to 3- to 10-μm sized particles to achieve the desired respiratory effects when dispersed as a solid aerosol. CS2 is CS containing a hydrophobic compound, Cab-O-sil, which improves the physical characteristics of CS by reducing agglomeration and hydrolysis. CS1 and CS2 are persistent and not used for civil disturbances.

The effects of CS start to occur at concentrations of about 5 mg/m^3. The estimated lethal dose is about 6,000 mg•min/m^3, but this is based on animal studies. Ocular symptoms may be found with concentrations as low as 4 μg/m^3.

Effects

General Symptoms of exposure to CS include profuse nasal and ocular discharge, intolerance to light, a burning sensation of all exposed mucous membranes, and conjunctival irritation. The intense ocular irritation causes the eyes to close. Patients experience significant lacrimation and rhinorrhea because of the irritation, hence the common name *tear gas*. The mucous membranes of the mouth will burn and the patient will experience excess salivation. A longer initial exposure may produce tightness in the chest, shortness of breath, malaise, and a feeling of suffocation.

A headache is common after even relatively brief exposure, and both malaise and headache may persist for several hours. Panic reactions are quite common and may be provoked by an intense desire to escape from the agent.

Pulmonary The most common route of absorption of CS is by inhalation. In a study using healthy human volunteers, low-dose exposure to CS had no acute effect on the lung mechanics or diffusing capacity.[1] Higher doses could irritate the bronchial mucosa and exacerbate chronic obstructive pulmonary disease and asthma.

Dermal Skin manifestations such as burns, ulcerations, and facial edema have been reported.[2] When applied directly to the skin, CS produces extreme irritation and erythema. This sensation is more pronounced in areas of fresh abrasions or recent shaving. When humidity is higher, the skin lesions produced are more severe. This is most likely related to the opening of sweat ducts in the increased humidity.

When the concentration of CS is high, the temperature is high, and the humidity is high, the patient may develop pronounced erythema, edema, and subsequent bullae and vesicles. (The patient may appear to have been exposed to a vesicant agent.) These lesions develop slowly, some 4 to 6 hours after exposure.[3] Firefighters in Washington, DC, were exposed to CS during the riots of April 1968. These minimally protected firefighters developed erythema and edema of periorbital skin and other exposed areas.[4] Similarly, soldiers equipped and trained with gas masks have developed delayed first-degree and second-degree burns on exposed skin in conditions of high heat and humidity.[5]

Prolonged Exposure Most individuals note marked effects at a concentration of 3 to 5 mg/m^3 and will attempt to leave the area immediately. Normally, the effects dissipate over 30 minutes after a brief exposure is terminated. The patient may have facial erythema and ocular irritation for 1 to 2 hours. If the patient is subjected to prolonged exposure, the effects become more severe and may include gagging, retching, and vomiting.

Decontamination and Personal Protection

Because CS is poorly soluble in water, aeration is the key to decontamination. CS tends to remain within clothing and thus may continue to cause symptoms. As with other lacrimator agents, the patient's clothing should be removed, because CA may remain within the clothing, causing continued symptoms and presenting risks to the medical provider. Skin can be decontaminated with soap and cold water. However, hot water or vigorous scrubbing may aggravate the injuries. Providers should wear Level C personal protection and use splash-proof garments and a protective mask for decontamination. Level A or B protection for those providers within the area of contamination is appropriate until the agent has been completely identified.

Outgassing (actually re-aerosolization of the fine particles) of CS occurs from exposed individuals and can cause symptoms in public safety personnel who are exposed to these particles. Indeed, in the confined space of a patrol car or the back of an ambulance, CS can literally make the atmosphere unbearable for the EMS workers or police officers within the vehicle.

Diphoterine is an active skin and eye decontamination solution that has been used to protect against CS exposure in an enclosed exposure chamber. It is not irritating to either skin or eye. It provides protection before exposure and decontamination after exposure. This agent promises much relief for law enforcement and medical workers who are exposed to CS. It has not been tested for any of the other riot control agents, but may also work for other agents.[6]

Tolerance

Tolerance develops in those who have been in regular contact with CS for a long period of time, such as trainers or laboratory workers.[7] Those who have developed such tolerance can stay in a concentration of CS that would render others incapacitated. These people may get CS on their clothing and become so accustomed to the effects that they unknowingly wear the contaminated clothing out of the work area and cause other people to complain. Tolerance to CS is decreased by warm and humid weather and increased by cold weather.

Complications

Significant contamination of the eyes with concentrated CS may lead to structural damage. Most eye damage from CS occurs when a weapon intended to disperse these agents is fired at close range. A blast injury may result, driving the agent deep into the tissue.

CN

CN is the standard tear gas used by local law enforcement agencies and is the active ingredient in many handheld gas projectors. CN was first synthesized in 1871. CN is a relatively volatile agent and produces a blue-white powder on release. Police in many countries adopted CN, which works primarily as an eye irritant, as a riot control agent between World War I and World War II. During World War II, many countries manufactured CN in large quantities.

Effects

CN is similar in effect to CS, though it is somewhat milder. The median incapacitating dose is slightly higher than CS, and the effects are less pronounced. During the 1950s, one limitation of CN became apparent. CN has such mild effects that determined demonstrators exposed to CN could continue to function by simply closing their eyes.

CN is toxic at 35 to 40 mg/m^3 and is 3 to 10 times more toxic than CS.[8] The maximum safe dosage (no significant complications) for short-term inhalation is 500 mg/m^3.[9] The lethal dose has been calculated at about 1,000 mg/m^3 from animal studies.

Allergic contact dermatitis requiring treatment with steroids has been noted after multiple exposures.[10,11] Rarely, blistering and dermal symptoms similar to those seen with CS are noted.

CN exposure has caused pulmonary edema, laryngospasm, and bronchospasm.[12] Bronchospasm and laryngospasm may be delayed for up to 24 to 36 hours after exposure. Pulmonary edema may occur up to 12 to 24 hours after exposure.[13]

Decontamination

Like CS, CN is poorly soluble in water, but aeration and vacuuming are generally sufficient for decontamination. If this is insufficient, CN can be decomposed with a 5% bicarbonate solution. As with other lacrimator agents, the patient's clothing should be removed, because CA may remain within the clothing, causing continued symptoms and presenting risks to the medical provider. The provider should utilize Level C personal protection. As with CS, re-aerosolization of CN particles can occur and cause symptoms in medical providers.

OC

OC is the concentrated, oily liquid extract of the cayenne pepper plant. Capsaicin is the active component of this extract. Unlike tear gas, which is an irritant, OC (also called pepper spray) is an inflammatory agent with profound lacrimation effects.

OC is often rated in Scoville heat units (SHU), named after Wilber Scoville, who developed a test for the irritation effects of the various forms of pepper and similar products. The pepper scale ranges from zero SHU for bell peppers to about 5,000 SHU for a jalapeno pepper to 200,000 to 300,000 SHU for a habanero pepper. Pure capsaicin extract is 15 million SHU. The more capsaicin content the spray has, the more effective the spray will be. Federal law limits consumer OC spray to 2 million SHU. Generally speaking, the sprays used by law enforcement agencies are five times more powerful than those sold to the general public.

Effects

OC causes effects immediately upon contact with the mucous membranes and eyes and causes irritation to the skin a few minutes later. It causes inflammation of the eyes, nose, mouth, upper respiratory system, and the skin. The patient will experience acute burning of these areas and involuntary eye closure. OC in the lungs forces rapid shallow breathing. The inflammation of the upper respiratory system may cause swelling of the mucous membranes, shortness of breath, and heavy coughing. The patient may also experience a choking sensation. The result of OC exposure is a temporary, nearly total loss of sight and a severe restriction of breathing. The effects of the agent begin to wear off within 10 to 15 minutes, but some dermal effects last up to 45 minutes. The patient may report some mild skin burning for a few hours that is not incapacitating.

Decontamination

OC is biodegradable, and extensive decontamination is unnecessary in most cases. As with other lacrimator agents, the patient's clothing should be removed, because OC may remain within the clothing, causing continued symptoms and presenting risks to the medical provider. Because it can be carried on skin, clothing, and transported from patient to medical provider, appropriate skin and respiratory protection are needed in handling patients who have been recently exposed and their personal effects. Level C protection will provide protection for ocular and respiratory effects. Gloves may be needed for handling casualties.

Complications

The FBI's Firearms Training Unit conducted extensive research on OC and feels that OC poses no identifiable, long-term health risks when used as a chemical agent. Although the official documentation for OC does not list any known specific lethal dose or lethal concentration, pepper spray has been implicated in anaphylactic reactions leading to death. Asthmatics appear to be at higher risk of having an adverse reaction to OC.

CR

CR is a relatively new and quite potent lacrimator agent developed in Great Britain in 1962 as an alternative to CS and CN.[14] CR is a crystalline powder that is the parent compound to the antipsychotic drug loxapine. It is capable of being deployed as either an aerosol or a liquid.

CR is much more potent than CS, though the two agents have quite similar effects. Despite this greater potency (5 to 10 times that of CS), toxic effects are less common with CR. The estimated concentration at which CR begins to create effects is about 1 mg/m³.

Effects

Eye irritation occurs at a concentration of 2 μg/m³. Exposure to even weak concentrations of CR produces an intense lacrimator reaction and causes blepharospasm. These effects last for at least 30 minutes after contact. The potential for serious eye damage is thought to be much less than that associated with CS or CN.[15]

A solution of CR splashed in the nose causes intense rhinorrhea and irritation. A splash in the mouth causes burning of the tongue and palate and increased salivation for 5 to 10 minutes. Contact with skin may produce the usual irritation, pain, and erythema. There is no delay of healing of skin injuries exposed to CR. Areas exposed to CR may become painful during showers (or other water contact) 24 to 48 hours after exposure.[16]

There have been no known lethalities associated with CR, but the estimated lethal dose is greater than 100,000 mg•min/m³ based on animal studies. The lethal dose for animals exposed to grenade-generated smoke was found to be greater than 150,000 mg•min/m³.

Decontamination

CR is insoluble in water and, like the other lacrimator agents, aeration is the primary means of decontamination. The patient's clothing should be removed, and the patient's skin should be washed with cold water and soap. Conjunctival irritation may require topical anesthesia, such as tetracaine, and irrigation with saline solution.

CA

CA is a highly irritating agent similar to CN. It has been used as a riot control agent. It was the last irritating agent introduced by the allies during World War I and is the most potent of the lacrimator agents. CA is unstable in iron and steel and therefore cannot be stored easily. It is sensitive to heat and degrades rapidly. Effects are similar to CN, but CA is much more toxic.

Decontamination

CA decontamination is similar to that of CN. Aeration is the primary means of decontamination. As with other lacrimator agents, the patient's clothing should be removed, because CA may remain within the clothing, causing continued symptoms and presenting risks to the medical provider. The patient's skin should be washed with soap and cold water.

Other Lacrimator Agents

CNC (chloroacetophenone dissolved in chloroform), **CNS** (chloroacetophenone and chloropicrin dissolved in chloroform), and **CNB** (chloroacetophenone in benzene and carbon tetrachloride) are other common lacrimator agents. These agents cause increased lacrimation and irritation of the skin. Because these tear compounds produce only transient casualties, they may be used for riot control and for situations where long-term incapacitation is unacceptable. When released indoors, they can cause serious illness and death.

CNC is used as a spray and causes effects identical to CN. CNS is also suitable for use as a spray, but it is longer lasting than CNC because of the chloropicrin additive.

CNB is another agent that causes effects that are similar to CN, but CNB is more potent. CNB is a slightly brown liquid with a benzene odor. CNB is quite flammable because of the benzene component. Like CN, CNB has a strong lacrimator effect, and it is similarly irritating to the skin. Because of the benzene component, CNB will penetrate clothing,

Decontamination

Lacrimator agents such as CNC and CNS should be decontaminated and treated in the same manner as CN or CS. Protection from them is the same as for CN. However, the use of an apron, gloves, facial protection, and a protective mask is the minimal recommended personal protection when dealing with CNB. As with other lacrimator agents, the patient's clothing should be removed, because CNB may remain within the clothing, causing continued symptoms and presenting risks to the medical provider.

Chloropicrin

Chloropicrin (PS) was first synthesized from picric acid (2,4,6-trinitrophenol) and calcium hypochlorite in 1848. Chloropicrin is a very stable compound and is insoluble in water, acids, or dilute alkalis such as bleach. When heated, chloropicrin undergoes thermal decomposition and can generate phosgene, nitrosyl chloride, chlorine, carbon monoxide, and various nitrogen oxides.

Chloropicrin was used as both an irritant and a lethal chemical during World War I. Although the toxicity of this chemical makes it a poor riot control agent, it is currently commercially used as a grain disinfectant and soil sterilizing agent. Despite its historical use in World War I, descriptions of chloropicrin's toxic manifestations remain poorly documented.

The effects of chloropicrin at various concentrations are shown in **Table 6-3**. Chloropicrin is known to cause profuse lacrimation and mucous membrane irritation at relatively low concentrations. Indeed, it is often added to other pesticides (such as methyl chloride) as a warning agent. Because it is produced in bulk for this and other uses, it is quite conceivable that an improvisational chemical weapon could be made from chloropicrin. Chloropicrin is toxic by all routes of entry.

Effects

Inhalation Exposure to a low concentration of chloropicrin leads to the effects of typical lacrimator agents, including profuse lacrimation and mucous membrane irritation. Theoretically, this effect should prompt the victim to remove him or herself from the potentially dangerous situation.

When exposed to higher concentrations, the victim may also have difficulty breathing, nausea, vomiting, cyanosis, and **chemical pneumonitis**. The victim who is exposed to a significant amount of chloropicrin may develop pulmonary edema, hence the dual classification as a pulmonary agent and a lacrimation agent. The pulmonary edema will be more severe and appear earlier if the victim engages in physical activity when exposed to this agent. Asthmatics will experience increased bronchospasm when exposed to chloropicrin. Auscultation of the lungs may reveal moist rales, but these may be present only in the most severe inhalation injuries.

Dermal Chloropicrin exposure causes reddened, irritated skin. The extent of the skin injury depends on the duration of the exposure and the concentration of the agent. Chloropicrin can cause burns of exposed mucosa, including the nose, mouth, and pharynx, and can also cause chemical burns or dermatitis.

Ocular Contact with the eyes causes pain, redness, and profuse tears. Prolonged exposure or high concentrations of chloropicrin can cause corneal damage and blindness.

Systemic Inhalation of chloropicrin can cause leukopenia with reduced **erythrocyte**, hemoglobin, and **hematocrits**. Exposure to high concentrations or ingestion will result in nausea, vomiting, tenesmus, colic, and diarrhea.

Personal Protection

Chloropicrin is not removed by standard organic vapor filters and can penetrate most masks. The provider should be protected with Level A protection if at all possible, because this agent also penetrates some protective clothing. The charcoal liner of military MOPP gear will provide protection from chloropicrin.

Decontamination

Chloropicrin can be removed by flushing the exposed area with water. Washing with soap and water may speed the decontamination process. Ensure that eyes are also flushed for at least 15 minutes. If irritation persists, repeat the irrigation.

Treatment

There is no antidote for exposure to chloropicrin. Treatment is entirely dependent on the symptoms. If there is a significant exposure, then the patient should be treated for an inhalation injury as if exposed to a pulmonary agent as described in Chapter 4.

Threat

Chloropicrin would be an easy weapon for a terrorist to acquire and deploy.[17] None of the chemicals used to make chloropicrin are particularly difficult to acquire, and chloropicrin itself is available in bulk quantities for industrial purposes.

■ Vomiting Agents

Vomiting agents are a class of riot control chemicals that are not often used in the United States. These agents are normally solids that vaporize with heating and then condense to form aerosols. They are included in most military summaries of chemical weapons; however, it is unlikely that these agents would be employed by a terrorist. They are somewhat difficult to procure and are not usually lethal.

The effects of the vomiting agents are quite similar to those of the lacrimation agents and include severe irritation of the eyes, nose, and throat. If the agent is inhaled for about 1 to 2 minutes, the patient will develop chest tightness and headache. The headache develops into nausea and vomiting in about 3 minutes.

DM

DM, also known as nausea gas or adamsite, was first discovered by German chemists working for F Bayer and Company in 1913. DM is a yellow-green, odorless, crystalline substance that is not very volatile. It is insoluble in water

Table 6-3 Symptoms Produced by Chloropicrin at Various Concentrations	
Concentration (ppm)	Symptom
0.29–1.0	Eye irritation and pain
4	Incapacitation
20	Pulmonary edema

and not particularly soluble in organic solvents. DM has been manufactured by many countries for use as a riot control agent, though, in recent years, it has been widely replaced in favor of CS and CN.

Effects

DM produces both the respiratory and skin irritant effects of the lacrimating agents in addition to profound nausea. In contrast to other riot control agents, the effects of DM do not appear immediately. The respiratory and skin effects appear only after a few minutes of exposure. Because of the absence of symptoms, a patient may not immediately don protective gear and may absorb a significant amount of agent. In addition, the delayed nausea and vomiting effects will often make the exposed person remove any protective gear.

DM may also cause substantial systemic effects, including depression, headache, chills, nausea, abdominal cramping, vomiting, and diarrhea. These effects may last several hours after exposure.

DM is substantially more toxic than the other lacrimator agents and is not used by US civilian law enforcement agencies. Despite limited military use in the United States, deaths have occurred during training with this agent.[18] The delayed presentation of the chemical increases the likelihood of severe injury when this agent is used.

Decontamination

The standard charcoal insert protective mask will work well for inhalation protection against DM. The skin irritation caused by this agent is relatively minor, and ordinary clothing will adequately protect against this agent. DM is poorly soluble in water, and aeration is the primary method of decontamination. As with other lacrimator agents, the patient's clothing should be removed, because DM may remain within the clothing, causing continued symptoms and presenting risks to the medical provider.

DC

DC is an irritating agent that causes the rapid onset of rhinorrhea and lacrimation symptoms associated with headache, nausea, and severe vomiting. The treatment and decontamination procedures are the same as for DM. Alkali solution or DS2 will suffice for decontamination in confined areas.

DA

DA is also classified as a vomiting agent. DA was first used by German troops in 1917. DA was considered to be a significant development in chemical warfare, because it could penetrate the activated charcoal gas mask filters used in World War I. DA was often deployed in combination with another agent, such as phosgene. The DA caused the exposed troops to remove their masks to sneeze, cough, or vomit, then the other agents deployed caused further casualties. DA causes a very rapid onset of both respiratory and skin irritations combined with severe nausea.

By 1967, the respiratory protection of military masks was sufficient such that the use of DA in combat was abandoned. This agent has been used in riot control and training, but it is not thought to be produced or currently stocked.

Decontamination

Dilute bleach solution is adequate for field decontamination of DA. Use of water for decontamination may not be appropriate. When mixed with water, DA produces diphenlyarsenious oxide and hydrogen chloride. The oxide is very poisonous if ingested. As with other riot control agents, the patient's clothing should be removed, because DA may remain within the clothing, causing continued symptoms and presenting risks to the medical provider.

The standard modern military charcoal insert protective mask will protect against inhalation of this agent. The skin irritation produced by DA is minor, and ordinary clothing will usually protect against it.

■ Incapacitating Agents

Incapacitating agents are chemicals that render the victim helpless and unable to make decisions or coordinated physical efforts. These nonlethal agents may be used as tools to diffuse hostage situations, or they may be used as tactical military tools.

Considering that the current crop of terrorists seems to favor lethal agents, it is unlikely that these incapacitating agents will appeal to them. Furthermore, they require relatively sophisticated devices to deploy en masse and significant skill to manufacture.

Only one chemical agent, BZ, has been advanced into documented production and use as an incapacitating weapon. One other agent, LSD, is easy to produce in large quantities and has been considered for use by credible terrorists as a possible chemical weapon in the 1950s. Undoubtedly, other classified agents exist and have probably been produced in restricted amounts.

LSD

LSD is a synthetic hallucinogenic (psychedelic) compound. LSD-25 is the 25th amide that was derived from rye fungus ergot in Sandoz laboratories by Dr Albert Hofmann and Dr Arthur Stoll in 1938. One of the codiscoverers was the first victim of an inadvertent "trip" (the nickname for the drug's effects), when he accidentally ingested a minuscule amount of LSD.

LSD is one of the most potent hallucinogenic drugs known. The average effective dose is about 75 μg, which is 5,000 times more potent than the drug mescaline.

LSD is typically not lethal, as the lethal dose is at least 1,000 times greater than the incapacitating dose. The onset of action occurs about 30 to 90 minutes after ingestion. LSD is rapidly metabolized and eliminated. There is no physical addiction to LSD and psychological dependence is quite rare. Long-term use does not appear to induce either psychosis or organic brain syndrome. There are no reported deaths from the direct effects of LSD.

As noted above, LSD is potent. The ingestion of only about 0.5 μg can produce an intoxication for up to 12 hours in a 70-kg person. In a typical dose of 20 to 400 μg, LSD causes alterations in perception, mood, and thinking.

LSD can be ingested orally or through mucous membranes. LSD can be administered in various forms: drops on blotter paper, on sugar cubes, or on other pills. LSD would probably be aerosolized if used as a weapon.

Effects

Perception changes caused by LSD are frequently reported. Sensory perception is particularly affected, with colors appearing brighter, smells sharper, and shapes and relations between objects noted more vividly. Patients also report alterations of time and space perceptions. Sometimes the patients will report that senses may be merged, with colors being felt or heard and sounds tasted or seen. Such hallucinations are a hallmark of LSD and are not found in any form of psychosis.[19]

Emotions are intensified and may change rapidly after exposure to LSD. The patient may become more suggestible or yielding or have two seemingly opposite feelings simultaneously. The patient may experience either distance from or empathy for other people.

Patients may also exhibit alterations in thinking, including feelings of depersonalization or out-of-body experiences. The sense of self may expand to include awareness of internal organs, and early childhood experiences may be vividly remembered.

Other signs and symptoms of LSD intoxication include dilation of the pupils, blurry vision, tremors, and **hyperreflexia**. Some of these effects result from a slight **sympathomimetic effect** and others result from anxiety induced by the trip.

LSD trips are sometimes confused with amphetamine or PCP reactions. Both have some sympathomimetic effects. The hallucinations of LSD are usually visual, whereas those of amphetamines are auditory. PCP causes prominent **nystagmus** (both vertical and horizontal) and hypertension.

Treatment

There is no antidote for LSD. The consequences of an unsuspecting LSD intoxication can be frightening to both the user and the medical provider, and may be dangerous or even fatal. The patient with LSD intoxication requires comfort, gentle reassurance, and careful monitoring.

If LSD is used as a weapon, the majority of patients will not recognize the effects of the drug and may well become panicked by the effects. Paranoid or suicidal behavior is common with a "bad" trip, so these patients should not be left alone. Rarely, agitation will not respond to verbal management, and sedation will be required. In these cases, oral diazepam (10 to 30 mg) may be effective. This may be repeated every 2 to 4 hours.

Threat

LSD is relatively easy and cheap to produce. Instructions on how to make LSD have been widely available since 1954, and LSD is readily available on the street market. LSD is not difficult to manufacture. It requires only about a year's worth of college chemistry skills to produce, as multiple students have demonstrated.

LSD was tested as a potential chemical warfare agent during the 1950s. The US military investigated the use of LSD spray as an incapacitating drug. LSD is not particularly stable and is often considered a poor choice as a chemical weapon. Because it can be produced cheaply in large quantities, it could conceivably be used by a terrorist, despite its drawbacks.

BZ and Agent 15

BZ is an incapacitation agent with a delayed onset of about 1 to 4 hours after exposure. BZ can be synthesized in laboratories, but it is commercially available as QNB and widely used in pharmacology research as a muscarinic receptor marker.

BZ was first studied as a therapeutic drug for gastrointestinal diseases, but the very frequent side effects of confusion and hallucinations caused it to be withdrawn from the study. BZ was then turned over to the US Army as a possible incapacitating agent.

BZ can be dissolved in propylene glycol, dimethyl sulfoxide, and many other solvents. However, BZ is stable in most solvents, with a half-life of 3 to 4 weeks in moist air. BZ is also quite stable in soil and water and will persist for weeks.

Little information is publicly known about Agent 15, except that it is either BZ or very closely related to BZ.

BZ, as a powdered compound, cannot be absorbed through the skin, although there is some military experience that suggests dimethyl sulfoxide can carry BZ through the skin in sufficient quantity. Propylene glycol also yields adequate skin absorption of the agent. When BZ is absorbed through the skin, the latent period is prolonged and may be as long as 24 hours.

Effects

The effects of BZ are similar to those caused by atropine. The provider should remember the saying, "dry as a bone, red as a beet, hot as hell, and mad as a hatter." BZ causes fast heartbeat, dizziness, vomiting, dry mouth, blurred vision, stupor, confusion, and unpredictable random behavior. A shrub within the vicinity of the exposed patient may appear to the patient as an immense danger and a threat. The affected patient may react as if drunk, may just sit quietly, or may become belligerent. Other effects of BZ and Agent 15 are listed in **Table 6-4**.

The onset of BZ and Agent 15 is slow, and the incapacitation is long in duration. BZ causes intoxication at doses of 0.5 to 5 mg. Effects are not experienced for 30 minutes to 24 hours after exposure. The performance decline is usually at a peak at 8 hours and subsides over 48 to 72 hours. The duration of incapacitation is about 24 hours. The patient may develop stupor and coma after high doses. Incapacitating aftereffects may remain 1 to 3 weeks after the poisoning. The various phases of effects resulting from BZ and Agent 15 exposure are listed in **Table 6-5**.

BZ is relatively safe, and the amount required to produce effects is more than 1,000 times less than the fatal dose. The ingested incapacitating dose is estimated to be 112 mg•min/m^3, and the lethal dose is estimated to be about 200,000 mg•min/m^3.

Table 6-4 Effects of BZ and Agent 15	
Peripheral effects	Blurred vision Dry mouth and skin Rapid heart rate (initially) Flushed skin
Central effects	Altered mental status Delusions and hallucinations (may be shared with others) Poor judgment and insight Shortened attention span Distractibility Impaired memory (particularly recent) Slurred speech Perseveration Disorientation Ataxia Alternating quiet and restless behavior (behavioral lability)

Table 6-5 The Course of Effects Resulting from Exposure to BZ and Agent 15	
Period or phase	Effect
Latent period: 30 minutes to 24 hours	No effect
First phase: 0–4 hr	Parasympathetic blockade and mild CNS effects
Second phase: 4–20 hr	Stupor with ataxia and hyperthermia
Third phase: 20–96 hr	Delirium that may fluctuate from moment to moment
Fourth phase: Resolution	Paranoia, deep sleep, automatism, eventual recovery

Detection

There is no currently available military or civilian detector that can detect BZ or Agent 15 in the environment. Confirmation of exposure would require specific laboratory analysis of specimens, and could not be conducted in a timely fashion. Urine drug screens do not detect BZ or Agent 15.

Treatment

The major threats to life in the BZ intoxicated patient are hyperthermia and injuries from the patient's own behavior or from the behavior of other similarly intoxicated patients. Monitor the patient's core temperature and maintain adequate fluids orally or intravenously.

Hyperthermia Hyperthermia is a serious effect of poisoning with BZ. Deterioration in the level of consciousness, hallucinations, and coma occur subsequently. Death from relatively low doses of anticholinergics such as atropine or BZ has occurred as a result of the impairment of sweating. The patient's body temperature can be reduced by wetting the patient's clothing and skin and placing the patient in the shade.

Physiostigmine The specific antidote to BZ is administration of another poison; that is, a nerve agent. Any compound that causes a rise in the acetylcholine concentration will restore normal function of the affected nerves. The drug of choice for this is the carbamate anticholinesterase physostigmine. Physostigmine is more effective than other similar compounds, because it penetrates the blood-brain barrier more easily.

The amount of physostigmine required is about 45 μg/kg per dose. Usually a test dose of 1 to 2 mg is used when the diagnosis is in doubt. If there is any improvement in the patient's condition, the routine dose can be administered. The improvement can be sustained by repeating the treatment in 1- to 4-hour intervals. (Physostigmine effects last only about 60 minutes after injection.) Physostigmine can be given orally with good effect, but the oral dose is about 1.5 times higher than the IM dose. The various doses of physostigmine are listed in **Table 6-6.**

Physostigmine is minimally effective during the first 4 hours after exposure, but it is quite effective after 4 hours. Physostigmine does not shorten the course of BZ poisoning, and relapses will occur if physostigmine is stopped prematurely.

Administration of physostigmine is not innocuous. Intravenous infusion may cause arrhythmias, excessive secretions, and convulsions. Indeed, IV administration may lead to a nerve agent–like syndrome. In addition, the sodium bisulfite in commercially available preparations of physostigmine can cause allergic responses in some individuals.

Decontamination

Decontamination of Agent 15 and BZ may be accomplished with water and soap or with dilute bleach. Decontamination is ineffective if the agent has already been absorbed. However, decontamination will help prevent further absorption from contaminated skin and clothing. Some patients will require physical restraint to protect both the provider and the patient from harm.

Protective garments are necessary during the decontamination phase. Protection of the medical staff from absorbed and systematically distributed BZ in the affected victim is unnecessary once the patient has been decontaminated. A chemical protective garment with either butyl rubber, Tyvek, or similar material provides appropriate protection against dermal exposure. The charcoal-filled MOPP gear will also provide protection.

A protective mask with charcoal filters is adequate to protect medical providers from inhalation exposure. Because this agent can be distributed in food, ingestion protection depends on the suspicion that the food or drink may be contaminated.

Table 6-6 Physostigmine Dose	
Intramuscularly:	45 μg/kg in adults, 20 mg/kg in children
Intravenously:	30 μg/kg slowly (1 mg/kg)
Orally:	60 μg/kg (use only in cooperative patients)

■ Calmative Agents

Pharmaceutical agents that are considered **calmatives** include compounds known to depress or inhibit the function of the central nervous system. These may include sedative hypnotic agents, anesthetic agents, opiate analgesics, antipsychotics, antidepressants, and **anxiolytics**.

These drugs have a range of effects that are dependent on the route of administration, dose, and duration of the drug administered. The physiological and behavioral effects include anxiety, sedation, hypnotic effects, coma, and even death.

These "knockout" chemical agents are not currently banned under international chemical weapons treaties and conventions, because they have been developed primarily for medicinal uses. The US Joint Non-Lethal Weapons Directorate defines a nonlethal chemical weapon as one that incapacitates 98% of the target population while causing fewer than 0.5% fatalities (JM Kenny, PhD, unpublished data presented by the Human Effects Advisory Panel of the National Academy of Sciences, 2001, Pennsylvania).

The ideal nonlethal calmative would have the following characteristics:

- Easy to administer
- Adaptable for administration by inhalation or by oral, subcutaneous, or intramuscular routes
- Rapid in onset
- Short in duration
- Able to produce (reliably) approximately the same amount of "calm" in all individuals of similar body mass and age
- Rapidly reversible (either by antidote or by rapid biodegradation of the compound)
- Free of prolonged toxicity
- Free of long-term side effects

Specific Calmative Agents

The spectrum of use of calmative agents ranges from knocking out armed hostage takers and terrorists to calming a group of hungry refugees who may be excited over the distribution of food and unwilling to wait for the distribution. Several classes of compounds have been identified as having a high potential for use as nonlethal calmative agents, including the following.

Opioid Receptors and Mu Agonists

Opioid receptors are classified into three different categories based on their pharmacologic profiles (mu, delta, and kappa receptors). (Opiates are drugs that are derived from opium. Opioids are drugs that are not derived from opium.) Because of their powerful analgesia-producing properties, mu receptors and mu receptor–selective agonists have been the focus of pain research and management. A rapidly acting and very powerful mu receptor agonist is fentanyl. Mu receptor agonists are easily reversed with naloxone or naltrexone.

Another similar and exceptionally fast-acting agent, which is not yet approved for human use, is carfentanyl. Carfentanyl is commonly used for sedating large animals.[20-22]

M99 is a widely available synthetic opiate that is more than 500 times more powerful than morphine. The lethal dose of M99 is only a few multiples of the effective incapac-

itating dose. (This is technically called a *narrow therapeutic window* and means that the dangerous dose is quite close to the desired dose. This is common with all anesthetic agents and is one of the reasons why anesthesiologists exist.) The weaponization and deployment of a fentanyl derivative (etorphine or M99—a potent anesthetic used to immobilize and capture big animals such as elephants, giraffes, and hippos), during a hostage crisis in Russia, came as a surprise to many chemical weapons experts and medical professionals.[23]

A patient exposed to an opioid-based agent would present with lethargy, bradypnea, apnea, and pinpoint pupils. In the only documented use of a knockout agent, M99, the casualties had typical opiate symptoms, including respiratory depression and apnea. What was alarming about the October 2002 hostage situation in Russia was the lethality of the supposed incapacitating agent used. Of the nearly 800 persons exposed to the gas, 117 were killed and close to 650 were hospitalized, including almost 50 in critical condition.

The Russian officials refused to identify the agent and any antidote until well after the incident. This delayed the proper care from being rendered to the patients and possibly led to many of the deaths.

Benzodiazepines

Benzodiazepines are often used as calming agents for treatment of anxiety, treatment of amnesia, and sedation for anesthesia. The major side effects of these agents are respiratory and cardiovascular depression. Newer, short-acting benzodiazepines are under investigation for use with panic attacks. These drugs may possibly be adapted for police or military use. Flumazenil is available as an antidote to benzodiazepines.

Neuroleptic Anesthetics

Short-acting agents such as propofol and ketamine have also been investigated as calming agents. As an intravenous agent with minimal side effects, propofol is used extensively

INCIDENTS IN Terrorism

The Moscow Theater Hostage Situation

On October 23, 2002, more than 50 radical Chechnyan terrorists held a crowded Moscow theater hostage. The terrorists, armed with weapons and wearing explosives, held the theater-goers hostage for three days, threatening to kill them all unless Russian troops withdrew from Chechnya. On October 26, fearing that the terrorists would carry out their threat, Russian special forces released an unidentified gas into the theater with the intent of incapacitating the terrorists. Unfortunately, this gas may have worked too well; close to 120 people died in the siege, most of them from the gas. Though the Russian government has been quiet about the gas used, it is widely assumed that the mystery gas was M99, a synthetic opiate that is 500 times stronger than morphine.

for sedation and anesthesia in the United States. This drug is a gamma-aminobutyric acid (GABA) receptor stimulant. Similar drugs may be developed that cause an equally rapid onset of effects and have better delivery systems for operational and tactical medicine.

Ketamine produces a state of unawareness without respiratory or cardiovascular depression. Because of their prolonged duration of action, ketamine and the quite similar PCP are not suitable as operational and tactical medicines. Similar drugs that have shorter durations of action are suitable for operational and tactical delivery.

Alpha$_2$-Adrenergic Agonists

Alpha$_2$-adrenergic agonists cause sedation, reduce anxiety, and enhance the effects of other anesthetic agents. A prototype agent of this class that is familiar to all EMS providers is the antihypertensive clonidine. Unfortunately, clonidine causes significant hypotension.

Another alpha$_2$-adrenergic agonist, dexmedetomidine, has been developed as a sedative-analgesic for veterinary medicine and adapted for human use. This agent also potentiates several anesthetic agents and reduces the dose requirements for these sedatives. This might reduce the dose-related side effects and increase the safety of the mixture.

An antidote for alpha$_2$-adrenergic agonists, fluparoxan, is under development. Fluparoxan permits the rapid reversibility of the drug-induced effects of alpha$_2$-adrenergic agonists.

Dopamine D3 Receptor Agonists

The D3 receptor agonists have been investigated as antidotes for PCP and cocaine.[24] There is no open-source literature that describes the use of these in operational and tactical medicine.

Selective Serotonin Reuptake Inhibitors

Selective serotonin reuptake inhibitors (SSRIs) are well known to emergency providers. Prozac (fluoxetine) is the prototype in this class. None of the current SSRI agents have an onset of action that is rapid enough for operational and tactical use.

Serotonin 5-HT1A Receptor Agonists

Serotonin 5-HT1A receptor agonists are also well known to the emergency provider. BuSpar/Wellbutrin (buspirone) is the prototype in this class. There is no known fast-acting Serotonin 5-HT1A receptor agonist.

Corticotropin-Releasing Factor Receptor Antagonists

Corticotropin-releasing factor is a peptide hormone that regulates the stress-induced release of hormones. When these receptors are blocked by a selective antagonist, anxiety reactions are subdued, and the patient experiences a calm behavioral state. There are no current drugs in this class approved for clinical use.

Cholecystokinin B Receptor Antagonists

The activation of cholecystokinin (CCK) receptors produces panic attacks. These effects are blocked with selective CCK-B antagonists. CCK-B receptor antagonists induce behavioral changes, whereby anxiety reactions are subdued, and the patient experiences a calm state.

There are no current drugs in this class approved for clinical use. The recent discovery of cell-penetrating peptides may open new possibilities for calming agents. With an appropriate delivery system and a powerful CCK-B antagonist, a safer calming drug suitable for operational and tactical applications may be found.

Dissemination

Although the use of calmative agents by terrorists has been rare, the Russian incident demonstrated that the deployment of these agents is possible. The agent used was described as a colorless and odorless gas. This state would be the most effective means for deploying a calmative agent within an enclosed space with a ventilation system that can be manipulated.

Major Problems With Calmative Agents

Unfortunately, seemingly nonlethal incapacitating agents can be quite lethal in actual use.[25] When the goal is to incapacitate everyone in a particular place (often an enclosed space), such as in a hostage rescue situation or in urban military operations, agent concentrations considerably higher than the 50% effective dose (ED$_{50}$) may be necessary. However, the result may be deadly.

If a pharmacologic agent considered to be very safe were used, the following would apply:

- ED$_{50}$ = 1 concentration unit (ED$_{50}$ is the dose that incapacitates 50% of exposed individuals)
- LD$_{50}$ = 1,000 concentration units (LD$_{50}$ is the dose that kills 50% of exposed individuals)

This describes an agent with a therapeutic index (TI) or safety margin of 1,000 (which is very good by almost any standards).

$$TI = LD_{50} / ED_{50}$$

If the commander of a task force wishes to immobilize all of the people in the enclosed space, the dose needed to incapacitate a given fraction of the target population is calculated as follows:

$$A_0 = ED_{50} / (1/f_1 - 1)$$

If we set f_1 to equal 0.99 and if the ED$_{50}$ is equal to 1, then A_0 will equal 99 concentration units or a concentration 99 times greater than the ED$_{50}$. How many people will this concentration kill? This is easily calculated using the LD$_{50}$:

$$f_l = 1/ (1 + LD_{50} / A_0)$$
$$f_l = 1/ (1 + 1000/ 99) = 0.09 \text{ or } 9\%$$

This means that 9% of the victims are going to die, even with an exceptionally high therapeutic index.

Remember that actual use of the agent may occur in a confined space where the initial concentration of the agent may be maintained for quite some time. The total dose to the victim continues to increase until the victim is evacuated. This overdosage can easily lead to concentrations 10 times the planned dose or more.

Operational factors may also cause an overdose. Higher than optimum concentrations may be deliberately used by the commander of the task force to compensate for an uneven distribution of the agent and to ensure that "enough stuff" is used. The potential costs of using too little drug (inadequate effect and consequential endangerment to the force and hostages alike) may be much greater than the costs of using too much drug (increased lethality in the target population). The requirement for faster incapacitation will require greater doses and may concomitantly inflict more deaths.

Considerably higher levels of lethality are encountered when pharmaceutical agents with therapeutic indices of 100 or less are used as incapacitating weapons. This is exactly what happened in the Moscow hostage rescue where 127 of the 750 hostages died (17%).

Treatment

The medical management of patients exposed to calmative agents should be geared towards the ABCs, particularly respiratory support. Patients who die as a result of exposure to these agents most often suffer from respiratory arrest.

At a minimum, the medical providers must do the following:

- Ensure that the patient did not go to sleep in a position that obstructs the airway.
- Ensure that the patient is still breathing.
- Evaluate injuries caused by a fall when the patient collapsed.
- Administer an antidote if available.
- Determine how long to monitor the patient and provide medical attention (this depends on the route of administration, dose of the agent, and available antidotes).

The challenge is to determine which drug has been used in the case at hand. Because opiate drugs have been used in the recent past, the use of naloxone is recommended as a first antidote. At all times, prudent management and good clinical judgment are essential tools in handling these patients.

■ Smoke and Similar Agents

White Phosphorus Munitions

Although technically not a chemical weapon, white phosphorus produces significant chemical weapons–like effects. White phosphorus is used extensively in the construction of military munitions and fireworks, is a component of insecticides and rodenticides, and is used as a screening smoke and incendiary munition. White phosphorus munitions of multiple sorts are currently stocked by most military units, both domestic and abroad. Because white phosphorous munitions are quite common, it is conceivable that a terrorist could use them against a civilian population.

White phosphorus, which is used primarily as a smoke agent, is also capable of causing serious burns. It is a waxy translucent substance that ignites spontaneously on contact with air. It is usually preserved under water and becomes liquid at 44°C/111.2°F.

Following an explosion of a white phosphorus munition, flaming droplets of white phosphorus are flung widely about, and dense clouds of white smoke with a garliclike odor are produced. The flaming pieces of phosphorus cause thermal tissue damage but may also cause high-speed projectile injuries.[26] The smoke can damage the lungs and skin. Also, some tracer bullets contain white phosphorus as a major component. Absorption of phosphorus fragments may result from either an explosion of a phosphorus-based shell or a bullet wound inflicted by a tracer bullet.[27]

Pieces of flaming white phosphorus remaining in patients' wounds should be extinguished by immersing the pieces in water. Surface particles and particles embedded in clothing should be promptly removed. During transport, the medical providers should cover the burned areas with moistened cloths to prevent further burning.

The military recommends washing these wounds with a 1% copper sulfate solution. This solution combines with the phosphorus to form copper phosphate, which can be readily identified as black particles.[28] These black pieces can be easily **debrided**. If the particles are not debrided, they will be absorbed, and systemic effects may occur.

Once debridement is completed, no further copper sulfate solution is needed. The copper sulfate solution should not be used for a prolonged period because of the risk of systemic copper poisoning, which is manifested by vomiting, diarrhea, decreased urine output (**oliguria**), intravascular hemolysis, blood in the urine (**hematuria**), liver tissue death (**hepatic necrosis**), and cardiovascular collapse.

To minimize copper absorption, the wound may be irrigated with a solution of 5% sodium bicarbonate and 3% copper sulfate suspended in 1% hydroxyethyl cellulose.[29] Wet dressings of copper sulfate in any form should never be applied to the wound.[30] Following debridement, the wound should be irrigated with large amounts of water to remove the copper salts.

Phosphorus is highly fat-soluble and is easily absorbed from particles in the subcutaneous tissues or from the gastrointestinal tract if ingested. The two most common systemic effects are hepatotoxicity and renal damage, but changes in blood phosphorus and calcium levels may also be noted. ECG changes including prolongation of the QT interval, ST segment depression, T-wave changes, and bradycardia can also be noted.[31] Sudden death has been reported in patients with reversed calcium-phosphorus ratios.[32] Monitoring for electrocardiographic abnormalities and changes in serum calcium and phosphorus is appropriate for patients with significant wounds. For patients in which systemic absorption is suspected, **blood urea nitrogen**, **creatinine**, serum phosphorus, and liver enzymes should be assessed frequently.

Phosphorus pentoxide, the white smoke associated with white phosphorus munitions, presents the same clinical picture as phosgene exposure. A patient can progress to pulmonary edema following the inhalation of phosphorus pentoxide smoke. This is managed symptomatically as phosgene toxicity.

INHOSPITAL INFO

■ General Treatment for Exposure to Lacrimator and Vomiting Agents

There is no antidote for exposure to lacrimator agents, and treatment is entirely supportive. All patients who have been exposed to a lacrimator agent will be in subjective distress (felt by the patient, but not apparent to the observer). In these situations, medical care should be reserved for those who are in objective distress (apparent to the observer). Most of these patients will recover without aftereffects with only decontamination as therapy. The effects from the agents are usually **self-limited** and of short duration.

Airway Care and Monitoring

Patients who have been exposed to one of these agents and are experiencing respiratory distress should receive oxygen, and the airway should be evaluated for edema. If a patient has prolonged dyspnea or objective signs of respiratory distress, the patient should be hospitalized and monitored carefully. Severe respiratory distress may be delayed for 12 to 24 hours. An intravenous line and cardiac monitoring are appropriate, but these may not be possible when faced with a mass exposure to these agents.

In severely symptomatic patients, arterial blood gases and chest radiographs should be obtained. Patients who experience respiratory distress after exposure is terminated should be observed for the development of bronchospasm. Worsening of respiratory distress may be delayed for 12 to 24 hours. Bronchospasm may be treated with the usual bronchodilator therapy. Pneumonia and pulmonary edema are late complications. Prophylactic antibiotics and steroids are controversial and probably not efficacious.

Decontamination

The second priority is decontamination and removal from exposure. Most patients will experience some measure of relief in 15 to 30 minutes by simple cessation of exposure. Significant decontamination may be achieved by simply undressing and showering the patient, even if the agents are not completely water-soluble.

Contaminated skin should be cleansed with soap and cool or tepid water. Warm or hot water may markedly worsen symptoms. Soap and water is more effective than simply showering, but may also cause an increase in the symptoms. Showers may also sweep hair contaminants onto eyes and skin, thus reactivating symptoms.

Ocular

The eyes should be examined and thoroughly flushed with water to remove any particles of the agent. The eyes may be treated with topical antibiotics and mydriatics (drugs that dilate the pupil) as needed. Topical antibiotics may be helpful while irrigating the eye. Eyes should be patched as for a chemical injury. Patients with severe lesions should receive a prompt referral to an ophthalmologist.

Dermal

Vesiculation and bullae should be treated as second-degree chemical injuries, and skin should be copiously irrigated with saline. Dermatitis may be treated with a topical steroid preparation. Oozing lesions have been treated with wet dressings, such as Burrow's solution. Vesicles have been successfully treated with cold silver nitrate compresses.

■ Summary

Nonlethal agents are intended to harass or cause temporary incapacitation. The intended target may be rioters, prisoners, hostage-takers, criminals, muggers, or rapists. These agents have little lethality (as the chapter title implies), but can cause fires, panic, and, in extreme cases, injuries and lethality.

The panic that nonlethal agents can cause in an unsuspecting populace combined with their ready availability make them quite useful for a terrorist. The devastating consequences resulting from the use of one of these agents in the appropriate situation would not be caused directly by the agent, but rather by the panic that it generates.

■ References

1. Beswick FW, Holland P, Kemp KH: Acute effects of exposure to ortho-chlorobenzylidenemalononitrile (CS) and the development of tolerance. *Br J Indust Med* 1972;29:298-306.
2. Petersen KK, Schroeder HM, Eiskjaer SP: CS taregasspray som skadevoldende middel: Kliniske aspecter. *Ugeskr Laeger* 1989;151:1388-1389.
3. Hellreich A, Doldman RH, Bottiglieri NG: *The Effects of Thermally Generated CS Aerosols on Human Skin.* Edgewood Arsenal, MD, Medical Research Laboratories (Technical Report No 4075), 1967, p 19.
4. Rengstorff RH, Mershon MM: *CS in Trioctyl Phosphate: Effects on Human Eyes.* Edgewood Arsenal, MD, Medical Research Laboratories (Technical Report No 4376), 1969.
5. Weigand DA: Cutaneous reaction to the riot control agent CS. *Military Med* 1969;134:437-440.
6. Viala B, Blomet J, Mathieu L, Hall A. Prevention of CS "tear gas" eye and skin effects and active decontamination with diphoterine: Preliminary studies in 5 French Gendarmes. *J Emerg Med* 2005;29:5–8.
7. Beswick FW, Holland P, Kemp KH: Acute effects of exposure to ortho-chlorobenzylidenemalononitrile (CS) and the development of tolerance. *Br J Indust Med* 1972;29:298-306.
8. Beswick FW: Chemical agents used in riot control and warfare. *Hum Toxicol* 1983;2:247-256.
9. Chapman AG, Whit C: Death resulting from lacrimatory agents. *J Forensic Sci* 1978;23:527-530.
10. Fuchs T, Ippen H: Kontallergie auf CN und CS: Tranengas. *Derm Beruf Umwelt* 1986;34:12-14.
11. Thorburn, KM: Injuries after use of the lacrimatory agent chloroacetophenone in a confined space. *Arch Environ Health* 1982;37:182-186.
12. Vaca FE, Myers JH, Langdorf M: Delayed pulmonary edema and bronchospasm after accidental lacrimator exposure. *Am J Emerg Med* 1996;14:402.

INHOSPITAL INFO

13. Stein AA, Kirway WE: Chloroacetophenone (tear gas) poisoning: A clinico-pathologic report. *J Forensic Sci* 1964;9:374-382.

14. Fine KC, Bassin RH, Stewart MM: Emergency care for tear gas victims. *J Am Coll Emerg Phy* 1977;6:144-146.

15. Ballantyne B: Riot control agents, in Scott RB, Frazer J (eds): *Medical Annual.* Bristol, England, Wright and Sons, 1977.

16. Holland P: The cutaneous reactions produced by dibenzoxazepine (CR). *Br J Dermatol* 1974;90:657-659.

17. Gonomori K, Muto H, Yamamoto T, et al: A case of homicidal intoxication by chloropicrin. *Am J Forensic Med Pathol* 1987;8:135-138.

18. *Medical Manual of Defense Against Chemical Agents.* London, England, Ministry of Defense, 1987.

19. Giannini AJ, Price WA, Giannini MC: Contemporary drugs of abuse. *AFP* 1986;33:207-216.

20. Cornick JL, Jensen J: Anesthetic management of ostriches. *J Am Vet Med Assoc* 1992;200:1661-1666.

21. Miller MW, Wild MA, Lance WR: Efficacy and safety of naltrexone hydrochloride for antagonizing carfentanil citrate immobilization in captive Rocky Mountain elk. *J Wild Dis* 1996;32:234-239.

22. Shaw ML, Carpenter JW, Leith DE: Complications with the use of carfentanil citrate and xylazine hydrochloride to immobilize domestic horses. *J Am Vet Med Assoc* 1995;206:833-836.

23. Wheeler J: Secret Russian gas identified. *The Washington Times,* http://www.washtimes.com/op-ed/20021029-26892395.htm (accessed March 20, 2003).

24. Witkin J, Gasior M: Dopamine D3 receptor involvement in the convulsant and lethal effects of cocaine. *Polish J Pharmacol* 1998;50(suppl):44-45.

25. Klotz L, Furmanski M, Wheelis M: Beware the siren's song: Why "non-lethal" incapacitating chemical agents are lethal. Federation of American Scientists Working Group on Biological Weapons, http://www.fas.org/bwc/papers/sirens-song.pdf (accessed March 20, 2003).

26. Konjoyan TR: White posphorus burns: Case report and literature review. *Milit Med* 1983;148:881-884.

27. Stewart C: *Environmental Emergencies.* Baltimore, MD, Williams & Wilkins, 1989.

28. Dempsy WS: Combat injuries of the lower extremities. *Clin Plast Surg* 1975;2:585-614.

29. Ben-Hur N, Appelbaum J: Biochemistry, histopathology and treatment of phosphorus burns. *Isr J Med Sci* 1973;9:40-48.

30. Stewart CE: Chemical skin burns. *Am Fam Physician* 1985;31:151-157.

31. Bowen TE, Whelen TJ Jr, Nelson TG: Sudden death after phosphorus burns: Experimental observations of hypocalcemia, hyperphosphatemia, and electrocardiographic abnormalities following production of a standard white phosphorus burn. *Ann Surg* 1971;174:779-784.

32. Bowen TE, Whelen TJ Jr, Nelson TG: Sudden death after phosphorus burns: Experimental observations of hypocalcemia, hyperphosphatemia, and electrocardiographic abnormalities following production of a standard white phosphorus burn. *Ann Surg* 1971;174:779-784.

Improvisational Chemical Warfare Agents

■ Introduction

Many articles have been written about the possible terrorist use of chemical weapons developed for use in warfare. A major question posed by EMS personnel, law enforcement agencies, government administrations, and probably the terrorists themselves is which agents can be obtained and effectively used by terrorists.

Several factors limit the use of recognized chemical weapons by terrorists, including limited access to the chemicals used to manufacture the agents, difficulty and danger associated with production of the agents, and problems associated with dispersion of the agents. Simply stealing a chemical agent from a government source would involve breaching the security surrounding the chemical agent stockpiles and would trigger recognition that the chemical agent presents an immediate threat.

State-sponsored terrorists or those with substantial financial resources or technical expertise, such as Aum Shinrikyo, may purchase or develop chemical weapons that are similar to those favored by military services. However, the process of manufacture and purchase of precursor chemicals is likely to draw unwanted attention, which could jeopardize a costly chemical weapons operation.

Although there is no question that the abundant stocks of "classic" chemical weapons or the ease of their manufacture makes their use attractive to terrorist organizations, there is no rule that mandates that a terrorist must use a recognized chemical warfare agent. Any potent toxin could be used for incapacitation or sabotage. Indeed, commonly available chemicals may be chosen because the standard military chemical agents may be difficult or dangerous to manufacture, access, or disburse. Hijacking a commercial tanker carrying several tons of hazardous materials is certainly easier and more practical for terrorists.

Many industrial chemicals capable of causing rapid, highly visible injuries are perceived by the public to be highly dangerous, are quite accessible, and are easily dispersed. Improvisational chemical weapons are made from these chemicals used in manufacturing and industry. Under the proper circumstances, these chemicals can be used as weapons. The emergence of apocalyptic or doomsday terrorist organizations with members who are willing to sacrifice their lives for a cause forces emergency providers to consider the misappropriation of industrial chemicals for use as improvisational weapons.

■ Threat

Steps required for the terrorist who desires to manufacture improvisational chemical weapons include the following:

1. Acquire the relevant expertise in chemical processes.
   - This is easily acquired through information that is available in the open-source literature.
2. Acquire the equipment and materials needed to produce the agent.
   - For some agents, the agent is directly available in large quantities and may simply be stolen during transportation or at a user's storage depot.
3. Produce agents in small quantities at a pilot plant.
4. Scale up to the required quantities by either purchasing multiple batches or producing them oneself.
   - The quantity required may be only a few liters, depending on the agent and the method of deployment, so this step is optional.
5. Develop a suitable delivery system.
   - This is the most critical portion of the deployment of a chemical weapon and is the sole portion of development in which Aum Shinrikyo failed.
   - Successful deployment may require test runs.
   - Documents found in **Taliban** classrooms and planning areas clearly showed that industrial chemicals, manufacturing sites, and multiple delivery mechanisms were being considered for additional terrorist activities.
   - Remember that a successful delivery system may require a suicidal operator. This presents no obstacle to some groups.
6. Deploy the agent for maximum effect.
   - Consider the timing of the initial device.
   - Choose an adequate location.
   - Consider the timing of a secondary or tertiary device. The detonation of a secondary or tertiary device, multiple simultaneous sites, or both may well increase the impact of a small amount of weapons.

A review of selected Environmental Protection Agency documents about chemical plant worst-case scenario calculations describes dozens of deadly possibilities[1]:

- A suburban California chemical plant routinely loads chlorine into 90-ton railroad cars that, if ruptured, could poison more than 4 million people in Orange and Los Angeles counties, depending on wind speed, wind direction, and the ambient temperature.
- The Atofina Chemicals plant outside Detroit projects that a rupture of one of its 90-ton railcars of chlorine could endanger 3 million people.
- A Philadelphia refinery keeps 180,000 kg of hydrogen fluoride that could asphyxiate nearly 4 million nearby residents.
- A chemical company in South Kearny, New Jersey, keeps 81,000 kg of chlorine and sulfur dioxide that could form a cloud that could threaten 12 million people.
- The West Virginia sister plant of the infamous Union Carbide Corp factory in Bhopal, India, keeps up to 90,000 kg of methyl isocyanate that could emit a toxic fog over 60,000 people near Charleston, South Carolina.

Although improvised chemical agents may be less toxic than military agents, the release of industrial chemicals at Bhopal shows that the casualties resulting from an improvised chemical attack could be equally horrendous. At least 123 plants in the United States keep amounts of toxic chemicals that, if released, could form toxic clouds that would put more than 1 million people in danger.[2] More than 700 US plants could put at least 100,000 people at risk, and more than 3,000 US plants could put at least 10,000 people at risk in the event of a chemical release.

The military feels that chemical pesticide plants are not easily convertible to the manufacture of nerve agents and that these agents are quite difficult for most terrorist groups to manufacture in "meaningful" quantities.[3] Because Aum Shinrikyo clearly was able to manufacture sarin in small quantities, and because the release of this small quantity was quite meaningful to the populace of Tokyo, terrorists may in fact reach their goals through the use of small quantities of an agent.

■ Potential Agents

Types of Chemicals

The US Department of Transportation Code of Federal Regulations (49 CFR 170–179) requires placards to be placed on all shipments of hazardous chemicals. These placards indicate the type of chemical being shipped and the hazard it presents **(Figure 7-1)**. Information published by the US Department of Transportation is a good beginning resource for the terrorist to work from, but it is vague.

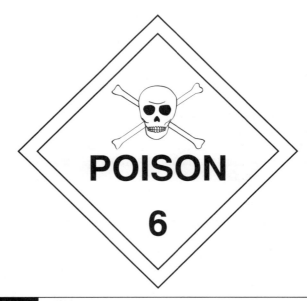

Figure 7-1 Placards are required on shipments of chemicals that could present a hazard.

Table 7-1 Chemical Agents Included on the CDC Threat List*

Type of agent	Specific chemical
Nerve agents	*Tabun* *Sarin* *Soman* *GF* *VX*
Blood agents (tissue toxins)	*Hydrogen cyanide* *Cyanogen chloride*
Blister agents	*Lewisite* *Nitrogen and sulfur mustards* *Phosgene oxime*
Heavy metals	Arsenic Lead Mercury
Volatile toxins	Benzene Chloroform Trihalomethanes
Choking agents	*Phosgene* *Chlorine* Vinyl chloride
Incapacitating agents	BZ
Pesticides, persistent and nonpersistent	Dioxins, furans, and polychlorinated biphenyls (PCBs)
Explosive nitro compounds and oxidizers	Ammonium nitrate combined with fuel oil Flammable industrial gases and liquids Gasoline Propane
Poison industrial gases, liquids, and solids	*Cyanides* Nitriles
Corrosive industrial acids and bases	Nitric acid Sulfuric acid

*Italics indicate that the chemical is well known and that appropriate protective gear is available, decontamination methods are outlined, and medical therapy is well studied.

Adapted from: Centers for Disease Control and Prevention. Biological and chemical terrorism: strategic plan for preparedness and response, recommendations of the CDC Strategic Planning Workgroup 2000. MMWR Morb Mortal Wkly Rep 2000; 49 (RR-4): 1-14.

The Centers for Disease Control and Prevention (CDC) has prepared a list of chemical and biological agents that might be used by terrorists. It is often used as a reference for training about how to manage these agents.[4] The chemical agents chosen by the CDC range from warfare agents to toxic chemicals commonly used in industry. Criteria used for determining an agent's inclusion on the CDC's lists of chemical agents include the following:

- The agent is already known to be used as weaponry
- The agent is available to potential terrorists
- Use of the agent is likely to cause major morbidity or mortality
- Use of the agent may cause public panic and social disruption
- The agent requires special action for public health preparedness

Categories of chemical agents included on the CDC threat list are listed in **Table 7-1**. The chemicals shown in italics are well known, and for these chemicals, appropriate protective gear is available for the soldier, decontamination methods are outlined, and medical therapy for victims is well studied. The remainder of the chemicals listed should be considered improvisational or expedient chemical weapons. Other common industrial chemicals that could be used as terrorist weapons include those listed in **Table 7-2**. Aromatic hydrocarbons, such as benzene, may be used as water supply contaminants.

Two other types of chemicals are also transported across country and stored in bulk **(Table 7-3)**. Although these are not chemical weapons, the destructive potential they represent is massive. These chemicals can easily be combined with **incendiary agents** to produce "fuel-air" explosives capable of massive destruction. The secondary products of these explosions may liberate more chemical toxins.

Compressed hydrocarbon fuels such as gasoline, kerosene, and jet fuel could be employed as incendiary materials. Gases such as LPG, propane, and isobutane could be used as incendiaries or simple asphyxiants.

Table 7-2 Common Industrial Chemicals That are Potential Terrorist Weapons

Type of agent	Specific chemical
Nerve agents	Multiple organophosphate pesticides and precursors Carbamate pesticides*
Blood agents (tissue toxins)	Analines Nitriles
Blister agents	Dimethyl sulfate
Choking agents	Ammonia Acrylates Aldehydes Isocyanates (effects already seen in Bhopal, India) Hydrogen sulfide

*Potential exists for use, but it is not known to have been used yet.

Table 7-3 Other Chemicals That are Potential Terrorist Weapons

Type of agent	Specific chemical
Oxidizers	Oxygen Butadiene Peroxides
Incendiary agents	Acetone Alkenes Amines Alkyl halides

It is likely that these chemicals will be deployed using available transportation such as tank cars, trucks, or even river barges. This would allow the terrorist an opportunity to deliver the chemical to the area of greatest importance or population concentration. Railway and highway delivery vehicles are particularly vulnerable, because they are not under security after leaving the staging areas. Indeed, during a recent visit to New Orleans, the author watched 35 tank cars slowly cross Canal Street. Many of the tank cars contained chemicals listed in the previous tables. The cars were moving slowly enough that a person could hop onto them quite easily. The scenario presented above is quite possible.

Remember that terrorists, in order to accomplish the terror objective, do not need to maximize casualties. They simply need to deploy the right agent at the right time to cause a few obvious casualties within a large population, and panic will do the rest. Hindering the responders' ability to work or identify additional hazards, by using a chemical that necessitates the use of protective gear, serves as another objective. Rendering an entire area uninhabitable for a length of time, which would have profound socioeconomic ramifications, serves as an additional objective.

The emergency provider must also remember that secondary devices are now quite common and may be delayed or **command detonated** from afar. These devices are intended to paralyze public service providers and enhance panic. The terrorist may not use the secondary device at the site of the incident, but may deploy it at a hospital, police rally point, or within an emergency service food and rest area.

Food and Water

Certain chemical agents can also be delivered covertly through contaminated food or water. The military does not consider ingestion to be a suitable route to employ chemical weapons, because the effects are too slow and unpredictable. The terrorist does not share the same mission profile. Ingestion is an attractive route of dissemination, and either water, food supplies, or both can be contaminated. Cyanides, heavy metals, and aromatic hydrocarbons such as benzene are quite suitable for this contamination.

Contamination of water supplies is often deemed unsuitable for a potential terrorism attack, because vast quantities of contaminating substances would be required to threaten a city's water supply. Although current decontamination and water purification techniques make contamination with biological substances unattractive as terrorism tools in municipal water supplies, the same could not be said of tank car loads of toxic pollutants.

In 1999, the vulnerability of the food supply was illustrated in Belgium, when chickens were accidentally given animal feed containing dioxin-contaminated fat.[5] This chemical contamination was not discovered for months. As a result, dioxin, a cancer-causing chemical that does not cause immediate symptoms in humans, was probably present in chicken meat and eggs sold in multiple parts of Europe during early 1999. This dioxin episode demonstrates how a covert act of food-borne chemical terrorism could affect commerce and human or animal health.

INCIDENTS INVOLVING Chemicals

The Belgian Poultry Dioxin Scare

In 1999, chickens from hundreds of Belgian farms were contaminated by dioxin, a serious cancer-causing agent. The chickens were inadvertently fed dioxin-contaminated feed after fat used in the feed was stored in tanks that had previously been used to hold industrial oil. Though the full effect of consumption of the contaminated eggs and meat will not be known for years, the economic effect on Belgium's agricultural industry was immediate, as a worldwide ban on the export of Belgian eggs, chickens, pork, and beef was temporarily instituted that year.

■ Security and Prevention

In many cities with chemical industries, there are already hazardous material control infrastructures and trained control response teams in place. This infrastructure may include detailed chemical information distributed in the local area, redundant automated control systems, vapor cloud suppression equipment, expanded evacuation routes, and earth barriers that surround chemical storage and manufacturing areas. This infrastructure would be effective in mitigating a deliberate or accidental chemical release.

Hazardous materials control response teams currently in place in chemical plants and adjacent cities in the United States are well trained and equipped. They are not equipped or trained, however, to perform their tasks in the potential combat situation of a terrorist attack. Given the suicidal nature of some terrorist groups, there is no reason to believe that a simple release would be planned. The hazardous materials teams must be aware that they may be targeted by snipers, subjected to dual or triple agent combinations designed to foil their protective gear, and further endangered by explosive devices, mines, and booby traps. These warlike devices may all be employed to delay mitigation, foil evacuation, and destroy the morale of the responders. These devices may be command detonated to increase the numbers of casualties.

There is also no guarantee that terrorists will act according to expectations and release the agent within the confines of an area covered by a well-trained hazardous materials control team. Considering that agents are transported in 90-ton railroad cars and 10-ton tank trucks, these agents can be delivered precisely where and probably when the terrorist chooses.

Even more worrisome is the fact that security for these potent chemicals is far from optimal. Although many comments have been made about airline security following September 11, 2001, there has been little focus on the security of the chemical workplace.

Chemical emergency response plans and worst-case scenario estimates for chemical manufacturing plants are required by federal law at the federal, state, and local government levels. Similar plans for the route taken by these hazardous materials are not available. Most state and local plans do not address chemical terrorism at all. Others only focus on the terrorist use of common military nerve and blister agents, but fail to address the much more accessible industrial chemicals.

In a recent survey of chemical plant security managers, these managers were very pessimistic about their ability to deter sabotage.[6] They had not implemented simple background checks for key employees, such as chemical process operators. None of the corporate security staff surveyed had been trained to identify combinations of common chemicals at their facilities that could be used as improvised explosives and incendiaries. (All were aware of individual chemicals with explosive, fire, and poison risks.)

Security for chemical transportation, in this study, ranged from poor to nonexistent. Chemical barges were left totally unsecured about the riverside of the facility. Railcars and trucks had no security beyond the staging areas. Railcars containing cyanide compounds, flammable liquid pesticides, liquefied petroleum gases, chlorine, and butadiene were transported through or even parked alongside residential areas.

The wise reader should already be aware that any division between the planned response before an attack and dealing with the consequences after an attack is both arbitrary and potentially misleading. Not only will the response have its own consequences, the response may play into the hands of the terrorist, as did the New York City Fire Department policy for establishing the location of the command center during the World Trade Center collapse (the command center was located at the base of the towers). Issues such as command centers, interagency cooperation, evacuation plans, the surge capacities of already strained hospital facilities, and the potential for secondary or even tertiary devices must be addressed before the terrorist strikes.

■ References

1. Grimaldi JV, Gugliotta G: Chemical plants feared as targets. *The Washington Post*, December 16, 2001:A01.
2. Grimaldi JV, Gugliotta G: Chemical plants feared as targets. *The Washington Post*, December 16, 2001:A01.
3. Technical aspects of chemical weapon proliferation, in *Technologies Underlying Weapons of Mass Destruction*. Washington, D.C., Federation of American Scientists.
4. http://www.bt.cdc.gov/AgentlAgentlist.asp (accessed February 10, 2002).
5. Ashraf H: European dioxin-contaminated food crisis grows and grows. *Lancet* 1999;353:2049.
6. Hughart JL, Bashor MM: Industrial chemicals and terrorism: Human health threat analysis, mitigation, and prevention. US Public Health Service, Agency for Toxic Substances and Disease Registry.

8 Introduction to Biological Warfare

■ Introduction

Biological warfare is the use of disease to harm or kill an adversary's military forces, population, food, or livestock. Biowarfare includes both the use of microorganisms (eg, bacteria, viruses, and **rickettsia**) and the use of the products of microorganisms (ie, toxins such as in botulism) **(Table 8-1)**.

A biological weapon is more than a pathogen or toxin. It is a system that is composed of four major components: the pathogen (payload), a container that keeps the pathogen virulent during the delivery (munitions), a means to deliver the agent (eg, a missile, a crop sprayer aircraft, or even an expendable soldier or martyr), and a dispersal mechanism (an explosive or spray device that will disperse the agent among the target population). Fortunately, the expertise required to develop the pathogen and the expertise required to deliver the munitions are not often found in the same person. Unfortunately, the expertise does exist, and terrorist applications may be far less demanding than military requirements.

The threat of an outbreak of disease caused by a biological weapon is credible, and, with advances in biotechnology and the current political climate, the question is not if an outbreak will occur, but when. To see why biological warfare is becoming more threatening, one only has to look at the current state of biotechnology and future possibilities. Successful genetic engineering is here. Daily, genetic codes are manipulated to create specialized organisms to produce insulin, **t-PA**, and a host of other substances. It is a small step to tailor an organism to produce vast quantities of a lethal toxin or to resist specific antibiotics. It is an even smaller step to tailor an organism to destroy livestock or crops.[1] This destruction can be achieved by disease or by toxins and can destroy a country's economy rather than killing its people. Furthermore, the resulting famine may be blamed on nature rather than a hostile action.

Biological weapons are much deadlier, pound for pound and dollar for dollar, than chemical agents **(Figure 8-1)** and even nuclear weapons **(Table 8-2)**. It has been estimated that 10 g of anthrax could kill as many people as a metric ton of the nerve agent sarin. Biowarfare weapons are inexpensive, easy to produce, and delivery devices may be disguised as agricultural sprayers or pest control devices. It is very difficult, if not impossible,

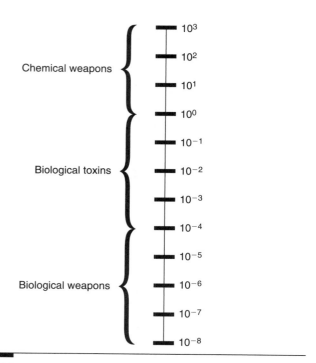

Figure 8-1 Estimated lethal dose of chemical and biological weapons (mg/person).

for an intelligence service to detect the research, production, or transportation of these agents. It is equally hard to defend against these agents once they have been employed.

There has been abundant posturing about preparedness for an attack with biological agents. Unfortunately, recent experiences with aircraft used as guided bombs have shown that the United States and other countries are not yet prepared to manage an attack with conventional weapons, much less an attack with biological weapons.

■ History of Biological Warfare

Biological warfare is not a 20th century development. The use of biological agents in warfare has a long and deadly history. Persian, Greek, and Roman authors note the use of animal cadavers to contaminate water supplies. According to the Greek historian Herodotus, fifth century Scythian archers dipped their arrows in blood mixed with manure or in decomposing cadavers.

In 1346, the Mongols catapulted corpses of plague victims into the city of Kaffa to infect the defenders. The disease spread rapidly in the besieged town, and the inhabitants were overcome. Not only did the city surrender, the resultant epidemic may have spread beyond the city of Kaffa. Medieval historians speculate that this action may have been the start of the Black Death. Between 1347 and 1351, a bubonic plague epidemic spread throughout Europe causing over 25 million deaths. Russian troops may have used the same tactic against Sweden in 1710.

During the French and Indian War, the British and early American settlers gave blankets used for victims of smallpox to the American Indians defending Fort Carillon. These Indians were thought to be loyal to the French. The resultant infection decimated the defenseless American Indian tribes. After the epidemic, Sir Jeffery Amherst and the British troops defeated the incapacitated force. Fort Carillon was subsequently renamed Fort Ticonderoga.

In 1861, Union troops advancing south into Maryland and other border states were warned not to eat or drink anything provided by unknown civilians for fear of being poisoned. Despite the warnings, there were numerous instances in which soldiers thought they had been poisoned after eating or drinking. Confederates retreating in Mississippi in 1863 left dead animals in wells and ponds to contaminate the water sources of the Union troops.

Germany may take the credit for opening the door to modern biological warfare during World War I. Covert operatives in Romania attempted to infect sheep destined for export to Russia. Containers with biological cultures

Table 8-1 Potential Biological Agents for Terrorism	
Category	Characteristics
Category A: high-priority agents	• Can be easily disseminated or transmitted from person to person • Cause high mortality with a potential for a major impact on public health • May cause public panic and social disruption • Require special action for public health preparedness
Category B: second-priority agents	• Are moderately easy to disseminate • Cause moderate morbidity and low mortality • Require specific enhancements of the CDC's diagnostic capacity and disease surveillance
Category C: third-priority agents (including organisms that are emerging pathogens that could be genetically engineered for mass dissemination)	• May be easily available • May be easily produced or disseminated • Have the potential for high morbidity and mortality and therefore may have a major impact on public health

Adapted from: Centers for Disease Control and Prevention. Biological and chemical terrorism: strategic plan for preparedness and response, recommendations of the CDC Strategic Planning Workgroup 2000. MMWR Morb Mortal Weekly Rep 2000; 49 (RR-4): 1–14.

Table 8-2 Criteria and Weighting Used to Evaluate Potential Biological Threat Agents*

[Agents ranked from highest threat (+++) to lowest (0)]

| Disease | Public health impact | | Dissemination | | Public perception | Special preparation | Category |
	Disease	Death	Dissemination potential[a]	Person-to-person transmissibility			
Smallpox	+	++	+	+++	+++	+++	A
Anthrax	++	+++	+++	0	+++	+++	A
Plague[b]	++	+++	++	++	++	+++	A
Botulism	++	+++	++	0	++	+++	A
Tularemia	++	++	++	0	+	+++	A
VHF[c]	++	+++	+	+	+++	++	A
VE[d]	++	+	+	0	++	++	B
Q fever	+	+	++	0	+	++	B
Brucellosis	+	+	++	0	+	++	B
Glanders	++	+++	++	0	0	++	B
Melioidosis	+	+	++	0	0	++	B
Psittacosis	+	+	++	0	0	+	B
Ricin toxin	++	++	++	0	0	++	B
Typhus	+	+	++	0	0	+	B
Cholera[e]	+	+	++	+/−	+++	+	B
Shigellosis[e]	+	+	++	+	+	+	B

[a]Potential for production and dissemination in quantities that would affect a large population, based on availability, BSL requirements, most effective route of infection, and environmental stability.
[b]Pneumonic plague.
[c]Viral hemorrhagic fevers due to filoviruses (*Ebola, Marburg*) or arenaviruses (eg, *Lassa, Machupo*).
[d]Viral encephalitis.
[e]Examples of food- and waterborne diseases.

*Particularly notable in the absence from this listing is the largest and most deadly epidemic recorded in history: the great influenza **pandemic** of 1912–1914. However, a similar strain of influenza could likely be engineered, cultivated, and released with comparable results. One only has to look at the latest SARS epidemic to understand how an epidemic can devastate a health care system.

Adapted from: Rotz LD, Khan AS, R. Scott et al. Public Health Assessment of Potential Biological Terrorism Agents. *Emerging Infectious Diseases.* Vol. 8, No. 2, February 2002; 225–230.

were confiscated from the German Legation in Romania. The Bucharest Institute of Bacteriology and Pathology identified anthrax in these vessels. At the same time, German saboteurs in France infected horses and mules with the same bacilli. A similar German operative in the United States, Dr. Anton Dilger, was successful in starting anthrax and glanders infections in horses and mules destined for the war front.

Anthrax was tested in 1941 by the Allies on Guinard Island off the shore of Scotland. Scientists used thousands of sheep to evaluate the effectiveness of the disease. As a result of the huge amount of anthrax spores dispersed on the island, the British could not effectively decontaminate the island after the program was stopped. The organism persisted in a virulent state until 1988, when the island was finally declared safe for unprotected humans.[2]

The Soviet Union started a biological weapons program in the late 1920s. By the beginning of World War II, the Soviet Union was able to manufacture weapons using tularemia, Q fever, and endemic typhus. They were working on techniques for producing weapons with smallpox, plague, and anthrax. There is anecdotal evidence that the Soviet Union used biological weapons in Russia in 1942

and 1943, with resultant infections of tularemia and Q fever among German troops.[3]

During World War II, on the Pacific front, the Japanese tested biological weapons on both civilians and prisoners of war in China in a program called Unit 731. Under the direction of Dr. Shiro Ishii until 1942 and Dr. Kitano Misaji from 1942 to 1945, the program employed a staff of more than 3,000 in over 150 buildings and 5 satellite camps. At least 10,000 prisoners died of "experimental infections" and scores more were executed after experiments to undergo autopsy. There were at least 12 field trials of biological agents, ranging from water supply contamination and food contamination to aerial sprays and vector releases. At least 11 Chinese cities were attacked with the biological agents of anthrax, cholera, shigellosis, salmonella, and plague.[4] By 1945, Unit 731 had stockpiled over 400 kg of anthrax spores to be used in specially designed bombs.

The Japanese also spread flea-infested debris over cities in mainland China, causing bubonic plague in both China and Manchuria. Unit 731 weaponized the plague in an interesting way. Plague-infected rats were fed upon by laboratory-grown fleas. The Japanese scientists collected the infected fleas, put them into containers, and released them over Chinese cities from low-flying aircraft.

Biological programs in both the United States and the former Soviet Union owe their germination to the work of Unit 731. The Russians captured the grounds of Unit 731 in Manchuria. Only after the agents of the Office for Strategic Services (OSS) discovered the activities of Unit 731 did the United States initiate its own offensive biological warfare program in late 1942. The United States later captured Shiro Ishii and Kitano Misaji in Japan and granted them immunity from prosecution if they divulged the details of their biological warfare program.

In recent times, the US military has examined the possibility of biological actions against the United States. The United States started an offensive biological warfare program at Fort Detrick in Frederick, Maryland, in late 1942. Ten years later, the defensive program began. Research and development facilities were located at Fort Detrick. A production facility was started in Terre Haute, Indiana, and testing areas were established in Mississippi and Utah. However, the production facility was considered to be unsafe and never put into service. A second production facility was opened during the Korean War in Pine Bluff, Arkansas. The type and amount of microorganisms produced are classified. By 1969, the United States had weaponized the agents causing anthrax, tularemia, botulism, brucellosis, Venezuelan equine encephalitis, and Q fever.[5]

During the Korean War, the United States developed an anti-crop bomb and delivered it to the US Air Force in 1951. This was designed to destroy the North Korean rice fields and would have caused a widespread famine in North Korea. North Korea repeatedly accused the United States of using biological agents during the Korean War. The United States denied the accusation, and no substantive proof has been found in the open-source literature.

The United States initiated a series of classified and quite controversial experiments to test the use of biological weapons dating from the Cold War. The American programs used supposedly nonpathologic bacteria as surrogates to demonstrate the deployment of more deadly organisms. The tests were shut down in 1969 and remain highly classified. Few details have been released.

In the 1950s, *Serratia* and *Bacillus* species were released from ships in the San Francisco Bay area and caused at least one death.[6] Declassified information indicates that, during the test, 5 to 10 times the normal respiratory infection rate was found in San Francisco areas that were sprayed.

Although the Soviet Union was a signatory to the 1972 Biological and Toxin Weapons Convention, the Soviet Union continued to maintain a high-intensity program to develop and produce biological weapons, at least through the early 1990s. The size and scope of this program were enormous. In the late 1980s and early 1990s, at least 60,000 people were employed by BioPreparat in the research, development, and production of biological weapons in the Soviet Union. Hundreds of tons of weaponized anthrax spores were stockpiled, along with dozens of tons of smallpox and plague. Many of these agents were reputed to have been specifically designed to be resistant to common antibiotics.

This program was remarkably robust and included research into genetic engineering, chimeras, binary biological compounds, and the development of an industrial capacity to produce these agents in quantity. The Russians considered the best biological agents to be those for which there was no prevention and no cure. When they developed an agent using a bacteria for which a vaccine or treatment existed, they also developed antibiotic-resistant or immuno-suppressive variants.

Nonmilitarized Bioterrorism

In 1984, the Paris police raided a residence suspected of being a safe house for the German Red Army Faction. During the search, they found documentation and a bathtub filled with flasks containing ***Clostridium botulinum***.[7]

The Aum Shinrikyo cult members (famous for the sarin gas attack in Tokyo subways) were also found to have anthrax and botulinum cultures. They had built dedicated laboratories and had purchased a helicopter equipped with spraying apparatus. They had also visited Zaire during the Ebola outbreak to collect specimens of the Ebola virus.[8]

Prior Bioterrorism in the United States

In the United States, there have been several verified releases of biological weapons by terrorists or deliberate sabotage in addition to those already mentioned.

- In September 1984, the Rajneesh cult in Antelope, Oregon, contaminated salad bars in local restaurants with typhoid bacteria. Over 750 people were poisoned. The cult stated that they did this to "influence the outcome of a local election."[9]
- A United States microbiologist named Larry Wayne Harris fraudulently ordered bubonic plague cultures by mail in 1995.[10] Harris has ties to militarist right wing groups in the United States. The ease with which he obtained these cultures prompted new legislation to ensure that biological materials are destined for legitimate medical and scientific purposes. He has subsequently become the author of a "civil defense" manual about biological warfare.
- In 1995, a Minneapolis jury convicted four members of a domestic extremist group called the Patriot's Council for violating the Biological Weapons Anti-Terrorism Act of 1989. The four members manufactured enough **ricin** to kill over 100 people. Their avowed intent was to kill law enforcement officers.
- Anthrax-contaminated letters were mailed to multiple politicians and media figures as detailed in the next chapter. The responsible party has yet to be discovered at the time of this publication.

Treaties

In the period between the world wars, the first attempt to limit the use of biological agents was written: the 1925 Geneva Protocol for the Prohibition of the Use in War of Asphyxiating, Poisonous, or Other Gases and Bacteriological Methods of Warfare. This protocol prohibited the use of bioweapons, but did not prevent research, production, or possession. There was no provision for inspection, and many countries stipulated that they had the right to retaliate with similar weapons if the weapons were first used by their enemies.

President Richard M. Nixon signed National Security Decisions 35 and 44 in November 1969 and February 1970. These decisions ended the United States offensive biological weapons program. These decisions mandated the destruction of the biological weapons stockpile, ended further research in biological weapons, and permitted only defensive research, such as chemotherapy, vaccines, and diagnostic tests.

At the same time in 1969, Britain submitted to the United Nations a proposal that included a prohibition on the development, production, and stockpiling of biological weapons. By 1972, the UN member nations had ratified the Convention on the Development, Production, and Stockpiling of Bacteriological and Toxin Weapons and Their Destruction. Among the 118 signatory nations are Russia, the United States, and Iraq. Research for "defensive" purposes is still allowed and continues across the globe.

Treaties are not guarantees that biological weapons will not be made or even used. Multilateral agreements cannot rid the world of chemical or biological weapons, which are simple, inexpensive, and produced by widely available technology. The new DNA technology brings the research tools to develop biological weapons into the realm of even modest-sized companies. The tools and techniques are not considered to be weapons or critical components of weapons and are therefore not restricted for international purchase or use. Even though some of the bacterial species considered are restricted, it is not difficult for a "legitimate" user to acquire most of these organisms.

■ Characteristics of Effective Biological Weapons*

Only a few of the vast numbers of bacterial or viral species in the environment consistently cause disease in a host. Because a major objective of the bacterium's existence is to reproduce, killing the host is not a survival characteristic. The most highly evolved pathogens are those that obtain the necessary nutrients to survive without killing the host until it has a chance to multiply. A good biological warfare agent would have the following characteristics:

- Potential to cause massive numbers of casualties
- Ability to produce lengthy illness requiring prolonged and extensive care
- Ability to spread via contagion
- Scarcity of adequate detection systems
- Incubation period that enables victims (and perpetrators) to widely disperse
- Nonspecific symptoms that complicate early diagnosis and mimic endemic infectious diseases

When microbiologists produce such bacteria for a biological weapon, they can choose to produce a liquid form or

*Adapted from USAMRIID's *Medical Management of Biological Casualties Handbook*, 4th Edition, February 2001.

a powdered form. For most biowarfare agents, the liquid form is easier to produce. The dry form, on the other hand, is easier to store, more stable in storage, and often easier to disperse. In some cases dispersal can be so easy that most military experts often forget that the terrorist does not need to go through all of the steps of producing the dry form in order to use the weapon effectively as a weapon of terror.

Liquid Biological Weapons

The steps for creating a liquid biological weapon are as follows:

- Procure a sample of the microorganism to be used.
- Culture the organism.
- Concentrate the cultured organism.
- Stabilize the culture.
- Disperse the culture in the desired population.

Dry Biological Weapons

A dry weapon is produced by drying the liquid culture and then grinding the powder into microscopic particles. The process of grinding the powder (called milling) can be quite complex in order to achieve the best particulate size to disseminate as an aerosol.

Deployment of the Weapon

The resulting biological weapon can then be deployed by several different methods.

Contamination of Food

This tactic has already been used on humans in Antelope, Oregon. Note, again, that this technique was also used to spread anthrax and **glanders** to livestock by Dr. Anton Dilger in Washington, DC, in the months preceding World War I. In both of these terrorist episodes, the liquid form of the agent was used to disseminate the disease.

Contamination of Water

Because the United States has good water purification systems, contamination of the water supply would be the least effective method for deploying a biological weapon in this country. If a terrorist could gain access to a postpurification water distribution system with an appropriate agent, then dissemination through the water supply would be possible.

Aerosol Spray

As the release of anthrax in the mail showed, inhalation of aerosol spray can be employed in a remarkably small way and still cause an exceptional disruption of the natural course of business. However, the maximum number of human casualties will be achieved if the particulate size in the aerosol is quite small (within 1 to 5 μm) as these transmit best to the alveoli **(Figure 8-2)**. Unfortunately, this does not mean that larger particles won't go into the alveoli, or that larger particles stuck in the trachea or bronchioles won't cause disease. Also, as recent events have shown, the distribution can be far from optimum and still cause disease, panic, and death.

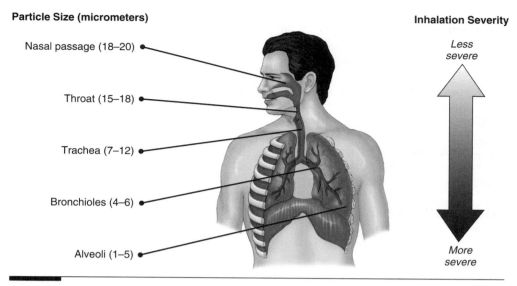

Figure 8-2 Aerosol and infectivity relationship.

Skin Contamination

Although this is a very ineffective form of transmission of a biological agent, the incidence of anthrax contamination of mail showed that it is quite possible for at least some infections to occur.

Infected Vectors

Infection can occur through the release of infected vectors such as mosquitoes or fleas, which then bite the victims, transmitting the microorganisms. As discussed, this technique was successfully used in China by the Japanese Unit 731 during World War II and the preceding years. This technique could also be used with infected humans as vectors of diseases that are easily transmitted from person to person. This, of course, may make a martyr of the infected person.

■ Initial Assessment and Treatment

The most likely indicator of a covert biological agent attack is an increased number of patients presenting with clinical symptoms caused by the featured disease agent. However, many diseases cause nonspecific clinical symptoms that can be difficult to diagnose and recognize as an outbreak resulting from a biological attack.

Suspicion

Health professionals should be watchful for a pattern to illnesses and diagnostic clues that might indicate an unusual disease outbreak associated with the intentional release of a biological agent. Unlike most chemical agents, the covert release of a biological agent may not have an immediate impact on the populace. The biological agent must replicate; hence, a significant delay (possibly days or even weeks after release) may occur between the victim's exposure and manifestation of the disease. The infectivity of the illness may closely resemble a naturally occurring outbreak of the disease.

Some indications of a potential release of a biological agent noted by emergency providers at all levels may include the following:
- Pathogens or toxins found in abandoned aerosol equipment or contaminants found in food or water. (This finding should trigger enhanced awareness of the suspect illness in surrounding geographic areas on the part of both police and emergency medical services.)
  - Discovery of abandoned specialized equipment
  - Spraying or other unusual activities prior to a public event
- An unusual temporal or geographic clustering of illness (such as persons who attended the same game, shopped in the same mall, or attended the same public event)
  - Simultaneous clusters of patients with similar illness without contiguous contacts or exposure
  - Ill patients presenting at nearly the same time from a point source
  - A lack of illness in persons not exposed to a suspect common ventilation system
  - Similar genetic type among pathogens isolated from sources that are separated in time or space
- Multiple patients with an unexplained febrile illness, particularly if this disease is associated with sepsis, pneumonia, respiratory failure, or unusual rash
- Endemic diseases with a sudden unexplained increase in incidence
- A higher than expected morbidity or mortality associated with a common disease or a failure to respond to usual therapy
  - Unusual age distribution for common diseases
  - Unusual disease presentation
  - Unusual patient distribution (geographic, seasonal, race, sex, or even blood type)

- Compressed epidemiologic curve (the rate of new cases is significantly higher than predicted, based on historical or modeling data)
- Unusual or unexplained clinical syndromes in the same patient
- A single disease caused by an uncommon agent
  - An unexplained botulism-like syndrome with flaccid muscle paralysis, particularly if this occurs in otherwise healthy persons (particularly if **bulbar paralysis** is present)
  - A large number of adult patients presenting with what appears to be a chickenpox-like illness
  - Unusual, atypical, genetically engineered, or antiquated strains of pathogens
- An unusual number of sick or dying animals
  - An unusual number of sick or dying pets. (Cats are particularly affected by plague.)
  - An unusual number of sick or dying wild animals

Event Discovery by Clinical Providers

Successful treatment of patients exposed to many of these pathogens or toxins is quite time dependent. There is a significant increase in mortality and morbidity when any delay occurs. Unless the terrorists declare the pathogen and the location prior to a release, medical providers are likely to be the first to identify a possible biological weapon deployment by a terrorist.

Unfortunately, many of the pathogens that are considered to be weapons have common early symptoms that mimic many naturally occurring diseases. Unless there is a significant and unusual number of patients who present with identical symptoms, these diseases may well be missed by the emergency provider in the first evaluation.

Of course, if suspicions have been raised by prior intelligence information, the clinician will be much more wary. Unfortunately, law enforcement officials at federal, state, and local levels are notoriously reluctant to share these data with other agencies or the public. The timely communication of intelligence with medical professionals at the front line may markedly cut response time for any possible epidemics. Conversely, if the medical provider is suspicious of a particular pathogen, this information should be rapidly passed to the proper authorities for further investigation and testing.

Astute first responders, emergency medical technicians, or dispatchers may also provide this first clue by noting multiple calls for similar reasons to a specific geographic location or noting calls for patients with similar complaints. Likewise, unusual activities, such as nighttime aerial spraying, may be noted by an astute paramedic responding to a call.

Approach to the Potential Victim

The approach to the victim depends on when the victim is found. If the victim has symptoms suggestive of an infectious biological agent, the approach to that victim should be different than that of a chemically contaminated victim. In this case, the exposure took place in the distant past (at least a few days ago), and cross-contamination of the provider from the patient is avoided by applying the principles of contagion and infection that the provider uses with all potentially infected patients.

Before medical personnel approach a potential biological agent casualty, they must ensure that they are appropriately protected. The rescuer will do little good if he or she fails to avoid infection and becomes a subsequent casualty. HEPA-filter masks will provide adequate protection against inhaled biological warfare agents and the respiratory spread of such diseases as plague or **tularemia**. Impermeable gowns and gloves complete the ensemble. Medical providers are already taught all appropriate infection control measures, including those associated with potentially lethal body fluid contamination. The application of these principles will protect the provider.

The initial assessment of the patient with a potential bioweapon infection is often hasty and may cloud the issue. As noted, in the early phases, many of these illnesses mimic common endemic illnesses. If the clinician neglects to consider how this patient may be different from other patients with similar illnesses, the patient's illness may be incorrectly identified, and the window for effective therapy may be missed.

Stabilization and Decontamination

Airway, breathing, and circulation problems should be addressed before any specific management is contemplated. Physical examination should concentrate on pulmonary, cardiac, and neuromuscular systems. Unusual dermatologic and vascular findings should be documented and photographed (if possible).

The incubation period of biological agents makes it unlikely that decontamination will be warranted. If the exposure is quite recent and known, then decontamination with soap and water or 0.1% bleach *may* be appropriate. (This kind of decontamination may be appropriate for exposure to a letter bomb of anthrax, for example.)

Diagnosis

Questions about food and water procurement sources, vector exposure, immunization history, travel history, occupation, and illnesses in other family members may offer clues and should be recorded in meticulous detail. The amount of expertise available to the emergency clinician will vary with the medical practice. At tertiary care centers, a full range of laboratory capabilities should help with a prompt diagnosis. At primary care centers, specimens should be obtained and forwarded through public health channels or reference laboratories.

Nasal swabs, blood cultures, serum cultures, sputum cultures, blood and urine toxin analyses, and throat swabs should be considered. If the patient has diarrhea, then stool specimens should be obtained. Nasal swabs may be used for both culture and PCR (polymerase chain reaction) analysis for common inhalation agents. The clinical laboratory should be notified that these specimens may represent biological warfare agents, so that the utmost precautions can be taken, and the use of optimum culture media can be planned.

While awaiting the results of the laboratory diagnosis, the clinician must formulate a clinical diagnosis. Anthrax, plague, tularemia, **Q fever**, **psittacosis**, and **SEB disease** may all present as pneumonia. Botulism and the encephalitis strains may present with neurological findings. Unfortunately, many of these diseases have early presentations of simple febrile illnesses.

Final treatment, including the proper protection for involved health care workers, must be predicated on an accurate diagnosis. The mobilization of national antidote stockpiles and additional help from state and federal resources also depend on an accurate diagnosis.

Of course, the ability to predict the spread of the disease, to give the patients and the public a prognosis, and to formulate public health responses also depends on a timely and accurate diagnosis. Specific agent identification may help law enforcement personnel attribute responsibility for the attack.

Treatment

Empiric therapy of pneumonia of **undifferentiated fever** should be considered. Patients with smallpox or other viral illness will not suffer significant harm from empiric antibiotics. Patients with plague, anthrax, or tularemia may well be saved by appropriate effective therapy. **Fluoroquinolones** or **doxycycline** may be considered for first-line empiric therapy, because these drugs are effective against most strains of anthrax, plague, and tularemia.

Notification

Hospital administration, public health officials, and law enforcement personnel must be notified about the possibility of a biowarfare incident. It is far better to call and activate systems early than to procrastinate and watch needless deaths because necessary supplies were unavailable.

■ References

1. Pellerin C: The next target of bioterrorism: Your food. *Environ Health Perspect* 2000;3:A126-A129.
2. Bernstein BJ: The birth of the US biological-warfare program. *Sci Am* 1987;Jun;256(6):116-121.
3. Alibek K: Testimony before congress. Washington, D.C., 1998.
4. Walker DH, Yampolska O, Grinberg LM: Death at Sverdlovsk: What we have learned. *Am J Pathol* 1994;144:1135-1141.
5. Christopher GW, Cieslak TJ, Pavlin JA, Eitzen EM Jr: Biological warfare: A historical perspective. *JAMA* 1997;278:412-417.
6. Cole LA: Cloud cover: The Army's secret germ warfare test over San Francisco. *Common Cause Magazine* 1988:14:16-37.
7. Douglas JD: *America the Vulnerable: The Threat of Chemical and Biological Warfare.* Lexington, MA, Lexington Books, 1987, p 29.
8. Flanagin A, Lederberg J: The threat of biological weapons: Prophylaxis and mitigation. *JAMA* 1996;276:410-411.
9. Cole LA: The specter of biological weapons. *Scientific American.com,* [December]1996, http://www.sciam.com/ 1296issue/1296cole.html (accessed March 7, 2004).
10. Horrock N: The new terror fear: Biological weapons. *US News and World Report,* May 12, 1997 found at http://static. highbeam.com/u/usnewsampworldreport/may121997/ thenewterrorfearbiologicalweapons/index.html URL (accessed March 7, 2004).

INHOSPITAL INFO

9 Live Bacterial Agents

■ Introduction

Bacteria are generally simple structures. Despite their simplicity, bacteria have an enormous range of metabolic capacities, and can be found in some of the most extreme environments on Earth. Only a small minority of bacteria cause disease, and a smaller minority is suitable for use in biological warfare. This section discusses some of the bacterial agents that could be employed in biological warfare or terrorism. This list is not all-inclusive.

The clinician at all levels must recognize that a terrorist may use diseases that do not pose obvious threats to humans. The use of genetic engineering to build bacterial resistance, enhanced virulence, or combinations of multiple characteristics from other bacterial species is also possible and must be considered.

Mechanisms of Pathogenesis

When examining the mechanisms that bacteria use to cause infections, it is important to point out that the fundamental object of both humans and bacteria is to multiply and prosper. Although there are a few bacteria that cause a succession of infections by passing from one susceptible host to another, most bacteria in the environment exist in us or on us without causing health problems. There are two important elements that control the interaction between bacteria (and other microorganisms) and humans. These two factors are the host defenses—or **immunity**—produced by the human hosts, and the **virulence factors** that are exhibited by the bacteria that enable them to produce infection. A major function of the weaponization of a bacterial disease is to either introduce the bacteria in such a way as to break down the human defenses, or increase the virulence factors of the disease to overcome the defenses.

Throughout this chapter, the following terms will be used:

- **Infection**: The organism enters the body, increases in number, and causes damage to the host in the process.
- **Pathogen**: An organism that is able to evade the normal defenses of the human host and cause an infection.
- **Prodrome**: The stage of infection where the patient has nonspecific symptoms such as headache, lethargy, or fever. It is the period before the development of a specific symptom complex that is suggestive of the classic infection. The patient may be quite contagious during the prodrome.

The course and severity of the disease depend on the balance between the organism's virulence and the success with which the immune system combats that organism. Clinical infection leads to a number of outcomes ranging from death to complete recovery.

Most patients will manifest the disease with classic signs and symptoms in a predictable pattern after exposure to a biological warfare agent. Some infections caused by biological agents may not be severe enough to produce clinical symptoms. These are called **subclinical** or **asymptomatic** infections. Patients with these infections may be capable of spreading the disease but do not contract a significant illness themselves. An example of this is a patient who has been previously vaccinated for smallpox who contracts very mild smallpox, but remains contagious during the course of the illness.

Other infections may produce **carriers** who are capable of tolerating the disease in their bodies without overt illness for long periods of time. These people can shed disease into food, drink, or water destined for others and spread the disease for a long period of time. The classic carrier is Typhoid Mary, who is described in the section on typhoid.

Once a bacterium enters the body, there are a number of ways in which it can cause disease. It may damage local tissues or injure distant structures using bacterial toxins. This distinction is not clear-cut, as there is nothing to stop toxins from acting locally as well. Many pathogenic bacteria suitable for biological warfare have both capabilities. Different therapy will be required to treat each of the two mechanisms.

Spore Formation

Some types of bacteria can transform into **spores** when faced with conditions that are harmful to life. The spore formed by the bacterial cell is more resistant to cold, heat, drying, chemicals, and radiation than the bacterium itself. Spores are a dormant form of the bacterium. Spores take on water and germinate when conditions are favorable for reproduction.

The first stage of spore formation is asymmetric cell division **(Figure 9-1)**. A septum or wall forms at one end of the cell and divides it into two parts: a small forespore and a larger mother cell. The two cells remain side by side during the process of producing a mature spore. The mother cell then engulfs the forespore so that it can produce coat proteins that surround and protect the forespore. At the end of the spore production, the mother cell breaks up (lyses) and releases the mature spore into the environment. The mature spore is durable because it has many layers of protection.

Spore formation makes the formation of a bacterial biological weapon quite a bit easier. When a bacterium forms spores, it has already established a durable and easily disseminated form of the organism. It is much more difficult to disseminate a bacterium that does not form spores, because the organism is much more fragile and hence may be destroyed by the environment or simple decontamination procedures prior to affecting the target. Organisms that do not form spores may not survive for long without special conditions of storage that may not be available to the terrorist. This is a major reason for the military's interest in anthrax; it forms hardy spores that can be kept in storage for a long time and are easy to disseminate.

■ Anthrax

Anthrax is caused by *Bacillus anthracis*. The species name comes from the Greek word *anthracis,* meaning coal, because the skin lesions produced by anthrax have black necrotic centers. Anthrax is considered to be a pathogen that can only grow inside a host organism **(Figure 9-2)**. It usually infects livestock after it is ingested as spores on vegetation or from the soil. The spores germinate inside the host and cause disease by forming vegetative cells that multiply and elaborate several toxins. When the animal dies and the carcass decomposes, the vegetative cells form durable dormant spores.

The formation of spores is repressed by high concentrations of carbon dioxide and low concentrations of oxygen in the host animal. The high concentrations of oxygen and low concentrations of carbon dioxide outside the animal appear to activate the spore-forming mechanism. Anthrax most readily forms spores in moist, alkaline soil with high organic content. These spores are long lasting and resistant to decontamination. Outbreaks of natural anthrax tend to occur after heavy rainfall followed by drought. The spores can last in the soil for decades.

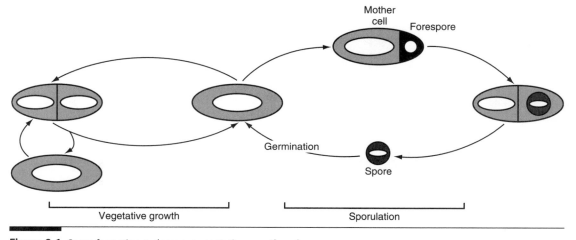

Figure 9-1 Spore formation cycle versus vegetative growth cycle.

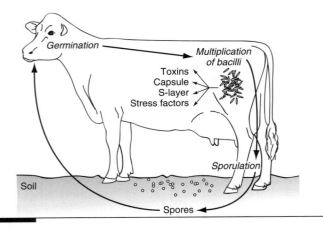

Figure 9-2 *Bacillus anthracis* cycle.

The infectious dose of anthrax by any route is not precisely known. Based on data from the studies of primates, the estimated infectious dose that will cause infectious anthrax is between 8,000 and 50,000 spores.[1,2] Between 2 and 45 days after inhalation exposure, the individual becomes acutely ill with a rapidly developing disease that normally results in about an 80% chance of mortality.

In the 1979 outbreak of inhalation anthrax in Sverdlovsk (now called Yekaterinburg or Ekaterinburg), cases were reported up to 43 days after exposure **(Figure 9-3)**. The duration of the disease is between 2 and 5 days. There is no known instance of human-to-human transmission.

Distribution and Epidemiology

Anthrax is primarily a disease of herbivores, which are exposed to the spores while grazing. Under usual (nonwartime) conditions, humans become infected by contact with infected or contaminated animal byproducts. Anthrax is found in the United States and Canada, but livestock vaccination programs have made outbreaks rare. Anthrax is endemic in West Africa, Spain, Turkey, Greece, Albania, Romania, and Central Asia **(Figure 9-4)**. In the United States, the disease tends to occur in late summer and early

fall in Texas, California, South Dakota, Nebraska, and Louisiana.

History

B anthracis is of profound historical significance. Descriptions of anthrax date to as far back as 3,500 years ago.[3] *B anthracis* was first described in 1850 by Davaine, a French parasitologist. Anthrax was the first bacterium recognized as pathogenic. The discovery of its life cycle by Koch led to the theory of infection, from which Pasteur developed the first attenuated vaccine.[4] Major outbreaks occurred in Germany in the 14th century and in Russia in the 17th century.

Whenever biological weapon threats are discussed, anthrax inevitably tops the list. The reasons are not merely alphabetical. Anthrax was investigated as a bioweapon by the Allies in World War II and by the communists in the former Soviet Union. The US Office of Technology Assessment estimated that a small private plane releasing 99 kg of anthrax spores over Washington, DC, on a windless night would kill between 1 and 3 million people and render the city uninhabitable for years. A US Department of Defense report of April 1996 noted that the Iraqis claimed to have manufactured over 8,300 L of anthrax.[5] Terrorists in other countries are certainly continuing to develop biowarfare capabilities with anthrax.

Indeed, an epidemic that caused at least 66 cases of human anthrax in the city of Sverdlosvk in spring of 1979 has been traced to an accidental release of a Russian bioweapon strain of anthrax. Note that 66 is the official casualty figure; a recently declassified US Department of Defense report placed numbers of casualties between 200 and 300. In this incident, the pathogen was airborne. Estimates of the amount of the release have varied from "only a pinch" to several kilograms of weaponized anthrax that blew through an opened ventilation port.[6] This accidental distribution of anthrax was not particularly effective as a bioweapon in terms of exposure and release technique. Nonetheless, the case-fatality rate was 86% for this exposure.

A massive disinformation campaign was conducted after the accidental release in Sverdlovsk. Concealment measures

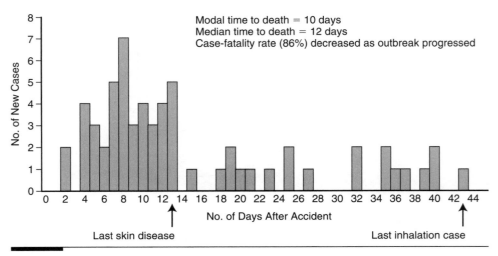

Figure 9-3 Deaths per day after anthrax release in 1979 in Sverdlovsk.

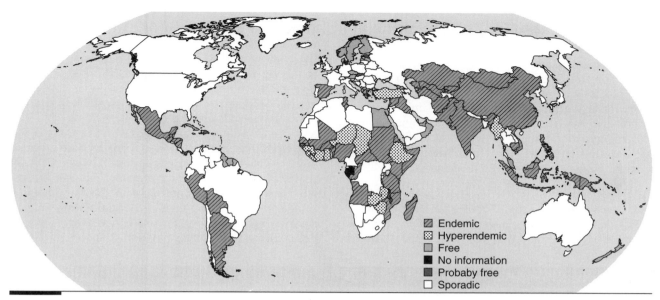

Figure 9-4 Anthrax worldwide distribution 2001-2002.

included the destruction of the medical records of the victims and the construction of an elaborate cover-up story that attributed the anthrax epidemic to contaminated meat. The cover-up story even involved the arrest of the peasant who supposedly sold the contaminated meat.[7]

Although medical records were confiscated by the KGB, investigators have pieced together the epidemiology and the source of the epidemic.[8] All of the cases occurred within a narrow zone that extended 20 km downwind in a southerly direction from a military microbiology compound called Compound 19. Following the epidemic, thousands of citizens were immunized against anthrax, the exteriors of the buildings and trees were washed by local fire brigades, and several unpaved streets were asphalted. Notably absent was a military component to the public health response.

In 1992, Russian President Boris Yeltzin admitted that the military was the source of the outbreak. Perestroika and the downfall of the former communist empire has led to a greater availability of information, but the staff of City Hospital 40, where the victims were cared for, remains quite sensitive about discussions regarding this event.

Presentation

There are three forms of anthrax: cutaneous, inhalation, and gastrointestinal. Almost all naturally occurring cases of anthrax are cutaneous or gastrointestinal. In the United States, only three cases of anthrax were reported between 1984 and 1993.[9] The case-fatality rate of cutaneous anthrax is 20% without antibiotic treatment and less than 1% with antibiotics. The case-fatality rate of gastrointestinal anthrax is estimated to be about 25% to 60%. In the United States, a case-fatality rate of 89% (16 of 18 cases) has been reported for inhalation anthrax. The case-fatality rate of the US letter-borne anthrax was less than 30% (5 of 22 cases). This is thought to be a result of improved intensive care units and rapid diagnosis as well as intravenous antibiotic therapy.

Anthrax spores germinate at the primary site of the infection. The bacillus causes local edema and necrosis and may cause inflammation. Bacilli are carried to lymph nodes and cause inflammation and bleeding in the lymph nodes. Spreading through the blood can cause septicemia, toxemia, and hemorrhagic meningitis. Uncontrolled intravascular multiplication of the bacilli resulting in fatal toxemia often occurs. Animal studies suggest that after the bacterial count reaches 10 million/mL, antibiotic therapy is futile.[10]

Cutaneous Anthrax

Over 95% of naturally occurring anthrax is cutaneous. The primary lesion is usually a painless pruritic papule on the head, neck, or extremities **(Color plate 9-1 A and B)**. This lesion appears about 3 to 4 days after exposure. Over the next day or so, this papule undergoes central necrosis and dries into a black eschar. The eschar sloughs in 2 to 3 weeks. The localized disease becomes systemic and fatal in about 5% to 25% of untreated cases. The excision of an eschar may cause this systemic dissemination.

Gastrointestinal Anthrax

Gastrointestinal anthrax is very rare and results from the ingestion of contaminated meat. Death results from peritonitis or anthrax toxemia.

Inhalation Anthrax

The inhalation form of anthrax is uncommon and particularly lethal. The naturally occurring form of inhalation anthrax is also known as woolsorter's disease. In its early stages of presentation, inhalation anthrax could be confused with a plethora of viral or bacterial respiratory illnesses. The patient progresses over 2 to 3 days and then suddenly develops respiratory distress, shock, and death within 24 to 36 hours. Dyspnea, strident cough, and chills are common during this inexorable downhill course.

The widening of the mediastinum and marked pleural effusions on the chest radiograph are common **(Color plate 9-2)**. Evidence of infiltrates on the chest radiograph is uncommon. Other suggestive findings include chest wall edema, hemorrhagic pleural effusions, and hemorrhagic meningitis.

Diagnosis

Diagnosis can be made with a culture of blood, pleural fluid, or cerebrospinal fluid. The blood culture is most often positive. In fatal cases, impressions of mediastinal lymph nodes or the spleen will be positive. Anthrax toxin may be detected in blood by immunoassay.

The victims in Sverdlosvk were diagnosed upon autopsy by a pathologist who noted a peculiar "cardinal's cap" meningeal inflammation typical in victims of anthrax (**Color plate 9-3**). All victims had hemorrhagic mediastinitis, which is also a basis for diagnosis in the United States.

Therapy

Penicillin is considered the drug of choice for the treatment of naturally-occurring anthrax. However, penicillin-resistant strains do exist in nature, and one may expect the strain of anthrax used as a biological weapon to be penicillin resistant. Tetracycline and erythromycin have been used for patients who are allergic to penicillin. The induction of resistance to these antibiotics via genetic manipulation is fairly easy. Consequently, warfare strains of anthrax should be presumed to be gentamicin resistant to these antibiotics until proven otherwise. Chloramphenicol and ciprofloxacin would be appropriate choices for initial therapy.

The US military and an AMA working group recommend oral ciprofloxacin or intravenous doxycycline for initial therapy.[11,12] This therapy is not supported by the FDA for those under 18 years of age or for pregnant females, but given the alternatives it may be appropriate.[13] Therapy should be continued for at least 60 days if the antibiotic-treated patient survives anthrax infection; this is necessary because of the possibility of delayed germination of spores.

Table 9-1 Treatment of Inhalation Anthrax	
Patient Category	**Recommended Therapy***
Adults	**Initial intravenous therapy:** Ciprofloxin, 400 mg every 12 hours OR Doxycycline, 100 mg every 12 hours OR One or two additional antimicrobials **Switch to oral therapy when clinically appropriate:** Ciprofloxacin, 500 mg twice daily OR Doxycycline, 100 mg twice daily **Continue for a total of 60 days (intravenous plus oral).** (There is a potential persistence of spores after an aerosol exposure, so extended therapy is important.)

Children	**Initial intravenous therapy:**
	Ciprofloxacin, 10 to 15 mg/kg twice daily
	OR
	Doxycycline,
	    > 8 years and > 45 kg: 100 mg every 12 hours
	    > 8 years and ≤ 45 kg: 2.2 mg/kg every 12 hours
	    ≤ 8 years: 2.2 mg/kg every 12 hours
	OR
	One or two additional antimicrobials
	Switch to oral therapy when clinically appropriate:
	Ciprofloxacin, 10 to 15 mg/kg twice daily (not to exceed 1 g/day)
	OR
	Doxycycline,
	    > 8 years and > 45 kg: 100 mg every 12 hours
	    > 8 years and ≤ 45 kg: 2.2 mg/kg every 12 hours
	    ≤ 8 years: 2.2 mg/kg every 12 hours
	Continue for a total of 60 days (intravenous plus oral).
	(There is a potential persistence of spores after an aerosol exposure, so extended therapy is important.)

Pregnant women	Use the recommended adult dose of antibiotics listed above. The risk of complications from the antibiotics is far less than the risk of death from inhalation anthrax.
Immunocompromised patients	Use the recommended adult or pediatric dose of antibiotics listed above as appropriate for the patient. The risk of complications from the antibiotics is far less than the risk of death from inhalation anthrax.

*Patients with gastrointestinal or oropharyngeal anthrax should be treated with a multidrug intravenous regimen, as if they have inhalation anthrax.

Adapted from: Henderson DA, Inglesby TV, Bartlett JG, et al: Anthrax as a biological weapon: Medical and public health management. *JAMA* 1999;281(18):1735-1745.

Supportive therapy for airway, shock, and fluid volume deficits are appropriate. Steroids may be considered as an adjunct therapy for patients with severe edema and for meningitis, based on experience with bacterial meningitis of other etiologies.

Other treatments include rifampin, vancomycin, penicillin, ampicillin, chloramphenicol, imipenem, clindamycin, and clarithromycin. Because of concerns about penicillin-resistant forms of anthrax, penicillin, and ampicillin should not be used alone. Initial therapy may be altered, based on the patient's clinical course. Ciprofloxacin or doxycycline alone may be adequate as the patient improves. If meningitis is suspected, then doxycycline alone is inadequate because of poor penetration into the central nervous system. The administration of 500 mg of amoxicillin for adults or 80 mg/kg for children given orally three times a day is an option after clinical improvement of the patient and antibiotic resistance testing of the anthrax.

The treatment of inhalation and cutaneous anthrax is listed in **Tables 9-1** and **9-2**, respectively.

Prophylaxis

Two types of anthrax vaccines for human use are available in the United States and the United Kingdom, albeit in totally insufficient quantities for a civilian biowarfare challenge.[14] The usual immunization series is six 0.5-mL doses over a span of 18 months. The military feels that a primary series of three 0.5-mL doses (0, 2, and 4 weeks) will be protective against both cutaneous and inhalation anthrax for about 6 months after the primary series.

These immunizations were given to many coalition troops during the Gulf War in 1991 in anticipation of Saddam Hussein's employment of this agent. Large quantities of antigen are presumed to be stockpiled for military use, because this agent has been considered a recurring threat. Since 1997, the US Department of Defense required anthrax immunization for all active duty service personnel, although only 33% of the personnel are currently immunized. Unless civilian immunizations start about 1 month prior to a terrorist attack, EMS and medical providers will be essentially unprotected.

Although minor reactions to the vaccine are common (6% of the immunized population), major reactions are uncommon. Obviously, the vaccine is contraindicated for those who are known to be sensitive to it and those who have already had clinical anthrax. The choice between immunization with some allergic reaction and no immunization in the face of a serious biowarfare threat will present a difficult clinical dilemma.

A live anthrax vaccine is used in Russia to immunize both livestock and humans. The Russians believe that this vaccine is superior at stimulating cell-mediated immunity.[15] There would be considerable resistance to the use of the Russian vaccine in Western countries because of concerns over the purity and residual virulence of a live vaccine.

There is no available nonclassified evidence that these vaccines will adequately protect against an aerosol attack.[16] New vaccines with highly purified protective antigens or designer attenuated strains have been used in laboratories but are not commercially available.[17,18]

Recent research has isolated components of the virulence factors associated with anthrax. Several approaches to

Table 9-2 Treatment of Cutaneous Anthrax	
Patient Category	Recommended Therapy*
Adults	**Preferred choices:** Doxycycline, 100 mg orally twice daily OR Ciprofloxacin, 500 mg orally twice daily **Continue for a total of 60 days.** (There is a potential persistence of spores after an aerosol exposure, so extended therapy is important.)
Children	**Preferred choices:** Ciprofloxacin, 10 to 15 mg/kg orally twice daily (not to exceed 1 g/day) OR Doxycycline, > 8 years and > 45 kg: 100 mg orally every 12 hours > 8 years and ≤ 45 kg: 2.2 mg/kg orally every 12 hours ≤ 8 years: 2.2 mg/kg orally every 12 hours **Continue for a total of 60 days.** The American Academy of Pediatrics recommends treatment of young children with tetracyclines for serious infections such as Rocky Mountain Spotted Fever.
Pregnant women	Use the recommended adult dose of antibiotics listed above. The risk of complications from the antibiotics is far less than the risk of death from cutaneous anthrax. Although tetracyclines are not recommended during pregnancy, their use is indicated for this life-threatening illness. Adverse effects on developing teeth and bones are dose related.
Immunocompromised patients	Use the recommended adult or pediatric dose of antibiotics listed above as appropriate for the patient. The risk of complications from the antibiotics is far less than the risk of death from cutaneous anthrax.

*Patients with extensive cutaneous lesions, lesions on the head or neck, or any systemic signs should be treated with intravenous antibiotics in a multidrug regimen, as if they have inhalation anthrax.

Adapted from: Henderson DA, Inglesby TV, Bartlett JG, et al: Anthrax as a biological weapon: Medical and public health management. *JAMA* 1999;281(18):1735-1745.

contracting these virulence factors have produced increased survival in animals infected with anthrax and promise better treatment agents in humans.

Antibiotic prophylaxis with ciprofloxacin (500 mg administered orally twice daily), or doxycycline (100 mg administered orally twice daily) is also recommended by the US military for an imminent attack with a biological weapon. Note that these are the same agents recommended for plague and tularemia. Although penicillin is the drug of choice for natural anthrax, it is presumed that terrorists will use anthrax that has been deliberately made resistant to penicillin. To date, this has not happened.

Other available fluoroquinolones (in the same group as ciprofloxacin) would probably be as effective as ciprofloxacin, but they have not been adequately tested. Should an attack be confirmed as anthrax, then antibiotics should be continued for at least 4 weeks for all who are exposed.

Children should receive prophylaxis with oral ciprofloxacin (10 to 15 mg/kg administered twice daily) or oral doxycycline (2.2 mg/kg administered twice daily).[19,20] Although these antibiotics are contraindicated for children, it is felt that the minimal damage to teeth, cartilage, connective tissue, or growth plates would be far easier on the child than infection with anthrax.

Those who have been exposed and have not been previously immunized should also be started on anti-anthrax vaccine according to the standard schedule (if it is available). Those who have received fewer than three doses of vaccine prior to exposure should receive a single booster injection. If a vaccine is not available, then antibiotics should be continued until the patient can be safely and closely observed when the antibiotics are discontinued. (Inhaled spores are not destroyed by antibiotics and may persist beyond the course of the antibiotics recommended.)

Biosafety

Standard body substance isolation should be employed when dealing with patients infected with anthrax. Animal carcasses should be burned, not buried, to prevent long-term environmental contamination. Human remains should be cremated at a high temperature if possible. **Table 9-3** summarizes biosafety information for anthrax.

Threat

Anthrax is likely to be disseminated as an aerosol of the very persistent spores. The incubation time is from 1 to 6 days, but as the Sverdlovsk incident demonstrated, anthrax may

have a prolonged incubation period of up to 2 months. The longer incubation periods occur most frequently when partial treatment has been given. The spores can be quite stable, even in the alveolus. The logistics of trying to provide antibiotics to tens or thousands or even hundreds of thousands of people who may have been exposed in an attack would be a formidable challenge.

■ Brucellosis

Brucellosis is also a zoonotic disease, meaning that it is transmissible from animals to humans, like anthrax. The brucellosis organism can survive in unpasteurized milk for days and in fomites (dust particles) for over 2 weeks.

Distribution and Epidemiology

The natural reservoir is domestic herbivores such as goats, sheep, cattle, and pigs. There are four species that are pathogenic in humans: *Brucella melitensis, B abortus* (cow), *B suis* (pigs), and *B canis* (dogs). Humans become infected when they ingest raw infected meat or milk, inhale contaminated aerosols, or become exposed through skin contact. Human infection is also called undulant fever.

Human-to-human transmission is rare, if it occurs at all. Infections in slaughterhouse and laboratory workers suggest that brucellosis is quite infective via the aerosol route. It is estimated that as few as 100 bacteria are sufficient to cause the disease in humans.

History

Sir David Bruce first identified brucellosis on the isle of Malta in 1887, when British soldiers contracted a frequently fatal febrile illness. It was later confirmed that the goats on the isle of Malta carried the disease.

Brucella species have been long considered as biological warfare agents because of the stability, persistence, and ease of infection without human-to-human transfer. Brucellosis can be spread by aerosol spray or by contamination of a food supply (sabotage). There is a long persistence of brucellosis in wet ground or food.

Presentation

Incubation Period

The incubation period is about 8 to 21 days but may be considerably longer or may be as short as a few days. The onset of the illness can be abrupt or insidious. When infecting humans, the bacteria localize in the **reticuloendothelial**

Table 9-3 Protection Against Anthrax		
Inactivation Requirements	**Decontaminating Agents**	**Personal Protection Requirements**
Heat at 250°F (121°C) for more than 30 minutes	2% glutaraldehyde	Wear gloves and a gown (tied at the wrists), preferably with a totally sealed garment.
	5% formalin (overnight)	Wear respiratory protection while handling potentially contaminated items.
		Utilize shower facilities.
		Change clothes.
		Dispose of contaminated products by incineration or steam sterilization.

Source: American Academy of Orthopaedic Surgeons, Stewart CE, Nixon RG. *Weapons of Mass Casualties Field Guide.* Jones and Bartlett Publishers, Boston; 2003.

system, particularly the lymph nodes, liver, spleen, and bone marrow. The severity of the subsequent infection depends on the strain of brucellosis involved.

Clinical Disease

The clinical disease is a nonspecific febrile illness with headache, fatigue, myalgia, anorexia, chills, sweats, and cough. The resultant fever often reaches 105°F/40.5°C. Cough and pleuritic chest pain occurs in up to 20% of infected patients. Gastrointestinal symptoms are common in adults, but less frequent in children.

Ileitis, colitis, and granulomatous or mononuclear infiltrative hepatitis may occur in up to 60% of infected patients. These patients may have both hepatomegaly and splenomegaly (about 30% to 40% of patients). Brucellosis can also cause hepatic abscesses or cholecystitis.

The disease may progress and include arthritis, lymphadenopathy, arthralgias, osteomyelitis, epididymitis, orchitis, and endocarditis. Infections may spread to both bone and joints. This may include vertebral osteomyelitis, intravertebral disk space infection, paravertebral abscess, and sacroiliac infections in a minority of patients. Some patients may develop meningitis or encephalitis.

Ocular symptoms of brucellosis occur in a minority of patients. Uveitis is the most common ocular symptom, but any part of the eye can be involved.[21] The uveitis is usually unilateral and may be granulomatous. It can vary markedly in severity. Vitreous exudates or retinal detachments may also be associated with brucellosis uveitis. Optic nerve involvement occurs in about 11% of patients. In one case of brucellosis, the patient's initial symptoms of the infection were blindness in one eye, intermittent fever, and headache.[22,23]

Meningitis is the most frequent complication of the central nervous system, but invasion of the central nervous system occurs in only about 5% of patients. Endocarditis occurs in less than 2% of patients but accounts for the majority of brucellosis-related deaths. Infected aneurysms of the brain, aorta, and other vessels can occur. Renal involvement is unusual. Orchitis has been reported in 20% of men with brucellosis. Epididymitis is also common. Disability is pronounced, but mortality is about 5% or less in usual cases. Mortality is highest in cases of endocarditis.

The disease may be followed by recovery and relapse. A relapse rate of 5% to 25% can be expected in patients treated for brucellosis, depending on the antibiotic regimen employed (**Table 9-4**). The duration of the disease is usually a few weeks, but brucellosis may last for years.

Diagnosis

Diagnosis of this disease is made by a blood culture, a bone marrow culture, or serology. The sensitivity of a single blood culture ranges from 15% to 70% depending on the method used and the length of incubation. Because *Brucella* organisms grow slowly, the cultures may require 4 weeks to mature. Cultures of bone marrow may be more sensitive than conventional cultures. There are no other laboratory findings that contribute to a diagnosis of brucellosis.

Presumptive diagnosis of brucellosis can be made by serologic studies that show specific *Brucella* IgG antibodies or the presence of IgM antibody to *Brucella*.[24-28] Standard serum agglutination tests do not detect antibodies to *B canis*, and serologic tests specific for that subspecies must be used. A molecular diagnosis using polymerase chain reaction has been developed, but it is not available for routine clinical use.[27]

Pulmonary symptoms may not correlate with radiographic findings. Chest radiographs are often normal, but may show lung abscesses, miliary nodules, pneumonia, enlarged hilar lymph nodes, or pleural effusion.

Therapy

Despite extensive studies over the past 15 years, the optimum antibiotic therapy for brucellosis is open to question. The US military and WHO recommend doxycycline (100 mg administered twice daily) plus rifampin (900 mg/day) for 6 weeks.[28,29] These antibiotics are generally available in sufficient quantities in the United States. An alternative therapy that has been proposed indicates doxycycline (100 mg administered twice daily) for 6 weeks and streptomycin (1 g/day) for 3 weeks.[30] TMP-SMX (Trimethoprim-sulfamethoxazole) or a floxacin

Table 9-4 Suggested Therapy for Brucellosis	
Preferred choices	**Adult dose:** Doxycycline, 100 mg intravenously twice daily for 6 weeks
	AND
	Gentamicin, 3 to 5 mg/kg/day intravenously in two divided doses for 2 to 3 weeks
	OR
	Streptomycin, 1 g/day intramuscularly for 2 to 3 weeks
	Additional information: Relapse occurs in about 6% of patients treated with this regimen. The use of this regimen is more labor intensive than the oral regime described below, but it is also more effective.
Alternative choices	**Adult dose:** Doxycycline, 100 mg orally twice daily for 6 weeks
	AND
	Rifampin, 600 to 900 mg orally twice daily
	Additional information: Relapse occurs in about 15% of patients treated with this regimen.
	Possibly, a fluoroquinolone may be used for treatment of brucellosis. Fluoroquinolones have demonstrated good activity against *Brucella* in vitro, but clinical results have been disappointing.

INHOSPITAL INFO

Table 9-5 Protection Against Brucellosis		
Inactivation Requirements	**Decontaminating Agents**	**Personal Protection Requirements**
Moist heat at 250°F (121°C) for more than 15 minutes Dry heat at 320° to 338°F (160° to 170°C) for more than 1 hour	Alcohol 1% bleach Iodophor Glutaraldehyde Formaldehyde	Wear gloves and a gown (tied at the wrists). Take secretion precautions. Decontaminate soiled items before disposal. Dispose of soiled items by steam sterilization, incineration, or chemical disinfection.

Source: American Academy of Orthopaedic Surgeons, Stewart CE, Nixon RG. *Weapons of Mass Casualties Field Guide.* Jones and Bartlett Publishers, Boston; 2003.

antibiotic have been given for 4 to 6 weeks but are thought to be less effective.[31] Relapse and treatment failure is common.

Although corticosteroid therapy has been recommended for treatment of brucellosis with central nervous system involvement, there are no controlled studies that validate this recommendation.

Prophylaxis

There is no information available about chemoprophylaxis for this disease. Human vaccines are not routinely available in the United States, but they have been developed by other countries. A live, attenuated variant of *B abortus,* S19-BA has been used in the former Soviet Union to protect occupationally-exposed groups. Efficacy is limited and annual revaccination is necessary. A similar vaccine is available in China using the 104M variant. Neither of these two vaccines would meet Western requirements for safety and effectiveness.[32]

Biosafety

Standard body substance isolation should be employed when dealing with patients infected with brucellosis. **Table 9-5** summarizes biosafety information for brucellosis.

■ Cholera

Cholera is a well-known diarrheal disease caused by *Vibrio cholerae* and acquired in humans through the ingestion of contaminated water. The organism causes a profound secretory "rice water" diarrhea (often over 1 L of diarrhea fluid per hour). This diarrhea causes a fatality rate of over 50% if untreated.

History

Cholera pandemics are a modern phenomenon; relatively rapid, global transportation and increased density of populations in large urban centers seem to have emerged at about the same time as pandemic cholera. It is believed that cholera has been endemic in India for many centuries. All the major cholera pandemics began in the subcontinent, often spreading along trade routes, among religious pilgrims, and among soldiers returning from foreign wars.

The first great cholera pandemic, probably originating near Calcutta in 1817, spread to Southeast Asia, Japan, and China and lasted until 1823. It is believed that an exceptionally cold winter in 1823 and 1824 kept the pandemic from reaching western Europe.

The second cholera pandemic began in Bengal and spread through India in 1826, reaching Afghanistan in 1827, Moscow in late 1830, England in 1831, New York by way of Canada in 1832, and from there throughout most of the United States. The second pandemic lasted until 1837.

The third major cholera pandemic reached Europe and the United States in 1848. The English physician John Snow observed during the 1848 London epidemic that the disease was spread by contaminated water. Snow made the connection that all of the infected households obtained drinking water from the same well.

The fourth cholera pandemic began in 1863 and spread first to the Middle East, and then into the Mediterranean. It spread to New York on a ship from France in October 1865. Before the pandemic ended in 1866, tens of thousands died; however, for the first time, public health reforms kept the death toll lower than it otherwise would have been. Another epidemic affected the Mississippi and Ohio valleys in 1873.

A fifth cholera pandemic began in 1881 and lasted until 1896. Improved sanitation kept it from reaching many European cities, and improved diagnosis and quarantine measures kept it from reaching the United States. During this wave, German physician Robert Koch discovered that *V cholerae* caused the disease.

A sixth pandemic that affected Asia began in 1899, but it failed to reach western Europe and the United States because of new technological developments in water treatment and sanitation.

The seventh, most recent pandemic began in Indonesia in 1961 and reached Peru and neighboring countries in 1991. It continues with periodic outbreaks in many areas of the world where clean water is not always available. The Peruvian outbreak coincided with a halt in that country's water chlorination program.

A cholera epidemic that began in 1992 in India and Bangladesh has spread to other countries in southern Asia. This outbreak was caused by a new strain of toxigenic *V cholerae* and is feared to be the beginning of the eighth cholera pandemic.

In 1915 the Germans released *V cholerae* in Russia and Italy in an attempt at biological warfare.

Dissemination

Although cholera can be spread by aerosols, the most likely terrorist or military dissemination would be achieved by the contamination of food or water supplies. There is negligible direct human-to-human transmissibility. The bacterium is only slightly persistent in food or pure water and is not persistent when applied by aerosols.

The host for cholera is the human. The organism is contracted by eating food or drinking water contaminated by the feces or vomitus of someone infected with cholera. Current research also implicates shellfish in an estuarine environment; this is as yet poorly understood but may involve the plankton on which the shellfish feed.

Presentation
Incubation

The incubation period is 1 to 5 days and the course of the illness is about 1 week. Cholera can cause a profuse watery diarrhea that causes hypovolemia and hypotension with the loss of more than 1 L of diarrheal fluid per hour. Without treatment, cholera can rapidly kill adults and children alike from severe dehydration and resultant shock. The patient may experience vomiting early in the illness. There is little abdominal pain associated with the disease.

Diagnosis

Gram staining of the stool sample will show few or no red or white cells. Renal failure may complicate severe dehydration. Electrolyte abnormalities are common with the profound fluid loss; generally, hypokalemia predominates.

Escherichia coli, rotavirus, and toxic ingestions, such as staphylococcal food poisoning, *Bacillus cereus*, or even *Clostridium* species can all cause similar watery diarrhea. The bacteriologic diagnosis of cholera diarrhea has been well studied for decades. *Vibrio* species can be seen and identified readily with darkfield or phase contrast microscopes. A culture will prove the diagnosis but is unnecessary for the treatment.

Therapy

Treatment of cholera is mostly supportive. Although most US emergency physicians are used to treating significant hypovolemia with intravenous fluid replacement, sufficient quantities of intravenous fluids are unlikely to be readily available if an epidemic of cholera is caused by a terrorist or enemy action. The World Health Organization (WHO) oral rehydration formula is appropriate, but it is generally not stocked in sufficient quantities in most cities. Certainly Pedialyte electrolyte maintenance solution and such sport drinks as Gatorade will provide interim oral hydration. If a

cholera epidemic is in place, then intravenous fluids should be reserved for those patients who are vomiting and are unable to tolerate oral rehydration, those patients who have more than 7 L per day of stool, and those patients who have such hypovolemia that they have shock.

Tetracycline and doxycycline have both been found to shorten the course of the diarrhea. Other effective drugs include ampicillin (250 mg every 6 hours for 5 days) and TMP-SMX (1 tablet every 12 hours). An appropriate scale should be used for pediatric doses. Concerns over tetracycline resistance have recently arisen and ciprofloxacin (500 mg every 12 hours), erythromycin (500 mg every 6 hours), or furazolidone (100 mg every 6 hours) have also been recommended.

Prophylaxis

The currently available vaccine is a killed suspension of *V cholerae*. It provides incomplete protection and lasts no longer than 6 months. It requires two injections with a booster dose every 6 months. The dose of vaccine varies with the patient's age and the route of administration. It may be given intradermally, subcutaneously, or intramuscularly. The poor track record of this vaccine has led most public health authorities to recommend against it. Improved vaccines are being tested but are not yet available.

Biosafety

Standard body substance isolation should be employed when dealing with patients infected with cholera. **Table 9-6** summarizes biosafety information for cholera.

Threat

The intentional use of cholera by terrorists would probably involve the contamination of food or water sources. Cholera is incapacitating, but with large numbers of casualties overwhelming available medical resources, quite a few deaths are possible.

■ Glanders and Melioidosis

Glanders and **melioidosis** are related diseases produced by bacteria of the *Burkholderia* species. The two diseases have similar symptoms and pathophysiology.

Table 9-6 Protection Against Cholera		
Inactivation Requirements	Decontaminating Agents	Personal Protection Requirements
Moist heat at 250°F (121°C) for more than 15 minutes Dry heat at 320° to 338°F (160° to 170°C) for more than 1 hour	70% ethanol 2% glutaraldehyde 8% formaldehyde 0.5% bleach 10% hydrogen peroxide for 30 minutes at 20°C/68°F	Wear gloves and a gown. Take secretion and enteric precautions. Wash hands frequently and carefully with soap and water. This is essential. Decontaminate equipment before disposal with standard decontamination solutions. In an outbreak, contaminated water and fresh fruits and vegetables must be avoided. Drinking water, as well as water used for bathing, washing utensils, and cooking, must be boiled or decontaminated with chlorine or iodine before use.

Source: American Academy of Orthopaedic Surgeons, Stewart CE, Nixon RG. *Weapons of Mass Casualties Field Guide.* Jones and Bartlett Publishers, Boston; 2003.

The causative agent of glanders is *Burkholderia* (formerly *Malleomyces*) *mallei*. This bacillus was formerly classified as a *Pseudomonas* species. Like anthrax, glanders is considered to be a zoonotic infection that usually affects only horses, donkeys, and mules. *B mallei* exists in nature only in susceptible hosts and is not found in water, soil, or plants.

There are four basic forms of disease caused by glanders in horses and mules. The acute forms are more common in mules and donkeys, with death typically occurring 3 to 4 weeks after the onset of the illness. The chronic form of the disease is more common in horses and causes a generalized disease of the lymph nodes, multiple skin nodules, and nodules in the local lymph nodes.

B pseudomallei, found in soil and water in tropical areas of Southeast Asia, causes a glanders-like disease called melioidosis. This disease may take a rather benign pulmonary form but may also develop into a rapidly fatal septicemia.

The course of melioidosis in humans ranges from a subclinical mild illness to an overwhelming septicemia. The septicemia causes a 90% mortality rate, and death usually occurs within 24 to 48 hours after the onset of the illness. Melioidosis, like tuberculosis, can reactivate years after the primary infection, resulting in another life-threatening illness.

History

In World War I, German forces reportedly spread glanders to debilitate enemy horses **(Figure 9-5)**. At that time, horses and mules were very important battlefield resources; they were used to bring supplies to the front and move artillery. Cultures confiscated from the German Legation in Bucharest, Romania, were identified as *B mallei*, and livestock were infected in Mesopotamia, France, and Argentina. Glanders, together with anthrax, was deliberately spread in the United States during World War I by Dr. Anton Dilger, a German-trained physician.

The Japanese deliberately infected horses, civilians, and prisoners of war with *B mallei* at the Pinfang Institute (which was operated by Unit 731) during World War II. In Mongolia, 5% to 25% of tested horses were reactive to *B mallei*, but few human cases were noted.

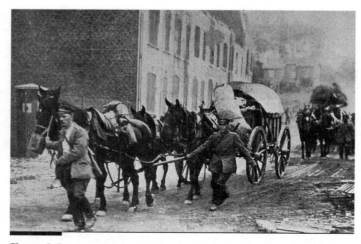

Figure 9-5 Horses were used extensively in World War I. This photo depicts the German Army.

Glanders was investigated by both the United States and the former Soviet Union as a biological warfare agent. In a single year in the 1980s, the Soviet Union produced more than 2,000 tons of dry agent for glanders. This production is a very good reason for the CDC to classify glanders as a potential biowarfare weapon.

B pseudomallei was also studied by the United States as a potential biological warfare weapon, but it was never produced as such. It has been reported that the Soviet Union was also experimenting with *B pseudomallei* as a biological weapon.

Glanders is a likely candidate for biological warfare and bioterrorism, in part, because only a few germs of *B mallei* can trigger disease.

Distribution and Epidemiology

Both glanders and melioidosis affect domestic and wild animals. Animals, like humans, acquire the diseases from inhalation or contamination to injuries. Human cases of glanders have primarily occurred in veterinarians, and horse and donkey handlers and breeders. Rarely, slaughterhouse workers contract the disease. There have been no naturally-acquired human cases in the last 60 years. According to the US Department of Agriculture, glanders was eradicated from the US animal population in 1934.

In contrast to glanders, melioidosis is widely distributed in the soil and water in the tropics. It is endemic in parts of Asia and northern Australia. In northeastern Thailand, *B pseudomallei* is one of the most common causes of septicemia. As a consequence of the long incubation period, it could be imported to the United States.

Presentation
Incubation Period

These organisms spread to humans by invading the nasal, oral, and conjunctival mucous membranes; by inhalation; and by invading abrasions on the skin. Military data show about a 46% infection rate in humans exposed to an aerosol of glanders, with an incubation period of about 10 to 14 days after exposure. An aerosol of glanders would be a deadly weapon.

The respiratory form of the disease is commonly referred to as glanders, while the cutaneous disease is known as farcy.[33] The pulmonary form may follow inhalation or result from the septicemic spread of the disease.

Clinical Presentation

There are three acute forms of glanders and melioidosis:

- **Pulmonary form:** Patients experience cough, nasal discharge, and acute or chronic pneumonia. This may be followed by necrosis of the tracheal-bronchial tree.
- **Localized cutaneous form:** Patients experience multiple purulent cutaneous eruptions, often following the lymphatic drainage system. This form causes pustular lesions that develop 1 to 5 days after bacteria break the skin.

    Acute infection of the oral, nasal, or conjunctival mucosa can cause a discharge of mucus and pus from the nose that is associated with mucosal or cutaneous lesions. The patient may develop nodules or ulcers in the septum and turbinates of the nose.

If systemic invasion occurs from mucosal or cutaneous lesions, the patient may develop a papular rash that turns into a pustular rash. The rash may be mistaken for smallpox.

- **Fulminant, rapidly fatal septicemic form:**
Evidence of sepsis and dissemination of the organism includes the presence of skin pustules, internal organ abscesses, and multiple pulmonary lesions. This form carries a high mortality rate, and most patients develop a rapidly progressing septic shock.

In the only reported case since 1945, the patient developed multiple splenic and hepatic abscesses. [34] He required ventilatory support for his pneumonia. Despite these potentially lethal complications, the patient survived after treatment with imipenem and doxycycline.

General symptoms of glanders include fever and headaches associated with rigors, muscle aches, muscle tightness, and pleuritic chest pain. The headache may be associated with photophobia. The examiner may find fever, enlargement of the lymph nodes (particularly cervical or proximal to pustular eruptions), enlargement of the spleen, and generalized papular or pustular eruptions.

Other symptoms vary according to how the organism enters the body—through the skin, eyes, nose, or respiratory tract—but include the following:

- Swollen lymph nodes
- Tearing of the eyes, light sensitivity
- Increased mucus in the eyes, nose, and respiratory tract
- Night sweats
- Diarrhea

Chronic Form

Cutaneous and intramuscular abscesses may be found in patients with chronic forms of glanders and melioidosis. These patients may also experience nasal discharge and ulceration (50% of patients). The chronic form is characterized by cutaneous and intramuscular abscesses on the extremities. The patient develops enlarged, indurated lymph nodes in the regional drainage area. The chronic form may well be asymptomatic, particularly in melioidosis, and is unlikely to be found within 14 days after an aerosol bioweapons attack.

Diagnosis

Labs

There is no specific laboratory test for glanders or melioidosis. Serologic tests can help confirm the diagnosis, but low titers and negative serology do not exclude the acute phase of the disease.

Methylene blue stain of nasal exudate or sputum may show the presence of scant small bacilli with a "safety pin" appearance. Standard cultures can be used to identify both *B mallei* and *B pseudomallei*. A sputum culture on standard media grows the organism after 48 hours at 37.5°C/ 199.5°F. The addition of 1% to 5% glucose, 5% glycerol, or meat nutrient mediums may accelerate the growth.

A complete blood count may show a mild leukocytosis with left shift. The chest radiograph may show miliary lesions, multiple small lung abscesses, or infiltrates involving the upper lungs. Consolidation and cavitation of these lesions may be noted.

Radiology

The chest radiograph may show either miliary nodules (0.5 to 1.0 cm), pneumonia, multiple small lung abscesses, or nodular necrotizing lesions. Miliary nodules represent small, multiple lung abscesses from glanders. The pneumonia resulting from glanders may be either bronchopneumonia or lobar pneumonia. Necrotizing nodular lesions are infrequently noted on chest radiographs. Complications of glanders include osteomyelitis, brain abscess, and meningitis.

Therapy

Glanders was thought to be uniformly fatal if untreated. However, even when treated, the disease has caused a high mortality rate (roughly 50%) in the few documented cases of human glanders.

Treatment protocols for glanders are not well developed because the disease is so rare. A variety of antibiotics have been used to treat glanders. In vitro, ceftazidime, gentamicin, imipenem, doxycycline, and ciprofloxacin all have reliable activity against *B. mallei*. [35] The current suggested therapy is listed in **Table 9-7**.

The limited number of infections in humans precludes evaluation of many of the antibiotic agents. Most antibiotic sensitivities are based on animal and in vitro studies. The clinician should note that various strains of both glanders and melioidosis have markedly different antibiotic sensitivities, and other antibiotics may be quite useful.

Prophylaxis

There is no vaccine available for glanders. Person-to-person airborne transmission is unlikely, although secondary cases may occur if infected secretions are improperly handled. Postexposure prophylaxis with Trimethoprim-sulfamethoxazole has been recommended, but there are too few human infections to adequately document the efficacy of this treatment.

Biosafety

Aerosols from cultures are quite contagious to laboratory workers. When working with these organisms in the laboratory, biosafety Level 3 containment practices are required. **Table 9-8** summarizes biosafety information for glanders and melioidosis. There is little evidence supporting human-to-human transmissibility of glanders and melioidosis, but it has been documented.

Threat

Aggressive control measures essentially eliminated glanders from the West. The only reported case in the United States since 1945 occurred in a military research microbiologist in 2000. [36] Despite the efficiency of spread in the laboratory setting, glanders has only caused sporadic disease in humans and no epidemics of human disease have been reported.

This agent was used by the Germans in World War I, the Japanese in World War II, and studied by the United States from 1943 to 1945. The former Soviet Union is thought to

INHOSPITAL INFO

Table 9-7 Suggested Therapy for Glanders and Melioidosis

Adults	**Preferred choices:** Amoxicillin/clavulanate, 60 mg/kg/day in three divided doses OR Tetracycline, 40 mg/kg/day in three divided doses OR Trimethoprim sulfa: TMP, 4 mg/kg/day; sulfa, 20 mg/kg/day in two divided doses **Additional information:** The patient should be treated for 60 to 150 days with one of these antibiotics.
Localized disease with signs of mild toxicity	**Preferred choices:** Amoxicillin/clavulanate, 60 mg/kg/day in three divided doses AND Trimethoprim sulfa: TMP, 4 mg/kg/day; sulfa, 20 mg/kg/day in two divided doses OR Tetracycline 40 mg/kg/day in three divided doses (not recommended for small children or pregnant women) **Additional information:** The normal duration of therapy for dual therapy is 30 days followed by monotherapy with either amoxicillin/clavulanate or trimethoprim sulfa for 60 to 150 days. If the patient has extrapulmonary suppurative disease, then therapy should be continued for 6 to 12 months. Surgical drainage of abscesses is often necessary.
Severe disease	**Preferred choices:** Ceftazidime, 120 mg/kg/day intravenously in three divided doses and trimethoprim sulfa: TMP, 4 mg/kg/day; sulfa, 20 mg/kg/day in two divided doses, intravenously **Additional information:** Intravenous therapy should be continued for 2 weeks, followed by 6 months of oral therapy. **Alternative choices:** Doxycycline, rifampin, and ciprofloxacin have been effective for experimental infection in hamsters.

Table 9-8 Protection Against Glanders and Melioidosis

Inactivation Requirements	Decontaminating Agents	Personal Protection Requirements
Moist heat at 250°F (121°C) for more than 15 minutes Dry heat at 320° to 338°F (160° to 170°C) for more than 1 hour	70% ethanol 2% glutaraldehyde 8% formaldehyde 0.5% bleach 10% hydrogen peroxide for 30 minutes at 20°C/68°F	Use biosafety Level 3 protection when working with cultures in the laboratory. Wear gloves, a gown, and an N95 particulate respirator when working with patients. Take contact and secretion precautions. Wash hands frequently with soap and water. Decontaminate equipment before disposal with standard decontamination solutions.

Source: American Academy of Orthopaedic Surgeons, Stewart CE, Nixon RG. *Weapons of Mass Casualties Field Guide.* Jones and Bartlett Publishers, Boston; 2003.

have investigated glanders as a potential bioweapon after World War II. Glanders is endemic in Africa, Asia, the Middle East, and Central and South America.

The occurrence of glanders outside of animal handlers is presumptive evidence of biowarfare intent, because this disease is not naturally-occurring in the United States. Obviously, an epidemic occurrence is attributable to biowarfare. There have been a few cases of meliodosis imported into the United States.

■ Plague

Plague is a zoonotic disease caused by *Yersinia pestis*. It is naturally found on rodents and prairie dogs and their fleas. Plague appears to have evolved from *Y pseudotuberculosis* relatively recently (1,500 to 20,000 years ago). Plague is found in every inhabited continent.

Plague is a stable, adaptable microorganism that spreads through host animals easily. At least 30 types of fleas and over 200 species of mammals serve as reservoirs for this disease. Plague can also adversely affect domestic pets, especially cats. An infected cat can readily transmit plague to its owners.

The plague bacillus can retain viability in water for 2 to 30 days, in moist areas for up to 2 years, and in near freezing temperatures for several months to a year. Person-to-person transmissibility is high and the bacterium is highly infective. The persistence is low, but the transmissibility is so high that this is immaterial.

Y pestis is a pathogen of rodents. The flea sucks up viable organisms into its intestinal tract when it bites an infected rodent. These organisms rapidly multiply in the flea and are regurgitated when the flea gets its next blood meal. Humans become infected when they are bitten by an infected flea.

The organism spreads explosively within the bloodstream and involves the liver, spleen, lungs, and often the meninges. The patient develops a bacterial pneumonia and starts to cough. The sputum contains large numbers of viable organisms that are spread into the air during fits of coughing.

The urban cycle of plague is an explosive, pandemic disease that causes high mortality. It killed 100 million people in the 6th century and 25 million people in the 14th century. During the urban cycle, human-to-human transmission of plague is caused by aerosol droplets or by infected fleas.

Epizootic plague occurs when sensitive or moderately-resistant hosts are infected by fleas or ingestion. It may also occur if the virulence of the microbe increases by mutation. This results in a highly visible die-off of rats, prairie dogs, rock squirrels, or other infected rodents. The fleas leave the dying hosts and move to the nearest available new host. If this die-off occurs in a city, then the fleas move to humans and infect the humans. This was the starting event in several recent plagues, including the Indian plague of 1996.

The sylvatic cycle of plague is the cause of almost all cases of plague since 1925. Currently, plague is endemic in rodents in the western United States. Resistant hosts maintain a stable rodent-flea infection cycle. Human infections are on the rise, but are limited to the western United States. (This may also be called enzootic plague.)

Humans may become infected through the bites of infected fleas or through direct contact with infected rodent tissues. Direct contact cases usually involve hunters who field dress infected squirrels without wearing gloves, allowing plague bacteria to enter the body through open cuts or abrasions in the skin.

Pets, particularly cats and occasionally dogs, may acquire infections through the bites of infected fleas or through the ingestion of infected rodent tissues. Domestic cats may also acquire plague by eating wild rodents. Pets may infect humans by bringing plague-infected fleas into the home. Humans may also become infected with plague by handling sick, infected pets. Cats with pneumonic plague, in particular, may cough infected droplets onto their owners. Plague can be found year-round but is most likely to occur in April through November when rodents are more active.

Distribution

In the United States, plague spread from the Pacific Coast inland and is now endemic in rodents as far east as the Mississippi River. Only Australia and Antarctica have no natural occurrence of plague. Worldwide, there are about 1,700 infections per year.

In the United States, 390 cases of plague were reported from 1947 to 1996. The cases reported from 1970 to the end of 2004 are represented in **Figure 9-6**. In the United States, most cases of plague are reported from New Mexico, Arizona, Colorado, and California **(Figure 9-7)**.[37]

History

The Black Death or plague has been one of the great epidemic scourges of humankind. For centuries, plague represented the epitome of disaster. Some populations were so devastated that there were not enough people left living to bury the dead. Plague outbreaks have caused intense panic in cities and counties where it has appeared—even in the 20th century after the advent of effective antibiotics.

Three great pandemics have been identified. They occurred in the 6th, 14th, and 20th centuries. Plague swept across Byzantine Asia and Europe in a series of devastating pandemics before and during the Middle Ages. The disease was responsible for the death of one third of the world's population (as many as 100 million people) in 541 and 542.

The second plague pandemic was probably imported along the trans-Asian "silk road" and again swept Europe between 1346 and the end of the century. It continued in France and Italy until the 18th century. During this time, at least 50 million more people died from the Black Death.[38]

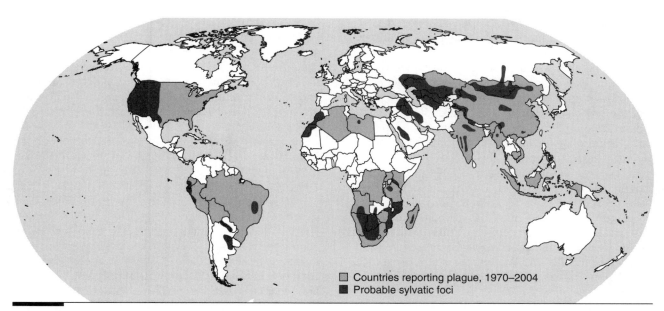

□ Countries reporting plague, 1970–2004
■ Probable sylvatic foci

Figure 9-6 Reported cases of plague from 1970 to 2004.

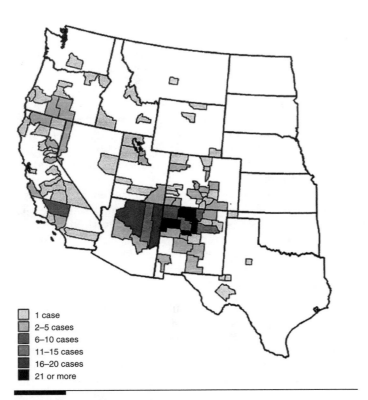

Figure 9-7 Reported human plague cases by US county from 1970 to 1997.

1 case
2–5 cases
6–10 cases
11–15 cases
16–20 cases
21 or more

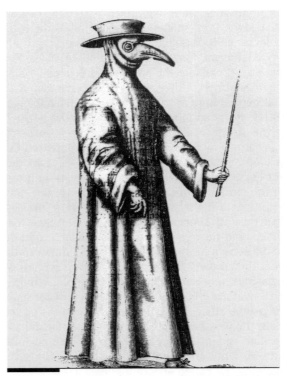

Figure 9-8 Medical protection worn in the Middle Ages to prevent infection with the plague.

The reasons that the first and second plague pandemics slowly died out are unknown. Many authors have advanced theories, including the following:

1. Fleas on humans were discouraged by the increased use of soap as the standard of living rose.[39]
2. The oriental rat flea *Xenopsylla cheopis* succumbed to a change in climate.[40]
3. The common black rat was displaced by the more aggressive Norwegian brown rat. The brown rat was less likely to live in close proximity to humans.[41,42]
4. The virulence of the *Yersinia* species changed. (Needless to say, a more virulent species can either emerge or be engineered.)[43]
5. A decreased ability to feed the population led to an increase in iron deficiency anemia; iron is needed for *Yersinia* species' virulence.[44]

One of the first uses of protective masks and garments by physicians was implemented during the second plague pandemic to avoid plague **(Figure 9-8).** The nosepiece of the mask contained herbs to ward off the infection.

The third plague pandemic began in 1894 in China and spread rapidly through the world. During the period from 1894 to the present, at least 15 million more people have died from plague, mostly in China, Hong Kong, Manchuria, and India. Plague was imported to the United States from this epidemic. It was found first in San Francisco in 1900, and later in New York City and Washington state. Rodents in the western United States were probably infected from this San Francisco source.

The modern epidemic was abated by general rat control and hygiene measures before the advent of antibiotics. Ur-ban plague is now quite uncommon. Nonetheless, small outbreaks of plague continue throughout the world.[45]

Dr. Alexander J. E. Yersin identified the causative agent of plague in Hong Kong in 1894 during the third plague pandemic. Because of its high lethality (about 200 million deaths throughout history), *Y pestis* has attracted attention as a possible biological warfare agent. Plague generates special concern because of its potential to cause panic, its contagiousness in the pulmonary form, its fulminating and highly fatal clinical course, and its ability to be genetically engineered for resistance.[46]

Plague could be spread by either infected vectors such as fleas or by an aerosol spray. Note that Unit 731 of the Japanese Imperial Army is reported to have dropped plague-infected fleas from aircraft over populated areas of China and caused multiple outbreaks of plague **(Figure 9-9).**

The US Army worked to develop *Y pestis* as a potential biowarfare agent in the 1950s and 1960s. Unclassified literature asserts that the United States was unable to develop a form of plague that could be spread through aerosol means (J. Hughes, Washington, DC, testimony before Congress, 1998).[47]

More than 10 institutes and thousands of scientists were reported to have worked with plague in the former Soviet Union.[48] In 1994, defectors revealed that the Russians had conducted research on *Y pestis* to make it more virulent and stable in the environment.[49] These weapons-grade species of *Yersinia* may be resistant to multiple antibiotics and may have increased virulence. These sources noted that plague has been weaponized by the Russians as an aerosol, which is the expected mode of delivery as a bioterrorist agent.[50]

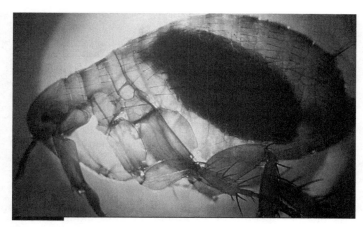

Figure 9-9 Flea.

A form of plague that remains stable over a long period was also apparently developed by the Soviet Union. The defectors noted that research was being conducted as part of a process to make plague more deadly. This development would destroy the early diagnosis and detection capability of many current bioweapons detectors.

With the breakup of the Soviet Union, these scientists often have difficulty finding employment and may be enticed by gainful employment offered by a well funded terrorist organization. Equally troublesome is the possibility that the stocks of weapons-grade plague developed by the Soviet Union may be released by unscrupulous individuals who gain access to them. There is also no question that native strains of plague may be harvested easily by a terrorist with only a modicum of training.

There is little unclassified information about the current actions of unaffiliated groups or individuals seeking to develop plague as a weapon. In 1995, in Ohio, a microbiologist with suspect motives was arrested after acquiring *Y pestis* by mail. With endemic plague in rodents in many parts of the country, there is no question that terrorists could still acquire plague and develop a weapon.

A WHO model of the release of 50 kg of *Y pestis* over a city of 5 million predicts 500,000 infections with over 100,000 deaths when both primary and secondary transmission of the bacteria are considered in the model **(Table 9-9)**.[51] In this scenario, the plague bacilli were assumed to remain

Table 9-9 WHO Plague Modeling Scenario (Circa 1970)

Results of 50 kg of plague released as an aerosol over a city of 5 million people:

- 150,000 cases of primary plague
- 36,000 deaths
- Hospitalization and isolation requirements for 80,000 to 100,000 people

Results of secondary spread of primary infection:

- Up to 500,000 additional cases
- Up to 100,000 additional deaths

Adapted from: World Health Organization. *Health Aspects of Chemical and Biological Weapons.* Geneva: World Health Organization, 1970.

viable as an aerosol for about an hour and expected to spread over 10 kilometers. Significant numbers of city inhabitants would likely attempt to flee and further spread the disease. Although this model was developed over 30 years ago, there is no reason to question its validity in modern times.

Indeed, with inevitable decreases in available hospital beds and medical resources in modern hospitals, the projection may well be quite conservative. If modern intensive care cannot be provided because of a lack of personnel and equipment, then mortality will surely increase.

Given the ability of natural plague to rapidly spread to rodents, it is quite possible that weapons-grade plague could be transmitted to rodents in the city and be a source of disease for years to come.

Presentation

Under normal conditions, three syndromes are recognized: pneumonic (inhalational), septicemic, and bubonic. The first infection is usually the bubonic form. Human plague normally occurs when plague-infected fleas bite humans who then develop bubonic plague. The onset of a human epidemic often starts when rodents die in large numbers. This causes the flea population to migrate from its natural rodent reservoir to humans (epizootic plague). Although most persons infected by this route develop bubonic plague, a small minority will proceed to sepsis without formation of a **bubo**—a tender, enlarged, inflamed lymph node, particularly in the upper chest, clavicle or groin area. This form of plague is termed primary septicemic plague. Neither bubonic nor septicemic plague spreads directly from person to person. A small percentage of patients with bubonic or septicemic plague will develop a secondary pneumonic plague. These victims can then spread the disease by respiratory droplets. Persons contracting the disease by the aerosol route will develop primary pneumonic plague.

Bubonic Plague

In bubonic plague, the incubation period is 1 to 10 days. The onset is acute with malaise, fever (often quite high), and subsequent purulent lymphadenitis. The initial lesion may form a bubo or a **carbuncle** at the site of the inoculation **(Color plates 9-4 and 9-5).**

The lymphadenitis is most often inguinal, but cervical and axillary nodes are also involved. As the disease progresses, the nodes become tender, fluctuant, and finally necrotic. Twenty-five percent of patients will develop various types of skin lesions; pustules, vesicles, eschars, and papules are all found in the lymphatic drainage of the bubo **(Color plate 9-6).** When the bubo is aspirated, the examiner will obtain serosanguineous fluids rather than pus.

INHOSPITAL INFO

Septicemic Plague

The bubonic form may progress to the septicemic form with seeding of the central nervous system and the lungs. Secondary septicemia is common, with over 80% of blood cultures testing positive in patients with the bubonic form. In the completely septic form, the patient will have neither pneumonia nor buboes, but the patient will have large numbers of organisms in the bloodstream. Septicemic plague without obviously diseased lymph nodes is difficult to diagnose because the manifestations are nonspecific and include elevated temperature, chills, abdominal pain, nausea, vomiting, diarrhea, tachycardia, tachypnea, and hypotension. Only about 25% of patients infected with bubonic plague will progress to clinical septicemia. Plague meningitis occurs in about 6% of patients.

Those patients with septicemia will experience symptoms similar to patients with other septicemia including chills, high fever, hypotension, vomiting, and diarrhea. The patient will appear quite toxic and may be prostrate, stuporous, or even comatose.

Plague septicemia can also cause thrombosis in the acral vessels. The first presentation is usually ecchymotic skin lesions. Black necrotic extremities and more proximal purpura may be seen. These reflect the development of intrastitial intravascular lesions that result in vascular obstruction. This causes necrosis and gangrene of the terminal vessels in the hands, feet, ears, and nose **(Color plate 9-7)**.

Sepsis with plague can result in the catastrophic physiologic consequences of compliment and cytokine cascade (systemic inflammatory response syndrome). The severity of the illness resulting from either septic or pneumonic forms of plague will require intensive medical care, including both respiratory and cardiovascular support, which may rapidly overwhelm hospital capacity in a local area.[52]

Pneumonic Plague

If the organisms are seeded to the lungs, then the pneumonic form follows, and the patient becomes contagious through coughing and droplet transmission. The course of the disease is 2 to 3 days, and the disease is quite lethal.

If the disease is disseminated as an aerosol, then the bulk of infections will be pneumonic plague. This is thought to be the mode of dissemination that appeals to most terrorist groups. Fortunately, it is relatively difficult to weaponize plague so that it can be easily spread by aerosol.

In primary pneumonic plague, the incubation period is 1 to 4 days. The onset is acute and fulminant and includes malaise, fever, chills, cough with bloody sputum, and toxemia. The pneumonia progresses rapidly to respiratory failure with dyspnea, stridor, and cyanosis. A catastrophic systemic inflammatory response ultimately occurs **(Color plate 9-8)**.

In untreated patients, the mortality rate is over 50% for the bubonic and septicemic forms. In the pneumonic form, the mortality rate approaches 100%. The terminal events are circulatory collapse, hemorrhage, and peripheral thrombosis in septicemic plague. In pneumonic plague, the terminal event is often respiratory failure as well as circulatory collapse. Multi-organ failure is common.

Ocular Plague

This rare form of plague occurs when the conjunctiva has been inoculated with *Y pestis*. The patient will develop severe conjunctivitis with lid edema and purulent drainage. Although this form is considered quite rare, if a populace has been exposed to an aerosol of *Y pestis*, a substantial number of people will receive bacteria into the conjunctiva. Ocular plague conceivably may be an indicator for the subsequent development of many cases of pneumonic plague.

Diagnosis

The characteristic sign of plague is the tender, swollen, very painful lymph node—the bubo. This finding, associated with fever, prostration, and a possible exposure to rodents should lead to the suspicion of plague. Once a human is infected, the illness is generally progressive and fatal unless specific antibiotic therapy is administered.

The presentation of plague following its use as a biological weapon would differ substantially from that of a naturally-occurring infection. The intentional dissemination of plague would likely be accomplished either with an aerosol of *Y pestis* or by the release of infected fleas as was done by Japan's Unit 731 in China. The former method would be more efficient for infecting large numbers of people simultaneously, but the latter might be more suitable for covert terrorist activity. The size of the outbreak would depend on several factors, including the quantity of the agent used, the characteristics of the strain used, the environmental conditions, and the method of aerosolization (if used). If an aerosol is used, then primary pneumonic plague is far more likely. If infected fleas are released, then primary bubonic plague is the first presentation likely to be seen by emergency providers.

Manifestations of plague include:

- General malaise, prostration, headache, and neck pain
- High fever with temperatures greater than 101.3°F (38.5°C)
- Pain or tenderness in regional lymph nodes
- Necrotizing pneumonia
- Septicemia
- Disseminated intravascular coagulopathy (a bleeding disorder with an abnormal reduction of clotting ability that leads to profuse hemorrhage in late stages)
- Convulsions (plague meningitis)
- Shock
- Diffuse hemorrhagic changes in the skin from the disseminated intravascular coagulopathy and cyanosis from the necrotizing pneumonia

Routine (Supportive)

A presumptive diagnosis can be made by finding the typical safety pin bipolar staining organisms in Giemsa or Romanovsky stained specimens. Appropriate specimens are lymph node aspirate, sputum, or cerebral spinal fluid.

Culture and virulence testing of this organism should be performed only in a biosafety Levels 3 or 4 containment facility by staff who have been thoroughly trained in the management of potentially fatal infectious diseases. Protective clothing and a full-face respirator should always be worn when working with this organism.

Although mouse inoculation is considered to be a supportive diagnostic test for plague, this is neither commonly available nor very sensitive. *Y pestis* is not a very biochemically reactive organism, so chemical profiles of the microbe are not particularly useful.

Nonspecific laboratory findings include leukocytosis with left shift. Increased fibrin split products are common and indicative of a low-grade disseminated intravascular coagulopathy. Blood urea nitrogen, creatinine, aspartate aminotransferase, alanine aminotransferase, and bilirubin may be elevated with multi-organ failure.

Routine (Confirmatory)

Standard classic microbiological diagnostic tests would be of limited value in a major bioterrorist event, because they are both time consuming and labor intensive. These standard confirmatory tests include a culture with phage lysis of the organisms. This may require 1 to 6 weeks for confirmation of the organism, but it is considered a gold standard. Likewise, an anti-F1 antigen is formed in patients who survive. A four-fold rise in this titer is considered confirmatory.

Specialized (Nonstandardized Testing)

Newer, rapid testing for this agent, such as antigen detection and DNA amplification has not been standardized and is not widely available. This includes enzyme immunoassay for both IgM (blocking for anti-F1 antigen) and polymerase chain reaction. Polymerase chain reaction is the basis for real-time assays including the Taqman™ and Smartcycler™ devices. Immunofluorescent staining is available and helpful if it is readily accessible.

Molecular characterization of the strain of *Y pestis* can accurately identify the origins of known organisms. This includes the examination of DNA of the capsule and plasmid profiles.

Therapy

Without treatment, the mortality rates of bubonic plague are up to 90%. Septicemic and pneumonic plague approach mortality rates of 100% without appropriate antibiotic treatment. The mortality rate of bubonic plague can be reduced to less than 5% with prompt therapy. The mortality rate of pneumonic plague is still over 50%, even with therapy. Survival is unlikely when treatment is delayed beyond 18 hours of infection.

Recommendations for the antimicrobial treatment of plague in a bioterrorist attack have been developed for both mass-casualty and contained-casualty situations. The principle recommended antibiotics are available in the National Pharmaceutical Stockpile.[53] **Table 9-10** lists the antibiotics recommended for treating plague. The penicillins and cephalosporins are not effective in treating plague, although these drugs may show activity in vitro.[54]

The efficient distribution of these antibiotics is complicated by the logistics problems previously discussed. Two of these antibiotics, ciprofloxacin and gentamicin, are not FDA approved for the treatment of plague.

Streptomycin, tetracycline, doxycycline, ciprofloxacin, and chloramphenicol are all useful if given within the first 24 hours after symptoms of pneumonic plague begin. Strep-

tomycin is considered to be the drug of choice, but it is not widely available. Gentamicin is considered an acceptable substitute.

The clinical deterioration of patients despite early presumptive therapy could indicate antimicrobial resistance and should be promptly evaluated. Note that *Y pestis* has the ability to acquire resistance and has apparently done so.[55-57] The Madagascar strain was resistant to chloramphenicol, streptomycin, sulfonamides, and tetracycline.

Incision and drainage of buboes is not recommended. Aspiration is safer and provides both diagnosis and symptomatic relief.

Supportive therapy of complications is essential. Patients with pneumonic plague will require substantial advanced medical supportive care. This may include both pulmonary and cardiovascular support. Complications of sepsis are expected, including disseminated intravascular coagulation, shock, adult respiratory distress syndrome, and multiorgan failure.

Tables 9-11 and **9-12** list the recommended treatment and prophylaxis for pneumonic plague in contained-casualty and mass-casualty situations.

Prophylaxis

The possibility of rapid death combined with both a vector (flea) transmission and a direct person-to-person transmission make plague an ominous biowarfare threat. Postexposure antimicrobial prophylaxis is recommended, but it will be difficult to identify the population at risk and administer the antibiotics to them in any timely fashion. The isolation and quarantine of exposed populations would be quite difficult to enforce and would likely create fear and chaos.

Postexposure Prophylaxis

Once plague is confirmed or strongly suspected in an area, anyone in that area with a fever of 101.3°F (38.5°C) or higher should be immediately treated with the appropriate antibiotics for a presumptive pneumonic plague. A delay of therapy markedly reduces the patient's chance of survival if plague is the cause of the fever. Postexposure prophylaxis should be given to household members, close contacts, hospital staff, first responders, EMS providers and law enforcement officers at the scene of a release, and epidemiologic interviewers.

Both ciprofloxacin and doxycycline are acceptable for prophylaxis for contact or possible exposure to plague aerosol. Note that these are the same agents recommended for anthrax and tularemia. Tetracycline and chloramphenicol are acceptable alternatives. Sulfonamides are recommended by the WHO for the treatment and prophylaxis of plague but have not been approved by the FDA for this indication. They may be useful for pediatric prophylaxis.

Asymptomatic persons who have had household, hospital, or other close contact with infected patients should be treated for 7 days and monitored for fever and cough. If symptoms occur, treatment antibiotics should be started. Persons who refuse prophylaxis should be carefully monitored for the development of fever or cough for the first 7 days after exposure and should be treated immediately if either occurs.

Historically, preparations of *Y pestis* have demonstrated a viability of only 1 to 2 hours after dissemination. Death and

Table 9-10 Antibiotics Recommended for Treating Plague
Parenteral:
• Aminoglycosides (gentamicin)
• Tetracyclines (doxycycline)
• Fluoroquinolones (ciprofloxacin)
Oral:
• Tetracyclines (doxycycline)
• Fluoroquinolones (ciprofloxacin)

Adapted from: Inglesby TV, Dennis DT, Henderson DA, et al: Plague as a biological weapon: Medical and public health management. *JAMA* 2000;283:2281-2290.

Table 9-11 Recommendations for the Treatment of Pneumonic Plague in Contained-Casualty Settings and for Postexposure Prophlaxis

Patient Category	Recommended Therapy*
Adults	**Preferred choices:** Streptomycin, 1g intramuscularly twice daily OR Gentamicin, 5 mg/kg intramuscularly or intravenously once daily or 2 mg/kg loading dose followed by 1.7 mg/kg intramuscularly or intravenously three times daily† **Alternative choices:** Doxycycline, 100 mg intravenously twice daily or 200 mg intravenously once daily OR Ciprofloxacin, 400 mg intravenously twice daily‡ OR Chloramphenicol, 25 mg/kg intravenously four times daily§
Children‖	**Preferred choices:** Streptomycin, 15 mg/kg intramuscularly twice daily (maximum daily dose of 2 g) OR Gentamicin, 2.5 mg/kg intramuscular or intravenously 3 times daily† **Alternative choices:** Doxycycline, ≥ 45 kg: administer the adult dosage < 45 kg: 2.2 mg/kg intravenously twice daily (maximum daily dose 200 mg) OR Ciprofloxacin, 15 mg/kg intravenously twice daily‡ OR Chloramphenicol, 25 mg/kg intravenously four times daily§
Pregnant women¶	**Preferred choice:** Gentamicin, 5 mg/kg intramuscularly or intravenously once daily or 2 mg/kg loading dose followed by 1.7 mg/kg intramuscularly or intravenously three times daily† **Alternative choices:** Doxycycline, 100 mg intravenously twice daily or 200 mg intravenously once daily OR Ciprofloxacin, 400 mg intravenously twice daily‡

*These are consensus recommendations of the CDC Working Group on Civilian Biodefense and are not necessarily approved by the FDA. See the "Therapy" section for explanations. One antimicrobial agent should be selected. Therapy should continue for 10 days. Oral therapy should be substituted when the patient's condition improves.

†Aminoglycosides must be adjusted according to renal function. Evidence suggests that gentamicin, 5 mg/kg intramuscularly or intravenously once daily, would be efficacious in children, although this is not yet widely accepted clinical practice. Neonates up to 1 week of age and premature infants should receive gentamicin, 2.5 mg/kg intravenously twice a day.

‡Other fluoroquinolones can be substituted at doses appropriate for the patient's age. Ciprofloxacin dosage should not exceed 1 g/day in children.

§Concentration should be maintained between 5 and 20 μg/mL. Concentrations greater than 25 μg/mL can cause reversible bone marrow suppression.

‖For children, ciprofloxacin dosage should not exceed 1 g/day, and chloramphenicol dosage should not exceed 4 g/day. Children younger than 2 years should not receive chloramphenicol.

¶For neonates, a gentamicin-loading dose of 4 mg/kg should be given initially.

Adapted from: Inglesby TV, Dennis DT, Henderson DA, et al: Plague as a biological weapon: Medical and public health management. *JAMA* 2000;283:2281-2290.

Table 9-12 Recommendations for the Treatment of Pneumonic Plague in Mass-Casualty Settings and for Postexposure Prophylaxis

Patient Category	Recommended Therapy*
Adults	**Preferred choices:** Doxycycline, 100 mg orally twice daily** OR Ciprofloxacin, 500 mg orally twice daily‡ **Alternative choice:** Chloramphenicol, 25 mg/kg orally four times daily§,††
Children‖	**Preferred choice:** Doxycycline,** ≥ 45 kg: administer the adult dosage < 45 kg: 2.2 mg/kg orally twice daily AND Ciprofloxacin, 20 mg/kg orally twice daily **Alternative choice:** Chloramphenicol, 25 mg/kg orally four times daily§,††
Pregnant women¶	**Preferred choice:** Doxycycline, 100 mg orally twice daily AND Ciprofloxacin, 500 mg orally twice daily **Alternative choice:** Chloramphenicol, 25 mg/kg orally four times daily§,††

*These are consensus recommendations of the CDC Working Group on Civilian Biodefense and are not necessarily approved by the FDA. See the "Therapy" section for explanations. One antimicrobial agent should be selected. Therapy should continue for 10 days. Oral therapy should be substituted when the patient's condition improves.

‡Other fluoroquinolones can be substituted at doses appropriate for the patient's age. Ciprofloxacin dosage should not exceed 1 g/day in children.

§Concentration should be maintained between 5 and 20 μg/mL. Concentrations greater than 25 μg/mL can cause reversible bone marrow suppression.

‖For children, ciprofloxacin dosage should not exceed 1 g/day, and chloramphenicol dosage should not exceed 4 g/day. Children younger than 2 years should not receive chloramphenicol.

¶For neonates, a gentamicin-loading dose of 4 mg/kg should be given initially.

#The duration of treatment of plague in mass-casualty setting is 10 days. The duration of postexposure prophylaxis to prevent plague infection is 7 days.

**Tetracycline could be substituted for doxycycline.

††Children younger than 2 years should not receive chloramphenicol. The oral formulation is available only outside of the United States.

Adapted from: Inglesby TV, Dennis DT, Henderson DA, et al: Plague as a biological weapon: Medical and public health management. *JAMA* 2000;283:2281-2290.

dissipation of the organism at the site of release would occur by the time the disease first presented to an emergency department. A risk of environmental contamination would occur if the organism seeded local rodents.

The bioengineered organisms, however, may not follow the historical model of *Y pestis*. Contamination with these gene-engineered organisms may require protocols similar to those developed for the longer lasting anthrax spores.

Vaccines

A plague vaccine is available, but it probably does not protect against an aerosol exposure and subsequent pneumonic plague. The usual dose is 0.5 mL given at 0, 1, and 2 weeks. Current whole-cell plague vaccines stimulate immunity against the bubonic form but are probably not ef-

Table 9-13 Protection Against Plague

Inactivation Requirements	Decontaminating Agents	Personal Protection Requirements
Moist heat at 250°F (121°C) for more than 15 minutes Dry heat at 320° to 338°F (160° to 170°C) for more than 1 hour	1% bleach 70% ethanol 2% glutaraldehyde Formaldehyde Iodines Phenols	Strictly isolate patients. Wear gloves, a gown, and a mask. (An impermeable protective garment is strongly recommended when dealing with this agent.) Wear a full-face respirator during the treatment of patients with pneumonic plague. Ensure protection from fleas. Decontaminate equipment before disposal with standard decontamination solutions.

Source: American Academy of Orthopaedic Surgeons, Stewart CE, Nixon RG. *Weapons of Mass Casualties Field Guide.* Jones and Bartlett Publishers, Boston; 2003.

fective against the pneumonic form.[58,59] In the United States, these preparations were discontinued in 1999 and are currently unavailable.

Plague vaccines providing protection against aerosol exposure are not yet available, but are under development.[60] One formulation shows promise for protection against aerosol delivery and protection against pneumonic plague.[61] Interestingly, an oral administration of a mutated *Salmonella typhimurium* bacterium protects mice against the subcutaneous inoculation of a virulent strain of plague.[62] These developments show great promise for an easily made and administered prophylaxis and treatment for plague.

Biosafety

This organism is quite easily spread by aerosol transmission. Secondary infection is very common, and respiratory droplet protection is mandatory for caregivers. Gowns, gloves, and eye protection should be worn by all persons caring for patients infected with pneumonic plague.

Routine testing should be conducted in a biosafety Level 2 laboratory, while any cultures should be grown in a biosafety Level 3 laboratory or better. Activities that generate a high potential for aerosol or droplet exposure (such as centrifuging, grinding, and studying animals) require biosafety Level 3 conditions. Bodies of patients who have died from plague should be handled with strict precautions. Aerosol-generating procedures, such as bone sawing, during postmortem examinations should be avoided or performed in a biosafety Level 3 facility.[63]

This disease is readily contagious, and strict isolation of the infected patients is essential. Both droplet and aerosol transmission is possible with pneumonic plague.[64] Patients infected with pneumonic plague should be isolated to at least protect against droplet transmission.[65] This isolation includes the use of surgical masks when standing within 1 meter of a patient, when other special ventilation precautions are not taken. The more stringent standard-of-care, which requires well-ventilated rooms with negative-pressure ventilation and class N95 respirators, is advocated by some.[66]

If large numbers of patients make isolation procedures impossible, pneumonic plague patients may be combined in one facility (cohorted). During transport to the facility, patients should be masked, and EMS personnel should wear gloves, a gown, and eye protection. After transport, emergency service vehicles and hospital rooms should be cleaned according to standard precautions. Linens and clothing used by patients may be disinfected with standard hospital protocols.

As noted earlier, pets are quite susceptible to plague.[67] Pet owners should be instructed to keep cats and dogs indoors or restrained within confines and to periodically treat them with antiflea medications. Because plague in cats is particularly contagious, persons caring for sick cats should take the same precautions as if they were treating a plague-infected human. **Table 9-13** lists biosafety information for plague.

■ Psittacosis

Psittacosis (also known as parrot fever, ornithosis, or chlamydiosis) is a bacterial zoonotic disease caused by *Chlamydia psittaci*. The term psittacosis was derived from the Greek word for parrot, psittakos, and was first used by Morange in 1892. The chlamydial organism is capable of being transmitted from birds to humans, but this rarely occurs despite the relatively high incidence of infection in birds. Waste material in birdcages may remain infectious for weeks. Person-to-person transmission has been reported when virulent avian strains are encountered.

Distribution and Epidemiology

C psittaci is found principally in psittacine birds (such as parrots, parakeets, and lovebirds), less often in pigeons and canaries, and occasionally in snowy egrets and some seabirds (such as herring gulls, petrels, and fulmars). Birds in the parrot family (such as parrots, macaws, cockatiels, and parakeets) are the most frequent source of infection. Other birds, particularly turkeys and pigeons, may also spread the disease. (The term ornithosis is often used to describe infection by nonpsittacine birds.) Some strains of *C psittaci* can infect sheep, goats, and cows and may cause chronic infection and abortion.

Both sick and apparently healthy birds may shed *C psittaci* bacteria, especially when stressed by crowding or shipping. Humans usually become infected by breathing dust from dried droppings or respiratory discharges that

INHOSPITAL INFO

have been put into the air. Because this disease is spread by birds in the parrot family, it is occasionally found in pet-store workers and people who have purchased an infected bird. It may also be found in farmers and slaughterhouse workers who process turkeys and other birds. Person-to-person transmission occurs rarely, if ever.

History

The largest natural epidemic of psittacosis occurred in 1930 and affected about 800 people. This epidemic led to the isolation of *C psittaci* in laboratories in Europe and the United States.

In the United States, reports of psittacosis occur about 200 times per year.[68] There is no known vaccine or prophylaxis for this disease. Because cultures of this disease are easily obtained, it may appeal to terrorists. Psittacosis could be easily aerosolized as a biowarfare agent.

Presentation

The incubation period is about 1 to 2 weeks. The longest observed incubation period was 54 days. After the incubation period, the course of the disease may range from a very mild presentation to severe pneumonia that requires mechanical ventilation. Psittacosis is usually a mild to moderate illness, but it can be severe, especially in untreated older individuals. A few infected individuals may develop acute respiratory failure, sepsis, and subsequent septic shock.

After the incubation period, the onset may be insidious or abrupt and may cause fever, chills, general malaise, and anorexia. Early symptoms include fever, nausea, vomiting, headache, and muscular pains. The patient's temperature gradually rises, and cough develops—initially dry but at times containing both mucus and pus. During the second week, pneumonia and frank consolidation may occur with secondary purulent lung infection. The patient's temperature remains elevated for 2 to 3 weeks, then falls slowly.

Relative bradycardia is common (the pulse elevation that normally occurs with fever is often absent). A progressive, pronounced increase in pulse and respiratory rates is an ominous sign. Mortality may reach 30% in severe untreated epidemics, and even higher rates are reported with virulent strains.

Patients may develop "Horder spots," which are rashes that resemble the "rose spots" of typhoid fever but appear on the face. Patients may also develop the rash of **erythema multiforme** and **erythema nodosum** (a subcutaneous skin nodule).

A prolonged convalescence may be likely in severe cases. Later in the course of the disease, the patients may experience delirium and disorientation. The course of the disease may last 3 to 4 weeks, causing a fatality rate of approximately 10%.

Psittacosis may be spread from human to human. This is more common with the virulent avian strains and would be expected to occur in strains selected for biowarfare. In general, the disease contracted by human-to-human transmission is more virulent.

The most common symptoms of infected patients are as follows:

- Fever (seen in 50% to 90% of patients)
  - Chills
- Malaise
  - Muscle aches
- Sore throat
- Epistaxis
- Cough, often nonproductive (seen in 50% to 90% of patients)
  - Rales and rhonchi
  - Dyspnea
- Headache
  - Photophobia
- Abdominal pain
  - Nausea and vomiting are uncommon

Diagnosis

INHOSPITAL INFO

There is no rapid diagnostic test for this disease. Blood tests at the start of the illness and 2 to 3 weeks later are usually necessary to confirm the diagnosis. Psittacosis is confirmed by recovery of the agent or by serologic complement fixation tests. (Complement fixation is not a specific test and may cross-react with other chlamydial species.)

Although a culture of *C psittaci* is possible, it may be hazardous to the laboratory workers. Biosafety Level 2 protection or greater should be used when handling the culture of this organism.

In the United States, serum specimens obtained early in the disease and in late convalescence may be submitted to the CDC. Acute-phase serum and convalescent-phase serum are examined 2 weeks after onset of the illness to confirm a fourfold or greater rise in the titer to *C psittaci*. This would be of little use in the acute management of a bioterrorist attack, but would confirm the agent.

Immunofluorescence and polymerase chain reaction studies are being investigated for the development of an early and specific test. Enzyme-linked immunosorbent assay (ELISA) and direct immunofluorescence are also experimental, but they have been used to diagnose psittacosis.

Clinical differentiation from other atypical pneumonias is difficult. Initially, psittacosis may be confused with influenza, typhoid fever, mycoplasmal pneumonia, legionnaires' disease, or Q fever.

Chest radiographs during the first week show pneumonitis radiating from the hilum; migratory lesions may be present. The most common finding is a unilateral, lower-lobe dense infiltrate or consolidation. Pathologic changes are those of a pneumonitis with a mononuclear cell exudate, as in other primary atypical pneumonias. Chest radiographs are abnormal for about 90% of patients and resolve in about 6 weeks.

Therapy

INHOSPITAL INFO

The administration of 1 to 2 g of tetracycline per day by mouth in divided doses every six hours or 100 mg of doxycycline by mouth, twice daily, is effective. Fever and other symptoms usually subside within 48 to 72 hours, but the antibiotic should be continued for at least 10 days. **Table 9-14** lists the suggested therapy for psittacosis.

Quinolones have been used for treatment of this disease, but quinolone failures have been observed. The use of Cipro and similar quinolones may not be appropriate.

Strict bed rest, supplemental oxygen, and control of the cough are appropriate. Severe cases may need intubation and respiratory support.

Table 9-14	Suggested Therapy for Psittacosis
Preferred choices	**Doxycycline** **Adult dose:** 100 mg orally twice daily for 2 to 3 weeks OR 4.4 mg/kg orally every 12 hours for severe cases **Pediatric dose:** 2 mg/kg/day orally or intravenously in two divided doses on the first day, then 1 to 2 mg/kg/day in two divided doses for 2 to 3 weeks, not to exceed 200 mg/day for children older than 8 years and/or over 45 kg (This drug is not recommended for children younger than 8 years.) OR **Tetracycline** **Pediatric dose:** 3 to 5 mg/kg/day intravenously in two divided doses for 2 to 3 weeks (Doxycycline is usually preferred.)
Alternative choices	**Erythromycin** **Adult dose:** 500 mg erythromycin stearate/base (or 800 mg ethylsuccinate) orally four times daily for 2 to 3 weeks (This may be increased up to 4 g per day depending on the severity of infection.) **Pediatric dose:** 30 to 50 mg/kg/day orally divided into 3 or 4 doses per day for 2 to 3 weeks (Double the dose for severe infections.) This is the drug of choice for children younger than 9 years and in pregnant women. As with all chlamydial species, related macrolides, such as azithromycin, would be expected to be effective. OR **Chloramphenicol** **Adult dose:** 500 mg intravenously four times a day for 2 to 3 weeks **Pediatric dose:** 50 to 100 mg/kg/day divided in four doses intravenously for 2 to 3 weeks (Hematologic complications of chloramphenicol are common, and blood studies should be performed every second or third day.)

Adapted from: Gregory DW, Schaffner W. Psittacosis. *Semin Respir Infect.* 1997 Mar;12(1):7-11.

Prophylaxis

Infection does not provide permanent immunity to psittacosis. There is no known immunization for this disease.

Biosafety

Standard body substance isolation should be employed when dealing with patients infected with psittacosis. Most household detergents and disinfectants, such as diluted household bleach (2% or 2 tablespoons of bleach mixed with one gallon of water), rubbing alcohol, or diluted Lysol disinfectant cleaner (1%), kill *C psittaci* bacteria.

Cultures of this organism may be hazardous to laboratory workers. Biosafety Level 2 or 3 is recommended for cultures. **Table 9-15** summarizes biosafety information for psittacosis.

■ Tularemia

Tularemia, also known as rabbit fever, is a widespread bacterial zoonosis caused by *Francisella tularensis*.[69] There are two strains of tularemia based on virulence testing (biovars):

- *F tularensis* biovar *tularensis* is recovered from rodents and ticks. It is highly virulent for rabbits and humans (hence the name *rabbit fever*). This more virulent *tularensis* biovar is prevalent in the United States.
- *F tularensis* biovar *palearctica* is more common outside the United States. It is not particularly virulent for either rabbits or humans. It is recovered from mosquitoes and aquatic mammals.

Tularemia is one of the most infectious pathogenic bacteria known.[70,71] As few as 10 organisms can cause disease in humans. Tularemia can infect humans through the skin, mucous membranes, gastrointestinal tract, and lungs. Humans can contract this disease naturally by the handling of an infected animal or by the bite of ticks, mosquitoes, or deerflies. The natural disease has a mortality rate of 5% to 10%.

Although tularemia does not form spores, it is quite hardy. Tularemia can remain viable for weeks in water, decaying animal carcasses, and soil. It is resistant for months to temperatures below freezing. As few as 10 organisms can cause disease in humans if inhaled. Many more are required for infection through ingestion. This organism can be produced in either a wet or dry preparation, and it can be employed similarly to other bacteria discussed in this publication. Tularemia can be spread in many ways.

Table 9-15	Protection Against Psittacosis	
Inactivation Requirements	Decontaminating Agents	Personal Protection Requirements
Moist heat at 250°F (121°C) for more than 15 minutes	Alcohol	Wear gloves, a gown, and a respirator.
	1% bleach	Decontaminate soiled items before disposal.
Dry heat at 320° to 338°F (160° to 170°C) for more than 1 hour	Glutaraldehyde	Decontaminate equipment before disposal with standard decontamination solutions.
	Formaldehyde	

Source: American Academy of Orthopaedic Surgeons, Stewart CE, Nixon RG. *Weapons of Mass Casualties Field Guide.* Jones and Bartlett Publishers, Boston; 2003.

Distribution and Epidemiology

The worldwide incidence of naturally-occurring tularemia is unknown. Tularemia occurs throughout the United States, Europe, the Middle East, Russia, and Japan. In Europe, tularemia has been reported most frequently in northern Europe, particularly in the Scandinavian countries and those of the former Soviet Union. It is rarely reported in the United Kingdom, Africa, Central America, and South America.

Tularemia is endemic in the United States and has been reported in every state except Hawaii. Most cases in the United States are reported in Arkansas, Illinois, Texas, Missouri, Virginia, and Tennessee. In the United States, tularemia occurs most frequently in June through September, when arthropod-borne transmission is most common. Winter cases are more common among hunters who handle infected animals.

The principle reservoir of tularemia in the United States is the tick, and more than 10 species have been identified as carriers of the disease. It is passed from generation to generation of ticks. It is probably transmitted to mammals via the tick's feces. (The bacterium is not found in the salivary glands of the tick.) In the United States, the most common mammal associated with tularemia is the rabbit.

In other areas of the world, particularly the former Soviet Union, tularemia is found in water rats and other aquatic mammals. During World War II, tularemia was epidemic in Russia because of the disruption of normal sanitation. Hundreds of thousands of troops and civilians contracted tularemia from contaminated water.[72]

History

Tularemia was discovered by Dr. G. W. McCoy in Tulare County, California, as the cause of a plaguelike illness in local ground squirrels, although the term tularemia was first described in 1921 by Dr. Edward Francis.[73-75] The first confirmed case was reported in 1914.[76]

Tularemia has long been considered to be a potential biological warfare weapon. It was one of the agents used by Unit 731 of the Japanese Army during World War II. Tularemia was investigated and then stockpiled by the United States during the 1950s and 1960s for use as a bioweapon. During the Cold War, a drug-resistant tularemia strain was developed by the Soviet Union. The Soviet Union may have developed a version of tularemia suitable for long-term storage and subsequent aerosol dispersion.

In 1970, the WHO used modeling techniques to develop a scenario of tularemia dispersion over a city of 5 million people. The WHO estimated that over 250,000 infections and 19,000 deaths would result from such a scenario. The model employed a preparation that remained viable for only 2 hours and was spread over only 20 km.

Presentation

F tularensis can infect humans through the skin, mucous membranes, gastrointestinal tract, and lungs. Natural tularemia can be spread by arthropods; direct contact; ingestion of contaminated food, soil, or water; handling infectious tissues of animals; or inhalation of infective aerosols.

Untreated, bacilli that are inoculated into the skin or mucous membranes will multiply and spread rapidly to regional lymph nodes. There, they will further multiply and may be disseminated to the target organs. The major target organs are the lymph nodes, lungs and pleura, spleen, liver, and kidney.

The onset of tularemia is rapid and includes a high fever of 100.4° to 104°F (38° to 40°C), headache, chills and rigors, body and lower back aches, coryza (acute inflammation of the mucous membranes of the nose), and sore throat. The pulse in tularemia may not reflect the fever measured. The patient may develop a dry or slightly productive cough. Substernal pain and tightness may be noted by the patient who is developing pneumonia. Nausea, vomiting, and diarrhea may occur. The patient may experience sweats, chills, progressive weakness, and anorexia.

In general, tularemia tends to be slower in development and tends to cause fewer casualties than either anthrax or plague.

Like plague, tularemia has a glandular form, a pneumonic form, and a septicemic form. It also has an ulceroglandular form, an oculoglandular form, and an oropharyngeal form, which are not seen with plague. The primary clinical forms vary in severity and presentation according to the virulence of the infecting strain, the dose of organism, and the site of the inoculum.

Ulceroglandular Tularemia

Ulceroglandular tularemia is the most common natural form of tularemia. Patients with ulceroglandular tularemia develop lesions on the skin or mucous membranes (including the conjunctival membranes), lymph nodes larger than 1 cm in diameter, or both **(Color plate 9-9)**. The ulceroglandular form occurs through inoculation of the skin or mucous membranes with blood or tissue fluids from an infected animal or human.

The resulting hardened, nonhealing, punched-out ulcer lasts about 1 to 3 weeks. The patient may experience fever, chills, headache, and malaise. Inflammation of the lymph nodes is common, and the lymph nodes may be fluctuant and drain spontaneously. The skin lesion is usually located on the fingers of the hand where contact occurred.

A cutaneous ulcer occurs in about 60% of naturally occurring tularemia infections and is the most common sign of tularemia. The ulcer may have a heaped-up edge.

Glandular Tularemia

Glandular tularemia is the second most common form. The most commonly infected nodes are the inguinal and femoral lymph nodes in adults and the cervical nodes in children. No skin ulcer is noted.

Oculoglandular Tularemia

Oculoglandular tularemia occurs when the inoculum is in the eye or periorbital skin. Patients develop painful purulent conjunctivitis. Preauricular and cervical adenopathy may be found.

Oropharyngeal and Gastrointestinal Tularemia

Oropharyngeal and gastrointestinal tularemia occurs when tularemia bacilli are ingested.[77] Abdominal pain and fever may result from the ingestion of contaminated water in endemic areas. It may also infect the oropharynx in about 25% of patients. The pharynx may be red or the patient may develop ecchymoses, ulcers, or exudates.

Septicemic Tularemia

The septicemic form can occur in 5% to 15% of natural cases. The clinical features include fever, prostration, and weight loss. The disease (also called typhoidal tularemia) has a mortality rate of between 30% and 60%. As few as 50 organisms can cause disease in humans if inhaled.

Pneumonic Tularemia

The primary pneumonic form may occur by inhaling naturally contaminated dusts or a deliberate aerosol. The onset will occur 3 to 5 days after the exposure to dust or aerosol. Fever, cough, headache, muscle aches, pharyngitis, and possibly gastroenteritis will occur prior to the onset of pneumonia.

Pneumonia may also occur with any of the other mentioned presentations of tularemia. Pneumonia is common when tularemia causes pharyngitis, probably reflecting a progression down the respiratory tract. The progression of tularemia from ulceroglandular disease to the pneumonic form occurs in 10% to 30% of patients. Up to 80% of septicemic cases progress to pulmonary involvement. The higher association of pneumonia with the septic form probably accounts for the higher mortality associated with this form of the disease.

The resulting pneumonia is atypical, variable, and may be fulminant. Hemorrhagic inflammation of the airways may be found early in the course of illness. Fever, headache, malaise, substernal discomfort, and cough are prominent. The cough is often nonproductive. The examiner may note objective signs of pneumonia, such as purulent sputum, dyspnea, tachypnea, pleuritic pain, and hemoptysis. Pleuritis with adhesion and effusion and mediastinal adenopathy (enlarged nodes of the mediastinum) are common.

Alternate Classification Scheme

Tularemia is divided by some authorities into the ulceroglandular form (75% of patients) and the typhoidal form (25% of patients), based on the clinical signs. As noted above, patients with ulceroglandular tularemia develop lesions on the skin or mucous membranes (including the conjunctival membranes), lymph nodes larger than 1 cm in diameter, or both. Patients with the typhoidal variant develop smaller lymph nodes; they do not develop cutaneous or mucous membrane lesions.

Diagnosis

The diagnosis of pneumonic tularemia will be difficult clinically, because there are several types of atypical pneumonia. The laboratory is unhelpful during the early stages of this disease. Rapid diagnostic testing for tularemia is not widely available. Respiratory secretions and blood should be collected. The laboratory should be alerted that there is a possibility of tularemia, so that appropriate precautions may be taken.

Bacterial agglutination or ELISA serologic testing will give the most diagnostic information. Microscopic demonstration of *F tularensis* can be performed using fluorescent-labeled antibodies in selected National Public Health Network labs. If the lab is alerted and prepared, results may be available within a few hours.

A culture of tularemia is the definitive means of confirming the diagnosis of tularemia. This may be best done on a cysteine-enriched media. Pharyngeal washings, sputum specimens, and fasting gastric aspirates are useful for cultures. White blood cell counts may be elevated. Lymphocytosis may be seen late in the disease. Blood cultures are not usually helpful.

A chest radiograph may or may not show pneumonia. About 50% of patients will develop pneumonia that can be seen on a chest radiograph. Patients with pneumonia may also have a pleural effusion.

Therapy

Recommended treatment is parenteral streptomycin or gentamicin for 10 to 14 days. Tetracycline and chloramphenicol are also useful, but the US military reports that there is a significant relapse rate with both tetracycline and chloramphenicol. The US military recommends that these agents be administered for a minimum of 14 days. A fully streptomycin-resistant strain of tularemia is known to exist. Ciprofloxacin is recommended for therapy and prophylaxis of both children and adults.

The clinician should be aware that drug-resistant organisms may be used by biological terrorists. Antimicrobial susceptibility testing should be conducted on all specimens. The clinical deterioration of patients despite early presumptive therapy could indicate antimicrobial resistance and should be promptly evaluated.

Tables 9-16 and **9-17** list the treatment and prophylaxis of tularemia in a mass-casualty situation.

Prophylaxis

Persons who begin treatment with an appropriate antibiotic during the incubation period of tularemia and continue this treatment for 14 days appear to be protected against symptomatic infection. Treatment for those who have been exposed is appropriate and may prevent many infections. Once tularemia is confirmed or strongly suspected in an area, anyone in that area with fever of 101.3°F (38.5°C) or higher should be immediately treated with the appropriate antibiotics for a presumptive tularemia infection. Postexposure treatment of close contacts is unnecessary, because tularemia does not spread from person to person.

Human-to-human transmission is unusual, and isolation is not required. Laboratory workers are at high risk of contagion, however. Laboratories should be alerted that tularemia is suspected. These specimens are best handled in a Level 3 laboratory, although, with extreme care, a Level 2 laboratory may be able to safely manage the samples.

A live vaccine strain is available to US military personnel and laboratory workers who handle this bacterium. This vaccine is delivered intradermally and provides protection against an aerosol challenge by the third week after immunization. However, protection is dependent on the inhaled dose of tularemia, and the inhalation of massive quantities of bacteria may overwhelm the protective effects of the vaccine.[78] Protection falls after 14 months, suggesting that a booster dose is appropriate. This vaccine is not routinely available for civilian use, but is under review by the FDA.

Table 9-16 Recommendations for the Treatment of Tularemia in Contained-Casualty Settings and for Postexposure Prophylaxis

Patient Category	Recommended Therapy*
Adults	**Preferred choices:** Streptomycin, 1g intramuscularly twice daily OR Gentamicin, 5 mg/kg intramuscularly or intravenously once daily† **Alternative choices:** Doxycycline, 100 mg intravenously twice daily OR Chloramphenicol, 15 mg/kg intravenously four times daily OR Ciprofloxacin, 400 mg intravenously twice daily†
Children	**Preferred choices:** Streptomycin, 15 mg/kg intramuscularly twice daily (not to exceed 2 g/day) OR Gentamicin, 2.5 mg/kg intramuscular or intravenously three times daily† **Alternative choices:** Doxycycline, $\geq$ 45 kg: 100 mg intravenously twice daily < 45 kg: 2.2 mg/kg intravenously twice daily OR Chloramphenicol, 15 mg/kg intravenously four times daily† OR Ciprofloxacin, 15 mg/kg intravenously twice daily‡
Pregnant women	**Preferred choices:** Gentamicin, 5 mg/kg intramuscular or intravenously once daily† OR Streptomycin, 1 g intramuscularly twice daily **Alternative choices:** Doxycycline, 100 mg intravenously twice daily OR Ciprofloxacin, 400 mg intravenously twice daily†

*One antibiotic (appropriate for the patient's age) should be chosen from among the alternatives. Treatment with streptomycin, gentamicin, or ciprofloxacin should be continued for 10 days; treatment with doxycycline or chloramphenicol should be continued for 14 to 21 days. Persons beginning treatment with intramuscular or intravenous doxycycline, ciprofloxacin, or chloramphenicol may switch to oral antibiotic administration when clinically indicated.

†This is not an FDA-approved use.

‡Ciprofloxacin dosage should not exceed 1 g/day in children.

Adapted from: Dennis DT, Inglesby TV, Henderson DA, et al. Tularemia as a biological weapon: Medical and public health management. Working Group on Civilian Biodefense. *JAMA.* 2001;285:2763-2773.

Table 9-17 Recommendations for the Treatment of Tularemia in Mass-Casualty Settings and for Postexposure Prophylaxis

Patient Category	Recommended Therapy*
Adults	**Preferred choices:** Doxycycline, 100 mg orally twice daily OR Ciprofloxacin, 500 mg orally twice daily†
Children	**Preferred choices:** Doxycycline, and $\geq$ 45 kg: 100 mg orally twice daily < 45 kg: 2.2 mg/kg orally twice daily OR Ciprofloxacin, 15 mg/kg orally twice daily‡
Pregnant women	**Preferred choices:** Ciprofloxacin, 500 mg orally twice daily† OR Doxycycline, 100 mg orally twice daily

*One antibiotic (appropriate for the patient's age) should be chosen from among the alternatives. Treatment with streptomycin, gentamicin, or ciprofloxacin should be continued for 10 days; treatment with doxycycline or chloramphenicol should be continued for 14 to 21 days. Persons beginning treatment with intramuscular or intravenous doxycycline, ciprofloxacin, or chloramphenicol may switch to oral antibiotic administration when clinically indicated.

†This is not an FDA-approved use.

‡Ciprofloxacin dosage should not exceed 1 g/day in children

Adapted from: Dennis DT, Inglesby TV, Henderson DA, et al. Tularemia as a biological weapon: Medical and public health management. Working Group on Civilian Biodefense. *JAMA.* 2001;285:2763-2773.

Postexposure prophylaxis with ciprofloxacine, doxycycline, or tetracycline is recommended when aerosol exposure is known. This should be started within 24 hours of the exposure and continued for 2 weeks. Note that these are the same agents recommended for plague and anthrax.

Biosafety

This organism is quite easily spread by aerosol transmission. Person-to-person transmission is very uncommon. However, gowns, gloves, and eye protection should be worn by all persons caring for pneumonic tularemia cases.

Routine testing should be conducted in the same way as for plague, in a biosafety Level 2 laboratory, while any cultures should be grown in a biosafety Level 3 laboratory or better. Activities that generate a high potential for aerosol or droplet exposure (such as centrifuging, grinding, studying animals) require biosafety Level 3 conditions. Bodies of patients who have died from tularemia should be handled with standard precautions. Aerosol generating procedures, such as bone sawing, during postmortem examinations should be avoided or performed in a biosafety Level 3 facility.

As noted, this disease is not very contagious through person-to-person transmission, and strict isolation of the patients is unnecessary. Contaminated linens and

Table 9-18 Protection Against Tularemia		
Inactivation Requirements	Decontaminating Agents	Personal Protection Requirements
Moist heat at 250°F (121°C) for more than 15 minutes Dry heat at 320° to 338°F (160° to 170°C) for more than 1 hour	1% bleach 70% ethanol Glutaraldehyde Formaldehyde	Strict isolation of patients is NOT required. (This agent is not very contagious by person-to-person transmission, but aerosol cough may be contagious from both animals and persons.) Wear gloves, a gown, and a mask. Wear a full-face respirator during the treatment of patients with pneumonic tularemia. Take secretion precautions when dealing with infected people or animals. Decontaminate equipment before disposal with standard decontamination solutions.

Source: American Academy of Orthopaedic Surgeons, Stewart CE, Nixon RG. *Weapons of Mass Casualties Field Guide.* Jones and Bartlett Publishers, Boston; 2003.

clothing can be decontaminated with standard hospital procedures.

Tularemia can survive for long periods in cold, moist conditions. It has been suggested that the public can be protected by being taught to avoid sick or dead animals and to take precautions against biting arthropods. If an aerosol release occurs while temperatures outside are cool, and if the area of release is known, then decontamination efforts may be quite appropriate even days or weeks after the event. A bleach solution of 0.5% would be expected to be quite effective in this regard. **Table 9-18** summarizes biosafety information for tularemia.

Typhoid Fever

Typhoid fever is caused by *Salmonella typhi*, which is also known a *S typhosa*. Typhoid fever is a different disease from typhus, which is caused by *Rickettsia typhi* (endemic typhus) and *R prowazekii* (epidemic typhus), both of which are spread by lice. (The latter two diseases are covered in Chapter 12: "Rickettsial Agents.")

Distribution and Epidemiology

The natural host of typhoid fever is the human. Typhoid is contracted by ingesting food or water that is contaminated by the stool of infected individuals. Common sources of such contamination are shellfish taken from sewage-contaminated waters and fruits and vegetables fertilized with human feces.

History

Major typhoid fever outbreaks have been associated with war, including outbreaks among the army of the Holy Roman Emperor Henry IV as he attempted to conquer Rome in 1081, the army of the first crusade in Syria in 1098 after the siege of Antioch, and the armies of the American Civil War from 1861 to 1865.

Typhoid fever is also notable because it can be spread by asymptomatic carriers. The best known of these carriers is the infamous "Typhoid Mary" Mallon, who worked as a cook in New York and Maine. Typhoid Mary was identified as the source of at least 28 infections, beginning around 1900 and lasting until 1907. Unofficially, she is also believed to be responsible for an epidemic in 1903 in Ithaca, New York, which spread to the community and caused 1,400 cases of typhoid fever. She was taken into custody by New York health officials and was placed in quarantine on March 20, 1907 after providing a stool sample that contained high levels of *S typhi*. In 1910, she was released from quarantine when she promised she would never prepare food for others. She also promised that she would return every 3 months to the New York Health Department laboratory.

These promises proved fruitless for the health authorities. She resurfaced again in 1915, using the name Mrs. Brown and working as a cook in Sloane Maternity Hospital in Manhattan. During her 3 months there, she spread typhoid to at least 25 doctors, nurses, and staff; two of them died.

She was quarantined at North Brother Island for the remainder of her life (23 years), alone in a one-room cottage. She was certainly not the only known typhoid carrier. In 1938, when she died, a newspaper noted that there were 237 others living under city health department observation.

Presentation
Incubation Period

The incubation period of typhoid fever is 1 to 3 weeks. Symptoms include fever, headaches, constipation (which is reported to occur more often than diarrhea in adults), fatigue, and transient rose-colored spots, particularly on the abdomen. The symptoms range from fleeting to quite severe. The fatality rate of untreated typhoid fever is about 10%.

Treatment

Treatment is summarized in **Table 9-19.**

Drug resistance began to emerge in the early 1970s in Mexico and Vietnam. Within a few years, 75% of cases in Vietnam were resistant. Multidrug-resistant typhoid is common in developing countries. These strains may be resistant to trimethoprim-sulfamethoxazole, amoxicillin, and ampicillin.

Table 9-19 Treatment of Typhoid Fever

Patient Category	Recommended Therapy
Adults	**Preferred choice:** Ciprofloxacin, 500 mg orally twice daily **Alternative choices:** Ceftriaxone, 1 to 2 g intravenously once daily for 5 to 7 days OR Trimethoprim-sulfamethoxazole, amoxicillin, ampicillin, or other third-generation cephalosporins
Children*	**Preferred choice:** Ceftriaxone, 50 to 80 mg/kg intramuscularly or intravenously once daily for 5 to 7 days **Alternative choices:** Trimethoprim-sulfamethoxazole, amoxicillin, ampicillin, or other third-generation cephalosporins
Pregnant women	**Preferred choice:** Ceftriaxone, 1 to 2 g intravenously once daily for 5 to 7 days **Alternative choices:** Trimethoprim-sulfamethoxazole, amoxicillin, ampicillin, or other third-generation cephalosporins

*Children younger than 18 years should not use ciprofloxin or similar drugs, as they can cause severe connective tissue and cartilage problems.

Adapted from: Parry CM, Hien TT, Dougan G, et al. Typhoid fever. *N Engl J Med* 2002;347:1770–1782.

Table 9-20 Protection Against Typhoid Fever

Inactivation Requirements	Decontaminating Agents	Personal Protection Requirements
Moist heat at 250°F (121°C) for more than 15 minutes Dry heat at 320° to 338°F (160° to 170°C) for more than 1 hour	70% ethanol 2% glutaraldehyde 8% formaldehyde 0.5% bleach 10% hydrogen peroxide for 30 minutes at 20°C	Wear gloves and a gown. Take secretion precautions. Wash hands frequently with soap and water. Decontaminate equipment before disposal with standard decontamination solutions.

Source: American Academy of Orthopaedic Surgeons, Stewart CE, Nixon RG. *Weapons of Mass Casualties Field Guide.* Jones and Bartlett Publishers, Boston; 2003.

Prophylaxis

Several vaccines are available and are equally effective in decreasing risk by 50% to 75%. Because vaccination does not offer full protection from infection, care should be used in selecting food and drink.

Biosafety

Table 9-20 summarizes biosafety information for typhoid fever.

Threat

Typhoid is easily obtained and easily cultured with commonly available media. It causes severe debilitation and is easily dispersed. It kills thousands of people yearly in third

Table 9-21 Potential Biological Agents for Terrorism

Category	Characteristics	Organism
Category A: High-priority agents	• Can be easily disseminated or transmitted from person to person • Cause high mortality with a potential for a major impact on public health • May cause public panic and social disruption • Require special action for public health preparedness	• Anthrax • Plague • Tularemia
Category B: Second-priority agents	• Are moderately easy to disseminate • Cause moderate morbidity and low mortality • Require specific enhancements of the CDC's diagnostic capacity and disease surveillance	• Brucellosis • Cholera • Shigella • *Escherichia coli* O157:H7 • *Salmonella* species • *Burkolderia mallei* (glanders)
Category C: Third-priority agents (including organisms that are emerging pathogens that could be genetically engineered for mass dissemination)	• May be easily available • May be easily produced or disseminated • Have the potential for high morbidity and mortality and therefore may have a major impact on public health	• Multidrug-resistant tuberculosis

Notes: Melioidosis is also a potential bacterium for biowarfare but is not categorized by the CDC

Many agents in category B have been used or considered as biological weapons.

Preparedness for category C agents requires ongoing research into disease detection, diagnosis, treatment, and prevention.

Adapted from: Khan AS, Morse S, Lillibridge S: Public health preparedness for biological terrorism in the USA. *Lancet* 2000;356:1179-1182.

world countries. Typhoid was used as a biological weapon in World War II by the Japanese.

Summary

Included in this chapter are all of the diseases considered to be threats by the CDC. Although these diseases have been proposed by the CDC, the US military, and others as possible biological warfare agents, there is no question that the chapter is neither exhaustive nor all-inclusive.

Considering the current stage of gene manipulation, it is easy to foresee a chimera-tailored bacterium that has the characteristics of a deadly disease, is resistant to all usual antibiotics, and yet is responsive to an unusual antibiotic that the designer has stockpiled. It is equally easy to imagine a tailored virus that has unusual mortality for a certain genetic profile, such as Anglo-Saxon males.

One does not have to imagine an increase in lethality in order to find substantial biowarfare applications. A rapidly spreading upper respiratory illness, such as the common cold, that merely causes 3 days of cough, fever, rhinorrhea, and malaise could be incapacitating if an entire army caught it simultaneously. A city's police force would be unable to deal with terrorists effectively if over 75% of the city's entire population had uncontrollable diarrhea for a two-day or three-day course.

The problems cited in dispersal, control, mutability, and side effects that were previously discussed in the section on chemical warfare and the introduction to biological warfare are entirely applicable for these live biowarfare agents. **Table 9-21** summarizes potential biological agents and lists those considered threats by the CDC.

References

1. Albrink WS, Goodlow RJ: Experimental inhalation anthrax in the chimpanzee. *Am J Pathol* 1959;35:1055-1065.
2. Brachman P: Inhalation anthrax. *Ann NY Acad Sci* 1980;353:83-93.
3. Shafazand S, Doyle R, Ruoss S, Weinacker A, Raffin TA: Inhalational anthrax: Epidemiology and management. *Chest* 1999;116:1369.
4. Laforce FM: Anthrax. *Clin Infect Dis* 1994;19(6):1009-1013.
5. Stephenson J: Confronting a biological Armageddon: Experts tackles prospect of bioterrorism. *JAMA* 1996;276:349-351.
6. Interview with Dr. Ken Alibek, first deputy director of Biopreparat (transcript). "Frontline." PBS, 1998, http://www.pbs.org/wgbh/pages/frontline/shows/plague/sverdlovsk/alibekov.html (accessed March 6, 2004).
7. Alibek K: Behind the mask: Biological warfare. *Perspective* 1998;9:1-6.
8. Meselson M, Guillemin J, Hugh-Jones M, et al: The Sverdlovsk anthrax outbreak of 1979. *Science* 1994;266:1202-1208.
9. Weir E: Anthrax: Of bison and bioterrorism. *CMAJ* 2000;163:608.
10. Laforce FM: Anthrax. *Clin Infect Dis* 1994;19(6):1009-1013.
11. Anonymous: *Handbook on the Medical Aspects of NBC Defensive Operations.* Washington, DC, US Government Printing Office (Field Manual 8–9), 1996.
12. Henderson DA, Inglesby TV, Bartlett JG, et al: Anthrax as a biological weapon: Medical and public health management. *JAMA* 1999;281(18):1735-1745.
13. Anonymous: Bioterrorism alleging use of anthrax and interim guidelines for management: United States, 1998; *Morb Mortal Wkly Rep* 1999;48:69-74.
14. Nass M: Anthrax vaccine: Model of a response to the biologic warfare threat. *Infect Dis Clin North Am* 1999;13:187-208.
15. Shlyakhov EN, Rubinstein E: Human live anthrax vaccine in the former USSR. *Vaccine* 1994;12:727-730.
16. Cohen HW, Sidel VW, Gould RM: Prescriptions on bioterrorism have it backwards. Letter. *BMJ* 2000;320:1211.
17. Coulson NM, Fulop M, Titball RW: *Bacillus anthracis* protective antigen expressed in *Salmonella typhimurium SL 3261*, afford protection against spore challenge. *Vaccine* 1994;12:1395-1401.
18. Ivins B, Fellows P, Pitt L, et al: Experimental anthrax vaccines: Efficacy of adjuvants combined with protective antigen against an aerosol *Bacillus anthracis* spore challenge in guinea pigs. *Vaccine* 1995;13:1779-1794.
19. Henderson DA, Inglesby TV, Bartlett JG, et al: Anthrax as a biological weapon: Medical and public health management. *JAMA* 1999;281(18):1735-1745.
20. Chemical-biological terrorism and its impact on children: A subject review. *Pediatrics* 2000;105:662-670.
21. Al-Kaff AS: Ocular brucellosis. *Int Ophthalmol Clin* 1995;35:139-145.
22. Elrazak MA: Brucella optic neuritis. *Arch Intern Med* 1991;151:776-778.
23. Akdurman L, Or M, Hasanreisoglu B, Kutar K: A case of ocular brucellosis: Importance of vitreous specimen. *Acta Ophthalmol* 1993;71:130-132.
24. Sanford JP: Brucella pneumonia. *Semin Resp Infect* 1997;12:24.
25. Solera J, Martinez-Alfaro E, Espinosa A: Recognition and optimum treatment of brucellosis. *Drugs* 1997;53:245.
26. Memish Z, Mah MW, Al Mahmoud S, et al: Brucella bacteremia: Clinical and laboratory observations in 160 patients. *J Infect* 2000;40:59.
27. Morata P, Queipo-Ortuno MI, Reguera JM, et al: Posttreatment follow-up of brucellosis by PCR assay. *J Clin Microb* 1999;37:4163.
28. Joint FAO/WHO Expert committee on Brucellosis. Sixth Report. World Health Organization Technical Report Series Number 740. Geneva: World Health Organization, 1986.
29. Hoover DL, Friedlander AM. Brucellosis, in Zaitchik R, Bellamy RF. *Medical Aspects of Chemical and Biological Warfare.* Borden Institute; Washington, DC, 1997.
30. Ariza J, Gudiol F, Pallares R, Rufi G, Fernandez-Viladrich P. Comparative trial of rifampin-doxycycline versus tetracycline-streptomycin in the therapy of human brucellosis. *Antimicrob Agents Chemother* 1985;28:548-551.
31. Akova M, Uzun O, Akalin HE, Hayran M, Unal S, Gur D. Quinolones in the treatment of human brucellosis; comparative trial of ofloxacin-rifampin versus doxycycline-rifampin. *J Antimicrob Chemother* 1993;37:1831-1834.
32. Corbel MJ: Vaccines against bacterial zoonoses. *J Med Microbiol* 1997;46:267-269.
33. Anonymous: AFIP Wednesday Slide Conference—No. 24. Armed Forces Institute of Pathology, 1999, http://www.afip.org/vetpath/WSC/wsc98/98wsc24.htm (accessed May 29, 2002).
34. Srinivasan A, Krause CN, DeShazer D. Glanders in a military research microbiologist. *NEJM* 2001;345;256-258.

35. Kenny DJ, Russell P, Rogers D, Eley SM, Titball RW. In vitro susceptibilities of *Berkholderia mallei* in comparison to those of other pathogenic *Burkholderia* spp. *Antimicrob Agents Chemother* 1999;43:2773-2775.

36. Srinivasan A, Krause CN, DeShazer D. Glanders in a military research microbiologist. *NEJM* 2001;345;256-258.

37. Anonymous: Fatal human plague: Arizona and Colorado, 1996. *Morb Mortal Wkly Rep* 1997;46:617.

38. Mee C: How a mysterious disease laid low Europe's masses. *Smithsonian* 1990;20:66-79.

39. Bayliss JH: The extinction of bubonic plague in Britain. *Endeavor* 1980;4(2):58-66.

40. Bayliss JH: The extinction of bubonic plague in Britain. *Endeavor* 1980;4(2):58-66.

41. Bayliss JH: The extinction of bubonic plague in Britain. *Endeavor* 1980;4(2):58-66.

42. McEvedy C: The bubonic plague. *Sci Am* 1988; Feb;258(2):118-123.

43. McEvedy C: The bubonic plague. *Sci Am* 1988; Feb;258(2):118-123.

44. Ampel NM: Plagues: What's past is present: Thoughts on the origin and history of new infectious diseases. *Rev Infect Dis* 1991;13:658-665.

45. Inglesby TV, Dennis DT, Henderson DA, et al: Plague as a biological weapon: Medical and public health management. *JAMA* 2000;283:2281-2290.

46. Galimand M, Guiyoule A, Gerbaud, G, et al: Multidrug resistance in *Yersinia pestis* mediated by a transferable plasmid. *NEJM* 1997;337:677-680.

47. Alibek K, Handyman S: Biohazard. New York, NY, Random House, 1999.

48. Alibek K, Handelman S: *Biohazard.* New York, NY, Random House, 1999.

49. Alibek K, Handyman S: *Biohazard.* New York, NY, Random House, 1999.

50. Inglesby TV, Dennis DT, Henderson DA, et al: Plague as a biological weapon: Medical and public health management. *JAMA* 2000;283:2281-2290.

51. Anonymous: *Health Aspects of Chemical and Biological Weapons.* Geneva, Switzerland, World Health Organization, 1970, pp 98-109.

52. Inglesby TV, Grossman R, O'Toole T: A plague on your city: Observations from TOPOFF. *Clin Infect Dis* 2001;32:436-445.

53. Inglesby TV, Dennis DT, Henderson DA, et al: Plague as a biological weapon: Medical and public health management. *JAMA* 2000;283:2281-2290.

54. Craven RB: Plague, in Hoeprich PD, Jordan MC, Ronald AR (eds): *Infectious diseases: A Treatise of Infectious Processes,* ed 5. Philadelphia, PA, JB Lippincott, 1994: 1302-1312.

55. McSweegan E: *Yersinia pestis,* antibiotic resistance: Madagascar. ProMED-mail, September 4, 1997.

56. Galimand A, Guiyoule A, Gerbaud G, et al: Brief report: Multidrug resistance in *Yersinia pestis* mediated by a transferable plasmid. *NEJM* 1997;337:677-681.

57. Dennis D, Hughes J: Multidrug resistance in plague. *NEJM* 1997;337:702-704.

58. Meyer KF: Effectiveness of live or killed plague vaccines in man. *Bull WHO* 1970:42:653-666.

59. Russel P, Eley SM, Hibbs SE, et al: A comparison of plague vaccine, USP and EV76 vaccine induced protection against *Yersinia pestis* in a murine model. *Vaccine* 1995;13:1551-1556.

60. Oyston PCF, Williamson ED, Leary SE, et al: Immunization with live recombinant *Salmonella typhimurium* aroA producing F1 antigen protects against plague. *Infect Immun* 1995;63:563-568.

61. Eyles JE, Sharp GJE, Williamson ED, et al: Intranasal administration of poly-lactic acid microsphere co-encapsulated *Yersinia pestis* subunits confers protection from pneumonic plague in the mouse. *Vaccine* 1998;16:698-707.

62. Titball RW, Howells AM, Oyston PCF, Williamson ED: Expression of the *Yersinia pestis* capsular antigent (F1 antigen) on the surface of an aroA mutant of *Salmonella typhimurium* induces high levels of protections against plague. *Infect Immun* 1997;65:1926-1930.

63. Nolte KB: Safety precautions to limit exposure from plague-infected patients. *JAMA* 2000;284:1648-1649.

64. Levison ME: Safety precautions to limit exposure from plague-infected patients. *JAMA* 2000;284:1648-1649.

65. Inglesby TV, Dennis DT, Henderson DA, et al: Plague as a biological weapon: Medical and public health management. *JAMA* 2000;283:2281-2290.

66. Nolte KB: Safety precautions to limit exposure from plague-infected patients. Letter. *JAMA* 2000;284:1648-1649.

67. Anonymous: Fatal human plague: Arizona and Colorado, 1996. *Morb Mortal Wkly Rep*1997;46:617-620.

68. Committee of the National Association of State Public Health Veterinarians: Compendium of measures to control *Chlamydia psittaci* infection among humans (psittacosis) and pet birds (avian chlamydiosis), 2000. *Morb Mortal Wkly Rep* 2000;49:3-17.

69. Dennis DT, Inglesby TV, Henderson DA, et al: Tularemia as a biological weapon: Medical and public health management. *JAMA* 2001;285:2763-2773.

70. Lake GC, Francis E: Six cases of tularemia occurring in laboratory workers. *Public Health Rep* 1922;37:392-413.

71. Burke DS: Immunization against tularemia: Analysis of the effectiveness of live *Francisella tularensis* vaccine in prevention of laboratory acquired tularemia. *J Infect Dis* 1977;135:55-60.

72. McCrumb FR Jr: Aerosol infection of man with *Pasturella tularensis. Bacteriol Rev* 1961;25:262-267.

73. McCoy GW: Plague-like disease in rodents. *Public Health Bull* 1911;43:53-71.

74. McCoy GW, Chapin CW: Further observations on a plague-like disease of rodents with a preliminary note on the causative agent, *Bacterium tularense. J Infect Dis* 1912;10:61-72.

75. Frances E: Tularemia (Francis 1921), I: The occurrence of tularemia in nature as a disease of man. *Public Health Rep* 1921;36:1731-1751.

76. Wherry WB, Lamb BH: Infection of man with *Bacterium tularense. J Infect Disease* 1914;15:331-340.

77. Karpoff SP, Anatoff NI: The spread of tularemia through water, as a new factor in its epidemiology. *J Bacteriol* 1936;32:243-258.

78. Hornick RB, Eigelsbach HT: Aerogenic immunization of man with live tularemia vaccine. *Bact Rev* 1966:30;532-538.

Viral Agents

■ Introduction

Viruses are intracellular parasites. The main purpose of a virus is to use the host cell to replicate itself. A complete virus particle is called a **viron**. More than 30,000 different viruses have been identified. These viruses have been grouped in more than 3,600 species, in 164 genera, and 71 families. Only 21 of these families are of medical importance.

A virus must enter living cells in order to replicate. A common source of cells for viral cultures is the egg, but laboratory animals and cell cultures designed for the replication of viruses are also frequently used. The user must be able to keep these cells viable in order for the virus to multiply.

■ How Viruses Cause Disease

Pathogenesis is the process by which a virus causes a disease. The pathogenic mechanisms of viral disease differ from those of bacterial disease and are as follows:

1. Implantation of the virus at the site of entry into the body
2. Local replication of the virus within a cell
   - Viruses disseminate through the blood after an initial replication, causing no significant signs or symptoms of illness.
3. Spread to target organs
   - The most common route of systemic spread is the circulation system. The virus may enter the target organs by multiplying in the capillaries, diffusing into the vessels, or being carried within a migrating white blood cell **(Figure 10-1)**.
   - Dissemination by the nervous system occurs with rabies, herpes, and poliovirus infections.
4. Virus multiplication in the target organ, which may be sufficient to cause disease and death, depending on the balance between the virus and the host defenses
   - Disease occurs when the virus replicates in a sufficient number of essential target cells and destroys them.
   - Subclinical infections may occur when the host defenses are sufficient to prevent widespread dissemination of the virus.
5. Spread to sites of **shedding**, where the virus is released into the environment
   - Although the respiratory tract, gastrointestinal tract, and blood are the most frequent sites of viral shedding, viruses may be shed in skin, saliva, semen, and urine.

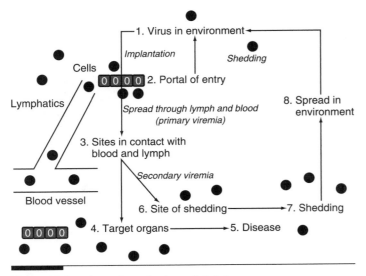

Figure 10-1 Pathogenic mechanisms of viral disease.

Virus	Examples
Table 10-1 Overview of Viruses Covered	
Influenza	
Paramyxoviruses	Nipah virus Hendra virus
Poxviruses	Smallpox Monkeypox
Togaviruses	**Alphaviruses** • Venezuelan equine encephalitis • Western equine encephalitis • Eastern equine encephalitis
Arboviruses	St. Louis encephalitis West Nile virus encephalitis
Hemorrhagic fever viruses	**Old World arenaviruses** • Lymphocytic choriomeningitis virus (LCM) • Lassa virus (causes Lassa fever) **New World arenaviruses** • Guanarito virus (causes Venezuelan hemorrhagic fever) • Junin virus (causes Argentine hemorrhagic fever) • Machupo virus (causes Bolivian hemorrhagic fever) • Sabia virus (causes Brazilian hemorrhagic fever) • North American Whitewater Arroyo virus **Bunyaviruses** • Hantavirus • Hemorrhagic fever with renal syndrome (HFRS) • Congo-Crimean hemorrhagic fever • Rift Valley fever virus **Filoviruses** • Ebola • Marburg **Flaviviruses (Flavaviruses)** • Yellow fever • Dengue

Because viruses cannot synthesize their genetic and structural components, they must rely on the host cell for these functions. The parasitic replication of a virus robs the host cell of energy and other important components. If enough cells in a vital organ are destroyed by this parasitism, the organ ceases to function, and the host dies.

The **incubation period** of a viral infection is the time between the exposure to the virus and the onset of clinical disease. During this time, the patient is often asymptomatic, but implantation, local multiplication, and spread of the virus are occurring.

The biological weapons variants of viral disease can be presumed to be far more dangerous than the natural variants. Although viruses can invade living cells through direct skin penetration and genital routes, the virus weapons most likely to be used by terrorists would be spread through the respiratory and gastrointestinal routes. These routes would most readily encourage the widespread dissemination of a disease.

The rest of this chapter discusses specific viruses, their signs and symptoms, and their treatment. The viruses covered in this chapter and the next one are summarized in **Table 10-1**.

■ Influenza

Pandemic **influenza** caused the worst single epidemic that occurred in the 20th century. It killed between 25 and 40 million people in a single year during the winter of 1918. In the United States alone, over 20 million cases were reported, resulting in over 1 million recorded deaths. In Philadelphia, 158 out of every 1,000 people died; in Baltimore, 148 out of 1,000; in Washington, DC, 109 out of 1,000. Sixty percent of the Eskimo population was wiped out in Nome, Alaska. Luxury ocean liners from Europe would arrive in New York with 7% fewer passengers than when they embarked. Known as Spanish flu or la grippe, the influenza epidemic of 1918 and 1919 was a global disaster. The 1957 Asian influenza pandemic and the 1968 Hong Kong influenza pandemic also killed millions, but they were far milder than the pandemic of the Spanish flu **(Figure 10-2)**.

The cause of the Spanish flu pandemic was a mutated swine virus. The actual killer was a pneumonia that accompanied the influenza infection. Eighteen months after the disease appeared, it vanished and has never shown up again. In 1997, the emergence of avian influenza in Hong Kong raised the specter of another global pandemic.

The astute clinician interested in biological terrorism should study this disease carefully. The spread of influenza, the measures used to control it, and the impact it can have on society reflect the issues that would be associated with any out-of-control bioterrorist agent (even if influenza were not used).

The influenza viruses are divided into three species (A, B, and C). These viruses cause influenza, which is usually a respiratory disease, but it often causes prominent systemic symptoms. Type A occurs in humans, birds, pigs, horses, and sea mammals. Types B and C are found only in humans.

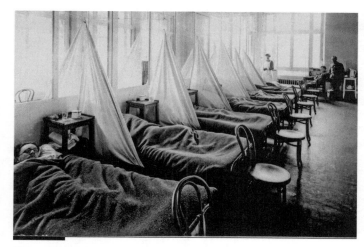

Figure 10-2 An emergency hospital for influenza patients.

Distribution

Influenza viruses differ from many other viral respiratory pathogens, because they cause annual epidemics that affect all age groups and also cause more serious pandemics (worldwide epidemics) that spread rapidly through populations. Epidemics of influenza A affect all age groups, but are especially dangerous to children and the elderly. They spread widely across regions and continents. Influenza B outbreaks usually take the form of a mild respiratory disease that tends to occur in children. Type B is associated with schools and other concentrated groups of children. Influenza C is an infrequent cause of mild respiratory illness in children.

History

As noted, type A viruses cause periodic pandemics. Both types A and B have caused recurring regional and local epidemics. Variations in influenza strains are responsible for the annual epidemics that occur between pandemics. Varied strains of influenza A and B viruses emerge and become predominant over about 2 to 5 years, only to be replaced by the next successful variant.

There have been three influenza pandemics during the 20th century. In 1918 and 1919, the Spanish flu caused over 1 million deaths in the United States and 25-40 million deaths worldwide. The Asian flu resulted in 70,000 US leaths in 1957 and 1958, and the Hong Kong flu resulted in 34,000 US deaths in 1968 and 1969.

Presentation

The clinical spectrum of influenza is broad. During some epidemics, the rate of asymptomatic infection may be as high as the rate of symptomatic infections. The severity of the disease may be equally variable, ranging from a mild stuffy nose to multisystem complications and death within hours.

Based on the clinical presentation, it is difficult to differentiate between influenza A and influenza B or between infections caused by different subtypes of influenza A. Influenza C generally causes a milder respiratory illness, but it can cause bronchitis and pneumonia. The elderly (over age 65); adults and children with chronic cardiopulmonary con-

ditions, renal failure, metabolic disorders, diabetes, hemoglobinopathies such as sickle cell disease, and immunosuppression; and pregnant women are at significantly higher risk from influenza. Influenza viruses are spread by small-particle aerosols of virus contained in respiratory secretions and propelled by coughing, sneezing, or even talking. Transmission by direct contact may also occur.

The classic influenza syndrome is a febrile illness of sudden onset with sore throat, tracheitis, and marked muscle pain. The patient suddenly develops headache, chills, fever, malaise, anorexia, and sore throat. The fever climbs rapidly to between 101° and 104°F (38.3° and 40°C). The respiratory symptoms then start with a nonproductive cough. Sneezing, rhinorrhea, and nasal congestion are common. The patient may experience photophobia, hoarseness, nausea, vomiting, diarrhea, and abdominal pain. The patient often appears ill and is usually coughing.

An examination of the lungs often reveals no signs of infection. The patient may develop minimal to moderate nasal congestion, nasal discharge, and pharyngitis. Many adults with influenza do not display the classic syndrome as described. Any given patient may have any or all of the symptoms with or without fever. The respiratory and systemic symptoms of influenza generally last 1 to 5 days. There are many complications of influenza, but an influenzal pneumonia with subsequent bacterial suprainfection is the most common.

Diagnosis

A definitive diagnosis of influenza can only be made after laboratory testing for the virus. If laboratory confirmation of influenza is available early in the course of infection, the patient may benefit from specific antiviral treatment as outlined subsequently in this chapter. Nasopharyngeal swabs alone or combined with throat swabs, nasopharyngeal aspirates, or nasal washes are useful specimens for a culture and for detection.

Virus isolation is the gold standard for the diagnosis of influenza. A rapid-culture technique using a monolayer of cells that can be stained for viral antigens with immunofluorescence or other methods reduces the time required to obtain a result.

Treatment

The four available drugs that can be used to treat influenza are as follows:

- Amantadine
- Rimantadine
- Zanamivir
- Oseltamivir

Amantadine and rimantadine can be used to both treat and prevent influenza A infections. These drugs interfere with virus uncoating and transport, so they block the ability of the virus to multiply. When administered for 10 days to the household contacts of a person with influenza, the drugs prevent infection up to 80% of the time. These drugs do not work against influenza B viruses.

Zanamivir and oseltamivir can be used to treat both influenza A and influenza B infections. Oseltamivir can also be used for the prevention of both of these infections.

INHOSPITAL INFO

INHOSPITAL INFO

Table 10-2 Comparison of Antiviral Drugs for Influenza

Drug	Brand Name	Influenza Virus Type	Approved Use	Treatment Age	Prevention Age
Amantadine	Symmetrel	A	Treatment and prevention	1 year or older	1 year or older
Rimantadine	Flumadine	A	Treatment and prevention	Adults	1 year or older
Zanamivir	Relenza	A and B	Treatment	7 years or older	n/a
Oseltamivir	Tamiflu	A and B	Treatment and prevention	1 year or older	13 years or older

Source: Courtesy of Centers for Disease Control and Prevention, http://www.cdc.gov/ncidod/diseases/flu/fluviral.htm. Accessed March 31, 2004.

Studies show that treatment with any of these drugs can shorten the time during which a person infected with influenza feels ill by approximately 1 day, if treatment is started during the first 2 days of illness. Common anti-influenza antiviral drugs are listed in **Table 10-2.** Recent strains of avian flu have shown marked resistance to amantadine, due to extensive use of this drug in avian feed in China.

Prophylaxis

Inactivated influenza virus vaccines have been used for about 40 years to prevent influenza infections. A given vaccine contains the strains of types A and B viruses that are thought to be most likely to spread during the following winter. The vaccine is administered in the fall. One or two doses may be required to treat, depending on the patient's immunization experience.

A vaccine's effectiveness against influenza varies from 50% to 90% in civilian population. It is not 100% effective, because the strains picked for the vaccine may not correspond exactly to the strains that spread. The annual use of inactivated influenza virus vaccine is currently recommended in the United States for persons at risk of developing pneumonia from this disease.

In order to give time for adequate vaccine stocks to be produced, a decision must be made, usually in August, as to which influenza A type to use for the coming winter's vaccine. There is a sophisticated worldwide epidemiologic monitoring system, which helps officials make these decisions.

Occasionally, type A viruses can change abruptly, and a new subtype will suddenly emerge. When this occurs, large numbers of people—sometimes an entire population— become vulnerable to infection without antibody protection. This results in a pandemic.

Biosafety

Because influenza is a respiratory illness, respiratory protection is very important. Particulate filter personal respiratory protection devices capable of filtering 0.3 μm particles (N95 masks) should be worn at all times when attending patients with suspected or confirmed influenza.

Handwashing is the most important hygiene measure for preventing the spread of infection. Gloves are not a substitute for handwashing. Hands should be washed before and after significant contact with any patient, after activities likely to cause contamination, and after removing gloves. Alcohol-based skin disinfectants formulated for use without water may be used in certain limited circumstances. Health care workers are advised to wear gloves for all patient handling. Gloves should be changed between patients and after any contact with items likely to be contaminated with respiratory secretions (such as masks, oxygen tubing, nasal prongs, and tissues). General information on influenza is summarized in **Table 10-3.**

Threat

Unfortunately, because influenza strains can vary quite a bit, the current vaccine may not be protective against a genetically engineered version of influenza or even against an unusual natural strain. Although it may be unexpected, the ability for influenza to create a worldwide pandemic makes it a potential bioterrorist weapon. The historical effects of the influenza pandemic of 1918 clearly show what an out-of-control biological weapon can do to our health care system.

Table 10-3 Summary of Influenza

Virus	Disease	Incubation	Location	Case-Fatality Rate	Treatment Available
Influenza	Spanish flu	3 to 7 days	Worldwide	2.5% to 25%	Historically, only supportive care was available.
Influenza	Influenza type A	3 to 7 days	Worldwide	The rate varies from strain to strain. Higher mortality occurs in children and elderly patients.	Supportive intensive care and respiratory therapy is particularly important for critically ill patients. Amantadine, rimantadine, zanamivir, or oseltamivir may be helpful.
Influenza	Influenza type B	3 to 7 days	Worldwide	The rate varies from strain to strain, but it is usually low.	Supportive intensive care and respiratory therapy is particularly important for critically ill patients. Zanamivir or oseltamivir may be helpful.
Influenza	Influenza type C	3 to 7 days	Worldwide	The rate varies from strain to strain, but it is usually low.	**There is no established therapy.** Supportive intensive care and respiratory therapy is particularly important for critically ill patients.

■ Paramyxoviruses: Nipah Virus

Nipah virus is a previously unknown paramyxovirus that has been identified primarily in pigs and humans. In humans, this virus causes fever, severe headache, muscle pain, and encephalitis. This encephalitis has a case-fatality rate of 50% in humans. The outbreak of Nipah virus infection in Malaysia and Singapore should serve as a reminder that known threats are not the only threats that are available to bioterrorists. The Nipah virus was first identified in horses in Australia in 1994. Nipah virus is closely related to, but distinct from, **Hendra virus**.

History

A Nipah epidemic of viral encephalitis, complicated by respiratory failure, occurred in Malaysia in 1998 and 1999, causing 265 cases of infection and 105 fatalities. Of those who became infected, 93% had occupational exposure to pigs. An associated outbreak among **abattoir** (slaughterhouse) workers in Singapore during March 1999 led to 11 cases of infection and 1 fatality. The causative agent, isolated from cerebrospinal fluid, was later named Nipah after the town that was most affected.

There have been three recognized outbreaks of the closely associated Hendra virus in Australia (1994, 1995, and 1999).[1] Three human cases of illness and 2 fatalities were noted in the 1994 and 1995 outbreaks. The mode of transmission to the three Australian patients is not understood, but all were in close contact with horses that were ill and later died.

Distribution

Currently, it is thought that some species of fruit bats are the natural hosts of both Nipah and Hendra viruses. These viruses and the bats are distributed across an area that encompasses the northern, eastern, and southeastern sections of Australia, Indonesia, Malaysia, the Philippines, and some of the Pacific Islands. It is unknown how the bat transmits the virus to humans.[2] Despite frequent contact between fruit bats and humans, there is no evidence of infection among humans that handle these bats.

For Nipah virus, the apparent source of infection for humans is direct contact with infected pigs. For Hendra virus, the apparent source of infection is direct contact with horses. For both viruses, evidence of infection in cats and dogs has also been found. Transmission of Hendra virus to humans is probably more difficult than transmission of Nipah virus. There is evidence that nosocomial transmission of Nipah is possible.

Presentation

The incubation period of both Hendra and Nipah is between 4 and 18 days. In most cases, this is followed by a mild or subclinical infection. In exceptional circumstances, the incubation period of Hendra can be as long as 12 months.[3,4] Animals are infectious during incubation. It is unknown whether humans are infectious during incubation, but this should be considered probable.

Clinical symptoms of Nipah range from mild to fatal. Nipah is characterized by 3 to 14 days of fever with sore throat, headaches, muscle pain, and respiratory symptoms.

Onset of the disease is usually flulike. This may be followed by drowsiness, dizziness, disorientation, and rapid progression into coma. The patient may develop flaccid paralysis and may require ventilatory support. Hypotension and bradycardia may precede death.

In the first two known cases of Hendra virus, respiratory symptoms predominated, and respiratory failure led to the death of one patient. The case-fatality rate of both viruses approaches 50%. Fifteen percent of surviving patients developed a persistent neurologic deficit.[5,6]

Diagnosis

CSF can be shown to contain Nipah virus by vero cell culture with a subsequent electron microscopy. Immunofluorescence and IgM ELISA have also been used to detect both Hendra and Nipah viruses in tissues of the central nervous system, lungs, and kidneys of both infected humans and swine.[7]

It has also been reported that magnetic resonance images of the brain in cases of Nipah virus encephalitis are significantly different from those associated with other viral encephalitis etiologies and that this may be useful for diagnosis.[8] This technology is unlikely to be readily available for any bioterrorist event; therefore, the utility of this diagnostic finding to the emergency provider is uncertain.

Treatment

No drug therapies have been proven to be effective for treatment of Nipah and Hendra virus infections. Intensive supportive therapy is the sole form of treatment. There is some experimental evidence that early treatment with the antiviral drug ribavirin can reduce the duration and severity of the infections. There have yet to be any controlled trials or large series of patients treated with this therapy.

Prophylaxis

There is no known vaccine or other prophylactic therapy for Nipah virus or Hendra virus. Because the related measles has a well developed and safe vaccine, it may be possible for a Nipah vaccine to be developed.

Biosafety

Two key features of the outbreak in Malaysia were the often fatal encephalitis and the nearly universal history of infected humans and other animals, including cats and dogs, having direct contact with infected pigs. The WHO states that the risk of transmission of Nipah virus from sick animals to humans is thought to be low and that transmission from person to person is yet to be documented. Only 6 of 1,412 military personnel developed antibodies to Nipah virus and only 2 of these developed clinical encephalitis.[9] (These soldiers were mostly protected with gloves, masks, gowns, and boots.) Family members of patients have remained uninfected. A survey of the physicians and nurses who had direct contact with infected persons found none with encephalitic illness or evidence of this infection. Despite this, the WHO recommends that this agent should be managed in a high-level biosafety laboratory. Previous work with related viruses, including measles and respiratory syncytial virus,

INHOSPITAL INFO

has demonstrated exceptional infectivity via the respiratory route. The emergency provider must be aware that this virus could be spread as an aerosol and infected patients would pose a significant hazard. **Table 10-4** summarizes biosafety information for Nipah. **Table 10-5** summarizes general information on Nipah and Hendra.

Threat

The potential for Nipah virus to be weaponized and used as a biological warfare agent exists. Such a virus may be grown in cell cultures or in embryonated chicken eggs. It could be used for terrorism, targeting either livestock or humans. The fact that the most affected livestock is pigs may make this virus appealing to a Muslim terrorist, because Islamic tradition forbids the consumption of pork.

■ Smallpox

Few diseases have caused as much human suffering and death as **smallpox**. A massive worldwide effort to rid the world of smallpox succeeded so well that no natural disease has been seen for 25 years. It is truly ironic that this agent is now a major biowarfare threat.

Smallpox affects primates, particularly humans. There are two types of smallpox: **variola major**, which has a mortality rate of 20% to 30% in unvaccinated individuals; and **variola minor**, which has a mortality rate of about 1%. Infection with variola minor protects against subsequent infection with variola major. All poxviruses cause pocks, which are elevated lesions of the skin.

History

Smallpox was described over 2,000 years ago and originated in India or western Asia and then spread to China. Around 700 AD, smallpox spread to Japan, Europe, and North Africa.[10]

European colonization of the Americas and Africa was associated with extensive epidemics of smallpox among native populations on those continents in the 1500s and 1600s.

The last naturally occurring case of smallpox was detected in Somalia in October 1977, and the last reported human infection occurred in a laboratory in 1978.[11] In 1980, the World Health Assembly recommended that all countries cease vaccination.[12] As a direct consequence, people stopped being immunized against smallpox and the world population's immunity has fallen dramatically. Until quite recently, vaccination was only recommended for laboratory workers. Recent vaccination efforts have included selected health care workers and the military because of an increased terrorist threat.

Smallpox was once considered an unlikely agent of biowarfare, because there was a high level of population immunity to the virus, there is an effective vaccine, and the use of the vaccine can rapidly control outbreaks.[13]

Theoretically, the virus now exists in only two laboratories in the world: in the United States and in Russia. As previously discussed, smallpox was a subject of investigation by BioPreparat in the former Soviet Union. The former associate director of this facility alleges that the Soviet Union produced large quantities of very potent smallpox. Other defectors from the former Soviet Union have confirmed this allegation. These people indicated that the laboratories deliberately produced more virulent and contagious recombinant strains. We simply do not know how much smallpox was made, was stockpiled, and yet remains from that biological warfare program. It has also been hypothesized that this modified smallpox virus has been combined with other dangerous pathogens for use as a biological weapon.

If smallpox virus were released as an act of terrorism, the results could be catastrophic. A large proportion of the adult population and all of the pediatric population lack any immunity. There is little available vaccine and no effective

Table 10-4 Protection Against Nipah		
Inactivation Requirements	Decontaminating Agents	Personal Protection Requirements
Heat at 212°F (100°C) for more than 10 minutes—boiling water Ultraviolet light	1% bleach 1% peracetic acid Formaldehyde Ethylene oxide (gas) Irradiation (This organism is not known to be particularly resistant to heat or chemicals. Routine cleaning is acceptable.)	Wear a facial visor. Wear gloves and a gown (secured at the wrists). Wash hands, using an antimicrobial agent, after taking off gloves. Take secretion precautions. Decontaminate soiled items before disposal. Dispose of soiled items by steam sterilization, incineration, or chemical disinfection.

Source: American Academy of Orthopaedic Surgeons, Stewart CE, Nixon RG. *Weapons of Mass Casualties Field Guide.* Jones and Bartlett Publishers, Boston; 2003.

Table 10-5 Summary of Nipah and Hendra					
Virus	Disease	Incubation	Location	Case-Fatality Rate	Treatment Available
Nipah	Nipah fever	3 to 16 days	Malaysia	Nearly 50%	**There is no established therapy.** Experimental therapies are all either marginal or ineffective.
Hendra	Hendra fever	Unknown	Unknown (potentially Philippines)	Unknown	**There is no established therapy.** Experimental therapies are all either marginal or ineffective.

treatment. The expected case-fatality rate is about 25% and many more would be critically ill. During the 1960s and 1970s as many as 10 to 20 second-generation cases were caused by a single case. Widespread panic could be expected even with outbreaks of as few as 100 people.

Distribution

Smallpox was once worldwide in scope **(Figure 10-3).** Thirty years ago, smallpox was endemic in 31 countries, affected 15 million people each year, and caused 2 million deaths per year. Survivors often remained disfigured or blinded for life. Before vaccination was introduced, virtually everybody contracted smallpox by adulthood.

Smallpox normally spread from person to person through the air or by direct contact with an infected person or an infected person's secretions. Contaminated clothing or bed linens can spread the disease. Smallpox is not spread by any known animal or insect vector. The infectious dose of smallpox is unknown but may be only a few virus particles.[14] In conditions of low temperature and low humidity, aerosolized smallpox is very stable and has resulted in widespread, hospital-based epidemics. The predominant means of transmission is usually airborne sputum, spread by cough or face-to-face contact.

The seasonal occurrence of smallpox is similar to chickenpox and measles. Its incidence is highest during the winter and early spring. This pattern is consistent with the duration of survival of the virus in aerosols and in low temperatures and low humidity. It is also consistent with the increased chances of successful inoculation in the close proximity of indoors. Large outbreaks in natural smallpox have been rare during the summer.

The transmission of smallpox is slow, because the disease is usually not infective until the patient has been confined to bed with a high fever and rash. The patient is most infectious from the onset of the rash through the first 7 to 10 days of the rash and is increased markedly in patients with a cough.[15]

Unfortunately, this also means that in-hospital infectivity is quite high. (In Germany, a smallpox patient with a cough, isolated in a single room, infected persons on three floors of a hospital.)[16] This infectivity is increased when diagnosis is delayed.

Presentation

Smallpox has a long incubation period of about 7 to 17 days, with an average of 12 days. The illness causes preliminary symptoms that occur for 2 to 3 days, including malaise, fever, headache, and backache. Over the next 7 to 10 days, all of the characteristic lesions erupt, progress from macules to papules to vesicles to pustules, and then crust and become scars.

Infection occurs following implantation of the virus on the oropharyngeal or respiratory mucosa.[17] The virus then spreads to the regional lymph nodes, and further multiplication of the virus occurs in the spleen, bone marrow, and distant lymph nodes. Around day 8, **toxemia** and fever occur.

At the end of the incubation period, the patient develops high fever, malaise, and prostration with headache and muscle pain, typically in the back muscles. The patient may also experience abdominal pain and delirium. A maculopapular rash then appears on the oral mucosa, pharynx, face, and forearms. The rash then spreads to the trunk and lower extremities.

Within 1 to 2 days, the rash becomes vesicular and progresses to pustules. These pustules are typically round, firm, and deeply embedded in the dermis. The pustules rupture and crust over on about the eighth or ninth day of the rash. As the scabs separate, they leave characteristic scars.

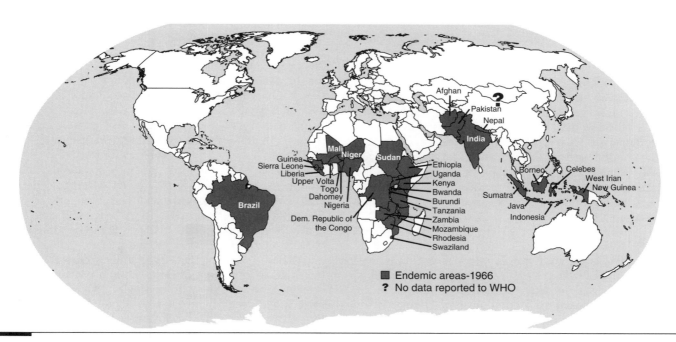

Figure 10-3 Incidence of smallpox in 1966.

The majority of smallpox-infected patients present with a typical rash that is densest on the face and extremities. The lesions appear during a 1- to 2-day period and evolve at the same rate. (In chickenpox, new lesions appear in crops, and lesions of different ages are present in adjacent areas of the skin. Chickenpox lesions are more numerous in the trunk than in the extremities.) Patients are most infectious during the first week of illness. The classic disease (variola major) is fatal in about 30% of cases.[18]

Complications

The most common result of smallpox is scarring, particularly on the face. Rarely, smallpox may cause blindness. Other complications include smallpox pneumonia and arthritis (which may cause permanent joint deformities). Bacterial infection is uncommon. Death often occurs during the second week of the illness. The patient may develop encephalitis that is indistinguishable from the encephalitis associated with measles, vaccinia, or chickenpox.[19,20]

Hemorrhagic Smallpox

Some patients will develop **hemorrhagic smallpox**, also called blackpox. Hemorrhagic smallpox is often fatal. The illness has a somewhat shortened incubation period and is accompanied by high fever and head, back, and abdominal pain. Shortly after the pain starts, the patient develops a dusky erythema, followed by petechiae and flank hemorrhages in the skin and mucous membranes. Death occurs by the fifth or sixth day after the rash.[21] Pregnant women are particularly susceptible to this variant of smallpox. Hemorrhagic cases of smallpox were frequently misdiagnosed as meningococcemia. There is some evidence that the hemorrhagic variant of smallpox was developed by the Russians in their BioPreparat facilities.

Malignant Smallpox

Another variant of smallpox is **malignant smallpox**, a "flat" smallpox associated with severe toxemia and high mortality. In the malignant form, the abrupt onset and shortened incubation period are similar to hemorrhagic smallpox. In malignant smallpox, the skin lesions develop slowly and do not progress to the pustular stage, hence the description as *flat*. The skin develops the appearance of a fine-grained, reddish-colored rubber. Hemorrhage is sometimes noted within the skin. The flat lesions disappear without scabs in survivors. Some patients will experience the shedding **(desquamation)** of large areas of affected skin. Diagnosis of this variant of smallpox may be quite difficult until viral studies are available. Malignant smallpox was frequently misdiagnosed because its appearance was atypical.

Variola Minor

The illness associated with variola minor is generally less severe and causes fewer systemic symptoms.[22] The rash is often sparse. This presentation may also be seen in those who have residual immunity from a prior vaccination. The evolution of the lesions may be more rapid. Variola minor causes only about 1% to 2% fatalities.

Monkeypox

Monkeypox has been reported in the Democratic Republic of the Congo (formerly Zaire) and other forested areas of Central and Western Africa.[23] In June 2003, monkeypox was imported into the United States in exotic animals. Human cases have been found in Illinois, Wisconsin, and Indiana.[24]

Monkeypox is caused by monkeypox virus, which belongs to the **orthopox** group of viruses (the same group that smallpox belongs to). Its clinical presentation is similar to smallpox (particularly variola minor). A major distinguishing factor of monkeypox is the presence of large cervical and **inguinal lymph nodes**. These are uncommon in both smallpox and chickenpox.

The mortality rate of verified monkeypox for patients who are not vaccinated is 11% (15% for children under 5 years of age).[25] Secondary bacterial pneumonia is common and associated with a 50% mortality rate. These statistics apply to remote areas of central and western Africa, where medical care is much less than optimum. In the recent cases of monkeypox in the United States (at time of this writing) there had been no fatalities.

Smallpox vaccine immunization seems to provide about 85% protection against monkeypox. As with smallpox, the disease is significantly milder in vaccinated persons. The CDC currently recommends smallpox immunization as prophylaxis for monkeypox for those who have been exposed.

Diagnosis

If the diagnosis of smallpox is seriously considered, immediate isolation is required, the CDC should be contacted, and all patient contacts should be identified and isolated.

ANY CASE OF SMALLPOX SHOULD BE CONSIDERED TO BE THE RESULT OF BIOTERRORISM UNTIL PROVEN UNEQUIVOCALLY OTHERWISE.

Like many viral diseases, the diagnosis of smallpox is best made by clinical impression. Smallpox has an incubation period of 10 to 14 days followed by the abrupt onset of fever, headache, malaise, and backache. Three to 4 days after the onset of symptoms, a characteristic rash appears on the oropharynx, face, forearms, and hands. The trunk and abdomen are usually spared. The rash evolves from macules, to papules, to vesicles, and finally to pustules. After 8 to 9 days, the pustules will rupture and crust over.

There is no widely available laboratory test to confirm smallpox infection. Routine labs are not helpful, although leukopenia is common. Clotting factors may be depressed and thrombocytopenia may be found. Sampling of pustular fluid should be performed only by people who have been recently vaccinated against smallpox. Samples should be handled by a biosafety Level 4 laboratory.

Diagnosis may be made with immunofluorescence, electron microscopy, or a culture. Orthopoxviruses are large, brick-shaped viruses with a single double-stranded DNA molecule. A recently developed polymerase chain reaction–based assay of the hemagglutinin gene allows classification of all of the species of the orthopoxvirus family.[26]

INHOSPITAL INFO

Table 10-6 Major Smallpox Criteria

Febrile preliminary symptoms	These occur 1 to 4 days before the onset of the rash. The fever is greater than 101°F (38°C) and at least one of the following is present: prostration, headache, backache, chills, vomiting, or severe abdominal pain.
Classic smallpox lesions	These appear as deep-seated, firm/hard, round, well-circumscribed vesicles or pustules. As they evolve, the lesions may become **umbilicated** or **confluent**.
Lesions in the same stage of development	On any one part of the body, the lesions appear at the same stage of development; that is, all are vesicles or all are pustules.

Adapted from: Evaluate a rash suspicious for smallpox. CDC website accessed at http://www.bt.cdc.gov/agent/smallpox/diagnosis/riskalgorithm/index.asp on March 7, 2004.

Table 10-7 Minor Smallpox Criteria

Centrifugal distribution	The greatest concentration of lesions is on the face and distal extremities.
Specific location of first lesions	The first lesions appear on the oral mucosa/palate, face, or forearms.
Toxic condition	The patient appears toxic or **moribund**.
Slow evolution	The lesions evolve from macules to papules to pustules over days, with each stage lasting 1 to 2 days.
Lesion spread	Lesions spread to the palms and soles.

Adapted from: Evaluate a rash suspicious for smallpox. CDC website accessed at http://www.bt.cdc.gov/agent/smallpox/diagnosis/riskalgorithm/index.asp on March 7, 2004.

Tables 10-6 and **10-7** list major and minor smallpox criteria. Differential diagnosis is listed in **Table 10-8**.

Response in Immunosuppressed Patients

There is little information about how individuals with induced immunosuppression (cancer chemotherapy and transplant patients, for example) and acquired immunosuppression (HIV and AIDS, for example) will respond to smallpox infection. Smallpox was eradicated before transplant surgery was extensively practiced and before HIV was identified. At least one authority feels that some of the cases of malignant and hemorrhagic smallpox resulted from defective immune responses.[27] Certainly, vaccinia can result in a continuing spreading lesion, viremia, and viral infection of multiple internal organs in the HIV-positive patient.[28] There is no reason to believe that the behavior of smallpox would be substantially different in the immunocompromised individual.

Therapy

Therapy is entirely supportive. Three compounds (**cidofovir**, its cyclic derivative, and ribavirin) demonstrate significant antiviral activity against smallpox.[29] These medications have not been used in the treatment of humans with smallpox and may or may not be effective.

Cidofovir is only available in an intravenous preparation and is an experimental drug. (It is currently licensed for treatment of cytomegalovirus retinitis.)[30] Cidofovir must be administered with concomitant hydration and **probenecid** to reduce the risks of **nephrotoxicity**.[31] It is only given once a week.

Cidofovir has demonstrated efficacy in monkeys against experimental infection with monkeypox. Monkeys exposed to large quantities of aerosolized monkeypox virus survived, provided that treatment with cidofovir was started within a few days after exposure.

Use of cidofovir should be strongly considered for patients with progressive vaccinia, severe eczema vaccinatum, generalized vaccinia, or extensive accidental inoculation of vaccinia. It should also be considered in severe cases of smallpox.

Ribavirin is active against smallpox. A single case report suggests that intravenous use of ribavirin was effective in an immunocompromised patient with progressive vaccinia.[32] There are no in vivo studies of ribavirin for poxvirus infections.

An emergency vaccination program should include all health workers at clinics or hospitals that may receive infected patients and all disaster workers, such as EMS, hospital staff, police officers, public health staff, and mortuary staff. These personnel should be vaccinated as soon as the first case is diagnosed, irrespective of prior vaccination status. Vaccination should also be considered for any other

Table 10-8 Differential Diagnosis of Smallpox

Contact dermatitis
Disseminated herpes simplex
Disseminated herpes zoster
Drug eruptions
Enteroviral infections (especially hand-foot-mouth disease)
Erythema multiforme (including Stevens-Johnson syndrome)
Impetigo
Molluscum contagiosum (another poxvirus that may disseminate in an immunocompromised person)
Monkeypox
Multiple insect bites, including fleas
Scabies
Varicella (chickenpox—primary infection with varicella-zoster virus)

Adapted from: Henderson DA, Inglesby TV, Bartlett JG, et al. Smallpox as a biological weapon: Medical and public health management. *JAMA.* 1999;281:2127-2137.

INHOSPITAL INFO

persons who would be responsible for patient care, investigation, and control of suspected outbreaks of smallpox.

Prophylaxis

Prophylaxis against smallpox has been available since 1796 and is well documented.[33] Because smallpox is presumed to have been eradicated worldwide, there is no recommendation or requirement for routine vaccination. Recent studies on tissue culture and experimental animals have suggested the possibility that cidofovir may be useful in the prevention of smallpox infection if it is administered within 1 to 2 days after exposure.[34]

Vaccinia

Vaccinia is an orthopox virus of uncertain origin. Edward Jenner first used vaccinia in 1796 as a prophylaxis against smallpox. The virus was thought to have been isolated from infected cows and, later, horses. The current smallpox vaccine is a suspension of live vaccinia virus, derived from the lymph of calves that have been inoculated with vaccinia virus. A vaccine produced by Acambis-Baxter Pharmaceuticals using the same strain of vaccinia virus, but which is grown in monkey kidney and human fibroblast cells, is expected to be available in sufficient amounts to vaccinate the entire US population in 2004.[35]

Vaccination within 5 years prior to or within 2 to 3 days after natural exposure provides almost complete protection against variola major. Vaccination administered within 4 days of first exposure has been shown to offer some protection against acquiring the infection and significant protection against a fatal outcome.[36]

Smallpox vaccine is administered by puncturing the skin with a split needle 15 times in a 5-mm diameter circle. The punctures are made with just enough pressure to produce a small amount of blood. Following successful inoculation with the vaccine, a papule forms over the course of 4 to 5 days. This papule often becomes intensely itchy and evolves over the course of 2 to 3 days into an umbilicated vesicle or pustule. The inflammatory response peaks after about a week with surrounding redness and hardness. Mild systemic symptoms, fever, and regional disease of the lymph nodes (**lymphadenopathy**) are quite common. The pustule frequently ruptures prior to scab formation. The scab separates and forms a scar at about 2 weeks. A successful vaccination will have a well formed pustule within 6 to 11 days after the vaccination. It leaves a scar that is about 1 cm in diameter.

The vaccination site should be covered with a nonocclusive dressing (a gauze pad) until the scab separates. Occlusive dressings can result in the softening of the tissue from moistness (**maceration**) and extensive local infection and should be avoided.[37-39] Semipermeable membrane dressings, such as OpSite dressings, are useful and may prevent the spread of the virus. Careful handwashing after contact with any drainage site is essential.

Prior Vaccination

The immune status of those who were vaccinated 20 years ago or more is not clear. Most experts believe that immunity after primary vaccination wanes substantially after 5 years, but residual protection against fatal disease may persist for many more years. Revaccination is considered likely to provide longer lasting immunity.

Epidemiologic studies during smallpox epidemics have shown that those who were vaccinated at some time in the past usually have an accelerated immune response, but are still likely to get a milder form of the disease. Those who have been previously vaccinated may be somewhat safer in situations with close patient contact.[40]

Vaccine Stocks

Adequate stocks of smallpox vaccine are probably not available for the emergency treatment of large portions of the population. The WHO retains about 500,000 doses of vaccinia, and 60 to 70 million doses are retained elsewhere. Not all of these doses may be properly stored or monitored for potency. These aging stocks of smallpox vaccine may not be sufficiently potent for the protection of the public. The United States may have adequate current stocks to vaccinate between 5 and 15 million persons.[41] (Properly sealed and stored vaccine has an almost indefinite shelf life.)

In November 2001, the US Department of Health and Human Services ordered 155 million more doses of smallpox vaccine to be delivered by the end of 2002. This order supplements the 15 million doses of vaccine currently in the stockpile and the 54 million doses previously ordered and scheduled for production in 2002. This will ensure that enough vaccine is available for generalized vaccination of the public, should this become necessary.

The current stocks of smallpox vaccine will be diluted in a 5:1 ratio in order to stretch the supply. Changes in the dilution process have caused the FDA to reclassify smallpox vaccine as an investigational drug. The new vaccine that is being manufactured by Acambis-Baxter Pharmaceuticals will also be classified as an investigational drug, because it is being grown in a cell tissue culture rather than on the skin of calves. As an investigational drug, all individuals who receive this vaccine must be told of the risks of the vaccine and give signed consent prior to use of the vaccine.

Prophylaxis Strategies

Studies about smallpox control and eradication efforts in the last 50 years have identified two available interventions: vaccination and quarantine (or both). There are three vaccination strategies that should be noted.

Quarantine (Isolation) Strategy This strategy implements the simple idea of isolating every case (and suspected case) of smallpox. It either kills off the population or makes them immune if they survive. This technique is brutal, but effective. However, isolation of all contacts of exposed patients would be difficult. Patients are not infective until the onset of the rash. A practical strategy is to take the temperature of all the contacts daily, preferably in the evening. A fever of 101°F (38°C) or higher should be cause for the isolation of the contact until a clinical or laboratory diagnosis is made. In a widespread dissemination of smallpox in multiple cities, this strategy may not be completely effective without the declaration of martial law and the use of troops to enforce the quarantine.

Whole Population Vaccination In this strategy, the entire population is vaccinated. Those with contraindications are not vaccinated (but will be exposed to vaccinia from those who have been vaccinated and are close contacts). This strategy depends on a useful vaccine that does not cause an unacceptable rate of complications. The acceptance of complications is in direct proportion to the potential lethality and perceived risk of the disease for which the vaccine is prepared. Our complete reliance on a single vaccine of unmodified vaccinia represents a serious potential vulnerability in this strategy, because weaponized strains can be modified, making the vaccine less effective.

Specific Individual Vaccinations In this strategy, health care providers, epidemiologists, law enforcement personnel, military personnel, and selected others are vaccinated against the disease. These people are expected to be in the forefront if there is an epidemic, and are therefore preprotected. Vaccination protection depends on the same variables as described above for complication rates and effectiveness.

Ring Vaccination Strategy In this strategy, epidemiologists identify and vaccinate contacts to provide a ring of immunity around each known case. This proposed strategy conserves available supplies of vaccine and minimizes the possibility of complications.[42]

This strategy requires the following:
1. A vaccine that prevents the spread of the disease
2. The ability to rapidly immunize those who have been exposed
3. A cadre of previously vaccinated health care providers who are able to administer the vaccine to the suspected population
4. An intact medical care system to support requirements 2 and 3

This technique was used during the later stages of the eradication campaign for smallpox with a good measure of success. This technique is currently advocated by the CDC for control of any smallpox infection. It may not have the same applicability for a weapons-grade smallpox release in a terrorist incident.

INCIDENTS INVOLVING Biological Agents

Pox Outbreak

In 1971, a small outbreak of smallpox occurred in Aralsk, Kazakhstan. This outbreak was unusual because Russia had most of its population immunized by 1971.[43] It was even more unusual because 7 of the 10 infections that occurred were in patients who had been previously immunized (some of them three times). All of the infected patients who were not previously immunized developed hemorrhagic smallpox and died.

It is strongly suspected that this infection was caused by an accidental release of a weaponized military strain of smallpox (blackpox). This illustrates a grave danger of the ring strategy of vaccination: if the vaccine does not prevent the disease, then the ring will not be a barrier to the spread of the disease.

Problems With the Vaccine

No one familiar with the currently available smallpox vaccine (prepared using 1950s or earlier technology) would be satisfied with this vaccine as the sole method of prevention of smallpox. This vaccine is controversial and possibly the least safe human vaccine. Complications can result from the vaccine to both the recipients and those who come into contact with the recently vaccinated. Risks posed by the vaccine have led physician groups, including the American Medical Association and the Infectious Diseases Society of America, to advise against a new broad-based campaign of vaccination unless disease is discovered in the United States.

The risks are serious and include **progressive vaccinia**, tissue necrosis, and encephalitis. Using data from the 1960s, the CDC calculated a death risk of 1 per 1 million people vaccinated. Indeed, among 5.5 million vaccinations administered during the 1961 and 1962 outbreaks of smallpox in the United Kingdom, vaccination caused at least 18 deaths.[44]

Complications Common adverse effects include nonspecific red or urticarial eruptions and erythema multiforme. The most common complication is accidental inoculation of a distant site on the patient. Infections of the face, eyes, and genitals are common. Ocular infections account for about 20% of the accidental infections and can result in permanent corneal injury.

Contraindications The routine contraindications for vaccination include immunosuppression (both HIV and transplant patients), eczema (and atopic dermatitis), pregnancy, household contact with individuals with known contraindications, and childhood. In addition, patients with other extensive skin diseases or inflammatory eye diseases should not be vaccinated. Pregnant patients may develop very rare congenital infections that are often fatal. In a smallpox epidemic, there are no contraindications to vaccination. The threat of the 30% or higher mortality rate of the disease far outweighs the possibility of a reaction.

Future Applications The frequency of complications of vaccinia is significant enough to recommend the development of another strain. Genetically engineered vaccinia strains are being investigated.[45,46] A human cell culture-derived vaccine is being developed at Fort Detrick. However, large-scale production of these vaccines is years away.

Biosafety

Smallpox is extremely infectious **(Table 10-9)**. A diagnosis of smallpox should mandate the immediate respiratory isolation of the patient (with or without consent). Place a mask on the patient at all times. Those who attend the patient should wear gowns, gloves, and National Institute for Occupation Safety and Health (NIOSH) particulate respirators (N95). All household and face-to-face contacts should be vaccinated and placed under surveillance. Because smallpox is spread rapidly by aerosol transmission, it poses a particular threat in hospitals that only have a few **negative pressure isolation facilities**.

Table 10-9 Mode of Acquisition of Smallpox in Europe (from 1950 to 1971)

Mode	Number of Cases	Percentage of Total Cases
Hospital transmission (includes hospital personnel)	359	54%
Work related	51	8%
Family and intimate contacts	129	20%
Casual contacts	63	10%
Miscellaneous	6	1%
Unpredictable	44	7%

Adapted from: Smallwood R. Health preparedness in Australia—Responding to Emergencies. Accessed at www.nationalsecurityaus.com/portalfiles/ white_paper/A02.pdf on March 7, 2004.

Because there is a serious threat of widespread dissemination of smallpox in hospitals, patients should be isolated in the home whenever possible. Home care is a very reasonable approach, considering that there is no effective therapy for this disease.

Objects that have been in contact with a contaminated patient need to be cleansed with live steam, sodium hypochlorite solution, or other standard disinfectants. The virus may remain viable for extended periods of time in clothing or linens. Bed linens and dressing material should be autoclaved before laundering or disposal.

Fortunately, aerosol vaccinia (and probably variola virus) is deactivated within 24 hours by ultraviolet light and heat. Therefore, if 24 hours have passed by the time patients present to the emergency department with clinical symptoms, these patients do not need to be decontaminated.

Biosafety information for smallpox is summarized in **Table 10-10.** The biosafety information for smallpox is the same as for hantavirus, with the exception of the smallpox vaccine.

Threat

Smallpox is a durable virus and can exist for long periods outside the host. It is remotely possible that smallpox is still living outside of the repository labs. Viable virus trapped within 13-year-old scabs was found by Dutch investigators. (It is unlikely that this virus, bound within the fibrin matrix, would be infectious in humans, but such a find may be able to be salvaged by a bioterrorist.)

The WHO proposed in 1986 that all laboratories destroy their variola stocks or transfer them to one of two WHO reference labs in Russia and the United States. All countries reported compliance. It is almost certain that Russia did not comply and that it has produced smallpox virus in large quantities for use in weapons. This should concern every health care provider, because funding in Russia is unstable at best. Consequently, existing expertise, equipment, or stocks of smallpox may be transferred to other countries or nongovernment entities as a result of financial influence. There is no question that smallpox should be high on the threat list for biological terrorism.

An aerosol release of variola virus would spread widely, because the virus is stable as an aerosol and the infectious dose is quite small. As noted, during epidemics in the 1960s and 1970s in Europe, as many as 10 to 20 additional people were infected by transmission from a single infected patient.[47] A clandestine aerosol release, even if it only initially infected 50 to 100 persons, would rapidly spread to cause 10 to 20 times more cases of infection from each individual case.

The average incubation period is 12 to 14 days. Therefore, a lapse of at least 2 weeks between the release and diagnosis of the first few infections may allow the terrorists to escape and may make tracking all of those who were exposed quite difficult.

General information on the poxviruses is summarized in **Table 10-11.**

■ Alphaviruses: Venezuelan Equine Encephalitis

Three viral meningitis-encephalitis syndromes are caused by the **alphaviruses**: **Venezuelan equine encephalitis** (VEE), **western equine encephalitis** (WEE), and **eastern equine encephalitis** (EEE). These similar viruses are quite difficult to distinguish clinically and share similar aspects of epidemiology and transmission. Natural in-

Table 10-10 Protection Against Smallpox

Inactivation Requirements	Decontaminating Agents	Personal Protection Requirements
Heat at 212°F (100°C) for more than 10 minutes Ultraviolet light	1% bleach	Wear respiratory protection with a fitted NIOSH N95 mask or better.
	1% peracetic acid	Wear gloves and a gown (secured at the wrists).
	Formaldehyde	Wash hands, using an antimicrobial agent, after taking off gloves.
	Ethylene oxide (gas)	Take secretion precautions.
	Irradiation	Decontaminate soiled items before disposal.
		Dispose of soiled items by steam sterilization, incineration, or chemical disinfection.

Source: American Academy of Orthopaedic Surgeons, Stewart CE, Nixon RG. *Weapons of Mass Casualties Field Guide.* Jones and Bartlett Publishers, Boston; 2003.

Table 10-11 Summary of the Poxviruses

Virus	Disease	Incubation	Location	Case-Fatality Rate	Treatment Available
Smallpox	Variola major	3 to 16 days	Currently stored in Russia, the United States, and potentially other places	30% among unvaccinated patients; 3% among vaccinated patients	**There is no established therapy.** Proposed therapies are all experimental, because this disease was last diagnosed in 1977. Cidofovir may be useful in the prevention of smallpox if it is used within 1 to 2 days after exposure. A good vaccine exists for known variants of this disease.
Smallpox	Variola minor	Assumed to be the same as for variola major	Assumed to be the same as for variola major	Less than 5%	Effective therapy is assumed to be the same as for variola major.
Smallpox	Hemorrhagic smallpox (blackpox)	Somewhat shorter than for smallpox	Assumed to be the same as for variola major	90% to 100%	It has been suggested that military strains of smallpox may have higher rates of hemorrhagic smallpox and somewhat less effectiveness (cross-reactivity) with vaccinia.
Smallpox	Flat smallpox	Assumed to be the same as for variola major	Assumed to be the same as for variola major	66% among vaccinated patients; 95% among unvaccinated patients	Effective therapy is assumed to be the same as for variola major.
Monkeypox	Monkeypox	About 1 week	Western and Central Africa (mostly in Zaire)	3% to 10%	**There is no established therapy.** Experimental therapies are all either marginal or ineffective. The current recommendation is to use smallpox vaccine for prophylaxis.
Cowpox	Cowpox, catpox; Rodents are thought to be the natural reservoir.	About 1 week	Europe and the former Soviet Union	The rate is undetermined. Infections in humans are rare, but fairly severe.[48]	**There is no established therapy.** Experimental therapies are all either marginal or ineffective. Infections have occurred in recently vaccinated adults.
Vaccinia	New York Board of Health strain most often used in the United States	3 to 5 days	Laboratory virus	Less than 1%	Vaccinia immune globulin is effective therapy for disseminated vaccinia. Supplies are limited.

fections are transmitted by the bites of a wide variety of mosquitoes. There is no evidence of human-to-human or horse-to-human direct transmission. However, the infective dose in humans is thought to be as little as 100 organisms. This means that neither the population density of mosquitoes nor the concentration of virus particles in an aerosol needs to be great for significant spread of VEE to occur.

History

From 1969 to 1971, a highly pathogenic strain of VEE moved from South America to the United States. In Mexico, over 17,000 people were infected without a single death.

Over 10,000 horses died in Texas alone. The vaccination of over 3.2 million animals and the control of mosquito populations along the Gulf Coast and the Rio Grande Valley finally controlled the epidemic.

VEE was tested as a biological warfare agent during the 1950s and 1960s. VEE is not particularly stable when spread by aerosol and does not persist for any length of time. The high infectivity of the virus is a principle reason why VEE was considered to be a potentially effective warfare agent.

VEE was part of the US stockpile of offensive biological weapons. The code name NU referred to weaponized VEE.

Presentation

VEE is a febrile incapacitating illness. Most infections are relatively mild. Only a small percentage of patients will develop encephalitis. The onset is sudden after an incubation period of 1 to 6 days. The acute phase runs about 24 to 72 hours and is characterized by chills, spiking fevers (often high), rigors, headache, malaise, photophobia, and muscle pain. Some patients may experience nausea, vomiting, cough, sore throat, and diarrhea. Patients may also develop conjunctivitis, **pharyngeal erythema**, and muscle tenderness. The disease may last for 1 to 2 weeks. About 4% of children and 1% or less of adults will develop signs of encephalitis. Of these, 10% of adults and up to 35% of children may die.

Diagnosis

Diagnosis of VEE, WEE, and EEE infections can be made by serologic techniques or by IgM ELISA after about 5 days of illness. An outbreak of VEE may be difficult to differentiate from influenza on clinical grounds. An increased number of neurologic cases or coexisting disease in horses may be the first clues of infection.

Therapy

There is no effective therapy for VEE and related illnesses. Treatment is entirely supportive and includes volume replacement and symptomatic care. Patients with encephalitis may require anticonvulsants.

Isolation is not required, because this disease is not transmitted from human to human. The patient should be treated in a screened room, because the disease is transmissible by a wide variety of mosquitoes. The virus is sensitive to all known disinfectants.

Prophylaxis

There is no vaccine available for humans. There are two investigational human vaccines. The first (TC-83) has been licensed for horses and used as an investigational vaccine for people who work in labs with VEE. The second (C-84) has been tested but not licensed for humans. This vaccine is used for those who do not respond to TC-83.

Biosafety

Biosafety for VEE, WEE, and EEE is the same as for smallpox, with the exception of the smallpox vaccine (see Table 10-10).

Threat

These viruses could be produced by relatively unsophisticated and inexpensive systems in large amounts. An aerosol of VEE would be highly contagious. VEE could also be spread by infected mosquitoes. The VEE complex is stable during transport and storage.

Because the mosquito vectors for VEE are widely dispersed in the United States, a bioterrorist event with VEE, in the appropriate locale and during the proper season, could pose a continuing threat.

■ Flaviviruses: St. Louis Encephalitis and West Nile Virus Encephalitis

Three viral meningitis-encephalitis syndromes are caused by the **flaviviruses**: **West Nile virus encephalitis** (WNV), and **St. Louis encephalitis** (SLE). These similar flaviviruses are quite difficult to distinguish clinically and share similar aspects of epidemiology and transmission. Natural infections are transmitted by the bites of a wide variety of mosquitoes. There is no evidence of human-to-human transmission.

History

WNV was first observed in the western hemisphere in New York City in 1999. This virus has rapidly spread throughout the eastern and southern United States. It is thought to have been imported in an infected bird.

SLE is widely distributed in the United States, and infections occur as periodic outbreaks of encephalitis in the midwestern, western, and southwestern United States. It has caused large summer outbreaks of encephalitis.

Presentation

SLE is a febrile incapacitating illness. Most infections are relatively mild. Only a small percentage of infected patients will develop encephalitis. The onset is sudden after an incubation period of 4 to 21 days. The disease can cause mild febrile illness, aseptic meningitis, or frank encephalitis. The acute phase runs about 24 to 72 hours and is characterized by chills, fever, headache, malaise, cough, and sore throat. Some patients may experience nausea, vomiting, headache, confusion, and disorientation. The disease may last for 1 to 2 weeks. A mortality rate of about 2% to 20% is recorded. SLE is more serious in older patients.

Diagnosis

Diagnosis of SLE and WNV infections can be made by serologic techniques or by IgM ELISA after about 5 days of illness.

Therapy

There is no effective therapy for WNV, SLE, and related illnesses. Treatment is entirely supportive and includes volume replacement and symptomatic care. Patients with encephalitis may require anticonvulsants.

Isolation is not required, because this disease is not transmitted from human to human. The patient should be treated in a screened room, because the disease is transmissible by a wide variety of mosquitoes. The virus is sensitive to all known disinfectants.

Biosafety

Biosafety for SLE and WNV is the same as for smallpox, with the exception of the smallpox vaccine (see Table 10-10).

Threat

Table 10-12 summarizes general information on the viral encephalitis agents.

Table 10-12 Summary of Viral Encephalitis Agents

Virus	Disease	Incubation	Location	Case-Fatality Rate	Treatment Available
Venezuelan equine encephalitis	VEE	1 to 5 days	South America	Less than 1%	**There is no established therapy.** Experimental therapies are all either marginal or ineffective.
Western equine encephalitis	WEE	1 to 4 days	The Plains regions of the Western and Central United States and Canada	Approximately 3%	**There is no established therapy.** Experimental therapies are all either marginal or ineffective.
Eastern equine encephalitis	EEE	4 to 10 days	Canada, North Central United States and along the Eastern and Gulf coasts of the United States, and Central and South America	30% to 60%	**There is no established therapy.** Experimental therapies are all either marginal or ineffective. There is a vaccine that will prevent this disease in horses.
St. Louis encephalitis (flaviviridae: group B arboviruses)	SLE	4 to 21 days	Most of the United States	3% to 20% (highest in the elderly)	**There is no established therapy.**
West Nile virus encephalitis (flaviviridae: group B arboviruses)	WNV	Unknown	First identified in the United States in New York City in 1999. It has rapidly spread across the United States	5% to 10% (highest in the elderly)	**There is no established therapy.**

■ References

1. Anonymous: *Nipah Virus Factsheet.* Geneva, Switzerland, World Health Organization (Fact Sheet No 262), 2001.
2. Yob JM, Rashdi AM, Morrissy C, et al: Nipah virus infections in bats (order chiroptera) in peninsular Malaysia. *Emerg Infect Dis* 2001;7:987-988.
3. Anonymous: *Hendra Virus and Nipah Virus Management and Control.* London, England, Department of Health, Social Services and Public Safety, 2000.
4. Mackenzie JS: Emerging viral diseases: An Australian perspective. *Emerg Infect Diseases* 1999;5:1-8.
5. Goh KJ, Tan CT, Chew NK: Clinical features of Nipah virus encephalitis among pig farmers in Malaysia. *NEJM* 2000;342:1229-1235.
6. Kerr JR: Nipah virus. *Infect Dis Rev* 2000;2:53-54.
7. Kerr JR: Nipah virus. *Infect Dis Rev* 2000;2:53-54.
8. Lim CC, Sitoh YY, Hui F, et al: Nipah viral encephalitis or Japanese encephalitis? MR findings in a new zoonotic disease. *Am J Neuroradiol* 2000;21:455-461.
9. Ali R, Mounts AW, Parashar UD, et al: Nipah virus infection among military personnel involved in pig culling during an outbreak of encephalitis in Malaysia, 1998-1999. *Emerg Infect Dis* 2001;7:759-761.
10. Fenner F, Henderson DA, Arita I, et al: *Smallpox and Its Eradication.* Geneva, Switzerland, World Health Organization, 1988.
11. Breman JG, Henderson DA: Poxvirus dilemmas: Monkeypox, smallpox, and biologic terrorism. *NEJM* 1998;339:556-559.

12. Anonymous: *The Global Eradication of Smallpox: Final Report of the Global Commission for the Certification of Smallpox Eradication.* Geneva, Switzerland, World Health Organization, 1980.
13. Henderson DA, Inglesby TV, Bartlett JG, et al: Smallpox as a biological weapon: Medical and public health management. *JAMA* 1999;281:2127-2137.
14. Wehrle PF, Posch J, Richter KH, Henderson DA: An airborne outbreak of smallpox in a German hospital and its significance with respect to other recent outbreaks in Europe. *Bull WHO* 1970;43:669-679.
15. Ellner PD: Smallpox: Gone, but not forgotten. *Infection* 1998;26:263-269.
16. Wehrle PF, Posch J, Richter KH, Henderson DA: An airborne outbreak of smallpox in a German hospital and its significance with respect to other recent outbreaks in Europe. *Bull WHO* 1970;43:669-679.
17. Fenner F, Henderson DA, Arita I, et al: *Smallpox and Its Eradication.* Geneva, Switzerland, World Health Organization, 1988, p 1460.
18. Mayers DL: Exotic virus infections of military significance. *Dermatol Clin* 1999;17:29.
19. Rao AR: *Smallpox.* Bombay, India, Kothari Book Depot, 1972.
20. Henderson DA, Inglesby TV, Bartlett JG, et al: Smallpox as a biological weapon: Medical and public health management. *JAMA* 1999;281:2127-2137.
21. Henderson DA, Inglesby TV, Bartlett JG, et al: Smallpox as a biological weapon: Medical and public health management. *JAMA* 1999;281:2127-2137.

22. Marsden JP: Variola minor: A personal analysis of 13,686 cases. *Bull Hyg* 1948;23:735-746.

23. Hutin YJF, Williams RJ, Malfait P, et al: Outbreak of human monkeypox, Democratic Republic of Congo, 1996-1997. *Emerging Infect Dis* 2001;7:434-438.

24. Anonymous: Preliminary report: Multistate outbreak of monkeypox in persons exposed to pet prairie dogs. Centers for Disease Control and Prevention, http://www.cdc.gov/nicidod/monkeypox (Accessed June 9, 2003).

25. Breman JG, Henderson DA: Poxvirus dilemmas: Monkeypox, smallpox, and biologic terrorism. *NEJM* 1998;339:556-559.

26. Ropp SL, Jin Q, Knight LC, et al: Polymerase chain reaction for identification and differentiation of smallpox and other orthopoxviruses. *J Clin Microbiol* 1995;33:2069-2076.

27. Henderson DA, Inglesby TV, Bartlett JG, et al: Smallpox as a biological weapon: Medical and public health management. *JAMA* 1999;281:2127-2137.

28. Redfield RR, Wright CD, James WD, et al: Disseminated vaccinia in a military recruit with human immunodeficiency virus (HIV). *NEJM* 1987;316:673-676.

29. Breman JG, Henderson DA: Poxvirus dilemmas: Monkeypox, smallpox, and biologic terrorism. *NEJM* 1998;339:556-559.

30. Bray M, Martinez M, Smee DF, et al: Cidofovir protects mice against lethal aerosol or intranasal cowpox virus challenge. *J Infect Dis* 2000;181:10-19.

31. Keating MR: Antiviral agents for non-human immunodeficiency virus infections. *Mayo Clin Proc* 1999;74:1266-1283.

32. Kesson AM, Ferguson JK, Rawlinson WD, Cunningham AL: Progressive vaccinia treated with ribavirin and vaccinia immune globulin. *Clin Infect Dis* 1997;25:911-4.

33. Diven DG: An overview of poxviruses. *J Am Acad Derm* 2001;44:1-14.

34. Henderson DA, Inglesby TV, Bartlett JG, et al: Smallpox as a biological weapon: Medical and public health management. *JAMA* 1999;281:2127-2137.

35. Anonymous: Smallpox vaccine. *Med Lett* 2003;45:1-3.

36. Henderson DA. Smallpox: Clinical and epidemiologic features. *Emerg Infect Dis* 1999;5:537-539.

37. McClain D: Smallpox, in Sidell F, Takifuji E, Franz D (eds): *Medical Aspects of Chemical and Biological Warfare.* Washington, DC, Borden Institute, Walter Reed Army Medical Center, 1997, pp 539-558.

38. Fenner F: Poxviruses, in Fields B, Knipe D, Howely P, (eds): *Fields Virology,* ed 3. Philadelphia, PA, Lippincott-Raven, 1996, pp 2673-2702.

39. Anonymous: *Vaccinia (Smallpox) Vaccine: Recommendations of the Advisory Committee on immunization practices.* Atlanta, GA, Centers for Disease Control and Prevention, 2001, p RR-10.

40. McClam E: Old smallpox vaccines may still help. Associated Press, http://dailynews.yahoo.com/h/ap/20011109/hl/smallpox_1.html (accessed on November 9, 2001).

41. Breman JG, Henderson DA: Poxvirus dilemmas: Monkeypox, small pox, and biologic terrorism. *JAMA* 1998;339:556-559.

42. Foege WH, Millar JD, Lane JM: Selective epidemiologic control in smallpox eradication. *Am J Epidemiol* 1994;4:311-315.

43. Tucker JB, Zilinskas RA: The 1971 Smallpox Epidemic in Aralsk, Kazakhstan, and the Soviet Biological Warfare Program CNS Occasional Papers: #9 May, 2002 by the Monterey Institute of International Studies, Monterey, CA. Accessed at http://cns.miis.edu/pubs/opapers/op9/ on March 7, 2004.

44. Baxby D: Vaccines for smallpox. Letter. *Lancet* 1999; 354:422-423.

45. Sutter G, Moss B: Novel vaccinia vector derived from the host range restricted and highly attenuated MVA strain of vaccinia virus. *Dev Biol Stand* 1995;84:195-200.

46. Moss B: Genetically engineered poxviruses for recombinant gene expression, vaccination, and safety. *Proc Natl Acad Sci USA* 1996;93:11341-11348.

47. Fenner F, Henderson DA, Arita I, et al: *Smallpox and Its Eradication.* Geneva, Switzerland, World Health Organization, 1988, p 1460.

48. Diven DG: An overview of poxviruses. *J Am Acad Derm* 2001;44:1-14.

Hemorrhagic Fever Viruses

■ Overview

Hemorrhagic fever is a clinical syndrome that causes fever, muscle pain **(myalgia)**, malaise, hemorrhage, and, in some patients, hypotension, shock, and death. These viruses produce vascular lesions with increased vascular permeability and hemorrhagic symptoms in severe cases. It would be quite difficult for the clinician to separate the various causes of these diseases, so the diseases are grouped together as the **viral hemorrhagic fever syndrome** (VHF).

There are four families of viruses that cause hemorrhagic fever: arenavirus, bunyavirus, filovirus, and flavivirus. The arenaviruses include Argentine, Bolivian, Brazilian, and Venezuelan hemorrhagic fevers, lymphocytic choriomeningitis, and Lassa fever. Bunyaviruses include hantaviruses, Congo-Crimean hemorrhagic fever virus, and Rift Valley fever (RVF) virus. Ebola and Marburg are the only known filoviruses. The flaviviruses include dengue and yellow fever, among others.

Each of these families share a number of features:

- **Arthropod** ticks and mosquitoes serve as natural vectors for some of these diseases.
- They all have a natural **reservoir** other than humans; the hosts of many of these diseases (such as Ebola and Marburg) are still unknown.
- Although the **distribution** of VHF is worldwide, these viruses are usually geographically restricted.
  - Exceptions include **hemorrhagic fever with renal syndrome** (HFRS) caused by Seoul virus which is carried by the common rat. Humans can get HFRS wherever the common rat is found.
  - Other infections can result from the introduction of animals from the usual geographic area to another area. This happened with Marburg hemorrhagic fever in Germany and Yugoslavia when monkeys were imported.
  - Travelers can bring home these diseases. In 1996, a medical provider became infected with Ebola and transmitted the disease to a nurse who became ill and died.
- Human outbreaks are irregular and sporadic. Humans can become infected in the following ways:
  - Receiving a bite from an infected arthropod
  - Handling an infected animal

- Contracting the virus from person-to-person transmission or by handling the infected body fluids of a patient
- There is no cure or established drug treatment for these diseases.

Many of these diseases are highly lethal and easily transmissible from person to person. Although **nosocomial** (in-hospital) transmission of Lassa fever and Ebola virus infection was prevented with simple universal precautions in Africa, the use of respiratory precautions has been advised by the CDC for medical workers who are in contact with patients who are infected with these diseases.

History

The hemorrhagic fever viruses have been evaluated and produced as biological weapons by the former Soviet Union and by the United States.[1-3] The Soviet Union produced large quantities of Marburg, Ebola, Lassa, and the New World arenaviruses (Junin and Machupo) until at least 1992. Yellow fever and RVF viruses were developed as weapons by the US offensive biological weapons program prior to its termination in 1969. The Aum Shinrikyo cult attempted to obtain specimens of Ebola in an effort to create biological weapons. There are reports that yellow fever has been developed for use as a weapon by North Korea.[4]

Transmission

Transmission of the VHF syndrome varies with the specific virus. For some of the viruses, human-to-human transmission is possible. All of these are potentially transmitted by aerosol. Several studies have demonstrated that the aerosol transmission of Ebola, Marburg, Lassa, and the New World arenaviruses has been accomplished by weapons researchers. Soviet Union researchers examined the aerosol infectivity of Marburg and determined that, in monkeys at least, only a few virus particles are necessary for an infection.[5,6]

Presentation

All of the VHFs begin with an acute febrile illness. Each disease has a short incubation period. The patient typically presents with an acute onset of fever, headache, muscle pain, nausea, and perhaps vomiting. Early in the course, the signs and symptoms are nonspecific and may include malaise and varying degrees of prostration. The patient may develop facial flushing, conjunctival injection, periorbital edema, and hypotension. Unfortunately, these initial symptoms are often seen with many benign illnesses.

The primary defect in patients with VHF is increased vascular permeability. After 3 to 5 days, the patient may develop petechiae **(Color plate 11-1)**, ecchymosis, **conjunctival injection** (reddened conjunctiva of the eye), and bleeding from the gums. Patients with severe cases of VHF often develop bleeding from body orifices, in internal organs, under the skin, or at the site of needle sticks and intravenous lines. As the disease progresses, diffuse bleeding and generalized mucosal hemorrhage develop. The patient may develop neurologic, hematologic, and pulmonary involvement. Vascular damage is often widespread. Diffuse bleeding may result. Severely ill patients may also experience shock, multisystem organ failure, coma, and seizures.

Ebola presents with the sudden onset of fever, weakness, muscle pain, headache, and sore throat. This nondescript onset is followed by vomiting, diarrhea, kidney and liver failure, and both internal and external bleeding. A rash is common with Marburg, Lassa, and Ebola. The only cutaneous manifestation of yellow fever is jaundice. Hepatic involvement is more common with Ebola, RVF, Congo-Crimean hemorrhagic fever, and yellow fever. Renal failure is a prominent feature of hantavirus infections.

The VHF syndrome should be suspected in any patient with a severe febrile illness and evidence of vascular involvement. However, it is important to note that not all infections caused by these viruses are associated with early hemorrhages. Fewer than 40% of Ebola and Lassa fever patients present with gum bleeding, petechia, hematemesis, or melena. Besides the nonspecific symptoms of high fever, muscle pain, headache, and nausea, the most predictive sign for Ebola and Marburg is abdominal pain accompanied by diarrhea. For Lassa fever, the patient will experience chest pain and sore throat. The hemorrhagic version of RVF begins with jaundice.

Diagnosis

Like many viral diseases, the diagnosis is best made by clinical impression. Routine labs are not helpful, although leukopenia is frequent. Clotting factors may be depressed, and thrombocytopenia may be found. Disseminated intravascular coagulopathy is common. Leukopenia is uncommon in Lassa, hantavirus, and some severe infections of Congo-Crimean hemorrhagic fever. **Proteinuria** and hematuria are common. High liver enzymes (particularly aspartate aminotransferase elevation) correlate with the severity of Lassa fever, and jaundice is a poor prognostic sign for patients with yellow fever.

Misdiagnosis of VHFs is common. Similar presentations are shared by a wide variety of tropical viral agents. Other tropical diseases include malaria, acute African trypanosomiasis, dysentery, typhus, typhoid fever, borreliosis, and leptospirosis. Also, hemorrhagic smallpox may present with significant bleeding **diathesis**. Any evidence of bleeding diathesis in multiple patients, or in a patient who has no significant risk factors for other diseases, is cause for the isolation and aggressive diagnostic testing of each suspect patient.

There is no commercially available laboratory test for the symptoms caused by these diseases. Diagnosis may be made with immunofluorescence, electron microscopy, or a culture. Specific serodiagnostic assays have been developed for each of these viral diseases, including ELISA, immunofluorescence assays, and virus neutralization assays. Reference laboratories such as the CDC detect specific antigens, sequence the genes of the virus, isolate the virus in a cell culture, examine it under an electron microscope, or detect IgM and IgG antibodies. Most patients are viremic at the time of presentation and a culture of the virus can make a definitive diagnosis in 3 to 10 days.

INHOSPITAL INFO

These tests are extremely dangerous to the laboratory worker. Because these diseases are highly contagious, the isolation of a viral agent with hemorrhagic symptoms should be conducted only in a reference laboratory with **P-4 containment capability**. Both the CDC and US Army Medical Research Institute for Infectious Diseases (USAMRIID) have diagnostic laboratories with a P-4 containment level. Laboratory specimens from infected patients should be double-bagged, and the outer bag should be decontaminated.

Remember that many illnesses can mimic a VHF. These diseases include bacterial or rickettsial sepsis, malaria, warfarin overdose, and other diseases that can cause severe bleeding.

Treatment

Because most physicians have little experience with these diseases, consultative assistance should be obtained as soon as possible. The CDC will provide emergency consultations by phone at (404) 639-1511 during the day and (404) 639-2888 at night.

Treatment is entirely supportive. Replacement of volume and blood loss is important. Because there is significant vascular permeability with these diseases, pulmonary edema may result from infusion. Colloids are recommended rather than crystalloids for volume expansion. Dopamine has been used for pressure support. The use of intravascular devices and invasive hemodynamic monitoring must be balanced against the risk of hemorrhage.

The management of bleeding should be the same as for any patient. Aspirin and other anticoagulant drugs should be avoided. Intramuscular injection may cause hemorrhage in the muscle used.

Lassa, Congo-Crimean, and HFRS may respond to prompt administration of **ribavirin**. Ribavirin is a nucleoside analogue that produces significant antiviral activity and may be useful for several of the VHF viruses. However, ribavirin has little antiviral activity against the filoviruses (Ebola and Marburg) and the flaviviruses (dengue and yellow fever). Most patients who survive the acute illness will recover.

Treatment with hyperimmune serum has been used with success in some patients infected with Ebola, Lassa, and Marburg. There are extremely limited quantities of hyperimmune serum obtained from survivors of Ebola. Experimental studies involving the use of hyperimmune sera on animals show that there is no long-term protection against the disease.

Argentinean hemorrhagic fever has responded to convalescent-phase plasma that was given within 8 days of onset. However, there are only limited quantities of this plasma available.

Prophylaxis

Yellow fever is the only hemorrhagic fever that has a vaccine. There are experimental vaccines for Argentine hemorrhagic fever, RVF, and Hantaan virus. The Hantaan virus vaccine is an experimental vaccinia-vectored vaccine available at USAMRIID. The vaccine for Argentine hemorrhagic fever appears to be effective for Bolivian hemorrhagic fever as well. It is available as an investigational new drug and was developed at USAMRIID. Some stocks of **sera** exist for Lassa, Ebola, and Marburg, which were obtained from survivors, but these stocks are adequate only for partial protection of a few people.

Ribavirin has been used for prophylaxis for Congo-Crimean hemorrhagic fever, HFRS, and Lassa fever virus exposure. Patients who receive ribavirin should be watched for breakthrough disease or disease after the cessation of therapy.

Biosafety

There are well documented infections in medical workers who have had no **parenteral** exposure to these viruses. Gloves, gowns, face shields, and respiratory protection with a fitted HEPA filtered respirator constitute the minimal protection for health care workers dealing with VHF patients. SCBA with positive-pressure garments may be appropriate in areas of high contamination.

These patients should be placed in isolation. The CDC has developed guidelines for the isolation of patients who may have VHF. Because most physicians have very little experience with these diseases, consultation should be called as soon as possible.

Any person who has contact with contaminated fluid or secretions, or who has had close physical contact with an infected patient, should be kept under strict surveillance. Close contacts or medical personnel exposed to blood or secretions from VHF patients should be monitored for symptoms, fever, and other signs during the established incubation period. Body temperature should be checked twice daily, and isolation should be imposed if the patient's temperature rises above 101°F (38.3°C). The surveillance of suspected patients should be continued for at least 3 weeks after the date of their last contact.

Bodies should be cremated or buried in leakproof material with minimal handling. **Table 11-1** summarizes biosafety information for the hemorrhagic fever viruses.

Threat

Hemorrhagic fever viruses cause high morbidity and high mortality. Some may replicate well enough in cell cultures to permit their use as a weapon. The filoviruses could be adapted as biowarfare agents because they are highly infectious, lethal, and can be stabilized for aerosol dissemination. Filoviruses have actually been considered to be too dangerous to use for biowarfare, because there are no therapeutic measures to protect the user. Because terrorists have been using suicidal weapons in other venues, this provides little assurance that filoviruses will be ruled out for use as biological weapons. Although technically difficult for terrorists to produce in large quantities, small-scale production suitable for terrorist use could be accomplished in the same space occupied by a two-car garage with only minimal modifications.[7]

The diagnosis of multiple cases of any VHF should be considered a bioterrorist event.

Table 11-1 Protection Against Hemorrhagic Fever Viruses

Inactivation Requirements	Decontaminating Agents	Personal Protection Requirements
Heat at 212°F (100°C) for more than 10 minutes	Common disinfectants	Wear respiratory protection with a fitted NIOSH N95 mask or better.
Low pH	70% ethanol	Wear gloves and a gown (secured at the wrists). This the minimum protection. A positive-pressure suit may be more appropriate for the management of VHF, but it has not been required by the WHO for its workers in infected areas.
Ultraviolet radiation	Commercial hypochlorite solutions such as 1% bleach	
Gamma radiation	2% glutaraldehyde	Wash hands, using an antimicrobial agent, after taking off gloves.
	Lipid solvents	Take secretion precautions.
	Detergents	Decontaminate soiled items before disposal.
		Dispose of soiled items by steam sterilization, incineration, or chemical disinfection.

Source: American Academy of Orthopaedic Surgeons, Stewart CE, Nixon RG. *Weapons of Mass Casualties Field Guide.* Jones and Bartlett Publishers, Boston; 2003.

Suspicion of a bioterrorist event should be quite high in a solitary case unless the patient handles primates that have been recently imported or has been recently traveling in a risk area. VHFs have a limited geographic distribution and an incubation period of less than 3 weeks. If the patient has documented VHF and has no travel history to a risk area or known exposure, consider bioterrorism.

■ Specific Hemorrhagic Fever Viruses

Old World Arenaviruses

The family name **arenavirus** comes from the Latin word, *arenaceous*, meaning sandy. Electron micrographs of the virus show that they have a granular or sandy surface, hence the name. Arenaviruses are spread by rats and mice.

The arenaviruses are often divided into two groups: the **New World arenaviruses** or **Tacaribe complex** and the **Old World arenaviruses** or LCM/Lassa fever complex. The New World arenaviruses will be discussed separately.

A new arenavirus has been found every 1 to 3 years since 1956. A number of these diseases cause hemorrhagic fever. These viruses often produce **chronic carrier states** in their hosts.

Distribution

Lymphocytic Choriomeningitis Lymphocytic **choriomeningitis** (LCM) is a rodent-borne disease that presents as an aseptic meningitis, encephalitis, or **meningoencephalitis**. It was isolated in 1933 during a study of epidemic St. Louis encephalitis. LCM is spread by the common house mouse. Mice can become chronically infected, after which they shed the virus in their urine.

LCM has been reported throughout the Americas, Europe, Australia, and Japan. Infections of the virus are often underreported, because many cases are clinically mild or inapparent. **Serologic studies** (studies of the antibodies present in the population) of this virus conducted in urban areas show that the prevalence of LCM virus infection may range from 2% to 10%.

Humans become infected by inhaling aerosolized particles containing rodent urine, feces, or saliva. Humans can also be infected by handling contaminated body fluids, blood, or body parts of either infected humans or mice. The ingestion of contaminated food can cause disease. Person-to-person transmission can occur from handling contaminated blood or body fluids. The infected pregnant woman can pass this disease to the fetus.

Although this disease is caused by one of the families of the viruses that cause hemorrhagic fever, it is not an agent of hemorrhagic fever, but of meningitis or encephalitis.

Lassa Fever Lassa fever is an acute viral illness most commonly found in West Africa. The illness was discovered in 1969 when two nurses died in Lassa, Nigeria.[8] The natural host for Lassa virus is the rat of the genus *Mastomys*. *Mastomys* rodents produce large numbers of offspring and are numerous in West, Central, and East Africa, and at least one species of this rat likes to live in human homes. Lassa fever is found in Guinea, Liberia, Sierra Leone, and Nigeria. It is **endemic** in these parts of West Africa. Because many of the rodents that carry the virus are found in additional sections of Africa, the disease may well be found in many other parts of Africa.

There are about 100,000 to 300,000 infections per year in West Africa. About 5,000 people die from this disease each year.[9] Unfortunately, the actual number of infections and deaths is estimated, because reporting in these countries is neither uniform nor reliable. In some areas of Sierra Leone and Liberia, as many as 10% to 16% of patients admitted to hospitals have Lassa fever.

Infection occurs in the same way as for LCM: from inhaling aerosolized particles from rodent urine, feces, or saliva. Because the *Mastomys* rodent is a food source for some populations, transmission can occur when preparing the rodent for food.

Presentation

The arenaviruses typically present with insidious onset, as opposed to a precipitous onset, as seen with other agents of VHF. Common findings on physical examination include ecchymosis (evidence of a diffuse capillary leak, such as edema at multiple sites), flushing, conjunctival injection, petechia, and shock.[10-13]

Lymphocytic Choriomeningitis The incubation period of LCM is about 8 to 14 days. Following incubation, the patient develops a characteristic **biphasic disease**. The initial phase, which lasts as long as a week, is quite nonspecific. The patient may experience an acute onset of fever, headache, muscle pain, nausea, and perhaps vomiting. Other, less common, symptoms include sore throat, cough, joint pains, chest pain, testicular pain, and salivary gland inflammation. Early in the course, the signs and symptoms are nonspecific and may include malaise and varying degrees of prostration.

Following a few days of remission, the second phase of the disease occurs. The patient starts to experience meningeal symptoms, including headache, fever, and stiff neck or symptoms of encephalitis, including drowsiness, confusion, sensory or motor disturbances, and paralysis.

LCM can also cause **hydrocephalus** that requires **ventricular shunting** to relieve the increased intracranial pressure. Rare complications include direct spinal cord infection (**myelitis**) and **myocarditis**.

Although LCM usually causes meningitis, it can also cause abortion, congenital defects, and mental retardation in the fetus when pregnant women are infected. Most patients who develop LCM make a complete recovery. No chronic infection has been described for LCM. However, when an infection in the nervous system occurs, there are frequent complications, including temporary or permanent neurologic damage.

Lassa Fever The incubation period of Lassa fever is 1 to 3 weeks. Following incubation, the patient develops a nonspecific fever, muscle pain, sore throat, nausea, vomiting, diarrhea, and conjunctivitis. The patient may also develop abdominal pain, chest pain, and facial swelling (**Color plates 11-2 and 11-3**). Because the symptoms of Lassa fever are varied and nonspecific, clinical diagnosis is difficult. Inflammation of the throat with white tonsillar patches is seen in patients infected with Lassa fever and is an important distinguishing feature.

Lassa fever is only slightly different in presentation from the New World arenaviruses. Lassa often causes somewhat less neurologic involvement and inconsistent changes in white blood cell components. Fewer bleeding abnormalities are present in Lassa fever than in the other hemorrhagic fever viruses. Lassa fever results in the greatest amount of edema in any of the hemorrhagic fever viruses.

Recovery typically takes about 10 days. If the patient develops edema, encephalopathy, tachypnea, hypotension, or bleeding manifestations, there is a poor prognosis.[14] About 15% to 20% of the patients hospitalized for Lassa fever die from their illness. Higher fatality rates occur in pregnant women.[15] The fatality rates are particularly high for women in the third trimester of pregnancy. About 95% of infected fetuses will die in utero, and spontaneous abortion is a serious complication of Lassa fever.

The most common long-term complication of Lassa fever is deafness. This occurs in about 33% of patients, and only 50% of these patients will recover some hearing after 1 to 3 months. Hair loss and loss of coordination may occur during recovery.

Diagnosis

Lassa fever is difficult to distinguish from severe malaria, sepsis, yellow fever, and other VHFs. Lassa fever is most often diagnosed with ELISA serologic assays for IgM and IgG antibodies. Laboratory specimens are extremely hazardous and must be handled with the utmost of care.

The virus may be cultured in 7 to 10 days in cell cultures. The virus can also be detected by reverse transcriptase-polymerase chain reaction (RT-PCR). Viral cultures should only be handled at a Level 4 biosafety laboratory, as this disease is quite hazardous.

Treatment

Ribavirin has been shown to be effective in vitro for several of the arenaviruses. Ribavirin has been studied as a treatment for Lassa fever in humans and has been shown to be effective therapy, if started within the first 6 days of the illness.[16,17]

Ribavirin is well tolerated with a mild **reversible hemolytic anemia** as the only consistent side effect in infected patients. The initial dose of ribavirin is 30 mg/kg given intravenously over 0.5 hour in saline or 2 g given orally. Ribavirin should be continued for 10 days.

Uterine evacuation improves survival in pregnant patients with Lassa fever. It is indicated because of the high likelihood of death of the fetus in these patients.

Prophylaxis

Immunity to reinfection occurs following infection, but the duration of this protection is unknown. Ribavirin has been recommended for postexposure prophylaxis of Lassa fever if the serum aspartate aminotransferase is greater than 150 IU/mL. There is little available information about efficacy of ribavirin in this situation.

Biosafety

Evidence of aerosol transmission of Lassa fever is limited, but aerosol transmission has contributed to nosocomial outbreaks. Transmission in hospitals has occurred when inadequate infection control measures were practiced. Lassa fever has caused the classic intrahospital progression of infecting the medical staff caring for a highly infective and lethal agent, as described in the following excerpt:

> On January 25, 1969, a 45-year-old nurse noticed a small cut on her finger as she cleared the secretions from the mouth of the first Lassa fever patient. Despite her immediate application of antiseptics to her finger, on February 3 she was suffering from chills, headache, severe back and leg pains, a sore throat, nausea, and a fever of 102°F. Four days later, she developed reddening of her pharynx and tender cervical lymph nodes. On February 10, she developed a rash that spread from her face to her neck, arms, trunk, and thighs. She had an inflamed and ulcerated throat, noisy breathing, coughing, chest pains, and a 104.8°F temperature. The symptoms got progressively worse as the days advanced. On February 12, the patient had a swollen face, rapid and weak heart rate. The patient died February 13, eleven days after the start of her illness. The results of the autopsy showed accumulated fluid and darkening of the lungs; enlarged, pale liver; congested heart, spleen, kidneys; and depleted lymphocytes.[18]

Biosafety for Lassa fever and LCM is the same as for all other hemorrhagic fever viruses (see Table 11-1). Patient excretions, sputum, blood, and all objects with which the patient has had contact should be disinfected with 0.5%

sodium hypochlorite solution or 0.5% phenol with detergent. Alternative methods of disinfecting include **autoclaving**, incineration, and boiling.

Serum may be heat-inactivated at 140°F (60°C) for 1 hour. Laboratory equipment used to carry out tests on blood should be disinfected as previously indicated.

Laboratory testing should be performed in high-containment facilities. If there is no such facility, specimen handling should be kept to a minimum and performed only by experienced technicians using gloves and **biosafety cabinets**.

All close contacts should be identified and observed for 3 weeks. The body temperatures of these patients should be checked at least twice daily. If a patient's temperature rises above 101°F (38°C), then the patient should be immediately hospitalized in isolation facilities as available.

Table 11-2 summarizes general information on Lassa fever and LCM.

New World Arenaviruses

The members of this family group that cause human disease are also called the Tacaribe complex of South American viruses.[19] This group includes the following viruses:

- **Guanarito virus**: causes Venezuelan hemorrhagic fever
- **Junin virus**: causes Argentinean hemorrhagic fever
- **Machupo virus**: causes Bolivian hemorrhagic fever
- **Sabia virus**: causes Brazilian hemorrhagic fever
- **North American Whitewater Arroyo virus**[20]

Distribution

As noted, both Old World and New World arenaviruses are spread by rats and mice.

Presentation

The New World arenaviruses cause less edema and variable amounts of petechiae, **purpura**, ecchymoses, **hyperemia** (congestion of blood in a body part), and mucosal hemorrhage. Minor bleeding, typically from the gum membranes, gastrointestinal bleeding, or oozing from needle stick sites, is seen in about 13% of Argentinean hemorrhagic fever patients and about 50% of Venezuelan hemorrhagic fever patients.[21,22]

Argentinean hemorrhagic fever is the most common and the most documented of the South American arenaviruses. It typically presents 6 to 14 days after exposure, but the incubation period ranges from 4 to 21 days. The onset is insidious with the usual fevers, chills, anorexia, muscle pain, and malaise. This progresses over several days to prostration, tremors, headache, abdominal pain, photophobia, and

vomiting and diarrhea. The patient does not usually develop sore throat, nasal congestion, or cough. An examination may reveal flushing of the face and upper body. An oral examination may show edema and hyperemia of the gums and oropharynx. Petechia of the oropharynx, small vesicles on the palate, and enlarged cervical lymph nodes are common. The patient may also develop conjunctivitis.

After the initial presentation, the patient develops neurologic disease within a week. The patient may develop a wide range of central nervous system dysfunction, including ataxia, dizziness, decreased deep tendon reflexes, and **hyperesthesia**.

About 75% of patients will improve over the second week of illness. The remaining 25% will manifest bleeding, progression of the central nervous system dysfunction, and shock. Development of bacterial infections, particularly pneumonia, is common. Coma, severe bleeding, seizures, and oliguria are associated with a poor prognosis. The mortality rate ranges from 15% to 30%.

Diagnosis

Appropriate laboratory diagnostic tests are not readily available for these viruses. In clinical specimens, the virus is either present in low concentrations or is difficult to isolate with common methods. Efforts are under way to evaluate whether specific detection of virus antigens in blood or tissues, presence of specific IgM in the serum of patients, or postmortem diagnostic tests (such as **immunohistochemistry**) can be added to virus isolation and RT-PCR for laboratory diagnosis of infection with these viruses.

Suspected cases should be reported to local and state health departments or to the CDC's Special Pathogens Branch, Division of Viral and Rickettsial Diseases—see this book's corresponding Website for contact information.

Treatment

Treatment with immune plasma, ribavirin, or both has reduced mortality rates to about 1%.[23,24] Convalescent patient serum (serum or plasma from patients who have recently survived an infection) has reduced mortality rates of the South American arenaviruses, but it is unavailable in the United States.[25] Use of this sera may also be associated with some late-onset neurologic diseases.[26,27]

Prophylaxis

A vaccine against Argentinean hemorrhagic fever has proven to be safe and effective in endemic areas. It also will protect monkeys against aerosol exposure to Bolivian hemorrhagic fever.[28]

Table 11-2 Summary of Lassa Fever and LCM					
Virus	Disease	Incubation Period	Location	Case-Fatality Rate	Treatment Available
LCM virus	Lymphocytic choriomeningitis	8–14 days	Worldwide	Less than 1%	Ribavirin has been studied for this disease but is not often used.
Lassa	Lassa hemorrhagic fever	5–16 days	West Africa	15%	Intravenous ribavirin should be used if serum glutamic-oxaloacetic transaminase is greater than 150 IU/mL. A vaccine is available, but it is experimental.

Preventative measures for arenavirus infections include control and exclusion of rodents in and around human buildings. Direct contact with rodents, their excretions, and nesting materials should be avoided.

Biosafety

Although person-to-person transmission has been documented for some New World viruses, it is rare. Nosocomial transmission can occur from direct contact with an infected patient's blood, urine, or secretions. Standard precautions should be taken during the treatment of patients with suspected arenavirus infections. Specific precautions against contact, droplets, and aerosol transmission should be taken for patients with severe clinical manifestations.

Bolivian hemorrhagic fever is associated with secondary person-to-person and nosocomial transmission. This occurs in a number of ways. Person-to-person transmission may occur as a result of direct contact with blood or other bodily fluids containing virus particles. Airborne transmission has also been reported. Contact with contaminated equipment or other objects may also be associated with transmission.

Argentinean hemorrhagic fever and Bolivian hemorrhagic fever appear to be less transmissible, but these viruses may be secreted in semen after recovery. This may result in the infection of an intimate partner.[29]

Specific biosafety and personal protection for each New World arenavirus will be summarized in the following sections on those specific viruses. General information on the New World arenaviruses is summarized in **Table 11-3**.

Bunyaviruses: Congo-Crimean Hemorrhagic Fever Virus

The **bunyaviruses** were named after Bunyamwera, Uganda, where the first species virus was isolated. All members of this group are spread by arthropods. The bunyaviruses discussed in this chapter are Congo-Crimean hemorrhagic fever virus and RVF virus. Congo-Crimean hemorrhagic fever virus is carried by ticks and causes a highly pathogenic form of VHF notable for aerosol transmission.

History

Congo-Crimean hemorrhagic fever virus was first observed in Crimea by Russian scientists in 1944 and 1945. At that time, human volunteers were used to determine that the virus could pass through filters and that the disease was transmitted by the bite of a tick. This agent was not maintained in the investigating laboratory and was lost. In 1956, the Congo virus was first isolated in Africa from the blood of a febrile patient in Zaire. In 1967, the Crimean virus was found to be indistinguishable from the Congo virus and the disease was renamed.

Distribution

Congo-Crimean hemorrhagic fever thrives in a wide endemic area with sporadic tick-borne outbreaks. There are frequent hospital-centered outbreaks that are marked by a high incidence of fatal infections in health care providers.[30,31] Outbreaks of Congo-Crimean hemorrhagic fever have occurred in Africa, Asia, and Europe. Outbreaks in Pakistan have highlighted the high mortality rate and the potential for person-to-person transmission of this disease.[32]

Presentation

Congo-Crimean hemorrhagic fever virus causes the most severe hemorrhage of all the hemorrhagic fever viruses. The infection is usually transmitted to a person by the bite of a tick. The incubation period is 2 to 7 days. The onset of the illness is sudden, and includes fever, chills, muscle pain, headache, and vomiting. The patient may experience epigastric and lumbar pain. Around the third to the fifth day, hemorrhages develop. These may present as petechial hemorrhages or purpura in the skin. The hemorrhages continue as bleeding from the mucous membranes, epistaxis, hemoptysis, hematuria, and melena develop. The patient may develop conjunctival injection and facial flushing. In fatal

Table 11-3 Summary of the New World Arenaviruses

Virus	Disease	Incubation	Location	Case-Fatality Rate	Treatment Available
Junin	Argentinean hemorrhagic fever	7–14 days	Argentina	15%–30%	Convalescent plasma is the established therapy. Intravenous ribavirin is effective. A vaccine is available.
Machupo	Bolivian hemorrhagic fever	7–14 days	Bolivia (province of Beni)	25%	**There is no established therapy.** Intravenous ribavirin is probably effective and should be used. The Junin vaccine may cross-protect.
Guanarito	Venezuelan hemorrhagic fever	7–14 days	Venezuela (state of Portuguesa)	40%	**There is no established therapy.** Intravenous ribavirin is probably effective and should be used.
Sabia	Brazilian hemorrhagic fever	Unknown	Brazil (state of Sao Paulo)	0.5%	**There is no established therapy.** Intravenous ribavirin is probably effective and should be used.

cases, death from massive hemorrhage occurs about 7 to 9 days after the onset of the illness.

Diagnosis

The diagnosis may be confirmed in the laboratory by intra-cerebral inoculation of baby mice with blood of the patient. The infected mouse will die in about a week. The virus can be identified by using known specific Congo virus antiserum in immunofluorescent antibody testing. ELISA and RT-PCR are available at the CDC's Special Pathogens Branch, Division of Viral and Rickettsial Diseases.

Prophylaxis

There are no vaccines available for human use in the United States.

Biosafety

Biosafety for Congo-Crimean hemorrhagic fever is the same as for all other hemorrhagic fever viruses, as listed in Table 11-1. **Table 11-4** summarizes general information on Congo-Crimean hemorrhagic fever.

Bunyaviruses: Rift Valley Fever

Rift Valley fever virus, or RVF, is a bunyavirus transmitted by mosquitoes. It is transmitted from animals to humans by bite or by exposure to infected animal tissues. A wide variety of mosquitoes may acquire the virus from feeding on infected animals, and infected female mosquitoes are capable of transmitting it to their offspring through the eggs. This provides a durable mechanism for maintaining the virus in nature, as these eggs may survive for several years in dry conditions.

Humans are highly susceptible to RVF virus infection and are readily infected by mosquitoes and aerosols. Humans can be a source of infection for mosquitoes and thus can introduce the disease to uninfected areas.

History

RVF was first described in the Rift Valley of Kenya in the early 1930s, but it is now endemic in restricted sites throughout much of sub-Saharan Africa.[33,34] Epidemics of the disease typically occur in cycles of 5 to 20 years.[35] There have been outbreaks in sub-Saharan and Northern Africa. In 1997 and 1998, there was a major outbreak in Kenya and Somalia. Major outbreaks hit Egypt in the late 1970s and Senegal and Mauritania in 1987.

Cases were found in Saudi Arabia and Yemen in 2000. Prior to this outbreak, the disease was confined to the African continent (Egypt, Kenya, Tanzania, and South Africa). Although some Western experts claim to have found the reservoir of the virus in wild rodents in the 1970s in Egypt, South African scientists contend that the reservoir is yet unknown.

The 1977 outbreak in Egypt affected 25% to 50% of all sheep and cattle. Among humans, 200,000 fell ill; 18,000 clinical cases were confirmed, including 598 deaths from hemorrhagic fevers. In 1987, RVF broke out in Mauritania following the opening of Diama Dam and resulted in more than 200 human deaths. The 1997 outbreaks in Kenya and Somalia have resulted in large losses of domestic animals as well as more than 300 human deaths. In September 2000, the disease crossed the boundaries of the African continent into Saudi Arabia and Yemen for the first time. Since then, 884 infections and 124 deaths were reported in Saudi Arabia, and 321 infections and 32 deaths were reported in Yemen.

In a pair of recent reports, NASA earth scientists have studied weather changes and subsequent outbreaks of two VHFs prevalent in Africa: RVF and Ebola. The diseases are dissimilar—Ebola only afflicts people in tropical forest areas, while RVF is deadly to livestock and occasionally to people in semiarid regions. But both are more likely to spread when the right climatic conditions exist—conditions which can be observed by satellite months in advance.

Outbreaks of RVF were linked to abnormally high and persistent rainfalls in semiarid Africa. Ensuing flooding creates the conditions necessary for the breeding of mosquitoes that transmit the virus, primarily to domestic cattle and frequently to people as well. Although the study on RVF was conclusive, the Ebola study was limited by the small number of Ebola outbreaks that occurred over the past 20 years.

Distribution

Many types of animals can be infected with RVF, and disease can be severe in many domesticated animals, including cattle, sheep, and goats. Sheep are more susceptible than cattle, and goats appear to be less susceptible.

Animals of different ages also differ in their susceptibility to severe illness. Over 90% of lambs infected with RVF may die, while only 10% of infected adult sheep die. The abortion rate among pregnant animals is very high, and a wave of unexplained abortions in livestock may signal the start of an epidemic.

Humans may become infected with RVF either by being bitten by an infected mosquito or by handling blood, fluids, or organs of infected animals. Inhalation by aerosol has caused infections in laboratory workers. It is possible that other blood-sucking insects, such as the sandfly and culicoides (commonly called no-see-ums or biting gnats), could

Table 11-4 Summary of Congo-Crimean Hemorrhagic Fever

Virus	Disease	Incubation	Location	Case-Fatality Rate	Treatment Available
Congo-Crimean hemorrhagic fever virus	Congo-Crimean hemorrhagic fever	3–12 days	Africa, Asia, Balkans, and Russia	30%	**There is no established therapy.** Intravenous ribavirin is effective in experimental animals. Clinical experience suggests that it may be useful.

act as vectors. Transmission could occur from the consumption of raw milk of infected animals, but consumption of meat of infected animals does not appear to be a common means of transmission.

Presentation

After infection, RVF virus is thought to move from the skin to draining lymph nodes, where it replicates. The virus is then spread throughout the body. The red blood cells and the liver are invaded by the virus.

The incubation period of RVF varies from 2 to 6 days. Some people show no symptoms. Others show a flulike illness that includes a sudden onset of fever of more than 101°F (38°C) for more than 48 hours, headache, weakness, nausea, muscle pain, backache, abdominal pain, and photophobia. The symptoms last for 2 to 7 days, after which the patient recovers. Although most patients with RVF develop a relatively mild case, a small proportion with RVF develop serious illness. Some patients also develop neck stiffness and vomiting. In these patients, meningitis may be suspected. The mortality rate of RVF is about 1%.

Eye Disease The most common complication associated with RVF is inflammation of the retina. Ocular lesions develop in 0.5% to 2% of RVF patients. The onset of the eye disease usually occurs 1 to 3 weeks after the onset of first symptoms. The patient presents with severe localized pain and blurring or loss of vision. As a result, approximately 1% to 10% of affected patients may experience some permanent vision loss. Death of patients with ocular disease is uncommon.

Meningoencephalitis The virus may also cross the blood-brain barrier and infect the central nervous system, causing meningoencephalitis. The onset occurs 1 to 3 weeks after the first symptoms appear. The presentation usually includes severe headache, vertigo, seizures, and/or coma. Meningoencephalitis appears in less than 1% of RVF patients. Death of patients with meningoencephalitis is uncommon.

Hemorrhagic RVF RVF may also manifest itself as hemorrhagic fever in less than 1% of RVF patients. Two to 4 days after the onset of illness, the patient shows evidence of severe liver disease. The patient may develop bleeding from the gums, jaundice, melena, bloody stools (**hematochezia**), purpura, and may vomit blood. In fatal cases, the patient hemorrhages and liver necrosis and vascular collapse occur, followed by shock and death. The fatality rate for hemorrhagic RVF is about 50%.

Diagnosis

Several approaches may be used to diagnose RVF. Serologic antibody tests, such as ELISA, can demonstrate the presence of specific IgM antibodies to the virus. The virus itself can be detected in blood during the **viremia** phase of the illness by virus propagation in cell cultures or experimental animals. It can also be identified by antigen detection testing or by RT-PCR detection of the viral genome.

Treatment

Most cases of RVF are mild and require no specific therapy. For the more severe cases, supportive therapy is appropriate. There is no established course of treatment for patients infected with RVF virus. The antiviral drug ribavirin has been shown to inhibit the viral growth of RVF in experimental animals, but it has not been evaluated in human populations.

Prophylaxis

A vaccine has been developed for human use, but it is not licensed or commercially available. The vaccine has been used to protect veterinary and laboratory personnel who are at high risk of exposure to RVF.

Other approaches to the control of disease include control of the mosquito population and protection of the human population from mosquito bites. Measures to control mosquitoes during outbreaks are appropriate and effective when access to the mosquito breeding sites is available.

Biosafety

Because many different species of mosquito are potential vectors for RFV virus, there is a potential for outbreaks in domestic livestock and associated epidemics in humans. Universal precautions are required when caring for patients with suspected or confirmed RVF. There are no reported cases of person-to-person transmission of RVF.[36] However, contact with blood and other body fluids of infected humans—especially during the later stages of illness, which are characterized by vomiting or hemorrhage—could spread the infection.

Airborne transmission during work with virus cultures or laboratory samples containing the virus was reported among laboratory workers.[37] Laboratory technicians are at risk of acquiring the disease by inhalation of these infectious aerosols generated from specimens. Samples taken for diagnosis from suspected human or veterinary cases of RVF should be carefully processed by trained staff in appropriately equipped laboratories.

At neutral or alkaline pH in the presence of protein such as serum, the virus can remain viable for up to 4 months at 39°F (4°C). Specimens stored below 32°F (0°C) will retain infectivity for 8 years. RVF virus in aerosols has a half-life in excess of 77 minutes at 77°F (25°C) and 30% relative humidity, so it is quite usable for bioterrorism.

RVF virus is inactivated by lipid solvents, detergents, and low pH. Contaminated surfaces should be washed to remove large amounts of organic matter and disinfected using strong solutions of sodium or calcium hypochlorite; residual chorine should exceed 5,000 ppm. Solutions having a pH of 6.2 (such as acetic acid) or lower are also effective.

Biosafety for RVF is the same as for all other hemorrhagic fever viruses, as listed in Table 11-1.

Threat

With the ready availability of this virus, there is no question that RVF has potential for bioterrorism. The lower mortality rate of this disease, however, would argue against its use. The high mortality of the hemorrhagic fever manifestation may make a selected strain of the virus more attractive to terrorists.

General information on RVF is summarized in **Table 11-5.**

Table 11-5 Summary of RVF					
Virus	Disease	Incubation	Location	Case-Fatality Rate	Treatment Available
Rift Valley fever virus	RVF	2–5 days	Sub-Saharan Africa	1% overall Approximately 50% for hemorrhagic fever	**There is no established therapy.** Intravenous ribavirin is effective in experimental animals. Clinical experience suggests that it may be useful. An investigational vaccine exists, but availability is doubtful.

Filoviruses: Ebola and Marburg

The name **filovirus** comes from the filamentous shape of the virus. **Ebola** and **Marburg** belong to this group. Ebola hemorrhagic fever is an acute, infectious hemorrhagic fever and arguably one of the most virulent diseases known to man. It can be spread by blood and blood products, by secretions, and by aerosol transmission.[38] It is highly lethal (with a mortality rate that is greater than 50%) and takes a rapid course. A closely related filovirus, Marburg, shares many characteristics. Marburg causes death in 50% to 90% of all clinically ill patients. Ebola virus has been covered significantly in popular literature and in several books and movies (such as *Outbreak*). The Aum Shinrikyo cult visited Zaire in 1982 to collect Ebola.[39]

History

Marburg was identified in 1967 in Marburg, Germany. A number of laboratory workers in Germany and Yugoslavia who were handling tissues from green monkeys developed hemorrhagic fever and died. A total of 31 infections and 7 deaths were associated with this outbreak. Marburg has caused a few sporadic cases of hemorrhagic fever since that time.[40]

Ebola virus was first identified in 1976 in Sudan and Zaire (now called the Democratic Republic of the Congo). In Zaire, there were 318 cases, resulting in 280 deaths over 2 months. Over 1,100 cases, resulting in more than 800 deaths, have been documented since the virus was discovered.

Distribution

Ebola Ebola hemorrhagic fever is encountered in the tropical forest areas of Africa, but despite its notoriety as a highly fatal disease, it remains a mystery in many respects. Ebola virus was described in 1976 after outbreaks of a febrile, rapidly fatal hemorrhagic illness was reported along the Ebola River in Zaire.[41] Sporadic outbreaks have continued since that time, usually in isolated areas of Central Africa. Though the first known Ebola epidemic occurred in Sudan in 1976, scientists still have not identified how the virus is transmitted or which animals host it.

An outbreak in Kikwit, Zaire, in 1995 led to 317 confirmed cases and an 81% mortality rate.[40-42] Over 60% of the patients were health care workers who were caring for infected patients. An outbreak in Uganda caused over 150 deaths, with similar demographics among health care workers. This means that any bioterrorist use of this agent would likely claim the lives of many health care workers.

One particularly fertile area for Ebola is the border of Kenya and Uganda in the Mount Elgon region. Visitors to the Kitum cave on top of Mount Elgon have contracted Marburg, while Ebola has been isolated from monkeys in Uganda, about 60 miles away.[43,44] Between 2% and 7% of the population of Central Africa have antibodies to Ebola or Marburg. Studies show that about 10% of all Asian and African monkeys have Ebola antibodies **(Color plate 11-4)**.

The natural reservoir for Ebola is unknown. Bats, monkeys, spiders, and ticks have all been investigated, but there are no definitive answers. Common factors indicate that the natural reservoir for Ebola is in part of rural Africa. Because the virus is as pathogenic in nonhuman primates as it is in humans, it is unlikely that monkeys are the natural reservoirs. It is speculated that a long-lived arthropod associated with the monkey is the natural reservoir.

Four subtypes of Ebola have been identified: Reston, Zaire, Sudan, and Ivory Coast. Although the Zaire and Sudan strains of Ebola are not usually passed between humans by aerosol, the Reston strain is easily transmitted by small-particle aerosol between monkeys and from monkeys to humans.

Secondary spread of both diseases is by contact with infected persons or contact with blood, secretions, or excretions of infected persons. The Marburg virus can be shed in semen for up to 3 to 4 months after illness, and sexual transmission of the disease has been documented in Germany.[45]

Marburg The endemic areas of Marburg appear to be in Central and East Africa. The natural reservoir for Marburg is unknown, but may be in Zimbabwe.

Presentation

Ebola virus causes hemorrhagic fever in humans and primates. Even so, little is known about how it causes infection. Studies of this virus have been hampered by the fact that it requires biosafety Level 4 containment and by the fact that no other similar, less lethal virus exists for study. The virus involves the heart, blood vessels, stomach, intestines, lymphoid tissues, and kidneys and causes organ failure and hemorrhage. The host usually dies before an immune response is achieved. As with Ebola, the exact mechanism by which the Marburg virus causes infection is unknown.

The incubation period is 2 to 21 days. The average incubation period for nosocomial transmission is 5 to 7 days. The average incubation period for close-contact transmission is 6 to 12 days. After the incubation period, the patient develops the sudden onset of fever and malaise coupled with extreme prostration **(Color plate 11-5)**. Ebola typically causes significant gastrointestinal symptoms, including nonbloody diarrhea in over 80% of patients and vomiting in over 60% of patients. Subsequently, the patient develops sore throat, abdominal and chest pain, and skin rash.

The filoviruses (both Marburg and Ebola) exhibit fairly characteristic rashes that are best seen in fair-skinned pa-

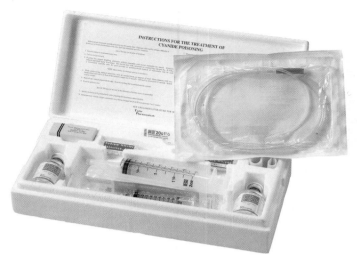

COLOR PLATE 2-1 Taylor Pharmaceuticals' cyanide antidote kit.

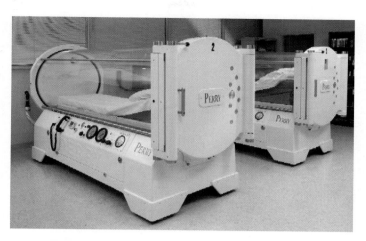

COLOR PLATE 2-2 Hyperbaric chamber.

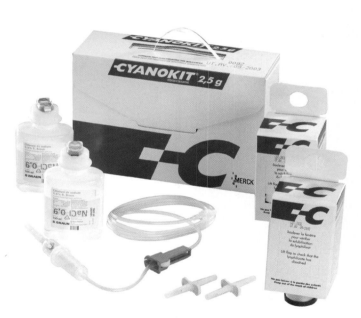

COLOR PLATE 2-3 Hydroxycobalamin cyanide antidote kit from France. Cyanokit® is a registered trademark of Merck Santé (France), an affiliate of Merck KGaA, Darmstadt, Germany. The product is not yet approved by the FDA in the U.S.

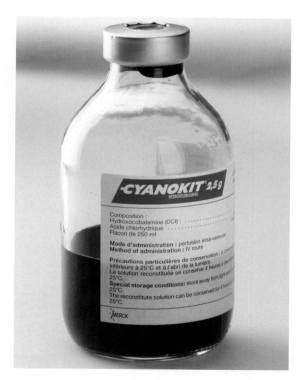

COLOR PLATE 2-4 Hydroxycobalamin. Cyanokit® is a registered trademark of Merck Santé (France), an affiliate of Merck KGaA, Darmstadt, Germany. The product is not yet approved by the FDA in the U.S.

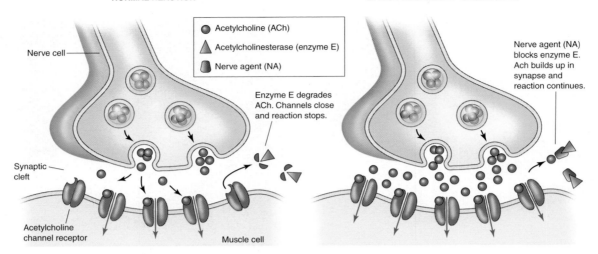

NORMAL REACTION | IN THE PRESENCE OF NERVE AGENT

- Acetylcholine (ACh)
- Acetylcholinesterase (enzyme E)
- Nerve agent (NA)

Nerve cell

Enzyme E degrades ACh. Channels close and reaction stops.

Nerve agent (NA) blocks enzyme E. Ach builds up in synapse and reaction continues.

Synaptic cleft

Acetylcholine channel receptor

Muscle cell

COLOR PLATE 3-1 A simplified picture of a cholinergic synapse. Acetylcholine is formed and released from the nerve cell. On the other side of the synapse, it binds to a muscle cell receptor for a brief time. The signal, at this stage, has been transferred from the nervous system to the performing muscle. The acetylcholine is then broken down by acetylcholinesterase. In the presence of nerve agent, acetylcholinesterase is inhibited and the acetylcholine is not broken down. It continues to send the signal to the receptor site and the muscle fatigues.

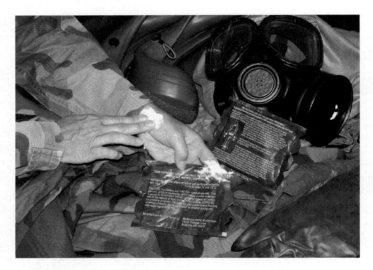

COLOR PLATE 3-2 Application of SERPACWA.

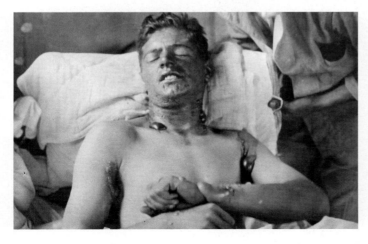

COLOR PLATE 5-1 World War I soldier with mustard burns bullae on exposed surfaces and axillae.

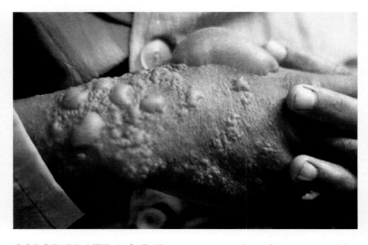

COLOR PLATE 5-2 Bullae on exposed surfaces caused by exposure to mustard.

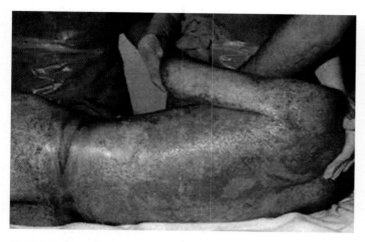

COLOR PLATE 5-3 Mustard skin burn damage.

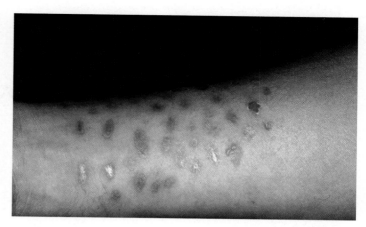

COLOR PLATE 5-4 Lesions caused by lewisite exposure.

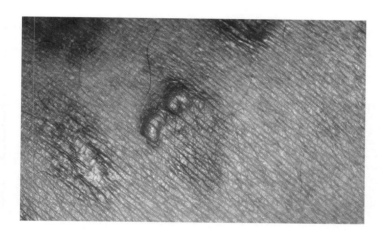

COLOR PLATE 5-5 Lewisite burns.

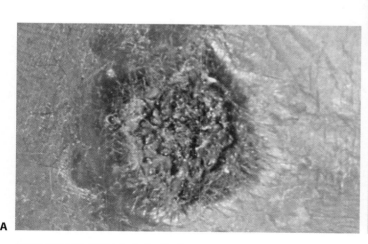

A

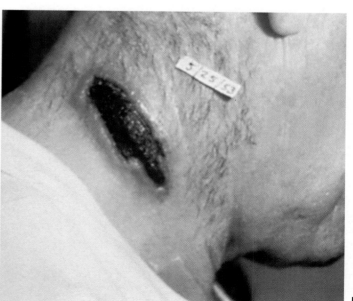

B

COLOR PLATE 9-1 A, B Cutaneous anthrax.

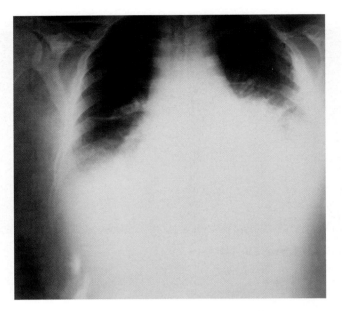

COLOR PLATE 9-2 Widened mediastinum caused by inhalation anthrax.

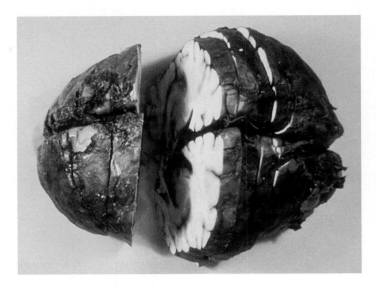

COLOR PLATE 9-3 Cardinal's cap meningeal inflammation.

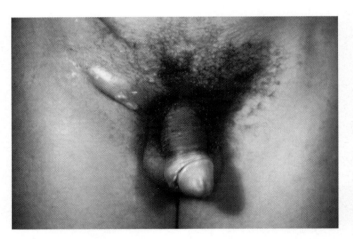

COLOR PLATE 9-4 Bubo of the groin.

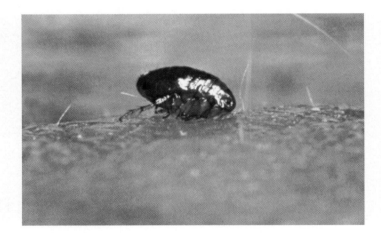

COLOR PLATE 9-5 Blood-filled biting flea.

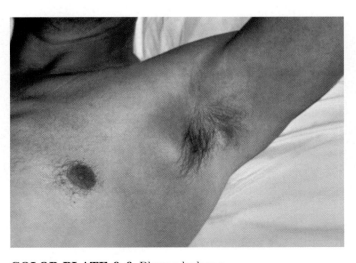

COLOR PLATE 9-6 Plague buboes.

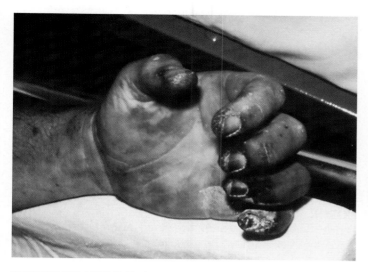

COLOR PLATE 9-7 Acral gangrene caused by plague.

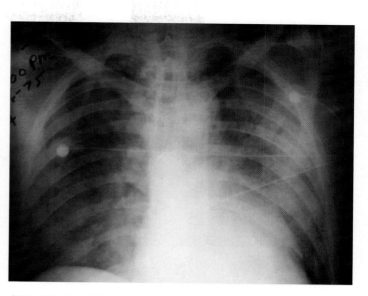

COLOR PLATE 9-8 Pneumonic plague chest radiograph. This chest radiograph was taken 24 hours before the patient expired. The patient had copious watery sputum with large numbers of organisms in it.

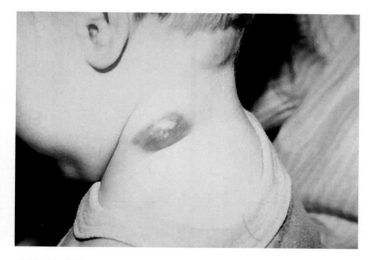

COLOR PLATE 9-9 Ulceroglandular form of tularemia.

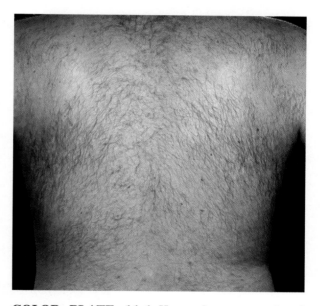

COLOR PLATE 11-1 Hemorrhages associated with dengue.

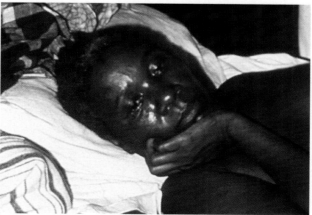

COLOR PLATE 11-2 Conjunctivitis and facial swelling associated with Lassa fever.

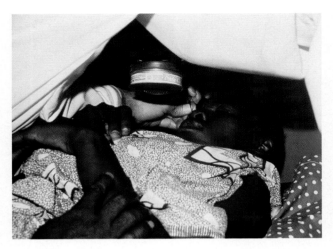

COLOR PLATE 11-3 Doctor taking eye scraping from a Lassa fever patient for testing in a Sierra Leone clinic.

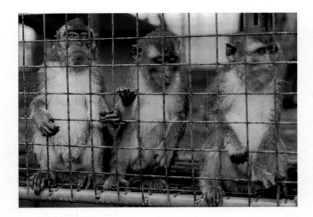

COLOR PLATE 11-4 Philippine macaque monkeys at the Fertile Scientific Research breeding farm in Laguna province south of Manila. The government ordered that all 640 monkeys at the facility be destroyed after an Ebola strain virus was found spreading in the area.

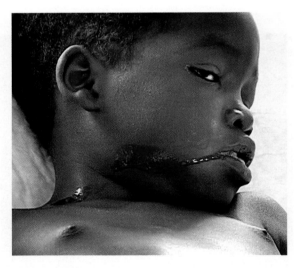

COLOR PLATE 11-5 Child with ebola.

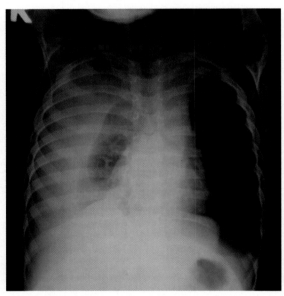

COLOR PLATE 11-6 A Chest x-ray showing a marked pleural effusion.

COLOR PLATE 11-6 B X-rays (4 days apart) of a young boy with dengue. Note the extensive pleural effusion from the plasma leakage.

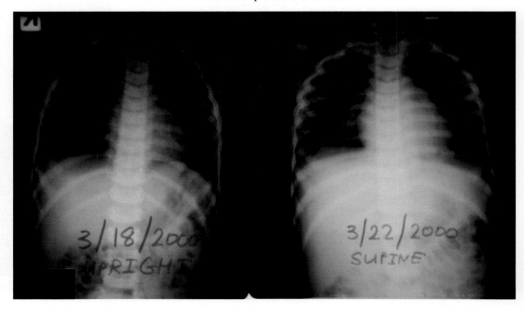

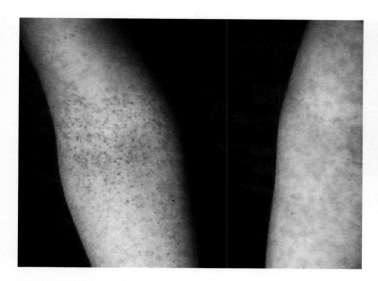

COLOR PLATE 11-7 Dengue positive tourniquet test.

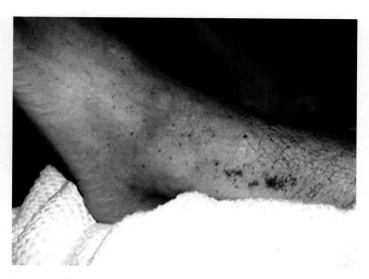

COLOR PLATE 12-1 Late (petechial) rash.

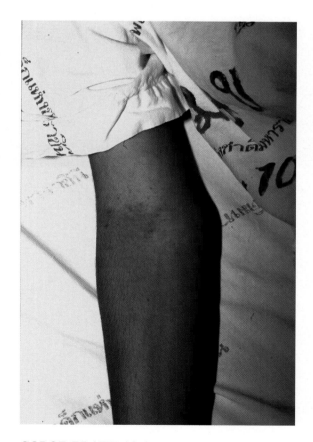

COLOR PLATE 12-2 Late (petechial) rash.

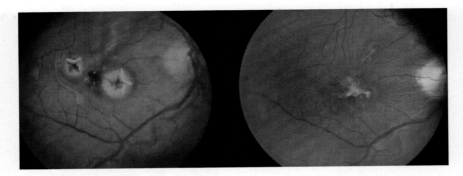

COLOR PLATE 15-1 Laser eye injury.

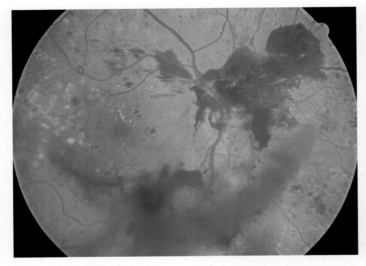

COLOR PLATE 15-2 Profuse hemorrhage into the vitreous humor.

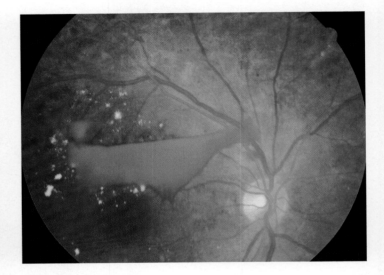

COLOR PLATE 15-3 Retinal hemorrhage.

tients. Hyperemia in the soft palate accompanies flulike symptoms and is followed, between the fifth and seventh days, by a nonitchy red rash with pinhead-sized bumps (**papules**). The rash is greatest on the chest and trunk and least on the extremities. Within 24 hours this rash develops into large hemorrhagic **macules** and papules. In severe cases, bleeding occurs from mucous membranes, needle stick sites, and all body orifices.

Ebola Ebola typically causes significant gastrointestinal symptoms, including nonbloody diarrhea in 80% of patients and nausea and vomiting in 60% of patients. Sore throat occurs in 66% of patients. The disease progresses in two phases, with apparent recovery after about 7 days. A minority of patients will gradually improve over the next 6 weeks with frequent aftereffects. The majority of patients will continue to worsen.

The patient's blood typically fails to clot, and the patient will begin to bleed from needle stick and injection sites and from the stomach, intestines, and other internal organs. Thirty-eight percent of patients develop bleeding from some site. Females may develop excessive uterine bleeding (**menometrorrhagia**). Patients who are at the greatest risk of death will develop extensive or diffuse hemorrhage into the skin, mucous membranes, gastrointestinal tract, and internal organs.

As the disease progresses, the patient may develop jaundice, interstitial pulmonary edema, and renal failure. Some patients develop hiccups. By the end of the first week of acute symptoms, the patient may bleed freely from the eyes, ears, and nose. A fall to normal body temperature may precede death.

Capillary leakage results in vascular collapse. Some patients experience coma and convulsions, followed by respiratory distress and death. Myocarditis, renal failure, and encephalitis are common, and the frequency varies depending on the specific Ebola strain.[46] Chest pain was a prominent feature in the Ebola-Sudan outbreaks, but is uncommon in Ebola-Zaire or Marburg disease.[47]

Marburg The patient will experience the sudden onset of fever, chills, and malaise with extreme prostration. The fever typically lasts 7 days. On the fifth day, the patient will develop a petechial rash that signals the start of hemorrhage. The rash is similar to the Ebola rash as previously described.

Other symptoms include headache, muscle pain, conjunctivitis, **gastritis**, and liver inflammation (**hepatitis**). The patient may develop both renal failure and pulmonary interstitial edema. Jaundice, meningitis, encephalitis, inflammation of the testicle (**orchitis**), and inflammation of the parotid gland (**parotitis**) may be noted in some patients.

Death from shock usually occurs 6 to 9 days after the onset of symptoms. Within 7 to 10 days, patients who will survive begin to recover. The recovery process can take 5 weeks or more. Patients may experience prostration, severe weight loss, and amnesia for the period of acute illness.

Diagnosis

The diagnosis of these diseases is confirmed by IgG ELISA. IgM ELISA can be used to separate acute infections from prior infection. Electron microscopy may be useful in distinguishing the filovirus, but it cannot distinguish between Ebola virus and Marburg virus. Ebola can be clearly diagnosed from the specimens obtained from deceased patients with virus isolation, immunohistochemistry, or polymerase chain reaction of blood or tissue specimens.

Laboratory findings include a reduction in the number of lymphocytes (lymphopenia) and an increased neutrophil count. The patient often has thrombocytopenia and a decreased platelet count. The serum aspartate aminotransferase is elevated and may be higher than the alanine aminotransferase.

Treatment

There is no specific treatment for Ebola or Marburg. Indeed, no currently available therapy, including **interferon**, antibody preparations, or any commercially available antiviral drugs, is effective against an infection of the filoviruses.[46-49] Several S-adenosylhomocysteine (SAH) hydrolase inhibitors have been studied that may provide some efficacy for Ebola or Marburg; however, these drugs are still under early development.[50-52]

The use of serum from recovering patients has been recommended by many as a possible therapy. During the 1995 Kikwit, Zaire, outbreak, eight Ebola patients received blood transfusions from Ebola survivors. Of these patients, seven survived. There was no clear evidence that directly linked their survival to this therapy, but the outcome demonstrated a remarkable reduction in the typical mortality rate of infected patients.

A new therapy has been developed by the U.S. Army Medical Research Institute that allowed increased numbers of animals injected with Ebola to survive. This therapy blocks coagulation factor VIIa.[53]

Prophylaxis

Exposure to Ebola does not provide subsequent immunity to another infection. A vaccine was recently demonstrated to be effective against Ebola virus in primates. However, there is currently no human vaccine available.

Biosafety

Ebola is classified as a biosafety Level 4 agent because of the extreme **pathogenicity** and the lack of any effective treatment. It is highly infectious by aerosol transmission of very few virus particles. The virus is sensitive to lipid solvents, detergents, commercial hypochlorite solutions, and phenol disinfectants. This virus is easily destroyed by ultraviolet or gamma radiation. Biosafety information for Ebola and Marburg is summarized in **Table 11-6**.

Threat

Dr. Ken Alibek, former deputy director of BioPreparat, avows that Russian scientists successfully produced a stable Marburg virus that could be delivered as a biological weapon. The use of these viruses should be considered as a potential doomsday operation. There is no guarantee that this virus would be able to be contained if it were spread to a modern city. The persistence is low, but the transmissibility is so high that the persistence is immaterial.

Table 11-6 Protection Against Ebola and Marburg

Inactivation Requirements	Decontaminating Agents	Personal Protection Requirements
Ultraviolet light Gamma radiation Heat at 140°F (60°C) for 1 hour 0.3% propiolactone for more than 30 minutes at 99°F (37°C)	Common disinfectants 70% ethanol Commercial hypochlorite solutions such as 1% bleach 2% glutaraldehyde 5% peracetic acid 1% formalin Lipid solvents Detergents	Wear respiratory protection with a fitted NIOSH N95 mask or better. Wear gloves and a gown (secured at the wrists). This is the minimum protection. A positive-pressure suit may be more appropriate for the management of these viruses, but it has not been required by the WHO for its workers in infected areas. Wash hands, using an antimicrobial agent, after taking off gloves. Take secretion precautions. Decontaminate soiled items before disposal. Dispose of soiled items by steam sterilization, incineration, or chemical disinfection.

Source: American Academy of Orthopaedic Surgeons, Stewart CE, Nixon RG. *Weapons of Mass Casualties Field Guide.* Jones and Bartlett Publishers, Boston; 2003.

Many texts note that the filoviruses are not spread by aerosol transmission, with the possible exception of Ebola-Reston. The data on the formal aerosol transmission of Ebola and Marburg indicate that these viruses are stable and infectious in small-particle aerosols.[53] This means that these viruses would be quite usable as agents of terrorism.

These viruses are well spread by body fluids, particularly blood. They are quite dangerous for the health care provider, because human-to-human contact will rapidly spread these diseases.

General information on Ebola and Marburg is summarized in **Table 11-7.**

Flaviviruses: Yellow Fever

The name **flavivirus** comes from the Latin word *flavus*, meaning yellow. This refers to the fact that this is the family of the **yellow fever** virus. Yellow fever is an acute, infectious hemorrhagic viral disease. It was the first human microbial disease that was discovered to be caused by an agent that was smaller than any known bacteria. The history of yellow fever is part of the history of the New World. Epidemics of yellow fever followed the trade ships from Africa to the Americas, and centuries of disease resulted from this transmission. It is postulated that the virus was imported to the New World in water casks and water barrels, where infected mosquitoes had laid their eggs.

Distribution

Yellow fever is found in West and Central Africa in the moist savanna zones. It is occasionally seen in urban African areas. It is uncommon in the jungle regions. Yellow fever is also found in South and Central America in woodland areas. The occasional remaining outbreak is seen among woodcutters and agricultural workers in wooded settings. There are no reported cases of yellow fever in Asia. It is thought that the high incidence of **dengue** (another flavivirus) in this area confers a limited protection against yellow fever virus. It may also be that the mosquitoes of Asia are not able to efficiently carry yellow fever virus.

The usual vector of yellow fever is the mosquito. Other insect vectors such as sand flies, horse mosquitoes, and common ticks have been shown to carry yellow fever. Mosquitoes become infected by feeding on infected monkeys. When the infected mosquito bites another host, such as a human, the virus is transferred in the mosquito's saliva to the new host. Infected humans then return to cities, where the virus is spread in the urban environment. Because of the mosquito breeding cycle, the incidence of yellow fever parallels the months of highest rainfall, temperature, and humidity. In Africa, the incidence of disease rises at the end of the rainy season.

Presentation

The incubation period of the disease is about 3 to 6 days. There are no significant symptoms during the incubation period. After the incubation period, yellow fever is characterized by a sudden onset of fever with paradoxical bradycardia (**Faget's sign**) and headache. In severe cases, the patient develops both hemorrhage and jaundice. A classic finding of yellow fever is black vomit (**hematemesis**). There are three main stages of yellow fever: invasion, remission, and intoxication.

Table 11-7 Summary of Ebola and Marburg

Virus	Disease	Incubation	Location	Case-Fatality Rate	Treatment Available
Ebola	Ebola hemorrhagic fever	3–16 days	Africa and Philippines	25%–90%	**There is no established therapy.** Hyperimmune serum has been successfully used in small numbers of humans in Russia.
Marburg	Marburg hemorrhagic fever	3–16 days	Africa and Philippines	25%–90%	**There is no established therapy.** Experimental therapies are under development.

Invasion The invasion stage lasts about 2 to 5 days and starts with the sudden onset of a fever of 102° to 104°F (39° to 40°C). Other symptoms include a flushed face, conjunctival injection, nausea and vomiting, epigastric pain, headache, muscle pain (particularly in the neck, back, and legs), prostration, restlessness, and irritability. Mild cases of yellow fever stop after 1 to 3 days of symptoms.

Remission The fever abruptly falls and the patient feels better during the remission stage. During this stage, the virus is replicating again. The remission may last several hours to several days.

Intoxication The fever and bradycardia recur during the intoxication stage. This stage lasts about 3 to 9 days. It is characterized by three distinct symptoms: jaundice, hematemesis, and renal failure. Other symptoms of yellow fever include mucosal hemorrhage, petechiae, ecchymosis, apathy, and confusion. The patient may develop melena, epistaxis, irregular uterine bleeding (**metrorrhagia**), hematemesis, dehydration, shock, hypothermia, hypoglycemia, and hiccups that cannot be cured. In terminal cases, the disease may also cause convulsions, coma, and death.

The mortality rate of yellow fever is about 10%. During epidemics, case-fatality rates may be as high as 50%.

Diagnosis

Mild cases of yellow fever are nonspecific enough that they cannot be distinguished from a variety of other conditions. Severe cases can be confused with other diseases that also cause jaundice, including viral hepatitis, malaria, typhoid, Q fever, other hemorrhagic fever viruses, typhus, and so on.

Diagnostic tests for yellow fever include antibody testing, antigen testing, and viral isolation and testing. Antibody testing includes hemagglutination inhibition (HI), complement fixation (CF), and neutralization antibodies, which appear about 7 days after the onset of the symptoms. Indirect immunofluorescence can detect antibodies when they appear. ELISA can detect antigen, even in poorly handled or contaminated specimens. RT-PCR detects the viral genome in serum.

Laboratory results may show leukopenia and thrombocytopenia. Clotting times may be prolonged, with elevated prothrombin times and some elements of disseminated intravascular coagulopathy in severe cases. In severe cases, decreased synthesis of vitamin-K–dependent coagulation factors, altered platelet function, and slightly elevated bilirubin may reflect the acute hepatic necrosis.

Treatment

Treatment of yellow fever is entirely supportive. Fluids must be carefully monitored for adequate blood volume. Transfusions may be required.

Prophylaxis

As mentioned, prior exposure to or infection with dengue appears to confer some protection against yellow fever. Likewise, infection with Wesselsbron virus and Zika virus has protected monkeys from yellow fever infections.

The 17D vaccine protects for about 10 years. This vaccine has a low incidence of side effects, including headache, muscle pain, and other minor symptoms. The vaccine is inappropriate for the following patients:

- Infants younger than 6 months (These infants have a high incidence of viral encephalitis.)
- Pregnant women (The live vaccine virus is passed through the placenta.)
- Patients with hypersensitivity to eggs (The vaccine is cultured in eggs.)
- Immunocompromised patients (There is an increased risk of adverse reactions.)

Biosafety

There are no reported cases of person-to-person transmission or nosocomial spread of the flaviviruses. However, the infection of laboratory personnel during cultivation of these viruses has been reported. This was apparently caused by the inhalation of aerosols generated from the culture media.[54] Biosafety information for yellow fever is summarized in **Table 11-8**.

Threat

As with RVF, there is a theoretical risk of flaviviruses becoming established in the environment after the infection of local arthropod vectors by a bioterrorist event. General information on yellow fever and other flaviviruses, which will be discussed next, are summarized in **Table 11-9**.

Table 11-8 Protection Against Yellow Fever		
Inactivation Requirements	**Decontaminating Agents**	**Personal Protection Requirements**
Heat at 212°F (100°C) for more than 10 minutes	Common disinfectants 70% ethanol 1% bleach 2% glutaraldehyde	Wear respiratory protection with a fitted NIOSH N95 mask or better if there is any chance of aerosol formation.
		Wear gloves and a gown (secured at the wrists).
		Wash hands, using an antimicrobial agent, after taking off gloves.
		Take secretion precautions.
		Decontaminate soiled items before disposal.
		Dispose of soiled items by steam sterilization, incineration, or chemical disinfection.

Source: American Academy of Orthopaedic Surgeons, Stewart CE, Nixon RG. *Weapons of Mass Casualties Field Guide.* Jones and Bartlett Publishers, Boston; 2003.

Table 11-9 Summary of Flaviviruses

Virus	Disease	Incubation	Location	Case-Fatality Rate	Treatment Available
Yellow fever	Yellow fever	3–6 days	Africa and South America	5%–20%	**There is no established therapy.** An excellent vaccine is available.
Dengue	DHF/DSS	3–16 days	Worldwide tropics and subtropics	1%	**There is no established therapy.** Proper fluid management is quite important because of massive capillary leak.
Kyasanur Forest disease virus	KFD	3–8 days	India (state of Mysore)	5%	**There is no established therapy.** A vaccine is produced in India.
Omsk HF virus	OHF	3–9 days	Western Siberia	5%–10%	**There is no established therapy.**
West Nile virus	WNV	5–15 days	Worldwide distribution	less than 1%	**There is no established therapy.**

Flaviviruses: Dengue

Another type of flavivirus causes dengue fever. Four types of dengue exist.

History

Dengue hemorrhagic fever (DHF) and **dengue shock syndrome** (DSS) were first described in 1954 in Southeast Asia. DHF has expanded from Southeast Asia to the Americas, China, and the Middle East.

Distribution

Dengue is the most common flavivirus infection of humans. Indeed, in some parts of Southeast Asia, the infection rate is 10% to 20% of the population.[55] There are an estimated 100 million cases of dengue each year. The disease is widespread and occurs in all tropical regions where *Aedes aegypti* mosquitoes are found. Dengue infections occur year-round, with a significant increase during the rainy season.

Dengue has appeared infrequently in the United States since the 1940s.[56] It remains a threat, because the mosquito vectors for dengue are widely dispersed in the United States, particularly in the states bordering the Gulf of Mexico.

Presentation

The four presentations of dengue fever are nonspecific febrile illness, classic dengue fever, DHF, and DSS. Several other dengue syndromes exist, including encephalopathy and cardiomyopathy.

Although dengue is considered to be comprised of four separate diseases from the epidemiologist's viewpoint, the clinician sees only one disease with four different presentations. Because there are four types of dengue, multiple sequential infections can occur.[57] Symptomatic illness is quite common with the first and second episodes of dengue. Subsequent infections tend to be mild or asymptomatic.

Dengue has an incubation period of 2 to 14 days. The patient usually experiences no symptoms during the incubation period. After the incubation period, the patient may develop a mild undifferentiated febrile illness or a severe and fatal hemorrhagic fever. During this time, the patient also develops **seroconversion** (the development of antibodies in the blood).

Nonspecific Febrile Illness The disease starts abruptly with high fever, chills, headache, back pain, anorexia, and nausea.[58] The patient often remembers the moment of onset of the first symptoms.[59] Fever, malaise, and a distinct macular rash occur and are quite like those seen in many less lethal diseases. These patients may never seek medical care.

Classic Dengue Fever The typical case of dengue fever is severe and may incapacitate the patient. The patient develops a high fever and chills. A diffuse red mottling of the skin may precede the fever. At the same time, the patient may develop a severe frontal and retro-orbital headache, diffuse muscle pain (particularly in the lower back, arms, and legs), joint pain (**arthralgia**, particularly in the shoulders and knees), profound weakness, and anorexia. Clinical findings also include facial flushing, sore throat, cough, conjunctivitis, and a slow pulse relative to the high fever.

The fever breaks on the third to fifth day and is associated with a diffuse maculopapular rash, resembling measles on the trunk. This rash spreads to the face and limbs and may burn or itch intensely. The soles and palms are often spared. Shedding of the skin may occur while the rash is healing.

Hemorrhagic symptoms may occur at about the time the fever falls. In milder cases, these can include petechiae, purpura, bleeding from the gums or nose, vaginal bleeding, and gastrointestinal bleeding. In classic dengue fever, susceptible patients may develop life-threatening gastrointestinal hemorrhage.[60]

The disease is milder in younger children.[61] In newborns, however, dengue fever varies in severity and may be lethal. Febrile seizures have been reported in children with this disease.[62] A high temperature without the usual tachycardia is more frequent in children than adults. Convalescence in children usually occurs without event.

The convalescent stage takes weeks to resolve. The patient continues to be weak, may have attention deficits, and may be depressed. The recovery of appetite and 2 to 3 days without fever or complications are good prognostic signs.

Dengue Hemorrhagic Fever and Dengue Shock Syndrome DHF and DSS are more severe forms of dengue, and were first described in the early 1950s. DHF is defined by the presence of fever thrombocytopenia and hemoconcentration.[63] DSS adds hypotension or profound shock.

Like classic dengue fever, DHF starts with the sudden elevation of body temperature. The disease appears to be similar to classic dengue until the second to fifth days, when the more severe symptoms start to appear.

Patients with DHF may have right upper quadrant tenderness and generalized abdominal pain. **Sonography** may show peritoneal fluid accumulations, indicating **acalculous cholecystitis**.

The hemorrhagic manifestations can be minimal or may dominate the clinical picture of these patients. Major hemorrhagic symptoms occur in 10% to 15% of infected patients. In milder cases, these symptoms can include petechiae, purpura, bleeding from the gums or nose, vaginal bleeding, and gastrointestinal bleeding. These patients may develop petechiae, ecchymoses, pleural effusions, and hypotension **(Color plates 11-6 A, B)**.

Massive plasma leakage into serous and interstitial spaces may occur for 12 to 48 hours. It is during this time that the most danger to the patient exists and the most fatalities occur. Plasma leakage may cause edema, hemoconcentration, and **hypoalbuminemia**.[64,65]

The patient who has DHF is also at risk for DSS. DSS occurs when the patient develops circulatory failure, including a narrowing of the pulse pressure (to less than 20 mm Hg), hypotension, or shock. The circulatory failure may develop rapidly and progress to death in 12 to 24 hours. The duration of the shock may be brief and may recur. If the patient experiences a recurrence of the shock, the prognosis is poor.[66]

Warning signs for DSS have been described by the WHO:
- Clinical
  - Severe abdominal pain
  - Prolonged and/or large volume vomiting
  - Abrupt change from fever to hypothermia, at times with syncope
  - Change in level of consciousness (including irritability and drowsiness)
  - Shock
- Laboratory
  - Progressively rising hematocrit
  - Progressively decreasing platelet count

Diagnosis

The diagnosis of dengue is clinical. The abrupt onset and muscle pain resemble those of influenza. The rashes resemble those of rubella, measles, and **meningococcemia**. The headache, prostration, and paradoxic bradycardia are similar to those found in typhoid fever. The rigors and chills that precede the infection are similar to those of malaria.

Dengue virus can be cultured on mosquito cell media. Diagnosis of dengue infections can be made by serologic techniques or by IgM ELISA after about 5 days of illness. All flavivirus species, including yellow fever, Japanese encephalitis, St. Louis encephalitis, West Nile, Murray Valley encephalitis, Kyasanur Forest disease, and tick-borne encephalitis viruses have common envelope proteins and cross-react in serologic tests. This makes unequivocal serologic diagnosis of infection by a flavivirus difficult. Identification of serotypes is possible by the use of serotype-specific antibodies. A fall in platelet count, associated with a rising hematocrit, suggests the development of DHF and the possibility of DSS.

One test that may be useful is the tourniquet test **(Color plate 11-7)**. Note that this test is not specific for dengue. This test is positive in over 50% of patients with DHF.
- *Method:* Inflate a blood pressure cuff to the median blood pressure (average of systolic and diastolic) in the patient's extremity for about 5 minutes or until positive.
- *Interpretation:* The test is positive when 3 or more petechiae per square centimeter or 20 per square inch appear. If the patient is in profound shock, the test may not be positive.

Treatment

There is no effective therapy for dengue. Ribavirin produces no activity against the flaviviruses. Most patients, however, do not require hospitalization for this disease.[67]

Treatment is entirely supportive and includes volume replacement and symptomatic care. The prognosis of patients with DHF/DSS depends on early recognition and treatment of the shock. Massive plasma leakage into serous and interstitial spaces may require equally massive fluid replacement. Generally, 10- to 20-mL/kg boluses of fluid are recommended every 30 to 60 minutes according to vital signs. These doses are quite suitable for children as well as adults. A patient should be considered critically ill if the clinician uses more than 60 mL/kg of fluids in boluses and the patient's condition fails to improve or continues to deteriorate. Further plasma loss may require colloidal solutions rather than crystalloids.

The critically ill patient should be monitored at least hourly for vital signs and urine output. Hematocrit should be checked every 2 to 4 hours. Patients with a declining hematocrit may benefit from transfusion, if it is available.

These patients may develop acute congestive heart failure, as the fluids given to maintain the pressure start to mobilize after 24 to 48 hours. To avoid **hypervolemia** and acute congestive heart failure after these massive fluid quantities, the intravenous fluids should be tapered at 1- to 2-hour intervals as soon as vital signs are stable. Despite all precautions, some patients will require diuretics and more invasive therapy for the congestive heart failure.

Aspirin and nonsteroidal anti-inflammatory drugs should be avoided because of the increased possibility of hemorrhagic complications. Steroids have been advocated but have no proven benefit.

Prophylaxis

The only measures currently available for the prevention of dengue are the personal protective measures taken to avoid mosquito bites and the public health measures taken to eliminate mosquito breeding sites. Ribavirin produces no activity against the flaviviruses and would be of no help in prophylaxis. A candidate vaccine is under development.[68,69]

Biosafety

Infection with dengue virus results in life-long specific immunity to that type of dengue. A cross-reactivity immunity lasts for 2 to 12 months, and individuals can theoretically become infected with all four serotypes of dengue.

As it naturally occurs, dengue requires a mosquito vector for transmission. There is no need for isolation procedures for patients infected with dengue. However, because diagnosis may be confused with other hemorrhagic fevers, these patients should be treated with strict isolation until the diagnosis is confirmed. Biosafety information for dengue is summarized in **Table 11-10.**

Threat

Dengue was excluded by the CDC Working Group on Civilian Biodefense, because it cannot be transmitted by small-particle aerosol, and because primary dengue only rarely causes VHF.[70] This may be overly optimistic. This virus is endemic in a large part of the world that does not always sympathize with the goals of the United States. Because the mosquito vectors for dengue are widely dispersed in the United States, a bioterrorist event with dengue, in the appropriate locale and during the proper season, could pose a continuing threat. Transmission by infected insects was used with moderate success in World War II by the agents of Japanese Army Unit 731. Dengue could be easily obtained and relatively easily disseminated with technology available since 1944.

Because dengue is a disease that is quite common in many parts of the world and has been documented in the United States, a solitary case of dengue should only raise suspicions of a bioterrorist event when circumstances do not fit the disease. If the patient has recently traveled to Texas, Louisiana, or south of the U.S. borders, a natural contraction of this disease is quite possible. If multiple cases of dengue occur in a small area in other parts of the country, then the practitioner should be quite suspicious of the involvement of bioterrorism.

Hantaviruses

The **hantaviruses** belong to the family of bunyaviruses. They are divided into Old World hantaviruses (such as the prototypical **Hantaan virus** of Korea), and New World hantaviruses. Rodents carry both types. Many hantaviruses are spread worldwide, causing two major syndromes: hemorrhagic fever with renal syndrome (HFRS) and **hantavirus pulmonary syndrome** (HPS).

History

A recent report from Argentina underscores the risk of secondary transmission of HPS and cites 15 cases resulting in 8 deaths.[71] In the southwestern United States, a previously undiscovered hantavirus, Sin Nombre virus, was the cause of an outbreak of highly lethal HPS in 1993.

Distribution

Epidemic and sporadic hantavirus associated diseases have occurred since the 1930s in Scandinavia and the northeastern part of Asia. Isolation of the first recognized hantavirus was reported in South Korea in 1978. Thousands of troops were infected with hantaviruses during the Korean War. Hantaviruses have been isolated from rodents in the United States. Acute disease was not reported in the Western hemisphere until 1993.

Presentation

The incubation period of HFRS is about 2 weeks. After the incubation period, the severity ranges from very mild illness to severe disease, with accompanying renal failure in the most severe cases.

Hantaviruses can cause a relatively distinctive rash with a petechial eruption around the neck and on the anterior and posterior axillary folds, the arms, and the trunk. A sunburnlike flush is often seen on the head, neck, upper chest, and back. This may be accompanied by facial edema. Oral and conjunctival surfaces may develop severe hemorrhages.

The illness begins with headache, malaise, muscle pain, and fever. Symptoms progress to vomiting, abdominal pain, and lower back pain. A blanching rash occurs about the torso and the face. Petechiae may be noted within the rash and on the palate.

The febrile period lasts about 3 to 7 days. At the end of the febrile period, many patients develop hypotension and shock. This period of hypotension may be accompanied by disseminated intravascular coagulopathy and bleeding diathesis. Renal failure with oliguria occurs in up to 70% of patients. Dialysis may be needed for therapy.

After the febrile period, the patient may begin a profound **diuresis** (increased excretion of urine). This fluid loss may cause life-threatening hypotension and electrolyte

Table 11-10 Protection Against Dengue		
Inactivation Requirements	Decontaminating Agents	Personal Protection Requirements
Heat at 212°F (100°C) for more than 10 minutes	Common disinfectants	Wear respiratory protection with a fitted NIOSH N95 mask or better.
Low pHs	70% ethanol	Wear gloves and a gown (secured at the wrists).
	1% bleach	Wash hands, using an antimicrobial agent, after taking off gloves.
	2% glutaraldehyde	Take secretion precautions.
		Decontaminate soiled items before disposal.
		Dispose of soiled items by steam sterilization, incineration, or chemical disinfection.

Source: American Academy of Orthopaedic Surgeons, Stewart CE, Nixon RG. *Weapons of Mass Casualties Field Guide.* Jones and Bartlett Publishers, Boston; 2003.

Table 11-11 Protection Against Hantaviruses

Inactivation Requirements	Decontaminating Agents	Personal Protection Requirements
Heat at 212°F (100°C) for more than 10 minutes Ultraviolet light	1% bleach 1% peracetic acid Formaldehyde Ethylene oxide (gas) Irradiation	Wear respiratory protection with a fitted NIOSH N95 mask or better. Wear gloves and a gown (secured at wrists). Wash hands, using an antimicrobial agent, after taking off gloves. Take secretion precautions. Decontaminate soiled items before disposal. Dispose of spoiled items by steam sterilization, incineration, or chemical disinfection.

Source: American Academy of Orthopaedic Surgeons, Stewart CE, Nixon RG. *Weapons of Mass Casualties Field Guide.* Jones and Bartlett Publishers, Boston; 2003.

abnormalities. Additional complications include pulmonary edema, cerebrovascular accidents, hemorrhage, and acidosis. The overall risk of death from this disease is about 5% to 7%, but this risk was 15% during the Korean War.

HFRS is caused by four strains of hantavirus. The most severe disease is caused by the Hantaan virus, which is distributed throughout the Far East, eastern Russia, and the Balkans, and by the Dobrava virus, which is also found in the Balkans. A milder form of disease is associated with the Seoul virus, which has worldwide distribution. The mildest form of the disease is associated with Puumala virus, which is found throughout Scandinavia, western Russia, and Europe.

HFRS is transmitted by the aerosolization of infected rodent dung. The peak rates of disease occur when rodent density and reproductivity are highest, in November and December. There may be up to 100,000 naturally occurring cases of HFRS each year. The majority occur in China.

Diagnosis

Hantavirus infection and HFRS can be diagnosed by culture, IgM ELISA, immunofluorescent antibody assays, or radioimmunoassay. HFRS is caused by a hantavirus that is difficult to culture. It is anticipated that polymerase chain reaction techniques will soon be available for these viruses. Laboratory findings include leukocytosis, thrombocytopenia, and proteinuria.

Treatment

Hantavirus infections have been treated effectively with intravenous and oral ribavirin. Because of this, ribavirin has been recommended as a potential treatment for other arenaviruses and bunyaviruses. This treatment is most effective when administered early in the clinical course. Patients with

HFRS should also receive ribavirin. The recommended loading dose is 33 mg/kg, followed by 16 mg/kg every 6 hours for 4 days, and then 8 mg/kg every 8 hours for 3 days.[72,73]

Other patient care is completely supportive. It is important to avoid injudicious use of intravenous fluids to avoid causing edema. Colloids or whole blood are appropriate to treat hemorrhagic shock. **Pressors** are appropriate for the treatment of hypotension. Dialysis can be lifesaving for patients with HRFS.

Prophylaxis

Ribavirin may be appropriate for postexposure prophylaxis. However, there are no controlled studies that address this. A vaccine against HFRS resulting from Hantaan virus has been developed, but this vaccine is not commercially available.

If the virus is spread by rodents, reducing the rodent population and avoiding contact with rodents is appropriate. By the time patients who have been deliberately infected with this disease present to an emergency department, it is unlikely that decontamination or isolation will be useful. As always, the isolation of a patient with hemorrhagic fever is appropriate until the virus is identified.

Biosafety

Biosafety information for hantaviruses is summarized in **Table 11-11.** Biosafety for HFRS is the same as for other hantavirus infections. **Table 11-12** summarizes general information on hantaviruses.

Threat

The Asian strains of the hantaviruses are not considered to be potential biological weapons at present. There is always the possibility of the genetic engineering of these agents.

Table 11-12 Summary of Hantaviruses

Virus	Disease	Incubation	Location	Case-Fatality Rate	Treatment Available
Hantaan Dobrava, etc	HFRS	9–35 days	Worldwide	5%–15%	**Supportive treatment including dialysis is critical.** Intravenous ribavirin may be useful.
Sin Nombre, Laguna Negra, Andes, etc	HPS	7–28 days	Americas	40%	**There is no established therapy.** Experimental therapies are all either marginal or ineffective. Supportive intensive care unit therapy is particularly important.

Table 11-13 Guidelines for VHF Isolation Precautions

Anyone presenting with fever and signs of bleeding such as the following, regardless of whether there is a history of contact with a suspected case:

- Bleeding from the gums
- Bleeding from the nose
- Red eyes
- Bleeding into the skin
- Blood or dark colored stools
- Vomiting blood

OR

Anyone living or deceased with the following:

- Contact with a suspected case of VHF

AND

- A history of fever, with or without signs of bleeding

OR

Anyone living or deceased with a history of fever and three of the following symptoms:

- Headache
- Vomiting
- Loss of appetite
- Diarrhea
- Weakness or severe fatigue
- Abdominal pain
- Generalized muscle or joint pain
- Difficulty swallowing
- Difficulty breathing
- Hiccups

OR

- Any unexplained death in an area with suspected cases of VHF

Adapted from: Borio L, Inglesby T, Peters CJ, Schmaljohn AL, et al. Hemorrhagic fever viruses as biological weapons: medical and public health management. *JAMA* 2002;287(18):2391-405.

Summary

Isolation precautions are paramount when dealing with highly pathogenic disease such as the VHFs. **Table 11-13** summarizes the conditions under which isolation precautions for VHFs must be taken.

■ References

1. Alibek K, Handelman S: *Biohazard: The Chilling True Story of the Largest Covert Biological Weapons Program in the World, Told From the Inside by the Man Who Ran It.* New York, NY, Random House, 1999.
2. Anonymous: Chemical and biological weapons: Possession and programs, past and present. Center for Nonproliferation Studies, November 2000, http://cns.miis.edu/research/cbw/possess.htm (accessed July 29, 2002).
3. Anonymous: A History of biological warfare. US Army Medical Research Institute for Infectious Diseases, http://www.au.af.mil/au/awc/awcgate/usamriid/bw-hist.htm (accessed July 29, 2002).
4. Anonymous: Country overviews North Korea: Biologic. Nuclear Threat Initiative, April 2003, http://www.nti.org/e_research/profiles/NK/Biological (accessed June 7, 2003).
5. Kortpeter MG, Parer GW: Potential biological weapons threats. *Emerg Infect Dis* 1999;5:523-527.
6. Peters CJ: Are hemorrhagic fever viruses practical agents for biological terrorism? in Scheld WM, Graig WA, Hughes JM (eds): *Emerging Infections,* ed 4. Washington, DC, ASM Press, 2000.
7. Peters CJ: Are hemorrhagic fever viruses practical agents for biological terrorism? in Scheld WM, Graig WA, Hughes JM (eds): *Emerging Infections,* ed 4. Washington, DC, ASM Press, 2000.
8. Frame JD, Baldwin JM Jr, Gocke DJ, Troup JM: Lassa fever, a new virus disease of man from West Africa. I. Clinical description and pathological findings. *Am J Trop Med Hyg* 1970;19(4):670-676.
9. McCormick JB, Webb PA, Krebs JW, Johnson KM, Smith ES: A prospective study of the epidemiology and ecology of Lassa fever. *J Infect Dis* 1987;155(3):437-444.
10. Bwaka MA, Bonnet MJ, Calain P, et al: Ebola hemorrhagic fever in Kikwit, Democratic Republic of the Congo: Clinical observations in 103 patients. *J Infect Dis* 1999;179(suppl 1): S1-S7.
11. Harrison LH, Halsey NA, McKee KT Jr, et al: Clinical case definitions for Argentine hemorrhagic fever. *Clin Infect Dis* 1999;28(5):1091-1094.
12. de Manzione N, Salas RA, Paredes H, et al: Venezuelan hemorrhagic fever: Clinical and epidemiological studies of 165 cases. *Clin Infect Dis* 1998;26(2):308-313.
13. Vainrub B, Salas R: Latin American hemorrhagic fever. *Infect Dis Clin North Am* 1994;8(1):47-59.
14. McCormick JB, King IJ, Webb PA, et al: A case-control study of the clinical diagnosis and course of Lassa fever. *J Infect Dis* 1987;155(3):445-455.
15. Price ME, Fisher-Hoch SP, Craven RB, McCormick JB: A prospective study of maternal and fetal outcome in acute Lassa fever infection during pregnancy. *BMJ* 1988;297(6648): 584-587.
16. McCormick JB, King IJ, Webb PA, et al: Lassa fever: Effective therapy with ribavirin. *N Engl J Med* 1986;314(1):20-26.
17. Huggins JW: Prospects for treatment of viral hemorrhagic fevers with ribavirin, a broad-spectrum antiviral drug. *Rev Infect Dis* 1989;11(suppl 4):S750-S761.
18. Unknown: Lassa fever: Pathology and pathogenesis. McMaster University, http://www.science.mcmaster.ca/Biology/Virology /18 /Sixnin.htm (accessed June 8, 2003).
19. Doyle TJ, Bryan RT, Peters CJ: Viral hemorrhagic fevers and hantavirus infections in the Americas. *Infect Dis Clin North Am* 1998;12(1):95-110.
20. Anonymous: Fatal illnesses associated with a new world arenavirus—California, 1999-2000. *Morb Mortal Wkly Rep* 2000;49(31):709-711.
21. Harrison LH, Halsey NA, McKee KT Jr, et al: Clinical case definitions for Argentine hemorrhagic fever. *Clin Infect Dis* 1999;28(5):1091-1094.
22. de Manzione N, Salas RA, Paredes H, et al: Venezuelan hemorrhagic fever: Clinical and epidemiological studies of 165 cases. *Clin Infect Dis* 1998;26(2):308-313.
23. Peters CJ, Buchmeier MJ, Rollin PE, Ksiazek TG: Arenaviruses, in Fields B, Knipe D, Howely P (eds): *Fields Virology,* ed 3. Philadelphia, PA, Lippincott-Raven, 1996, pp 1521-1551.
24. Enria D, Bowen MD, Mills JN, Shieh W, Bausch DG, Peters CJ: Arenavirus infections, in Guerrant RL, Walker DH, Weller PF (eds): *Tropical Infectious Diseases: Principles, Pathogens, and Practice.* New York, NY, WB Saunders, 1999, pp 1191-1212.

25. Borio L, Inglesby T, Peters CJ, Schmaljohn AL, et al. Hemorrhagic fever viruses as biological weapons: Medical and public health management. *JAMA* 2002;287(18):2391-2405.

26. Enria DA, Briggiler AM, Fernandez NJ, Levis SC, Maiztegui JI: Importance of dose of neutralising antibodies in treatment of Argentine haemorrhagic fever with immune plasma. *Lancet* 1984;2(8397):255-256.

27. Maiztegui JI, Fernandez NJ, de Damilano AJ: Efficacy of immune plasma in treatment of Argentine haemorrhagic fever and association between treatment and a late neurological syndrome. *Lancet* 1979;2(8154):1216-1217.

28. Jahrling PB: Viral hemorrhagic fevers, in Sidell FR, Takafuji ET, Franz DR (eds): *Medical Aspects of Chemical and Biological Warfare.* Falls Church, VA, Office of the Surgeon General, Department of the Army, United States of America, 1997, pp 591-602.

29. Enria D, Bowen MD, Mills JN, Shieh W, Bausch DG, Peters CJ: Arenavirus infections, in Guerrant RL, Walker DH, Weller PF (eds): *Tropical Infectious Diseases: Principles, Pathogens, and Practice.* New York, NY, WB Saunders, 1999, pp 1191-1212.

30. Isaacson M: Viral hemorrhagic fever hazards for travelers in Africa. *Clin Infect Dis* 2001;33(10):1707-1712.

31. Weber D, Rutala W: Risks and prevention of nosocomial transmission of rare zoonotic diseases. *Clin Infect Dis* 2001;32(3):446-456.

32. Anonymous: Outbreak news. *Wkly Epidemiol Rec* 2002;77:1-9

33. Daubney R, Hudson JR, Garnham PC: Enzootic hepatitis or Rift Valley fever: An undescribed viral disease of sheep, cattle, and man from East Africa. *J Pathol Bacteriol* 1931;34:545-579.

34. Findlay GM: Rift Valley fever or enzootic hepatitis. *Trans Royal Soc Trop Med Hyg* 1931;25:229-262.

35. Davies FG, Linthicum KJ, James AD: Rainfall and epizootic Rift Valley fever. *Bull World Health Organ* 1985;63:941-943.

36. Jouan A, Coulibaly I, Adam F, et al: Analytical study of a Rift Valley fever epidemic. *Res Virol* 1989;140:175-186.

37. Smithbum KC, Mahaffy AF, Haddow AJ, et al: Rift Valley fever, accidental infections among laboratory workers. *J Immunol* 1949;62:213-227.

38. Jaax N, Jahrling P, Geisbert T, et al: Transmission of Ebola virus (Zaire strain) to uninfected control monkeys in a biocontainment laboratory. *Lancet* 1995;356:1669-1671.

39. Anonymous: A case study on the Aum Shinrikyo. Senate Government Affairs Permanent Subcommittee on Investigations, October 31, 1995, http://www.fas.org/irp/congress/1995_rpt/aum/part08.htm (accessed June 8, 2003).

40. Borio L, Inglesby T, Peters CJ, Schmaljohn AL, et al. Hemorrhagic fever viruses as biological weapons: Medical and public health management. *JAMA* 2002;287(18):2391-2405.

41. Kahn AS, Tshioko FK, Heymann DL, et al: The reemergence of Ebola hemorrhagic fever: Democratic Republic of the Congo, 1995. *Journal of Infect Dis* 1999;179(suppl 1): S76-S86.

42. Amblard J, Obiang P, Edzang S, Prehaud C, Bouloy M, Guenno BL: Identification of the Ebola virus in Gabon in 1994. *Lancet* 1997;349(9046):181-182.

43. Le Guenno B, Formenty P, Boesch C: Ebola virus outbreaks in the Ivory Coast and Liberia, 1994-1995. *Curr Top Microbiol Immunol* 1999;235:77-84.

44. Georges AJ, Leroy EM, Renaut AA, et al: Ebola hemorrhagic fever outbreaks in Gabon, 1994-1997: Epidemiologic and health control issues. *J Infect Dis* 1999;179(suppl 1):S65-S75.

45. Anonymous: Facts on Ebola. Centers for Disease Control and Prevention, http://www.cdc.net/~gildrnew/fil/filo12.html (accessed June 7, 2003).

46. Bwaka MA, Bonnet MJ, Calain P, et al: Ebola hemorrhagic fever in Kikwit, Democratic Republic of the Congo: Clinical observations in 103 patients. *J Infect Dis* 1999;179(suppl 1):S1-S7.

47. Sanchez A, Peters C, Zaki S, Rollin PE: Filovirus infections, in Guerrant RL, Walker DH, Weller PF (eds). *Tropical Infectious Diseases: Principles, Pathogens, and Practice.* New York, NY, WB Saunders, 1999, pp 1240-1252.

48. Jahrling PB, Geisbert TW, Geisbert JB, et al: Evaluation of immune globulin and recombinant interferon-α2b for treatment of experimental Ebola virus infections. *J Infect Dis* 1999;179(suppl 1):S224-S234.

49. Mitchell SW, McCormick JB: Physicochemical inactivation of Lassa, Ebola, and Marburg viruses and effect on clinical laboratory analyses. *J Clin Microbiol* 1984;20(3):486-489.

50. Mupapa K, Massamba M, Kibadi K, et al: Treatment of Ebola hemorrhagic fever with blood transfusions from convalescent patients. International Scientific and Technical Committee. *J Infect Dis* 1999;179(suppl 1):S18-S23.

51. Huggins JW. Prospects for treatment of viral hemorrhagic fevers with ribavirin: A broad-spectrum antiviral drug. *Rev Infect Dis* 1989;11(suppl 4):S750-S761.

52. Huggins J, Zhang Shen-Xi, Bray M: Antiviral drug therapy of filovirus infections: S-Adenosylhomocysteine hydrolase inhibitors inhibit Ebola virus in vitro and in a lethal mouse mode. *J Infect Dis* 1999;179(suppl 1):S240-S247.

53. Peters CJ, LeDuc JW: An introduction to Ebola: The virus and the disease. *J Infect Dis* 1999;179(suppl 1):ix-xvi.

54. Banerjee K, Gupta NP, Goverdhan MK: Viral infections in laboratory personnel. *Indian J Med Res* 1979;69:363-373.

55. Mayers DL: Exotic virus infections of military significance. *Derm Clinic* 1999;17:29.

56. Fauci AS: Infectious diseases: Considerations for the 21st century. *Clin Infec Dis* 2001;32:675-685.

57. Halstead SB: Pathogenesis of dengue: Challenges to molecular biology. *Science* 1988;239:476.

58. Geisbet TW, et al: Treatment of Ebola virus infection with a recombinant inhibitor of factor VIIa/tissue factor: a study in rhesus mon. *Lancet* 2003; 362(9400):1953-1958.

59. Sabin AB: Research on dengue during World War II. *Am J Trop Med Hyg* 1952;1:30.

60. Isturiz RE, Gubler DJ, del Castillo JB: Dengue and dengue hemorrhagic fever in Latin America and the Caribbean. *Infect Dis Clin North Am* 2000;14:121.

61. Sumarmo HW, Wulur H, Jahja E, et al: Encephalopathy associated with dengue infection. *Lancet* 1978;1:449-450.

62. Isturiz RE, Gubler DJ, del Castillo JB: Dengue and dengue hemorrhagic fever in Latin America and the Caribbean. *Infect Dis Clin North Am* 2000;14:121.

63. Anonymous: Regional guidelines on dengue/DHF prevention and control. Geneva, Switzerland, World Health Organization, 1982.

64. Anonymous: Technical guide for diagnosis, treatment, surveillance, prevention, and control of dengue hemorrhagic fever. Geneva, Switzerland, World Health Organization, 1982.

65. Halsted SB: Dengue: Hematologic aspects. *Semin Hematol* 1982;19:116-131.

66. Halstead SB: Dengue hemorrhagic fever: A public health problem and a field for research. *Bull WHO* 1980;58:1-21.

67. Isturiz RE, Gubler DJ, del Castillo JB: Dengue and dengue hemorrhagic fever in Latin America and the Caribbean. *Infect Dis Clin North Am* 2000;14:121.

68. Patt HA, Feigin RD: Diagnosis and management of suspected cases of bioterrorism: A pediatric perspective. *Pediatrics* 2002;109:685-692.

69. Brandt WE: Development of dengue and Japanese encephalitis vaccines. *J Infect Dis* 1990;162:577-583.

70. Bhamarapravati N, Yoksan S, Chayaniyayothin T, et al: Immunization with a live attenuated dengue-2 virus candidate vaccine (16681-PDK 53): Clinical immunological and biological responses in adult volunteers. *Bull WHO* 1987;65:189-195.

71. Peters CJ, Jahrling PB, Khan AS: Patients infected with high hazard viruses. *Arch Virol Suppl* 1996;11:141-168.

72. McGovern TW, Christopher GW, Eitzen EM Jr: Cutaneous Manifestations of Biological Warfare and Related Threat Agents. *Arch Dermatol* 1999;135:311-322.

73. Huggins JW: Prospects for treatment of viral hemorrhagic fevers with ribavirin, a broad-spectrum antiviral drug. *Rev Infect Dis* 1980;11(suppl 4);S750-S761.

74. Huggins JW, Hsiang CM, Cosgriff TM, et al: Prospective, double-blind, concurrent, placebo-controlled clinical trial of intravenous ribavirin therapy of hemorrhagic fever with renal syndrome. *J Infect Dis* 1991;164:1119-1127.

Rickettsial Agents

■ Introduction

The rickettsia are a diverse collection of obligate intracellular parasites of humans and animals. Rickettsia replicate in the cytoplasm and nucleus of the host cell. They have apparently evolved in such close association with their normal arthropod hosts that they can no longer grow without enzymes provided by the host animal's cells. This means that laboratories cannot cultivate rickettsia on agar plates or on broth, but must culture them in a viable host cell, such as cell cultures, embryonated eggs, or susceptible animals.

The family Rickettsiaceae has four genera: *Rickettsia, Ehrlichia, Rochalimaea,* and *Coxiella.* Although they were once thought to be related and part of the same family, they are now considered to be unrelated bacteria. Each of these genera is associated with significant diseases. There are five diseases or disease groups caused by these organisms. *Coxiella burnetii* is the causative organism for Q fever, a species of *Rochalimaea* causes trench fever, while species of *Ehrlichia* cause ehrlichiosis. The genus *Rickettsia* is generally further divided into three groups: the spotted fever group, the typhus group, and "other."

Rickettsia may be spread by the bite of ticks, lice, mites, chiggers, and fleas. These zoonotic pathogens cause infections that disseminate in the blood to many organs. In humans, rickettsia live and multiply within cells that line the small- to medium-sized blood vessels and cause damage or death of the cells. This causes blood to leak through tiny holes in vessel walls into the adjacent tissues. Rickettsia do not elaborate any toxins or cause distant effects.

Rickettsial organisms are important causes of human disease in the United States and abroad. Rocky Mountain spotted fever, Q fever, murine typhus, sylvatic typhus, ehrlichiosis, and rickettsialpox are found within the United States. Q fever, murine typhus, Rocky Mountain spotted fever, scrub typhus, epidemic typhus, boutonneuse fever, and other spotted fevers are caused by rickettsial organisms in other parts of the world. Of these, Rocky Mountain spotted fever and Q fever are relatively common.

Rickettsial infections have played a significant role in history. Epidemic typhus has been documented since the 16th century and has long been associated with famine and war. The outcome of several wars has been influenced by epidemic typhus. Over 100,000 casualties resulted from typhus during World War I and World War II.

Rickettsial diseases are difficult to diagnose, both clinically and in the laboratory. As noted, a rickettsial culture requires a viable host cell, such as an antibiotic-free cell culture, embryonated eggs, or a susceptible animal. Confirmation of the diagnosis usually requires both acute and convalescent serum antibody titers or newer DNA-based diagnostic techniques, such as ELISA.

■ Q Fever

Q fever is a rickettsial zoonotic disease caused by *C burnetii*. The animals that are usually affected are sheep, cattle, and goats. Q fever is also known as query fever, Balkan influenza, Balkan grippe, pneumorickettsiosis, and abattoir fever.

C burnetii is spread to humans by aerosol particles in nature and is contracted by inhalation. The usual sources of infection are heavily infected placentas of sheep and other mammals. Human infection with this bacterium is possible, because the urine, feces, milk, and amniotic fluid of these animals contain high concentrations of the bacterium. When dried, the aerosol particles can be inhaled. *C burnetii* is also spread in nature by the brown dog tick, *(Rhipicephalus sanguineus)*, the Rocky Mountain wood tick *(Dermacentor variabilis)*, and the lone star tick *(Amblyomma americanum)*.

C burnetii varies in size and has an **endospore**-like form. The endospore form of *Coxiella* is resistant to heat and drying and is highly infectious by the aerosol route. A single inhaled organism can cause clinical illness. A biological warfare attack would produce disease similar to the natural illness. This mode of dissemination makes it a potential biological weapon.

History

Q fever was first identified and described in Queensland, Australia.[1] The United States manufactured quantities of Q fever for potential use as a warfare agent in the 1960s. Q fever was an official part of the US stockpile until 1972. *C burnetii* was referred to by the US military by the code name OU. The former Soviet Union also developed a weaponized form of Q fever.

Presentation

Q fever is a self-limiting febrile illness of 2 days to 2 weeks. The incubation period is about 10 to 20 days. The bacteria proliferate within the **endothelial** cells of the blood vessels,

Table 12-1 Suggested Therapy for Q Fever	
Preferred Choices	Dosage and Additional Information
Doxycycline	**Adult Dose:** 100 mg orally twice daily for 2–3 weeks OR 4 mg/kg/d intravenously every 12 hr for severe cases (often given for 5–7 days and then switched to oral as above) **Pediatric Dose:** 4 mg/kg/d orally or intravenously in two divided doses on day 1, then 1–2 mg/kg/d in two divided doses for 2–3 weeks, not to exceed 200 mg/d for children over 8 years and/or over 45 kg **Additional Information:** The usual course is 3 days after fever subsides and/or unequivocal clinical improvement—usually about 5–10 days. Severe or complicated disease may require longer treatment courses. Doxycycline is not usually considered a preferred drug for pregnant women because of possible fetal birth defects.
Tetracycline	**Adult and Pediatric Dose:** 3–5 mg/kg/d intravenously in two divided doses for 2–3 weeks (Doxycycline is usually preferred.) **Additional Information:** Tetracycline is not usually considered a preferred drug for pregnant women because of possible fetal birth defects.
Alternative choice	
Chloramphenicol	**Adult Dose:** 500 mg intravenously four times daily for 2–3 weeks **Pediatric Dose:** 50–100 mg/kg/d intravenously in four divided doses for 2–3 weeks **Additional Information:** Hematologic complications of chloramphenicol are common, and blood studies should be performed every second or third day. There is no drug that is completely safe during pregnancy that is available to treat this disease. Chloramphenicol may be the safest for the pregnant patient. Use extreme caution in term pregnancy because of the potential toxic effects on the fetus (grey baby syndrome).

Note: See text for other possible alternative antibiotics.

causing increased permeability and intravascular coagulation. The disease causes a sudden onset of flulike symptoms, with fever and headache predominating.

The patient usually experiences illness, but uneventful recovery is the rule. Q fever pneumonia is a frequent complication and may be noted only on radiographs in most cases. Some patients will develop nonproductive cough and **pleuritic chest pain**. About 33% of patients will develop an acute hepatitis. This can present with both fever and abnormal liver function tests, in the absence of pulmonary signs.

The ocular symptoms of inhalation Q fever include conjunctival injection, eye pain, papillae on the conjunctiva, petechiae, iritis, retinitis, and possible optic nerve edema. The ocular symptoms result from a vasculitis caused by the rickettsia.

Other complications are uncommon but may include chronic hepatitis, endocarditis, meningitis, encephalitis, and osteomyelitis. Patients who develop these complications will pose a challenge to the clinician's diagnosis. The complications may overshadow the original Q fever and further delay diagnosis.

Diagnosis

Q fever's presentation as a febrile illness with an atypical pneumonia is similar to many other atypical pneumonias, including **Mycoplasma pneumoniae infection**, **legionnaires' disease**, **Chlamydia pneumonia infection**, psittacosis, or hantavirus. More rapidly progressive Q fever cases may resemble tularemia or plague.

The diagnosis can be confirmed serologically and other laboratory findings are unlikely to be helpful. It is difficult to isolate rickettsia, and Q fever is no exception. ELISA testing is available at reference laboratories.

Q fever is a significant hazard to laboratory personnel who work with the organism. Refer to the sections on biosafety for detailed information and protective equipment.

Most patients with Q fever will have slightly elevated liver enzymes. A leukocytosis may be present. Sputum examination is often unhelpful.

The chest radiograph is abnormal for 50% of the patients. Chest radiograph abnormalities include patchy infiltrates typical of a viral or mycoplasma pneumonia. Hilar adenopathy may be noted.

Therapy

As with other rickettsial diseases, such as Rocky Mountain spotted fever, the treatment of choice is tetracycline, doxycycline, or chloramphenicol. Erythromycin has been shown to be effective. Although not tested, azithromycin and Biaxin (clarithromycin) would also be expected to be effective. Ciprofloxacin and other quinolones have been shown to be active and should be administered to the patient who is unable to take the other recommended medications. The specifics of therapy for Q fever are listed in **Table 12-1.**

Prophylaxis

Person-to-person transmission of Q fever has been reported only rarely. A formalin inactivated whole-cell vaccine is available as an investigational drug in the United States and has been used for those who are at risk of occupational infection with Q fever.[2] One dose will provide immunity for an aerosol challenge within 3 weeks. Protection lasts for at least 5 years. Another Q fever vaccine is licensed in Australia. Skin testing is required to prevent a severe local reaction in previously immune individuals. A live attenuated strain (M44) has been used in the former Soviet Union to confer immunity.[3] Q fever is a significant hazard to laboratory personnel who work with the organism.

Prophylaxis is not uniformly effective. Tetracycline or doxycycline has been recommended for prophylaxis (using the same doses as oral therapy and continued for 5 days). **Table 12-2** summarizes biosafety information for Q fever.

Threat

The organism that causes Q fever is found worldwide, is relatively easy to acquire, is hardy, and is resistant to drying. Intentional release by a terrorist group would presumably involve aerosolization. Because Q fever has a low mortality rate, it would have relatively little impact as a weapon of terrorism. However, it may be employed as an incapacitating agent.

Table 12-2 Protection Against Q Fever		
Inactivation Requirements	Decontaminating Agents	Personal Protection Requirements
Moist heat at 250°F (121°C) for more than 15 minutes	Most disinfectant solutions, including:	Wear gloves, a gown, goggles, and NIOSH N95 respiratory protection or better.
Dry heat at 320°–338F° (160°–170°C) for more than 1 hr	Alcohol	Decontaminate soiled items before disposal.
	0.5% bleach	Decontaminate equipment with standard decontamination solutions before disposal.
	Glutaraldehyde	Patients exposed to Q fever by the aerosol route do not present a risk for secondary contamination or re-aerosolization.
	Formaldehyde	
	Soap and water	Sporelike forms of *Coxiella burnetii* may withstand quite harsh conditions and may persist in the environment for long periods of time. There is little information about the hazard to humans entering an area contaminated with an intentional release of Q fever.
		Q fever is a significant hazard to laboratory personnel who work with the organism.

Source: American Academy of Orthopaedic Surgeons, Stewart CE, Nixon RG. *Weapons of Mass Casualties Field Guide.* Jones and Bartlett Publishers, Boston; 2003.

■ Rocky Mountain Spotted Fever

Rocky Mountain spotted fever is the most severe and frequently reported rickettsial illness in the United States.[4] The disease is caused by *Rickettsia rickettsii,* which is usually spread by ixodid (hard) ticks. Rocky Mountain spotted fever was first recognized in the Snake River Valley of Idaho and was first called black measles because of the characteristic rash. It was a dreaded disease that was frequently fatal prior to antibiotics. By the 1900s, this disease was found in Washington, Montana, California, Colorado, and Idaho and as far south as Arizona and New Mexico.

The name Rocky Mountain spotted fever is a bit of a misnomer. Rocky Mountain spotted fever is now distributed throughout the United States, and it is found in Canada, Central America, Mexico, and parts of South America. It has been reported in all states in the United States except Hawaii, Maine, Vermont, and Alaska.

Howard T. Rickets was the first to identify the organism that causes this disease. He and his colleagues also identified the vector as being a tick and identified a complex natural cycle of transmission. Humans were found to be accidental hosts and were not involved in this complex transmission cycle involving ticks and mammals. The rickettsia are maintained in nature by transmission from an infected female tick to ova that hatch into infected larval offspring.

Presentation

The incubation period of Rocky Mountain spotted fever is about 5 to 10 days. The early clinical presentation of the disease is quite nonspecific. The initial signs and symptoms of the disease include a sudden onset of fever, headache, and muscle aches. This is followed by the development of the typical rash. Initial symptoms may include the following:

- Fever (94% of patients develop a temperature greater than 102°F/38°C.)
- Severe headache (86% of patients will report a headache.)
- Muscle pain (85% of patients will report myalgias.)
- Nausea
- Lack of appetite
- Vomiting

Later signs and symptoms include the following:

- Rash (60% to 90% of patients will develop a rash and 10% to 15% of patients will develop no spots.)
- Encephalitis (25% of patients will develop confusion and/or lethargy. This may progress to stupor, seizures, or coma.)
- Respiratory distress (Pulmonary findings can be consistent with a focal pneumonia or with pulmonary edema.)
- Abdominal pain
- Joint pain
- Diarrhea (often positive for blood)

General Manifestations

Rocky Mountain spotted fever is a multisystem disease. Severe manifestations of the disease include respiratory, central nervous system, gastrointestinal system, or renal complications. In any one patient, a single organ system may be more affected than the rest. The clinical gravity of Rocky Mountain spotted fever is the result of severe damage to blood vessels by the organism. *R rickettsii* is unusual among the rickettsia in its ability to spread and invade vascular smooth muscle cells as well as endothelial cells. Damage to the blood vessels in the skin leads to the characteristic rash. The body's attempt to plug the vascular walls consumes platelets and leaves the patient open to other clotting problems.

Skin Manifestations

The rash usually appears 2 to 5 days after the onset of fever. The rash is often very subtle in the early course of the disease. Younger patients develop the rash sooner than older patients. A spotless fever does not indicate that the disease is milder, because a substantial number of deaths occur in patients who do not develop a rash.

The rash begins as small, flat, pink, non-itching macules on the wrists, forearms, and ankles. When pressure is applied to these spots, they blanch (turn pale).

The characteristic red, spotted, petechial rash of Rocky Mountain spotted fever is usually seen after the sixth day of symptoms **(Color plates 12–1 and 12–2)**. The rash is more common on the palms or soles of the feet (50% to 80% of patients with a rash). This typical rash is seen in 35% to 60% of patients with the disease, but as many as 10% to 15% of patients will never develop a rash. In as many as 35% to 80% of the patients with Rocky Mountain spotted fever, the rash will be atypical.

Cardiovascular and Pulmonary Manifestations

A systemic increase in vascular permeability leads to edema, decreased blood volume, and a decrease in the serum albumen, as this protein is lost through the porous blood vessels. Severe pulmonary involvement leads to a noncardiogenic pulmonary edema, interstitial pneumonia, and the development of respiratory distress syndrome. The development of pulmonary complications indicates a poor prognosis for the patient.

Central Nervous System Manifestations

Central nervous system involvement includes both a direct encephalitis caused by the organism, and a meningoencephalitis caused by the vascular injury. Central nervous system complications are common.

Renal Manifestations

Renal disease also includes both direct damage from the organism and indirect damage resulting from vasculitis within the kidney. Renal manifestations include acute renal failure and **prerenal azotemia** resulting from hypovolemia.

Acute renal failure increases the chances of death by a factor of 17 or more. Acute renal failure is more common with advanced age, decreased platelet count, increased bilirubin, or the presence of neurologic involvement.

Gastrointestinal Manifestations

Gastrointestinal involvement includes abdominal pain, nausea, vomiting, and diarrhea. Stools may test positive for blood. Death from massive gastrointestinal bleeding has been reported. Hepatic failure does not appear to occur frequently, but nearly 40% of patients will develop a **focal hepatocellular necrosis** with elevated liver enzymes.

Host Factors Affecting Morbidity and Mortality

Host factors that are associated with a more serious illness include alcoholism, advanced age, male sex, African-American race, and **glucose-6-phosphate dehydrogenase deficiency**.

- Patients with glucose-6-phosphate dehydrogenase deficiency often follow a clinical course that is fatal within 5 days of the onset of the illness.
- Patients who are treated more than 4 days after the onset of symptoms have three times the mortality rate of patients treated at 4 days or earlier.
- On average, patients who died received antibiotics 2 days later than patients who lived.
- Mortality in patients who are older than 60 years is about double that of younger patients.

Late Complications

Long-term health problems following infection with Rocky Mountain spotted fever include partial paralysis of the lower extremities, hearing loss, incontinence of bowel or bladder, **vestibular** and motor dysfunctions, movement disorders, language disorders, and stroke. These complications are more frequently seen in patients with more serious or prolonged illness.

Some patients will develop permanent skin lesions at the site of **focal cutaneous necrosis**. Distal circulation may be impaired, and the patient may develop gangrene in distal portions of the toes, nose, or fingers. Gangrene that requires amputation is rare. About 4% of patients will develop skin necrosis or gangrene.

Diagnosis

There is no rapidly available laboratory or diagnostic test for early Rocky Mountain spotted fever. Treatment decisions should be based on clinical suspicion and should not wait for laboratory confirmation. Routine clinical laboratory findings of Rocky Mountain spotted fever may include a normal white blood count, thrombocytopenia, **hyponatremia**, or elevation of the liver enzymes.

Isolation of *R rickettsii* is possible from the blood of infected patients. However, most laboratories do not perform this culture, because recommended precautions include biosafety Level 3 laboratory facilities or better.

Serologic assays are now available and are frequently used, but they usually require specimens to be sent to a reference laboratory. The indirect immunofluorescence assay is the most commonly used. An alternative approach is to use immunostaining from a skin biopsy.

Immunofluorescence assay can be used to detect either IgG or IgM antibodies to Rocky Mountain spotted fever. This test requires both acute (early in the disease) and convalescent (late in the disease) serum for confirmation. Antibody titers may persist for years after an original exposure, so both acute and convalescent sera are needed for an accurate diagnosis. Direct immunofluorescence staining of cutaneous biopsy specimens is the only timely method of diagnosis during an acute disease.

Immunostaining has significant error rates and may not detect the disease in as many as 30% of cases. The assay may be used to test autopsy results in otherwise unexplained deaths. If the suspicion is high, patients should be treated even if the test is negative.

Therapy

Before the discovery of tetracycline and chloramphenicol in the late 1940s, this disease was fatal in about 30% of cases. Despite the availability of antibiotics and advanced medical care, about 3% to 5% of victims who become ill with Rocky Mountain spotted fever still die with this infection. A significant portion of the persistent mortality of Rocky Mountain spotted fever is thought to be caused by delays in diagnosis and therapy.

Antibiotic treatment should be started immediately, whenever there is a suspicion of Rocky Mountain spotted fever. *Treatment should NOT be delayed for laboratory confirmation.*

Doxycycline may be administered in doses of 100 mg orally twice daily for 2 to 3 weeks or 4 mg/kg intravenously every 12 hours for severe cases. The usual course of treatment is 3 days after fever subsides and/or the patient shows unequivocal clinical improvement—usually about 5 to 10 days. Severe or complicated disease may require longer treatment courses.

Chloramphenicol has been used with success as well. It is administered in an initial loading dose of 50 mg/kg, followed by 50 mg/kg/day divided into 3 or 4 doses. Chloramphenicol is continued until the patient is afebrile for 24 hours.

Most broad-spectrum antibiotics, including macrolides (such as erythromycin), penicillins, cephalosporins, and sulfa-containing antimicrobials, are *ineffective treatments* for Rocky Mountain spotted fever. There are no human data to support the use of fluoroquinolones in Rocky Mountain spotted fever. In almost all clinical situations, including disease in children younger than 8 years, the antibiotic of choice is doxycycline.

Doxycycline is used infrequently by physicians as initial therapy for children who present with signs and symptoms of a rickettsial illness, because the use of tetracyclines in young children has been strongly discouraged because of the potential for tooth discoloration. Tetracycline's staining of teeth is *dose related,* and available data suggest that one course of doxycycline for presumed Rocky Mountain spotted fever does not cause clinically significant staining of permanent teeth. The use of doxycycline should be reserved for patients who are strongly suspected of having a rickettsial illness. Because the disease and its complications are so serious, the possible complications of doxycycline are outweighed by the necessity of treatment.

The specifics of therapy for Rocky Mountain spotted fever are listed in **Table 12-3.**

Prophylaxis

No vaccine exists for the prevention of Rocky Mountain spotted fever. Some general guidelines for preventing Rocky Mountain spotted fever (and other tick-borne diseases) include the following:

Table 12-3 Suggested Therapy for Rocky Mountain Spotted Fever

Preferred Choices	Dosage and Additional Information
Doxycycline	**Adult Dose:** 100 mg orally twice daily for 2–3 weeks OR 4 mg/kg intravenously every 12 hours for severe cases **Pediatric Dose:** 4 mg/kg/d orally or intravenously in two divided doses on day 1, then 1–2 mg/kg/d in two divided doses for 2–3 weeks, not to exceed 200 mg/day for children older than 8 years and/or over 45 kg **Additional Information:** This drug is the drug recommended by the CDC for children even younger than 8 years, although this is open to some debate because of possible tooth staining. The usual course is 3 days after fever subsides and/or unequivocal clinical improvement—usually about 5–10 days. Severe or complicated disease may require longer treatment courses. Doxycycline is not usually considered a preferred drug for pregnant women because of possible fetal birth defects.
Tetracycline	**Adult and Pediatric Dose:** 3–5 mg/kg/d intravenously in two divided doses for 2–3 weeks (Doxycycline is usually preferred.) **Additional Information:** Tetracycline is not usually considered a preferred drug for pregnant women because of possible fetal birth defects.
Alternative choice	
Chloramphenicol	**Adult Dose:** 500 mg intravenously four times daily for 2–3 weeks **Pediatric Dose:** 50–100 mg/kg/d intravenously in four divided doses for 2–3 weeks **Additional Information:** Chloramphenicol is distinctly inferior to doxycycline. Thirty percent of patients given chloramphenicol will require hospitalization, compared to only 11% of patients given doxycycline. Hematologic complications of chloramphenicol are common and blood studies should be performed every second or third day. There is no drug that is completely safe during pregnancy that is available to treat this disease. Chloramphenicol may be the safest for the pregnant patient. Use extreme caution in term pregnancy because of the potential toxic effects on the fetus (grey baby syndrome).

- Ticks cannot bite through clothing, so wear the following:
    - Light-colored clothing (makes spotting the tick easier)
    - Long-sleeved shirts tucked into pants (with sleeves buttoned for best protection)
    - Socks and closed-toe shoes
    - Long pants with legs tucked into socks
- Check often for ticks in the following places (at least twice daily):
    - Areas where ticks are commonly found: belly button, in and behind the ears, neck, hairline, and the top of the head
    - All parts of the body that bend: behind the knees, under the arms, and around the groin
    - Areas of pressure points such as belt lines and underwear lines
    - All other areas of the body and hair (Check visually and run fingers gently over the skin.)
- Other helpful measures include the following:
    - Walk on cleared paths and pavement through wooded areas and fields when possible.
    - Shower after all outdoor activities are over for the day. It may take up to 6 hours for ticks to attach firmly to skin. Showering may remove any loose ticks.
- Consider using insect and tick repellent:
    - Products that contain DEET repel ticks, but they do not kill ticks and are not 100% effective.
    - Treat clothing with a product that contains permethrin, which will kill ticks on contact. Do not use permethrin on skin.
- If a tick is attached, remove it immediately with tweezers:
    - Gently grasp the tick as close as possible to the skin and slowly pull it away.
    - Do not use petroleum jelly, hot objects such as matches, or other methods.
    - After handling ticks, be sure to wash the hands thoroughly.

Table 12-4 Protection Against Rocky Mountain Spotted Fever

Inactivation Requirements	Decontaminating Agents	Personal Protection Requirements
Moist heat at 250°F (121°C) for more than 15 minutes Dry heat at 320° to 338°F (160° to 170°C) for more than 1 hour	Most disinfectant solutions, including: Alcohol 1% bleach Glutaraldehyde Formaldehyde	Wear gloves, a gown, goggles, and NIOSH N95 respiratory protection or better. Decontaminate soiled items before disposal. Decontaminate equipment with standard decontamination solutions before disposal.

Source: American Academy of Orthopaedic Surgeons, Stewart CE, Nixon RG. *Weapons of Mass Casualties Field Guide.* Jones and Bartlett Publishers, Boston; 2003.

Biosafety

The normal disease is spread to humans by contact with the tick; it is not spread from one person to another. Once a person has had Rocky Mountain spotted fever, that person cannot be reinfected. No specific recommendations have been given by any governmental agency regarding Rocky Mountain spotted fever.

Most household detergents and disinfectants, such as diluted household bleach (2% or 2 tablespoons of bleach mixed with one gallon of water), rubbing alcohol, or diluted Lysol disinfectant cleaner (1%), kill *R rickettsii* bacteria. **Table 12-4** summarizes biosafety information for Rocky Mountain spotted fever.

Threat

The use of *R rickettsii* as a biological warfare or terrorist agent has not been documented in the open-source literature. The organism is not particularly hardy, and it is easily destroyed by common disinfectants. However, the CDC continually includes this agent in its list of biological agents, so it must be supposed that it has been covertly developed as a biological agent by at least one state-sponsored agency known to the federal government.

Similar agents such as rickettsialpox and boutonneuse fever also have high mortality rates and are more widespread. These organisms would be candidates for terrorism. They would presumably respond to similar antibiotics as Rocky Mountain spotted fever.

■ Epidemic Typhus

Epidemic typhus, caused by *R prowazekii*, is a different disease from typhoid fever. It was once designated by the US military code name YE. Epidemic typhus is transmitted by human body lice. Unlike other rickettsial diseases, the primary reservoir for epidemic typhus is the human. Epidemic typhus occurs mostly among people in overcrowded and unsanitary conditions, such as refugee camps found in wars, famines, and natural disasters. The other natural hosts of epidemic typhus are flying squirrels and their fleas. Unlike the vectors of other rickettsial diseases, the louse does not have transovarian transmission of the bacteria to the eggs.

When an infected louse bites a human, it defecates, and the bacteria are expelled in the feces. Irritation of the bite causes the person to scratch and inoculate the skin with the bacteria from the fecal contamination.

Brill-Zinsser disease is a recurrence of epidemic typhus. It may occur decades after the initial infection. The clinical course of the disease is similar to epidemic typhus but it is milder, without skin rash, and recovery is faster.

Presentation

The incubation period of epidemic typhus is 6 to 15 days, with an average of 8 days. The disease presents with a sudden onset of fever, muscle and joint aches, headaches, and weakness. About 7 days after the onset of the fever, the patient develops a rash. This rash is often maculopapular, but it can also be petechial or hemorrhagic. Unlike the rash of Rocky Mountain spotted fever, the rash of epidemic typhus develops first on the trunk and then spreads to the extremities.

The patient may develop stupor and delirium as the disease progresses. The mortality rate is quite high (usually 30%) if untreated. This can vary, and some epidemics have mortality rates of 60% to 70%.

Diagnosis

Isolation of the organism is possible but is considered dangerous. Indirect fluorescent antibody and latex agglutination tests are available at reference laboratories. Acute and convalescent serology can provide a diagnosis, but it is too slow for emergency care of the patient.

Therapy

As with the other rickettsial diseases, the treatment of choice for epidemic typhus is doxycycline or tetracycline. An alternative is chloramphenicol. The dose is the same as for treatment of Rocky Mountain spotted fever. Recovery from this disease may take months.

Prophylaxis

A vaccine exists for epidemic typhus, but it is not readily available.

Biosafety

The normal disease is spread to humans by contact with the louse; it is not usually spread from one person to another. No specific recommendations have been given by any governmental agency regarding epidemic typhus as a bioweapon. For the natural disease, louse control measures are important and effective.

Most household detergents and disinfectants, such as diluted household bleach (2%), rubbing alcohol, or diluted Lysol disinfectant cleaner (1%), kill *R prowazekii* bacteria.

Table 12-5 Protection Against Epidemic Typhus

Inactivation Requirements	Decontaminating Agents	Personal Protection Requirements
Moist heat at 250°F (121°C) for more than 15 minutes Dry heat at 320°–338°F (160°–170°C) for more than 1 hour	Most disinfectant solutions, including: Alcohol Bleach (1%) Glutaraldehyde Formaldehyde	Wear gloves, a gown, goggles, and NIOSH N95 respiratory protection or better. Decontaminate soiled items before disposal. Decontaminate equipment with standard decontamination solutions before disposal. Isolation of the organism is dangerous.

Source: American Academy of Orthopaedic Surgeons, Stewart CE, Nixon RG. *Weapons of Mass Casualties Field Guide.* Jones and Bartlett Publishers, Boston; 2003.

Table 12-5 summarizes biosafety information for epidemic typhus.

Threat

The use of *R prowazekii* as a biological warfare or terrorist agent has not been documented in the open-source literature. The organism is not particularly hardy, and it is easily destroyed by common disinfectants. However, the CDC continually includes this agent in its list of biological agents.

■ Summary

Table 12-6 summarizes information on rickettsial diseases discussed in the text as well as other similar rickettsial diseases.

Table 12-6 Rickettsial Diseases

Disease	Organism	Geographic Distribution	Basis of Injury	Rash	Serologic Diagnosis
Boutonneuse fever	*Rickettsia conorii*	The Mediterranean basin, Africa, and the Indian subcontinent	Microvascular damage	97%	IFA, LA, CF
Cat scratch fever	*Bartonella henselae*	Presumably worldwide	Vascular proliferation and granulomas	Rare	IFA, EIA
Ehrlichiosis	*Ehrlichia canis* or *E chaffeensis*	North America, Europe, and Africa	Microvascular damage, pneumonia, and granulomas	40%	IFA
Epidemic typhus	*Rickettsia prowazekii*	Africa, South America, Mexico, and the eastern United States	Microvascular damage	100%	IFA, IHA, EIA
Murine typhus	*Rickettsia typhi*	Worldwide	Microvascular damage	50%	IFA, IHA, EIA
North Asian tick typhus	*Rickettsia sibirica*	Russia, China, Mongolia, Siberia, and Pakistan	Microvascular damage	100%	IFA, CF
Oriental spotted fever	*Rickettsia japonicas*	Japan	Microvascular damage	100%	IFA, CF
Oroyo fever/verruga peruana	*Bartonella bacilliformis*	South America	Acute hemolysis and chronic vascular proliferation	None	EIA
Q fever	*Coxiella burnetii*	Worldwide	Pneumonia, encephalitis, hepatitis, conjunctivitis, endocarditis, and osteomyelitis	None	IFA, EIA, CF
Queensland tick typhus	*Rickettsia australis*	Australia	Microvascular damage	90%	CF
Rickettsialpox	*Rickettsia akari*	North America, Europe, and Korea	Microvascular damage	100%	IFA, CF
Rocky Mountain spotted fever	*Rickettsia rickettsii*	North, Central, and South America	Microvascular damage	90% (only about 60% have a classic rash)	IFA, LA, IHA
Scrub typhus	*Rickettsia tsutsugamushi*	Asia, the South Pacific, and Australia	Microvascular damage	50%	IFA, EIA
Trench fever	*Bartonella quintana*	North America, Europe, and Africa	Perivesiculitis	May occur	IHA, EIA, CF

CF: Complement fixation

EIA: ELISA or enzyme-linked immunosorbent assay

IFA: Immunofluorescent antibody testing

IHA: Indirect hemagglutination assay

LA: Latex agglutination

■ References

1. Abelson MB, Parver L, Fink K, Welch D: Biological terrorism: What ophthalmologists may see. *Rev Ophthalmol* 2002;9:52-54, 55-59.
2. Ackland JR, Worswick DA, Marmion BP: Vaccine prophylaxis of Q fever: A follow-up study of the efficacy of Qvac (CSL) 1985–1990. *Med J Aust* 1994;160:704-708.
3. Genig VA: Experience on mass immunization of human beings with the M-44 live vaccine against Q fever. Report 2. Skin and oral routes of immunization. *Vopr Virusol* 1965;6:703-707.
4. Anonymous: Rocky Mountain spotted fever, introduction. Centers for Disease Control and Prevention, http://www.cdc.gov/ncidod/dvrd/rmsf/Index.htm (accessed August 29, 2002).

13 Possible Biotoxins

■ Introduction

Toxins are effective and specific poisons produced by living organisms. These toxins may be produced by numerous organisms including bacteria, fungi, algae, and plants. Many of them are extremely poisonous, with a toxicity that is several orders of magnitude greater than the nerve agents.

At one end of the spectrum are the bacterial toxins such as botulinum toxin and staphylococcal enterotoxin, both of which have been stockpiled as biological weapons. These are high molecular weight proteins that can be produced only by processes of industrial microbiology. In the middle of the spectrum are the snake poisons, insect venoms, plant alkaloids, and a host of other substances, such as ricin, which have been used as weapons. At the far end of the spectrum are the small molecules, such as cyanide, that can be easily synthesized by chemical processes, even though they are also produced by certain living organisms. (This means that cyanide falls within the legal definition of a "toxin.")

Political and scientific events have moved toxins to a more prominent medical and social position. Popular media have highlighted the possible uses of many of these toxins. The discovery that some of these toxins have been used as agents in warfare or have been stockpiled to use in warfare have given some health care providers an impetus to learn more about the effects and production of toxins for biological warfare.

Toxins can be classified by the organism that produces the toxin or by the mechanism of toxicity:

- Cytotoxins cause cellular destruction; ricin is an example.
  - Enterotoxins affect the digestive tract; staphylococcal enterotoxin B is an example.
  - Hemorrhagic toxins cause bleeding; mycotoxin T-2 is an example. The RCA associated with ricin is another example of a hemorrhagic toxin.
  - Hepatotoxins cause liver damage.
  - Nephrotoxins cause kidney damage.
  - Others inflame skin and mucous membranes; mycotoxin T-2 and oleoresin capsicum fit in this category.
- Neurotoxins affect the central nervous system.
  - Presynaptic and postsynaptic neurotoxins; botulinum toxin, tetanus toxin, and saxitoxin are examples.
  - Ion-channel and sodium-ion binding toxins; tetrodotoxin is an example of an ion-channel neurotoxin.

- Ionophores; pardaxin, a toxin secreted by the Red Sea Moses sole fish, is an example. These toxins cause an increase in intracellular activation of calcium and intracellular release of neurotransmitters, particularly dopamine. The release occurs because of increased membrane pore formation.[1] Another ionophore is found in recluse spider venom.[2]

Mixed toxins are toxins that show multiple mechanisms from different categories.

The Biological and Toxin Weapons Convention of 1972 prohibits the development, production, and stockpiling of toxins as weapons. The 1925 Geneva Protocol prohibiting the use of chemical and bacteriological weapons also covers the use of weapons based on toxins. Because the definition of chemical weapons includes toxins, they are also covered by the Chemical Weapons Convention.

In the late 1970s, there was a rapid development of gene technology and biotechnology. This led to the threat of toxins for use as chemical weapons agents. It became possible to produce greater amounts of many toxins more easily, in some cases, even synthetically. Gene technology can be used to modify the toxin genes so that the end product has new properties; for example, a modified toxin may be less sensitive to sunlight.

There are literally thousands of toxins that could be used or adapted for use as weapons or terrorist agents. Although this chapter discusses some of the commonly used toxins, many, many more exist and have been evaluated as weapons. A list of those that have been evaluated for use as weapons is included at the end of this chapter.

Because toxins are not volatile as are chemical agents, the terrorist would have to expose targets to an aerosol or put the toxin into foodstuffs or beverages in order for the toxin to be effective. The use of food or beverages would generally result in a slow exposure involving far fewer people.

The use of an aerosol would complicate the task of the terrorist to some degree by limiting the number of toxins that could be considered for use. The use of these toxins in closed-space environments, such as an auditorium or shopping mall, would enhance the effects of any toxin. The more confined the military or terrorist target (for example, inside shelters, buildings, ships, or vehicles), the greater the list of toxins that might be effective. Fortunately, they are more easily removed from air-handling systems than chemical agents. **Table 13-1** compares the lethality of toxins to the lethality of certain chemical weapons.

■ Botulinum Toxins

Botulism is the paralytic disease caused by the neurotoxins of *Clostridium botulinum* and related bacteria. These gram-positive spore-forming anaerobic bacteria can be found in soil and marine sediments throughout the world.

Botulinum neurotoxin is among the most potent toxins known.[3,4] A single gram of crystalline toxin, evenly dispersed and inhaled, would probably kill more than 1 million people. Fortunately, there are multiple technical factors that make such a dissemination quite difficult. The minimum lethal dose of botulinum toxin for humans is unknown, but it can be estimated from primate studies to be about 0.70 to

Table 13-1 Comparative Lethality of Toxins and Selected Chemical Weapons

Agent	LD$_{50}$ (μg/kg)	Source
Botulinum toxin	0.001	*Clostridium botulinum*
Shiga toxin	0.002	Bacterium
Tetanus toxin	0.002	*Clostridium tetani*
Abrin	0.04	Plant (rosary pea)
Diphtheria toxin	0.10	*Clostridium diphtheriae*
Maitotoxin	0.10	Marine dinoflagellate
Palytoxin	0.15	Marine soft coral
Ciguatoxin	0.40	Fish/marine dinoflagellate
Textilotoxin	0.60	Elapid snake
Clostridium perfringens toxins	0.1 to 5.0	Bacterium
Batrachotoxin	2.0	Arrow-poison frog
Ricin	3.0	Plant (castor bean)
Conotoxin	5.0	Cone snail
Taipoxin	5.0	Elapid snake
Tetrodotoxin	8.0	Puffer fish
Tityustoxin	9.0	Scorpion
Saxitoxin	10.0 (inhalation: 2.0)	Marine dinoflagellate
VX	15.0	Chemical agent
SEB (Rhesus/Aerosol)	27.0 (ED$_{50}$)	Bacterium
Anatoxin-A(s)	50.0	Blue-green alga
Microcystin	50.0	Blue-green alga
Soman (GD)	64.0	Chemical agent
Sarin (GB)	100.0	Chemical agent
Aconitine	100.0	Plant (monkshood)
T-2 Toxin	1,210.0	Fungal mycotoxin

Adapted from: The Virtual Naval Hospital, http://www.vnh.org/DATW/chap1.html (accessed August 10, 2003).

0.90 μg inhaled or 70 μg ingested. The lethal dose for mice is less than 0.1 ng per 100 g of mouse weight. It is over 275 times more toxic than cyanide.

Botulinum toxin was used to assassinate Reinhard Heydrich, a Nazi leader and probable successor to Hitler. The Czechoslovakian underground used a grenade impregnated with botulinum toxin made by English researchers in Porton. Although Heydrich's wounds were relatively minor, he died unexpectedly several days after the attack.[5]

The major source of botulinum toxin is the organism *C botulinum. C butyricum* and *C baratii* also produce botulinum toxin, but they are much less frequently found. There are seven serotypes of toxin produced by *Clostridium* species: A, B, C, D, E, F, and G. Of these, A, B, and E cause most botulism in humans.[6] The toxin types serve as epidemiologic markers. Type G has not been shown to cause neuroparalytic disease but has been associated with sudden death.

Upon entering the body, botulism toxin travels to the nerves by the bloodstream and irreversibly binds to nerve receptors at the peripheral synapses. The toxin breaks down the nerve cell proteins that moderate the release of the

IN HOSPITAL INFO

synaptic transmitter acetylcholine and inhibits the subsequent release of acetylcholine. The effects are quite similar to the nerve agent's inhibition of acetylcholinesterase. The result is a flaccid muscle paralysis (**Figure 13-1**).

Effects

Botulism was first described by Mueller (1735–1793) and Kerner (1786–1862) in Germany. They associated the disease with the ingestion of insufficiently cooked "blood sausages" and described death by muscle paralysis and suffocation. In the early 1900s, botulism occurred commonly in the United States and nearly destroyed the canned food industry.[7]

Three natural types of poisoning occur commonly: foodborne botulism, wound botulism, and infant botulism. A fourth natural form of the disease, adult intestinal colonization botulism, has recently been identified, but it is quite rare. The fifth form, inhalational botulism, is not natural at all. The effects of the different types of botulism are the same. Fewer than 200 cases of botulism are reported in the United States each year. All forms of botulism result from the absorption of the toxin from a mucosal surface in the gut, mouth, or lung, or from a wound.

As noted, once botulinum toxin is absorbed, it is carried to the peripheral neuromuscular junction, where it binds irreversibly. *This means that all forms of human botulism will have identical neurologic signs.* Disease manifestation may differ in pace and extent among patients exposed to identical amounts of toxin. The rapidity of onset and the severity of paralysis depend on the amount of toxin absorbed in the system. Some patients may have mild disease, and others may require months of ventilatory assistance.

Ocular findings are crucial to a diagnosis of botulism. Botulism causes a **descending flaccid paralysis**, so ocular manifestations are often the first indications of toxicity. After intoxication with botulinum toxin, cranial nerve **palsies** with eye symptoms, such as blurred vision, **diplopia** (double vision), **ptosis**, and photophobia, are prominent.

Patients who developed ptosis, slow-reacting dilated pupils, and a **medial rectus paresis** had a 73% chance of developing respiratory dysfunction within 6 to 12 hours.[8] If none of these three signs was present, the patient had only a 3% chance of developing respiratory insufficiency. This set of symptoms may provide a predictive aid to emergency clinicians in determining how severe the patient's affliction is likely to become.

Dysphonia and dysphagia follow. The mouth may appear dry and the pharynx reddened. Gag reflexes may be lost. The victim then develops decreased bowel function and muscle weakness that can progress to a flaccid paralysis. The patient will generally be awake, oriented, and afebrile.

The development of respiratory failure may be quite rapid after initial symptoms develop. The progression from the onset of symptoms to respiratory failure may take as little as 24 hours in cases of foodborne botulism. When severe respiratory muscle paralysis is present, the patient may be cyanotic or may have carbon dioxide retention.

In the untreated patient, death occurs by airway obstruction caused by the flaccid muscles of the pharynx and upper airway or by inadequate respiratory gas exchange. Intubation and ventilation are literally lifesaving.

The classic signs of botulism are as follows:
1. Symmetric descending flaccid paralysis
   a. Prominent bulbar involvement (4 Ds)
      i. Diplopia (double vision)
      ii. Dysarthria (difficulty walking caused by descending skeletal muscle paralysis)
      iii. Dysphonia (difficulty speaking)
      iv. Dysphagia (difficulty swallowing)
2. Afebrile patient
3. Clear sensorium

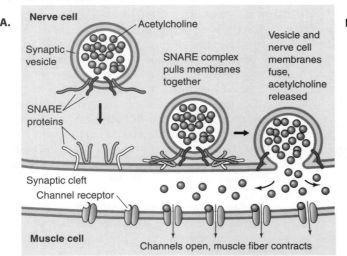
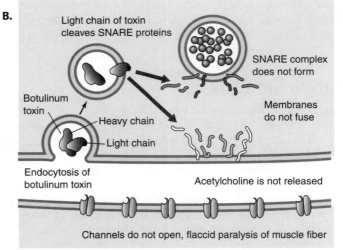

Figure 13-1 **A.** Normal neurotransmitter release. **B.** Exposure to botulinum toxin.

Botulinum toxin causes permanent damage to the nerves. (Sensory nerves are not affected.) Recovery from botulinum intoxication results when new motor nerves sprout to reinnervate paralyzed muscle fibers. This process may take weeks or months to occur.

Foodborne Botulism

In the first type of botulism, food tainted with *Clostridium* species is stored or processed in a way that allows the anaerobic organisms to grow and multiply. As they grow, they produce and release toxin. If the food is not subsequently heated to destroy the toxin, clinically significant amounts can be consumed. The toxin passes through the gut into the general circulation and is distributed throughout the body.

Although the neurologic signs of botulism are always the same, foodborne botulism may be preceded by nausea, vomiting, abdominal cramps, and diarrhea. These gastrointestinal symptoms may be caused by other bacterial metabolic products present in the food. It is unknown if purified botulinum toxin intentionally placed in food or aerosols will cause these symptoms.

In cases of foodborne botulism, patients with an early onset of clinical symptoms and patients over the age of 60 experience a longer clinical course and fare worse than younger patients who have a later onset of the disease. The case-fatality rate of foodborne botulism is about 7.5% overall, but type A toxin causes 10% fatalities, while type B causes only 5%. The case-fatality rate for patients over 60 years of age is 30%.

Infant Botulism

In cases of infant botulism, the organisms colonize and produce their toxin in the gut. In a child who is younger than 1 year, the normal intestinal flora may not have developed enough to prevent the colonization of these organisms. Fifty percent of all cases of infant botulism are reported in California. The case-fatality rate of infant botulism is 1.3%, but there is a 5% relapse rate.

Wound Botulism

Wound botulism is caused by the systemic spread of toxin produced by bacteria introduced into a wound. It is associated with trauma, subcutaneous drug injection, and sinusitis from intranasal cocaine use. The case-fatality rate of wound botulism is 10%.

Adult Intestinal Botulism

Adult intestinal botulism is similar in pathology to infant botulism. Adult intestinal botulism occurs in the presence of colitis, in patients with recent bowel surgery, or in association with other conditions that create a disruption of the normal bowel flora. Jejunoileal bypass, surgery of the small intestine, and Crohn's disease are also predisposing factors for adult intestinal botulism. This is a rare disease, with less than 10 reported cases in the medical literature.

Inhalational Botulism

Inhalational botulism results from aerosolized botulinum toxin. This mode of transmission has been demonstrated experimentally in primates and has been the intended outcome of at least one country's (Iraq's) specially designed artillery shells and missiles.[9] Inhalational botulism has occurred accidentally in humans at least once.[10]

The CDC notes that the onset of symptoms from inhalational botulism usually occurs from 12 to 36 hours after exposure. It varies according to the amount of toxin absorbed and could easily be shorter after a biowarfare attack. When a low dose of toxin is inhaled, the symptoms may take a longer time to develop.

Differential Diagnosis

It is difficult to distinguish organophosphate nerve agent poisoning from botulism. The copious secretions caused by the nerve agent will be the significant clue. Any group of patients with a significant disorder of the cranial nerves should bring botulism intoxication to mind. Isolated cases have a wider differential diagnosis, including Guillain-Barré syndrome, **myasthenia gravis**, and tick paralysis.

In cases of intoxication with a nerve agent, inhibition of acetylcholinesterase causes an accumulation of acetylcholine. In cases of botulism, the problem is a lack of a neurotransmitter in the synapse. The use of anticholinergic agents, such as atropine, would cause a worsening of symptoms. Nerve agents cause copious respiratory secretions, whereas botulism would likely decrease secretions.

Detection

The occurrence of an epidemic of afebrile patients with symmetric progressive neurologic disorders that end in flaccid paralysis strongly suggests terrorism by botulinum intoxication. Individual cases maybe confused with neuromuscular disorders, such as Guillain-Barré syndrome or tick paralysis.

Myasthenia gravis may be easily confused with botulinum intoxication because the edrophonium or Tensilon test may be transiently positive in botulism. If a lumbar puncture is initiated, the spinal fluid will be normal in botulism, which distinguishes it from all of the viral and bacterial meningitis and encephalitis infections.

Current laboratory tests are not helpful in the clinical course. The treatment of botulism must be started before the laboratory can return the positive diagnosis.

The clinician may collect serum, stool, gastric aspirate, vomitus, and any suspect foods, if available. About 30 mL of blood collected in a "tiger-top" or red-top tube is required for an adult. Gastric aspirate may be useful for the detection of an inhalational botulinum toxin. (With the longer latent period before symptoms, fecal samples may also be useful in inhalation cases.) Nasal swabs and induced respiratory secretions may possibly be used for toxin assays to prove inhalation of the agent. These samples must be obtained before therapy with antitoxin begins.

Detection of botulinum may be achieved by mouse bioassay or by liquid chromatography. The standard diagnostic test for clinical specimens and food is the mouse bioassay. In this test, type-specific antitoxins protect the mouse against any botulinum toxin in the specimens. The mouse bioassay can detect as little as 0.03 ng of botulinum toxin, but it takes from 6 to 96 hours to perform.

The use of radioimmunoassay and radioreceptor assays have also been reported. A DNA probe has been designed for the detection of botulinum toxin, which would markedly expedite diagnosis.[11] The detection of toxin in clinical or environmental samples is sometimes possible with ELISA or similar testing.

INHOSPITAL INFO

Prophylaxis and Treatment

Treatment is supportive for paralyzed patients. The rapid use of antitoxin is recommended for suspected patients who are not yet paralyzed. Respiratory failure will require prolonged (weeks to months) ventilatory support. If ventilatory support is available, then fatalities are likely to occur in less than 5% of the exposed population. Full recovery may take up to a year.

Antitoxin

The available equine antitoxin may be of some help in both foodborne and aerosol botulism. This is available from the CDC and protects against A, B, and E toxins. It has been used for treating ingestion botulism and should be administered as soon as the diagnosis is made. It does not reverse paralysis, but it does prevent progression of the disease. There is no human-based antitoxin currently available, but human-based antitoxin testing is now in progress. Obviously, it will not help for types C and D intoxication.

The usual dose is two vials of equine trivalent antitoxin as soon as the diagnosis is made, prior to laboratory confirmation. This dose administers about 10,000 units of antibodies against each of toxin types A, B, and E. Therapy is most effective within 24 hours after the onset of illness. The antitoxin has a circulating half-life of 5 to 7 days. Nine percent of patients have an adverse reaction, with 3.6% having serum sickness, 2.6% having urticaria, and 1.9% having anaphylaxis.

A heptavalent antitoxin against types A through G is available in limited supply at USAMRIID in Frederick, MD. Obviously, logistics would preclude most use of this antitoxin, because limited quantities are available, typing is necessary before release, and the antitoxin must be delivered to the area in need. This antitoxin was used with good effect in a large Egyptian outbreak of type E foodborne botulism in 1991.

Supportive Care

Botulism patients require significant resources for care. The ventilated patient requires not only airway care, but also feeding and the treatment of secondary infections. All patients with suspected botulism should be watched carefully for respiratory distress.

The average duration of respiratory support for those who require mechanical ventilation is 6 to 8 weeks, but it may be as long as 7 months. Intubation is required for up to 66% of patients with type A botulism, 50% of patients with type B, and about 40% of patients with type E. The survivors completely recover within 1 year after exposure to type A, and 2 years after exposure to type B.

Botulinum patients who are not ventilated should be placed in a reverse Trendelenburg position (of about 20 to 25 degrees) with cervical vertebral support. This position has been helpful in pediatric botulism patients, but has not been tested in adults. This position decreases the aspiration of oral secretions and increases diaphragmatic excursions.

Airway obstruction or aspiration usually proceeds hypoventilation in botulism. When respiratory obstruction starts to deteriorate, the clinician should intubate the patient before hypoxia or aspiration is noted. The incidence of intubation ranges from 20% for foodborne botulism to over 60% for infant botulism. The incidence of intubation is unknown for inhalational botulism.

Spirometry, pulse oximetry, and arterial blood gas measurements can be monitored. Vital capacity is an easy bedside measurement that can help predict respiratory failure. Intubation should be considered when the vital capacity is less than 30% of the predicted capacity. This is more likely when the patient has either hypercarbia or has rapidly progressive paralysis with hypoxemia.

Penicillin and other antibiotics have been recommended, but the use of antibiotics is controversial. Aminoglycoside antibiotics and clindamycin are contraindicated, because they will exacerbate neuromuscular blockade by blocking neuronal calcium entry. The release of toxin in the gut may worsen neurologic symptoms through lysis of bacterial cells in the gut or wound.[12] Antibiotics would be ineffective if the disease is caused by a direct toxin release such as found in inhalational botulism. The use of antibiotics may be appropriate for wound botulism, because the bacteria grow in the wound.

Toxoid

A **toxoid** is a vaccine that prevents botulism by inducing an immune reaction to a denatured toxin. The most commonly used toxoid is tetanus toxoid. The tetanus shot uses a deactivated toxin (the toxoid) to induce an immune response to tetanus toxin. Survivors will probably not develop an antibody response because of the minuscule amount of toxin that is lethal.

Botulinum toxoid vaccine is available.[13,14] A pentavalent toxoid of types A, B, C, D, and E is available for preexposure prophylaxis. This toxoid is distributed to laboratory workers at high risk of exposure to botulinum toxin and to the military for the protection of troops against attack. The military believes that F and G type toxins are unlikely to be used in warfare, because the strains of *C botulinum* that produce toxins F and G are difficult to grow in large quantities. If new techniques allow the production of toxins F and G in large quantities, the pentavalent toxoid will be useless.

The pentavalent toxoid is available as an investigational drug only. This product has been given to several thousand volunteers and workers who are at risk because of their occupations. It induces sufficient serum antitoxin levels. It requires three injections and a yearly booster for complete protection. The quantities are quite limited, and it is expected that this toxoid will be reserved for groups judged to be at very high risk of exposure (such as investigative agents).

All of the available antitoxins are derived from horse serum. Patients should be tested for possible allergic reaction to horse serum before administering the antitoxin.

Biosafety

The toxin does not penetrate intact skin, and there is no threat of secondary aerosol from exposed patients. Despite its extreme potency, botulinum toxin is easily destroyed. Heating to about 185°F (85°C) for at least 5 minutes will destroy all botulinum toxin in contaminated food or drink. Although the spores of *C botulinum* survive for 2 hours at 212°F (100°C), the **exotoxin** is not nearly as hardy.

Depending on the weather, aerosolized toxin will decay at about 1% per minute. The toxins are easily **denatured**. Sunlight deactivates the toxins within 1 to 3 hours, and standard water treatment chemicals inactivate the toxin within 20 minutes. Complete inactivation of the toxin could

INHOSPITAL INFO

Table 13-2 Protection Against Botulinum Toxin		
Inactivation Requirements	Decontaminating Agents	Personal Protection Requirements
Moist heat at 185°F (85°C) for more than 5 minutes	1% bleach Formaldehyde Soap and water (for contaminated clothing and skin)	Strict isolation of patients is NOT needed. This agent does not breach intact skin. **Respiratory protection is needed when dealing with the agent.** Respiratory protection with a fitted NIOSH N95 mask or better will probably suffice, although more effective protection is safer. Providers caring for casualties will likely not need protection, because the incubation period is 18 to 36 hours after release, and substantial degradation is expected during this time frame. A toxoid is available from the CDC for types A, B, C, D, and E, but it is restricted to military and laboratory workers.

Source: American Academy of Orthopaedic Surgeons, Stewart CE, Nixon RG. *Weapons of Mass Casualties Field Guide.* Jones and Bartlett Publishers, Boston; 2003.

take as long as 2 days, so this agent should be considered to be relatively persistent.

Contaminated objects or surfaces can be cleaned with 1% bleach. Biosafety information for botulinum toxin is summarized in **Table 13-2.**

Threat

There is no question that botulinum toxin should be considered to be a major bioterrorist threat. The toxin can be spread by either inhalation or ingestion of food or water that is contaminated with the toxin. This makes it a particularly good potential biological weapon.

Terrorists have already used botulinum toxin as a weapon. Aerosols of botulinum toxin were dispersed at multiple sites in downtown Tokyo, Japan, and at US military installations in Japan on at least three occasions between 1990 and 1995 by the Japanese cult Aum Shinrikyo.[15] Aum Shinrikyo is also believed to have attempted attacks with the toxin on the US embassy in Tokyo. The reason why these attacks failed is uncertain. It may be because of faulty microbiological technique, deficient aerosol generating equipment, or even internal sabotage.

The German Red Army Faction was found to have manufactured the toxin in a safe house in Paris in the 1980s.

The toxin was considered for use as a weapon by the United States, Britain, and Japan. The head of the Japanese biological warfare unit (Unit 731) admitted to feeding prisoners botulinum toxin in the 1930s.[16] There are suggestions that it was used by the Japanese to poison streams used by the Russians for water sources in Manchuria. (In fact, cholera was used by the soldiers of Unit 731 for this purpose.)[17]

The United States produced botulinum toxin during World War II. (The US military designator for botulinum toxin is agent X). More than 1 million doses of antitoxin were available for Allied troops preparing to invade Normandy on D-Day. Although the public reason was because of concerns that Germany had weaponized botulinum toxin, private speculation was that the United States was prepared to use botulinum toxin if chemical agents were used against allied forces in the invasion.

Although both Iraq and the Soviet Union signed the 1972 Biological and Toxin Weapons Convention, both produced botulinum toxin for use as a weapon. Botulinum toxin was one of several agents tested on Vozroshdeniye

Island at the site Aralsk-7. Dr. Ken Alibek, former deputy director of BioPreparat, reported that the Russians had attempted to splice the botulinum toxin-producing gene from *C botulinum* into other bacteria.

Iraq has declared to the United Nations the production of concentrated botulinum toxin. 19,000 liters of botulinum toxin were produced by Iraq, and 10,000 liters were loaded into military weapons.[18,19] Of these, over 3,000 liters were unaccounted for by the United Nations Special Commission's report to the Security Council of the United Nations on October 11, 1995. Since the invasion of Iraq in 1993, this toxin has not been located. It is possible that some of this botulinum toxin could find its way into the hands of terrorists. Three other countries listed by the United States as "state sponsors of terrorism" (Iran, North Korea, and Syria) have developed or are believed to be developing botulinum toxin as a weapon.[20-22]

Some contemporary analysts discount the use of botulinum toxin as a weapon of terrorism, because there are significant constraints in concentration and stabilization that make production of the toxin difficult in a form suitable for aerosol distribution. Because the multiple sources listed above have already produced active botulinum toxin, these arguments are specious. The technology already exists to produce this toxin, and it is in the hands of those who have been known to sponsor terrorism.

As noted, botulinum toxin can be spread by either inhalation or ingestion of food or water that is contaminated with the toxin. A point-source release of botulinum toxin could incapacitate or kill 10% of persons downwind of the release.[23] Contamination of food could either produce a widespread outbreak of botulism from a single meal, or it could produce episodic, widely spread outbreaks. Botulinum toxin is colorless, odorless, and very probably tasteless in a solution. This makes botulinum a particularly good potential biological weapon.

Any multipatient outbreak of botulism should be suspected as an act of terrorism. The absence of a common dietary exposure should make the clinician particularly suspicious.

Features of an outbreak that suggest a terrorist release of botulinum toxin include the following:[24]

- Outbreak of a large number of cases of botulism
  - Acute flaccid paralysis with prominent cranial nerve palsies

INHOSPITAL INFO

- Pupils are often dilated or unreactive (50%)
- Outbreak of an unusual type of botulinum toxin
  - Type B in the western United States
  - Type A in the eastern United States
  - Type C, D, F, or G
  - Type E toxin that is not associated with aquatic foods
- Outbreak with a common geographic factor, but no common food
  - Airport, stadium, or public event
  - Features suggestive of an aerosol attack
- Multiple simultaneous outbreaks without a common source

Other Clostridial Toxins

INHOSPITAL INFO

Tetanus neurotoxin is secreted by *Clostridium* species in similar fashion to botulinum. The intoxication occurs at extremely low concentrations of toxin, is irreversible, and, like botulism, requires activity of the nerve to cause toxicity to that nerve. *C perfringens* also secretes at least 12 toxins and can produce gas gangrene (clostridial myonecrosis), **enteritis necroticans**, and clostridial food poisoning. One or more of these toxins could be produced as a weapon. The alpha toxin is highly toxic and could be lethal when delivered as an aerosol.

Effects

Whereas botulinum toxin causes a flaccid paralysis, tetanus causes **spastic paralysis**. The tetanus neurotoxin migrates up the nerve fiber and reaches the spinal inhibitory neurons, where it blocks neurotransmitter release and thus causes a spastic paralysis. Despite the seemingly different actions of tetanus and botulism, the toxins act in a similar way at the appropriate cellular level. The effect in humans is well documented and includes twitches, spasms, **rictus sardonicus**, and convulsions.

Tetanus toxin is one of the three most virulent poisons known to man. Mortality rates vary from 40% to 78% in the literature.[25] Death from tetanus usually results from interference with respiratory mechanics.

C perfringens alpha toxin causes vascular leaks, pulmonary damage, thrombocytopenia, and hepatic damage. Inhaled *C perfringens* causes serious respiratory distress.

INHOSPITAL INFO

Detection

Acute serum and tissue samples should be collected for further testing. Specific immunoassays are available for both *C perfringens* and *C tetani*. Bacteria may be readily cultured. As with most of these toxins and diseases, specific laboratory findings may be too late to be of clinical use.

Blood for serum assays should be collected in tiger-top or red-top tubes. Urine may be collected for immunoassays. Nasal swabs and induced respiratory secretions may be used for toxin assays to prove inhalation of the agent.

Prophylaxis and Treatment

C perfringens and *C tetani* are generally sensitive to penicillin, and this is the current drug of choice. There are some data that indicate that treatment with either clindamycin or rifampin may decrease *C perfringens* toxin production and produce better results.

Every medical provider is aware of the schedule for tetanus immunizations. The use of tetanus as a weapon is thought to be unlikely in the United States because of widespread tetanus immunization.[26] This may not be true, as there has been no published literature about clinical syndromes caused by overwhelming amounts of inhaled tetanus toxin. Although the CDC experts appear to discount this toxin, it is so easy to produce and spread and is so lethal that it may make a useful biological toxin. Because there is no evidence that these immunizations will protect against a large inhaled dose of tetanus toxin, this disease cannot be easily dismissed as a potential weapon of terrorism.

Because of the widespread use of tetanus toxoid for prophylactic immunization, fewer than 150 cases per year occur in the United States. Most US cases occur in individuals over the age of 60, so waning immunity is a significant risk factor. The disease is still a significant problem in the rest of the world, with over 300,000 occurrences per year. Most cases of tetanus, worldwide, occur from a small puncture wound contaminated with *C tetani* that causes a small localized infection.

There is no specific prophylaxis against most of the *C perfringens* toxins. Some toxoids for enteritis necroticans are available for humans. Veterinary toxoids are widely used. **Table 13-3** summarizes biosafety information for other clostridial toxins.

Table 13-3 Protection Against Other Clostridial Toxins

Inactivation Requirements	Decontaminating Agents	Personal Protection Requirements
Moist heat at 185°F (85°C) for more than 5 minutes	1% bleach Soap and water (for contaminated clothing and skin)	Isolation of patients is NOT needed. This agent does not breach intact skin. **Respiratory protection is needed when dealing with the agent.** Respiratory protection with a fitted NIOSH N95 mask or better will probably suffice, although more effective protection is safer. Providers caring for casualties will likely not need protection, because the incubation period is 18 to 36 hours after release, and substantial degradation is expected during this time frame.

Source: American Academy of Orthopaedic Surgeons, Stewart CE, Nixon RG. *Weapons of Mass Casualties Field Guide.* Jones and Bartlett Publishers, Boston; 2003.

■ Ricin

The seeds from the castor bean plant, ***Ricinus communis***, are poisonous to people, insects, and animals. One of the main toxic proteins is **ricin**, named by Stillmark in 1888 when he tested an extract of the beans on red blood cells and noted agglutination of the red blood cells.[27] Ricin is produced by the castor bean plant and secreted in the castor seeds.

A castor bean is a not a true bean, but a derivative of the spurge family (*Euphorbiacea*) that is manifested by seed-producing deep-rooted perennials. The castor bean plant is actually a tall, leafy plant that originated in tropical South Africa and is found in many tropical and temperate climates worldwide **(Figure 13-2).** The plant produces clusters of spiny pods, each of which contain an average of three poisonous seeds **(Figure 13-3).** The seeds are black or brown in color and strongly resemble ticks.

There are many medicinal and practical uses for the castor bean. For instance, the bitter-tasting castor oil has been used for years as an antidote for various digestive problems. This naturally occurring oil is also a common ingredient in such things as paint, varnish, and high-performance motor oils.

Castor beans are available worldwide. Ricin can be extracted cheaply and in large quantities from these beans, using low technology. The toxin is quite easy to extract from the mash left by pressing castor oil from the castor beans. (The remaining mash contains about 5% ricin by weight).[28] It can be prepared as a liquid, crystals, or as a dry powder. It can be disseminated as an aerosol, injected into a victim, or used to contaminate food or water on a small scale.

A related toxin, abrin, is produced from the bean of *Abrus precatorius*, which is called the jequirity plant or rosary pea.

Although ricin is only a natural product of the castor bean plant, ricin has been produced from transgenic tobacco using gene transfer principles. Large amounts of toxin could be produced easily by this transgenic method.[29]

The toxins found within the castor bean are ricin and ***Ricinus communis agglutinin***, or RCA. Ricin is composed of two toxins: RCL III and RCL IV. Ricin is a strong **cytotoxin**, meaning that it targets the cells of a particular organ, while RCA is a member of the **hemagglutinin** class, a toxin that specifically targets the red blood cells.

Because of the high toxicity of ricin and the extreme ease of its production, ricin was considered as a biological weapon by the United States. The military code name for ricin was compound W. Work with the British resulted in the development of a W bomb during World War II, which was tested but never used in battle. Although ricin is 1,000 times less toxic than botulinum toxin, it is still more lethal than the nerve gases.

At least one fatality has been documented as a direct result of ricin employed in biowarfare. In 1978, Georgi

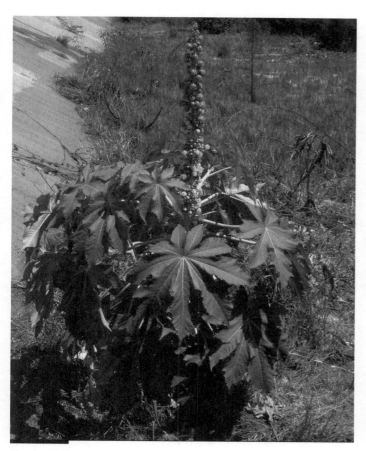

Figure 13-2 The castor bean plant.

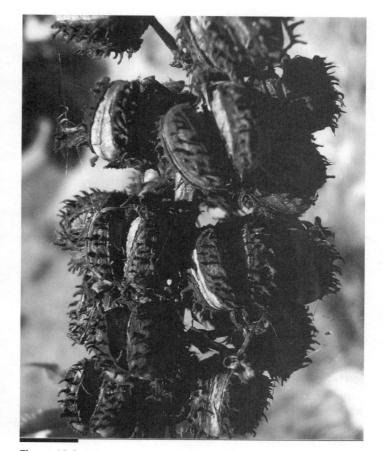

Figure 13-3 Seed pods on the castor bean plant.

Markov and Vladimar Kostov were shot by ricin-impregnated pellets fired from an umbrella. The pellets were coated with wax that was designed to melt at body temperature and release the ricin. At least six other assassinations have been attempted using the same technique according to intelligence sources.

Effects

The clinical picture depends on the route of exposure. The toxin is quite stable and extremely toxic by many routes of exposure, including inhalation. Perhaps 1 to 3 mg of ricin can kill an adult, and the ingestion of one seed can probably kill a child.

Oral

Although all parts of the castor bean are actually poisonous, it is the seeds that are the most toxic. Castor bean ingestion causes a rapid onset of nausea, vomiting, abdominal cramps, and severe diarrhea, followed by vascular collapse. Death usually occurs on the third day in the absence of appropriate medical intervention.

Ricin is least toxic by the oral route. This is probably a result of poor absorption in the gastrointestinal tract, some digestion in the gut, and, possibly, some expulsion of the agent as caused by the rapid onset of vomiting. Ingestion causes local hemorrhage and necrosis of the liver, spleen, kidney, and gastrointestinal tract. Ricin does not cause lung irritation when it is administered by routes other than inhalation.

Signs and symptoms of ricin ingestion are as follows:
- Latent period of 4 to 8 hours
- Fever
- Chills
- Headache
- Myalgias (muscle aches)
- Nausea
- Vomiting
- Diarrhea
- Tenesmus (profound abdominal cramping)
- Dehydration
- Gastrointestinal bleeding
- Necrosis of liver, spleen, kidneys, and gastrointestinal tract

Inhalation

Inhalation of ricin causes nonspecific weakness, cough, fever, hypothermia, and hypotension. Symptoms occur about 4 to 8 hours after inhalation, depending on the inhaled dose. The onset of profuse sweating some hours later signifies the termination of the symptoms.

Lethal human exposures have not been described. In animals, respiratory symptoms, including necrosis and alveolar infiltrates, are followed by cardiovascular collapse about 24 to 36 hours after inhalation. Death will occur about 36 to 48 hours after inhalation. Large doses of ricin by inhalation appear to produce severe enough pulmonary damage to cause death. (Inhalation of ricin by rats causes diffused necrotizing pneumonia with interstitial and alveolar inflammation and edema.)

Signs and symptoms of ricin inhalation are as follows:
- Latent period of 4 to 8 hours
- Fever
- Chills
- Nausea
- Local irritation of eyes, nose, and throat
- Diaphoresis (profuse sweating)
- Headache
- Myalgias
- Nonproductive cough
- Chest pain
- Dyspnea
- Pulmonary edema
- Severe lung inflammation (alveolar infiltrates)
- Cyanosis
- Convulsions
- Respiratory failure

Injection

Ricin has been used as an injectable toxin for assassinations, as previously described. Although the injection of ricin would not be a widespread method of terrorism, the emergency provider could conceivably care for a patient with this syndrome. When injected, ricin can cause disseminated intravascular coagulopathy. Microcirculatory failure and multiple organ failure follow.

Detection

ELISA, for blood or histochemical analysis, may be useful in confirming ricin intoxication. Ricin causes a marked immune response, and sera should be obtained from survivors for the measurement of antibody response. Polymerase chain reaction can detect castor bean DNA in most ricin preparations. Standard laboratory tests are of little help in the diagnosis of ricin intoxication. The patient may have some leukocytosis, with neutrophil predominance.

Blood for serum assays should be collected in tiger-top or red-top tubes. Urine may be collected for immunoassays. Nasal swabs and induced respiratory secretions may be used for toxin assays to prove the inhalation of the agent.

The pleomorphic picture of ricin intoxication would suggest many respiratory pathogens and may be of little help in diagnosis. The chest radiograph may show bilateral infiltrates. Arterial blood gases may show hypoxemia, and a leucocytosis rich in neutrophils may be noted.

Prophylaxis and Treatment

Treatment

Treatment is supportive and includes both respiratory support and cardiovascular support as needed. Early intubation, ventilation, and positive end expiratory pressure, combined with treatment of pulmonary edema, are appropriate. If oral ingestion is suspected, then **lavage**, followed by **cathartics**, is appropriate. Because ricin is a large molecule, charcoal is of little use for ingestions, although it is commonly recommended. Intravenous fluids and electrolyte replacement are useful for treating the dehydration caused by profound vomiting and diarrhea.

INHOSPITAL INFO

Because ricin acts rapidly and irreversibly, therapy after exposure is difficult. There is a large ongoing effort to look for an agent to treat ricin poisoning, but nothing has been found thus far.

Prophylaxis

There is no approved immunologic or chemoprophylaxis at this time. Animal studies have shown that immunization is very effective protection. These immunization techniques have been used to treat animals, but are not currently available for humans. There is an ongoing effort to produce both active immunization and passive antibody prophylaxis by means that are suitable for humans.

Active prophylaxis through an immunization against the ricin toxin is the only potentially effective medical countermeasure. Either a toxoid of the native ricin toxin or a preparation of the purified A-chain will produce protection against the inhalation of multiple lethal doses of ricin toxin.[30] This formalin-treated toxoid has been submitted to the FDA as an investigational drug.

The use of passive prophylaxis or therapy (if the therapy is given within a few hours after exposure) has also been studied. In this study, animals were protected with aerosolized immunoglobulin G (specific for ricin). This treatment completely protected the animals that inhaled the passive immune agent 1 hour *prior* to the exposure. These studies also point out that intravenous injection or aerosol inhalation of a specific antibody *after* exposure provided little or no protection.

Respiratory protection will prevent inhalation exposure and is the best prophylaxis currently available. Ricin does not cause any dermal activity and does not penetrate the skin.

Table 13-4 summarizes biosafety information for ricin.

Threat

In recent years, ricin has become a favorite threat of extremist individuals and groups. In 1995, two tax protestors were convicted of possession of ricin as a biological weapon. This was the first case of prosecution under the 1989 Biological Weapons Anti-terrorism Act.[31] This agent has been used in at least one assassination and has been developed by many countries for use as a weapon. Ricin's appeal to terrorists stems from its ready availability, its ease of production in relatively large quantities, and its popularization by the media.

In January 2003, three men were charged with producing ricin in their apartment in London. Although the men were suspected of being part of a terrorist plot, only traces of the toxin were found in their apartment, with no reported deployable quantities. This may suggest that the toxin had been removed prior to the arrival of authorities.

The development of multiple cases of very severe pulmonary distress in a previously healthy population should prompt the emergency clinician to consider ricin. Of course, other pulmonary toxins, such as phosgene and similar agents, should also be considered.

■ Staphylococcal Enterotoxin

Staphylococcus toxins are a common cause of diarrheal food poisoning after the ingestion of improperly handled or refrigerated foodstuffs. Because they normally exert their effect on the gut, they are often called **enterotoxins**.

There are at least five distinct forms of staphylococcal enterotoxins (SEA, SEB, SEC, SEE, and toxic shock syndrome toxin–1). Staphylococcal enterotoxin B (SEB) is the best studied of these toxins. SEB is excreted by staphylococcal bacteria and has a primary effect on the gastrointestinal tract. SEB is a protein that consists of 239 amino acids, is easily soluble in water, and is relatively stable. It can withstand boiling for 2 minutes, and when it is placed in a freeze-dried state, it can be stored for more than 1 year. When contracted by inhalation, it causes a clinical syndrome that is markedly different and often more disabling than when it is ingested.

SEB has been studied by the United States and other countries as an incapacitation agent. Indeed, this toxin was part of the US stockpile prior to its destruction in 1972. (The military designator for SEB is PG.) The median disabling dose for humans by inhalation is estimated at 0.0004 ng/kg. The lethal dose is about 50 times the disabling dose (30 ng/kg).

SEB can be dispersed as an aerosol or as a food contaminant. As noted, the toxin is markedly different in action when it is inhaled, as opposed to when it is ingested. When

INHOSPITAL INFO

Table 13-4 Protection Against Ricin		
Inactivation Requirements	**Decontaminating Agents**	**Personal Protection Requirements**
Moist heat at 185°F (85°C) for more than 5 minutes (The heat stability of this toxin decreases with increasing moisture content.)	0.1% bleach (1 part household bleach added to 49 parts water) Soap and water (for contaminated clothing and skin)	Isolation of patients is NOT needed. This agent does not breach intact skin. **Respiratory protection is needed when dealing with the agent.** Respiratory protection with a fitted NIOSH N95 mask or better will probably suffice, although more effective protection is safer. **Providers caring for casualties will need respiratory protection,** because the incubation period is 4 to 8 hours after aerosol release, and substantial degradation is NOT expected during this time frame.

Source: American Academy of Orthopaedic Surgeons, Stewart CE, Nixon RG. *Weapons of Mass Casualties Field Guide.* Jones and Bartlett Publishers, Boston; 2003.

inhaled, SEB causes symptoms at very low doses in humans (less than one one-hundredth of the dose necessary to cause symptoms when ingested).

No matter which route is used to disseminate staphylococcal enterotoxin, the resulting illness would cause symptoms in up to 80% of those who are exposed to it. In a large target population, the subsequent demand on emergency services would rapidly overwhelm the system.

The organism that produces this agent is readily available and could be tailored to produce large quantities of the toxin. Related toxins include the toxic shock syndrome toxin-1 and exfoliative toxins (staphylococcal-mediated exfoliative dermatitis).

Effects

Oral

Patients exposed to oral SEB fall ill after a few hours and develop typical food poisoning symptoms, such as stomach cramps, diarrhea, and vomiting. In cases of foodborne SEB, fever and respiratory involvement are absent and the gastrointestinal symptoms predominate. Fluid losses resulting from vomiting and diarrhea may be substantial.

Inhalation

The disease caused by inhalation of the toxin begins 1 to 12 hours after exposure, and includes the sudden onset of fever, chills, headache, myalgia, and a nonproductive cough. The cough may progress to dyspnea and substernal chest pain. In severe cases, pulmonary edema may be found. Nausea, vomiting, and diarrhea are common (as in the poisoning familiar to health care providers). Gastrointestinal symptoms may accompany respiratory exposure; these result from an inadvertent swallowing of the toxin after inhalation. As in the oral form, the fluid losses may be significant.

With the exception of dehydration and postural hypotension, the results of a physical examination are often normal. The only physical finding of note is conjunctival injection. In very severe cases, the chest radiograph may show infiltrates.

The patient frequently recovers from the nausea and vomiting without special treatment within 24 hours. The fever may last up to 5 days and may rise to 106°F/41.1°C. The patient may experience chills, rigors, and prostration. The cough may persist for up to 4 weeks. Sickness may last as long as 2 weeks, and severe exposure may cause fatalities.

Signs and symptoms of staphylococcal enterotoxin ingestion are as follows:

Latent period of 3 to 12 hours
- Fever
- Chills
- Headache
- Myalgias
- Nausea
- Vomiting
- Diarrhea
- Tenesmus
- Dehydration
- Shock

Signs and symptoms of staphylococcal enterotoxin inhalation are as follows:
- Latent period of 4 to 10 hours
- Fever
- Chills
- Headache
- Myalgias
- Nonproductive cough
- Chest pain
- Dyspnea
- Nausea and vomiting (if the toxin is ingested as well)
- Diarrhea (if the toxin is ingested as well)
- Pulmonary edema
- Respiratory failure
- Shock from fluid losses

Detection

The diagnosis of inhalation SEB intoxication is clinical. The lab is not helpful. A nonspecific rise in the white blood cell count may be seen and erythrocyte sedimentation rate may be elevated, but these are nonspecific findings. A chest radiograph is usually normal, but it may show increased intrastitial markings and possibly pulmonary edema.

Epidemiology of this agent is relatively easy. With the rapid onset and equally rapid inactivation in the nature of the toxin, all intoxicated patients should be present within a single 24-hour period. Infections would present over a more prolonged period of time.

Patient samples may be unlikely to test positive for the toxin following aerosol exposure unless the exposure is large and the samples are obtained rapidly. Blood for serum assays should be collected in tiger-top or red-top tubes. Urine may be collected for immunoassays. Nasal swabs and induced respiratory secretions may be used for toxin assays to prove the inhalation of the agent.

The differential diagnosis for this agent is vast. An epidemic of influenza, parainfluenza, adenovirus, or mycoplasma could also cause fever, nonproductive cough, muscle aches, and headache in large numbers of patients within a short time. The early clinical manifestations of SEB intoxication are also similar to those seen in inhalation anthrax, tularemia, plague, and Q fever. The stability of the patient after a few hours would argue against any bacterial infection. Chemical agents, such as phosgene, may also have a similar presentation.

Prophylaxis and Treatment

Treatment

There is no significant treatment regimen available. Supportive therapy has proven to be adequate in cases of accidental respiratory exposure to SEB aerosol. Therapy is entirely supportive, and includes attention to fluid status, oxygenation, and the development of respiratory failure. In severe cases, where pulmonary edema develops, ventilation with positive pressure and diuretics may be of value. The value of corticosteroids is unknown.

Table 13-5 Protection Against Staphylococcal Enterotoxins

Inactivation Requirements	Decontaminating Agents	Personal Protection Requirements
Moist heat at 185°F (85°C) for more than 5 minutes (Note that this toxin is relatively stable and can withstand boiling water for a few minutes.)	0.5% bleach for 10 to 15 minutes Soap and water (for contaminated clothing and skin)	Isolation of patients is NOT needed. This agent does not breach intact skin. **Respiratory protection is needed when dealing with the agent.** Respiratory protection with a fitted NIOSH N95 mask or better will probably suffice, although more effective protection is safer. **Providers caring for casualties will need respiratory protection,** because the incubation period is 4 to 10 hours after release, and substantial degradation is NOT expected during this time frame. All potentially exposed or contaminated foods should be destroyed.

Source: American Academy of Orthopaedic Surgeons, Stewart CE, Nixon RG. *Weapons of Mass Casualties Field Guide.* Jones and Bartlett Publishers, Boston; 2003.

Prophylaxis

There is no current prophylaxis or human vaccine available for immunization against SEB. A vaccine candidate is in advanced development for testing.[32] Naturally acquired immunity has been noted, but does not confer complete protection, even for natural gastrointestinal disease. Passive immunity has been demonstrated, but there is no current immunotherapy available.

Because this is an intoxication and not an infection, no isolation of the patient is needed. SEB does not penetrate intact skin. Secondary aerosols are not a hazard. Decontamination is accomplished with soap and water. All potentially exposed foods should be promptly destroyed. **Table 13-5** summarizes biosafety information for staphylococcal enterotoxins.

◼ Tetrodotoxin

Tetrodotoxin is another potent neurotoxin, which is produced by the puffer fish (also called the globefish or blowfish).[33] The tetraodon puffers are equipped with four large teeth, which are nearly fused, forming a beaklike structure that is used for cracking mollusks and other invertebrates, as well as for scraping corals and general reef grazing.

Many species of the family *Salamandridae* and a group of Central American toads, the harlequin frogs, also possess the toxin, but tetrodotoxin is even more widely distributed. It appears in trigger fishes, ocean sunfishes, globefishes, porcupine fishes, some parrot fishes, a goby, xanthid crabs, sea stars, an angelfish, a horseshoe crab, a number of marine snails, a flatworm, a South Atlantic sea squirt, ribbon worms, and a marine red alga **(Figure 13-4).**

All organs of the fresh water puffer are toxic, with the skin having the highest toxicity, followed by the gonad, muscle, liver, and intestine. In saltwater puffers, the liver is the most toxic organ.

It was a mystery why such a diverse group of unrelated organisms would all evolve the same toxin until researchers discovered that a bacteria is harbored in these animals that produces tetrodotoxin.[34] Because this toxin is produced by a bacteria, it could be genetically engineered into other bacteria. Likewise, the yield of the target bacteria could be improved.

It is noteworthy that tetrodotoxin and saxitoxin are unusual, because there are few potent nonprotein toxins. The lethal dose of tetrodotoxin is only 5 mg/kg in the guinea pig. In humans, the lethal dose is 334 mg/kg by ingestion. The lethal dose by inhalation is unknown.

Puffer intoxication is a serious public health problem in Japan, and over 50 people each year are intoxicated. Raw puffer fish, commonly called fugu, is a delicacy in several Southeast Asian countries, including Japan. The consumption of fugu causes mild tetrodotoxin intoxication, which produces a pleasant peripheral and perioral tingling sensation. Improperly prepared fugu may contain a lethal quantity of tetrodotoxin. Fatalities have gradually decreased because of the increased understanding of the toxin and careful preparation of the puffer for food.[35] Cooking the food will not dissipate the toxin. Tetrodotoxin is heat stable.

There are several microbial sources of tetrodotoxin including *Pseudomonas*, *Vibrio*, *Listonella*, and *Alteromonas* species. Although there is only one known bacterium that has produced tetrodotoxin toxicity in humans, there is a significant potential for the genetic alteration of common species of bacteria to produce tetrodotoxin.[36]

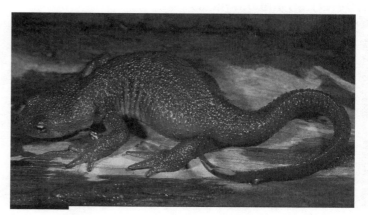

Figure 13-4 The rough-skinned newt (*Taricha granulosa*) ranges from California to British Columbia. An adult contains enough tetrodotoxin in its tissues to kill several adult humans.

Tetrodotoxin is well known for its ability to inhibit neuromuscular function by blocking the axonal sodium channels.[37] Tetrodotoxin binds to the sodium channel of the nerve and prevents the passage of the nerve impulse. Although the target is similar to that of saxitoxin, the two appear to act independently.

Tetrodotoxin is quite specific in blocking the sodium ion channel and the flow of sodium ions without having any effect on potassium ions.[38] Binding within the channel is relatively tight. The hydrated sodium ion binds reversibly and is cleared within nanoseconds. Tetrodotoxin, much larger than the sodium ion, acts like a cork in the channel. It diffuses out of the sodium channel in tens of seconds, long enough for fatal nerve paralysis.

Effects

The clinical symptoms and signs of tetrodotoxin poisoning are similar to those of the acetylcholinesterase poisons.[39] Clinical symptoms include nausea, vomiting, vertigo, perioral numbness, unsteady gait, and extremity numbness. Clinical symptoms begin within 30 minutes of ingestion. The speed of onset depends on the quantity of the toxin ingested. Death can occur within 17 minutes after the ingestion of tetrodotoxin.

Because tetrodotoxin does not cross the blood-brain barrier, the patient remains conscious until hypoxia intervenes. There are reports of fugu poisoning survivors who were completely lucid during the entire event, recovering to tell the tale.

The symptoms progress to muscle weakness, chest tightness, diaphoresis, dyspnea, chest pain, and finally paralysis. Hypotension and respiratory failure are seen in severe poisonings. Patients will frequently complain of a sensation of cold or chilliness. Paresthesias spread to the extremities, with symptoms often more pronounced distally.

Death from tetrodotoxin is thought to be caused by hypoxic brain damage from prolonged respiratory paralysis. Patients who survive 24 hours usually make a complete recovery. **Diabetes insipidus** has been reported in critically ill patients.

Detection and Diagnosis

There is no test for tetrodotoxin available in the acute clinical situation. Detection of tetrodotoxin is accomplished by mouse bioassay or by liquid chromatography. Use of radioimmunoassay and radioreceptor assays has also been reported, but these are not yet widely available. An in vitro colorimetric cell assay against a rabbit antiserum has been developed and may be more rapid than older methods, but it is not yet publicly available.[40]

Blood for serum assays should be collected in tiger-top or red-top tubes. Urine may be collected for immunoassays. Nasal swabs and induced respiratory secretions may be used for toxin assays to prove the inhalation of the agent.

Prophylaxis and Treatment
Treatment

At present, there is no known antidote for tetrodotoxin intoxication. There are numerous anecdotal treatments of survivors with supportive therapy alone. Certainly, respiratory support and airway management will be lifesaving for a majority of these patients. Gastric lavage will remove unabsorbed toxin from the gut and is used for puffer fish intoxication. Activated charcoal has been reported to effectively bind the toxin and may be employed for ingestions.

4-Aminopyridine has been used to treat tetrodotoxin intoxication in laboratory animals.[41] 4-Aminopyridine is a potent potassium channel blocker, and it enhances impulse-evoked acetylcholine release from presynaptic motor terminals. There have been no human studies of its use as an antidote. 4-Aminopyridine can cause muscle fasciculation and seizures in a dose-dependent phenomenon.

Naloxone has been proposed as a possible antidote, because the opiates and tetrodotoxin have similar molecular configurations.[42] However, there are no reports of its use as an antidote for tetrodotoxin intoxication in either laboratory or clinical settings.

Prophylaxis

Active and passive immunization is possible for tetrodotoxin. Although this has been demonstrated in laboratory animals, there is no known available human immunization for tetrodotoxin.[43] Tolerance does not develop after repeated puffer fish exposure. Monoclonal antibodies have been produced, and they have protected laboratory animals against lethal doses of tetrodotoxin.[44,45] **Table 13-6** summarizes biosafety information for tetrodotoxin.

Threat

The dangers of tetrodotoxin poisoning were known by the ancient Egyptians (2400 to 2700 BC). Although relatively little is known about tetrodotoxin as a possible weapon, it was evaluated by Japanese Unit 731 during World War II. It is included in the **Australia Group** lists of biotoxins because of its toxicity. (The Australia Group is an informal consortium of 33 nations that are determined to address the growing problem of the proliferation of biological and chemical warfare weapons.) It is not known to be made in quantities that could be used in weapons. Little or nothing is available in the open-source literature about its inhalation toxicity.

There is no confirmed terrorist acquisition or attempted use of tetrodotoxin. As noted, besides puffer fish, the presence of tetrodotoxin has been detected in a wide range of animals, including frogs, the blue-ringed octopus, and the California newt. The Nobel Prize was awarded, in part, to Dr. R. B. Woodward for a successful synthesis of tetrodotoxin in 1965.[46] This synthesis is quite difficult and would be unlikely to appeal to a terrorist.

INHOSPITAL INFO

INHOSPITAL INFO

Table 13-6 Protection Against Tetrodotoxin

Inactivation Requirements	Decontaminating Agents	Personal Protection Requirements
Moist heat at 185°F (85°C) for more than 5 minutes	1% bleach Soap and water (for contaminated clothing and skin)	Strict isolation of patients is NOT needed. This agent is slowly absorbed through intact skin. **Protective garments are recommended.** Simple overgarments, such as gloves and a water-permeable gown, should suffice. **Respiratory protection is needed when dealing with the agent (but not with patients who have been decontaminated).** Respiratory protection with a fitted NIOSH N95 mask or better will probably suffice, although more effective protection is safer. **Providers caring for casualties will need respiratory and skin protection,** because the incubation period is only moments after release, and NO substantial degradation is expected during this time frame.

Source: American Academy of Orthopaedic Surgeons, Stewart CE, Nixon RG. *Weapons of Mass Casualties Field Guide.* Jones and Bartlett Publishers, Boston; 2003.

■ Saxitoxin

Saxitoxin is a toxin that is responsible for paralytic shellfish poisoning during red tides. It is also found in several species of puffers and other marine animals. It was originally discovered in 1927.[47]

Red tides occur when warm weather and ocean conditions allow for an abundant overgrowth or bloom of phytoplankton. Several of the phytoplankton (dinoflagellates of *Alexandrium, Gynmodium,* and *Pyrodinium*) are known to produce saxitoxin.

Saxitoxin is collected from the tissues of butter clams and other shellfish that ingest the dinoflagellates and concentrate the toxin. When the shellfish are consumed by birds or mammals, paralysis occurs. The green shawl crab, found in the Great Barrier Reef in Australia, concentrates enough saxitoxin to kill 3,000 people.[48] Saxitoxin can also be synthesized, with some difficulty.

Saxitoxin is one of the most potent nonprotein toxins known to man. Saxitoxin is about 1,000 times more toxic than a typical synthetic nerve gas, such as sarin, and about 50 times more potent than **curare**. The minimum lethal dose is between 0.5 and 12.5 mg. In children, the minimum lethal dose is estimated to be 25 ng/kg.

The toxin is water soluble and stable, so dispersal as an aerosol is feasible. The toxin is heat stable and is not destroyed by cooking. Saxitoxin was developed by the US military and the CIA as a potential weapon. The military designator for saxitoxin is SS. It is also known as mytilotoxin.

Effects
Oral

Saxitoxin is similar in effects and treatment to tetrodotoxin. The onset of symptoms occurs within 10 to 60 minutes of exposure. Numbness and tingling of the lips and tongue (from local absorption) spreads to the face and neck. This may be followed by a prickling feeling in the fingers and toes, which spreads to the arms and legs. Motor activity is reduced. The patient's speech becomes garbled and incoherent, because of paralysis of the muscles of speech, and respirations become labored. Other symptoms include a sensation of floating, headache, ataxia, muscle weakness, and **cranial nerve dysfunction**. Gastrointestinal symptoms are less common and may include nausea, vomiting, diarrhea, and abdominal pain.

Victims die from paralysis of the respiratory muscles. Death may occur within 2 to 24 hours. If the patient survives, then normal functions are regained within a few days. The estimated lethal dose for humans is 9 to 10 mg/kg for ingestion of saxitoxin.

Inhalation

There are no human cases of inhalation of saxitoxin reported in the medical literature. Animal experiments suggest that the entire syndrome is compressed, and death from respiratory paralysis may occur within minutes. The estimated lethal dose for inhalation for humans is 2.0 mg/kg.

Detection

There is a standardized mouse assay available for routine surveillance. A mouse unit is the minimum amount of toxin that will kill a 20-g mouse within 15 minutes. It is unlikely that this assay will help the emergency clinician.

Saxitoxin can also be detected using ELISA and high performance liquid chromatography. Direct human serum assays for the shellfish toxins are not available.

Blood for serum assays should be collected in tiger-top or red-top tubes. Urine may be collected for immunoassays. Nasal swabs and induced respiratory secretions may be used for toxin assays to prove the inhalation of the agent.

Prophylaxis and Treatment

There is no antidote for saxitoxin, so symptomatic treatment is appropriate. The toxin is normally cleared rapidly from the body by urinary excretion. Victims who survive for 12 to 24 hours will usually recover. Antibodies for

INHOSPITAL INFO

Table 13-7 Protection Against Saxitoxin		
Inactivation Requirements	Decontaminating Agents	Personal Protection Requirements
Saxitoxin maintains its activity in water heated to 120°F (49°C).	1% bleach Soap and water (for contaminated clothing and skin)	Isolation of patients is NOT needed. This agent does not breach intact skin. **Respiratory protection is needed when dealing with the agent.** Respiratory protection with a fitted NIOSH N95 mask or better will probably suffice, although more effective protection is safer. **Providers caring for casualties will need respiratory protection,** because the incubation period is only moments after release, and no substantial degradation is expected during this time frame. There is no outgassing, but the significance of re-aerosolization from contaminated clothing is unknown.

Source: American Academy of Orthopaedic Surgeons, Stewart CE, Nixon RG. *Weapons of Mass Casualties Field Guide.* Jones and Bartlett Publishers, Boston; 2003.

tetrodotoxin will frequently protect against saxitoxin.[49] There is no vaccine for saxitoxin exposure for human use. **Table 13-7** summarizes biosafety information for saxitoxin.

Threat

Saxitoxin was extensively evaluated by the US military and the CIA as a military agent, an assassination agent, and a rapidly acting suicide agent for covert operatives. Apparently, saxitoxin was selected for use in suicide capsules for U2 pilots, because it was faster and surer than cyanide. It was assigned the military designator SS. It may be administered by ingestion, injection, or inhalation. Today, saxitoxin is classified as a Schedule I chemical warfare agent per the Schedule of Chemicals from the Convention on the Prohibition of the Development, Production, Stockpiling, and Use of Chemical Weapons and on Their Destruction. The only other naturally occurring toxin that is so classified is ricin.

According to public knowledge, saxitoxin remains only a potential threat and has not been employed as a military weapon or as a terrorist agent. Nonetheless, it is an agent that is quite toxic in small amounts and attainable without substantial difficulty. It would be difficult to differentiate the effects of the inhalational use of saxitoxin from the use of botulinum toxin in a mass-casualty situation.

■ Trichothecene Mycotoxins

The **trichothecene mycotoxins** are a group of over 40 compounds produced by fungi (specifically, *Fusarium*, a common grain mold). The toxins were inadvertently discovered when contaminated flour was used to make bread; the poisoned victims developed a severe gastrointestinal disease that caused a high mortality rate. The effects of the toxins can occur after ingestion, inhalation, or skin contact. The toxins achieved fame in the 1970s, when they were considered to be the best candidates for the infamous "yellow rain" found in Laos, Cambodia, and Afghanistan. Naturally occurring trichothecenes have caused moldy corn toxicosis in animals. Two of the better-known toxins are **T-2** and **deoxynivalenol** (or vomitoxin).

Trichothecene mycotoxins are potent inhibitors of protein synthesis. They inhibit mitochondrial respiration, impair DNA synthesis, and destroy cell membranes. They cause bone marrow suppression and suppress mucosal protein synthesis.

Trichothecene mycotoxins constitute the only class of biological toxins that causes skin damage. They cause blisters, **pruritus**, vesicles, necrosis, and sloughing within minutes to hours after skin exposure. The toxins are nonvolatile compounds that are extremely stable in the environment. Hypochlorite solution does not inactivate these toxins. They retain their bioactivity even when autoclaved.

Effects

Symptoms caused by the toxins are wide ranging and include vomiting, diarrhea, ataxia, and hemorrhaging. The consumption of trichothecenes causes weight loss, vomiting, bloody diarrhea, and diffuse hemorrhage. This was discovered by the Russians, when contaminated bread was ingested and caused **alimentary toxic aleukia**. Within days, the gastrointestinal symptoms progressed to bone marrow depression with **neutropenia** and secondary sepsis. Survivors developed bleeding from all body orifices and diffuse bleeding into the skin.

The onset of the illness occurs within hours, and death may occur within 12 hours in cases of significant inhalation exposure. Early symptoms include eye pain, tearing, eye redness, and a foreign body sensation in the eye. The patient may develop nasal itching, nasal burning, nasal blistering, epistaxis, and bloody rhinorrhea. Mouth and throat exposure causes

INCIDENTS INVOLVING Toxins

Yellow Rain

One of the most enduring controversies regarding the use of biological weapons stems from the alleged yellow rain incidents of the 1970s and early 1980s. During this time period, Soviet Union aircraft reportedly showered villages in Laos, Khmer, and other Southeast Asian villages with an unknown yellow substance. Those exposed to the attacks reportedly experienced eye pain, blurred vision, headache, dizziness, chest pain, breathing difficulties, and diarrhea. Sources report that between 10% and 20% of those directly exposed died. Although the exact nature of yellow rain is unknown, many have speculated that it is aerosolized T-2 mycotoxins.

pain and blood tinged saliva and sputum. Skin exposure may result in burning skin pain, erythema, blistering, tenderness, and a progression to skin necrosis with a blackening and sloughing of skin surfaces. Inhalation exposure adds respiratory distress and failure to the picture. The patient may start with dyspnea, wheezing, and cough before progressing to respiratory distress.

Systemic toxicity occurs with any route of exposure. The patient develops weakness, prostration, dizziness, ataxia, and loss of coordination. The symptoms progress to tachycardia, hypotension, and shock. A late effect is bone marrow depression with pancytopenia and secondary sepsis and bleeding.

Detection

INHOSPITAL INFO

There is no readily available diagnostic test, although reference laboratories may be able to help with gas-liquid chromatography. There are some polyclonal and monoclonal antibodies for detection in liquid or solid samples.

Pathologic specimens should include blood, urine, lung washings, stool samples, and stomach contents. Urine samples are most useful for this purpose, because the metabolites can be detected in urine for as long as 28 days after exposure to the agent. Blood for serum assays should be collected in tiger-top or red-top tubes. Nasal swabs and induced respiratory secretions may be used for toxin assays to prove the inhalation of the agent.

The symptoms will be similar to those of a chemical agent attack. The clinician must ensure that mustard or other vesicant agents are not present.

Prophylaxis and Treatment

There is no specific treatment that is generally recommended for these agents. Ascorbic acid has been proposed to decrease the lethality of the toxins. This has been studied in animals only, but, because ascorbic acid has few side effects and is cheap, it should be used in all suspected cases. Dexamethasone (1 to 10 mg intravenously) has also been shown to decrease lethality as late as 3 hours after exposure to these toxins.

The eyes should be irrigated with normal saline or water to remove toxin. The skin should be thoroughly washed with soap and water. In a case of ingestion, charcoal or superactivated charcoal will absorb remaining toxin and decrease lethality.

The only recommended protection is an appropriate mask with protective clothing. **Table 13-8** summarizes biosafety information for trichothecene mycotoxins.

Other fungal toxins include the following:
- Mycotoxin F2: A mycotoxin produced by numerous species of *Fusarium*. It inhibits fertility.
- Aflatoxin B1: A mycotoxin produced by *Aspergillus flavus*, a fungus that can grow on many grains and nuts. Aflatoxin B1 causes liver cancer. Aflatoxin was produced by Iraq as a biological weapon.

Threat

The T-2 mycotoxins are the most likely agents to have been employed in the Soviet Union's yellow rain, which was used in Afghanistan, Laos, and Cambodia from 1974 to 1981. In accounts of these attacks, a yellow cloud of dust or a mist was sprayed from aerial sprayers. The liquid form rapidly dried to a powder.

Although these agents are not readily available like ricin, they can be cultured using standard fungal culture techniques. It should be presumed that the technology used to build these toxins did not disappear after the breakup of the Soviet Union, and may well be in terrorists' hands. The skin toxicity of the agent may make the agent especially appealing to terrorists, because it could be confused with a vesicant like mustard. It is the only toxin with such properties.

■ Bioregulators

During recent years, the use of **bioregulators** as chemical weapons agents has been evaluated. These types of substances do not belong to the group of toxins, but they are, nonetheless, grouped with them, because their possible use

Table 13-8 Protection Against Trichothecene Mycotoxins		
Inactivation Requirements	Decontaminating Agents	Personal Protection Requirements
Extreme heat at 1,500°F (857°C) for 30 minutes 5% bleach with an exposure time of 6 to 10 hours (Reusable equipment should be soaked for at least 1 hour in a 1% bleach solution that also contains 0.1M of sodium hydroxide.)	Although the trichothecene mycotoxins require more stringent means to *deactivate* them, they can be removed from the skin with simple soap and water wash. Washing the skin with soap and water within 1 hour of exposure may prevent skin toxicity, and washing within 5 to 6 hours may reduce tissue damage. If the eyes are exposed, flush with large amounts of saline.	Strict isolation of patients is NOT needed. Outgassing is not a hazard during patient exposure, but contact with the patient's contaminated clothing can cause exposure. This agent can breach intact skin, and **impermeable garments are needed when dealing with this agent.** **Respiratory protection is needed when dealing with this agent.** Respiratory protection with a fitted NIOSH N95 mask or better will probably suffice, although more effective protection is safer. **Providers caring for casualties will absolutely need protective garments and respiratory protection, because this agent is quite stable.**

Source: American Academy of Orthopaedic Surgeons, Stewart CE, Nixon RG. *Weapons of Mass Casualties Field Guide.* Jones and Bartlett Publishers, Boston; 2003.

is similar. Bioregulators are related to regulatory substances normally found in the body that control blood pressure, heart rate, and other critical functions. They may be algogenic (pain-causing) or anesthetic, or they may influence blood pressure. Bioregulators are active in extremely low doses and frequently take rapid effect.

One example of this group of substances is Substance P, a polypeptide that is active in doses of less than 1 μg. Substance P causes, for example, a rapid loss of blood pressure, which may cause unconsciousness. Another example within this group of substances is histamine. Healthcare providers are familiar with the properties of histamine in the wheal, flare, and inflammatory response of an acute allergic reaction. Histamine is clearly a human bioregulator, yet it is also an active ingredient in wasp venom, for example. Although histamine may not be made into an effective weapon, the principle may guide investigators to other research that does yield weapons.

Now that large-scale production processes for biologically active peptides and similar substances are in commercial development, bioregulators and other toxins have become a field rich in potential for weapons as well as for pharmaceuticals. These may become weapons of intense disabling or incapacitating power. Using the latest recombinant-DNA techniques, scientists might modify bioregulators to enhance their potency and effect.

Bioregulators almost certainly would evade current biological agent detectors. They may cause immediate effects and thus be used to disrupt police or military actions. Finally, they may be far more potent than traditional chemical agents. Given the complexity of development and dispersal, the use of bioregulators by terrorists is hardly imminent, but cannot be dismissed.

Table 13-9 lists toxins that have been evaluated as potential chemical weapons by the CDC.

Table 13-9 CDC Restricted Select Toxins

• Abrin	• C botulinum toxin E	• T-2 toxin
• Abrin A	• C botulinum toxin F	• T-2 toxin tetraol
• Abrin B	• C perfringens epsilon toxin	• T-2 hemisuccinate
• Abrin C	• Conotoxins	• Tetrodotoxin
• Abrin D	• Diacetoxyscirpenol	• Tetrodotoxin citrate, 2-hydroxy
• Abrin reconstituted (A+B mix)	• Ricin	• Tetrodotoxin 4,9-anhydro
• Aflatoxins	• Ricin A	• Tetrodotoxin 4,9 anhydro, 8,3-diacetate
• Aflatoxin 495	• Ricin A-chain	• Tetrodotoxin 4-amino-4-deoxy
• Aflatoxin B	• Ricin B	• Deoxytetrodotoxin
• Aflatoxin B1	• Ricin C	• Methoxytetrodotoxin
• Aflatoxin B1 mixed with G1	• Ricin D	• Ethoxytetrodotoxin
• Aflatoxin B1 dichlorides, oxides, epoxides	• Ricin D alanine-chain protein	• Recombinant organisms and molecules:
• Aflatoxin B2 dihydro B1	• Ricin D isoleucine-chain reduced	1. Genetically modified microorganisms or genetic elements from organisms listed previously that are shown to produce or encode for a factor associated with a disease
• Aflatoxin G1	• Ricin nitrogen	
• Aflatoxin G2 dihydro G1	• Ricin, reduced	
• Aflatoxin M1 4-hydroxy B1	• Ricin, total hydrolysate	
• Aflatoxin M2 4-hydroxy B2	• Ricin toxin, Con A	2. Genetically modified microorganisms or genetic elements that contain nucleic acid sequences coding for any of the toxins listed previously or their toxic subunits
• Aflatoxin P1	• Saxitoxin	
• Aflatoxin Q1	• Saxitoxin hydrate	
• Aflatoxin Ro	• Saxitoxin dihydrochloride hydrochloride	
• Botulinum toxins	• Saxitoxin p-bromobenzenesulfonate	*Exemptions:* Toxins for medical use that are inactivated for use as vaccines and toxin preparations for biomedical research use at a lethal dose for vertebrates of more than 100 ng/kg are exempt. National standard toxins required for biological potency testing are exempt.
• Clostridium botulinum	• Shigatoxin	
• C botulinum neurotoxin	• Shigella shigae neurotoxin	
• C botulinum toxin A	• Staphylococcal enterotoxins	
• C botulinum toxin B	• Staphylococcal enterotoxin A	
• C botulinum toxin C1	• Staphylococcal enterotoxin B	
• C botulinum toxin C2	• Staphylococcal enterotoxin F	
• C botulinum toxin D	• Tetrodotoxin	

Adapted from: Schedule of Chemicals from the Convention on the Prohibition of the Development, Production, Stockpiling, and Use of Chemical Weapons and on Their Destruction. http://www.mitretek.org/home.nsf/homelandsecurity/CWCDefSched (accessed April 1, 2004.)

■ References

1. Rademaker C: A scientific look at the Red Sea Moses sole's nurotoxin: Pardaxin. George Mason University. http://mason.gmu.edu/~crademak/Neurotoxin.html (accessed July 28, 2003).

2. Yoshioka M, Chiba T, Matsukawa M, et al: Diversity of Joro spider toxins. The Ministry of Education, Science, Sports and Culture Japan. http://neo.pharm.hiroshima-u.ac.jp/ccab/2nd/mini_review/mr121/yoshioka.html (accessed July 28, 2003).

3. Gill MD: Bacterial toxins: A table of lethal amounts. *Microbiol Rev* 1982;46:86-94.

4. Anonymous: *Registry of Toxic Effects of Chemical Substances (R-TECS)*. Cincinnati, Ohio, National Institute of Occupational Safety and Health, 1996.

5. Mobley JA: Biological warfare in the twentieth century: Lessons from the past, challenges for the future. *Mil Med* 1995;160:547-553.

6. Caya JC: Clostridium botulinum and the ophthalmologist: A review of botulism, including biological warfare ramifications of botulinum toxin. *Survey Ophthalmol* 2001;46:25-34.

7. Meyer KF: The status of botulism as a world health problem. *Bull World Health Organ* 1956:15:281-298.

8. Terrenova W, Palumbo JN, Breman JG: Ocular findings in botulism type B. *JAMA* 1979;241:475-477.

9. Anonymous: *Tenth Report of the Executive Chairman of the Special Commission Established by the Secretary-General Pursuant to Paragraph 9(b)(1) of Security Council Resolution 687 (1991) and Paragraph 3 of Resolution 699 (1991) on the Activities of the Special Commission.* New York, NY, United Nations Security Council, 1995, p S;1995:1038.

10. Holtzer VE: Botulism from inhalation. *Med Klin* 1962;57:1735-1738.

11. Minton NP: Molecular genetics of clostridial neurotoxins. Molecular genetics of clostridial neurotoxins, p 161-194, in Montecucco C (ed.), *Clostridial neurotoxins: The Molecular Pathogenesis of Tetanus and Botulism.* Berlin, Germany, Springer, 1995.

12. Hatheway CL: Botulism: The present status of the disease. *Curr Top Microbiol Immunol* 1995;195:55-75.

13. Anonymous: *Biological Defense: Vaccine Information Summaries.* Frederick, MD, US Army Medical Research Institute for Infectious Diseases, 1994.

14. Wiener SL: Strategies for prevention of a successful biological warfare aerosol attack. *Mil Med* 1996;161:251-256.

15. Arnon SS, Schechter R, Inglesby TV, et al: Botulinum toxin as a biological weapon: Medical and public health management. *JAMA* 2001;285:1059.

16. Arnon SS, Schechter R, Inglesby TV, et al: Botulinum toxin as a biological weapon: Medical and public health management. *JAMA* 2001;285:1059.

17. Anonymous: *Botulism: Current, Comprehensive Information on Pathogenesis, Microbiology, Epidemiology, Diagnosis and Treatment.* Center for Infectious Disease Research and Policy, http://www.cidrap.umn.edu/cidrap/content/bt/botulism/biofacts/botulismfactsheet.html (accessed July 28, 2003).

18. Anonymous: *Tenth Report of the Executive Chairman of the Special Commission Established by the Secretary-General Pursuant to Paragraph 9(b)(1) of Security Council Resolution 687 (1991) and Paragraph 3 of Resolution 699 (1991) on the Activities of the Special Commission.* New York, NY, United Nations Security Council, 1995, p S;1995:1038.

19. Zilinskas RA: Iraq's biological weapons: The past as future? *JAMA* 1997;278:418-424.

20. Anonymous: *Patterns of global terrorism, 1999.* United States Department of State (Publication No 10687), April 2000, http://www.state.gov/global/terrorism/annual_reports.html (accessed October 1, 2001).

21. Bermudez JS: *The Armed Forces of North Korea.* London, England, IB Tauris, 2001.

22. Cordesman AH: *Weapons of Mass Destruction in the Gulf and Greater Middle East: Force Trends, Strategy, Tactics, and Damage Effects.* Washington, DC, Center for Strategic and International Studies, 1998, pp 18-52.

23. Arnon SS, Schechter R, Inglesby TV, et al: Botulinum toxin as a biological weapon: Medical and public health management. *JAMA* 2001;285:1059.

24. Arnon SS, Schechter R, Inglesby TV, et al: Botulinum toxin as a biological weapon: Medical and public health management. *JAMA* 2001;285:1059.

25. Bleck TP: Tetanus: Pharmacology, management, and prophylaxis. *Dis Month* 1991;37:551.

26. Lebeda FJ. Deterrence of biological and chemical warfare: A review of policy options. *Mil Med* 1997:162:156-161. Op Cit.

27. Stillmark R: Ueber Ricen. Arbeiten des Pharmacologicshen Institutes zu Dorpat. 1989 iii. Cited by Flexner J: The histologic changes produced by ricin and abrin intoxications. *J Exp Med* 1987;2:197-216.

28. Wanemacher R, Hewetson J, Lemley P, et al: Comparison of detection of ricin in castor bean extracts by bioassays, immunoassays, and chemistry procedures, in Gopalakrishnakone P, Tan C (eds): *Recent Advances in Toxinology Research.* Singapore, National University of Singapore, 1992, pp 108-119.

29. Sehnke PC, Pedrosa L, Paul AL, et al: Expression of active processed ricin in transgenic tobacco. *J Biologic Chem* 1994;269:22473-22476.

30. Hewetson J, Rivera V, Lemley P, et al: A formalinized toxoid for protection of mice from inhaled ricin. *Vaccine Research* 1996;4:179-187.

31. Sharn L: Probe aims at the sale of deadly bacteria. *USA Today,* July 11, 1995:2A.

32. Kortepeter M, Christopher G, Cieslak T et al (eds) *Medical Management of Biologic Casualties Handbook.* Frederick, MD, US Army Medical Research Institute for Infectious Diseases, 2001.

33. Lange WR: Puffer fish poisoning. *Amer Fam Phys* 1990;42:1029-1033.

34. Light WH: Eye of newt, skin of toad, bile of pufferfish. California Academy of Science. http://www.calacademy.org/calwild/sum98/eye.htm (accessed August 29, 2002).

35. Laobhripatr S, Limpakarnjanarat K, Sanwanloy O, et al: Food poisoning due to consumption of the freshwater puffer *Tetradon fangi* in Thailand. *Toxicon* 1990:28:1372-1375.

36. Nozue H, Hayashi T, Hasimoto Y, et al: Isolation and characterization of Shewanell alga from human clinical specimens and emendation of the description of S. Alga Simidu et al. *Int J Syst Bacteriol* 1990:42;628-634.

37. Tambyah PA, Hui KP, Gopalakrishnakone NK, Chin TB: Central nervous system effects of tetrodotoxin poisoning. *Lancet* 1994;343:538-539.

38. Noda M, Ikeda T, Kayono T, et al: Tetrodotoxin: Mode of Action. *Nature* 1986;320;188.

39. Mackenzie CF, Smalley AJ, Barnas GM, Park SG: Tetrodotoxin infusion: Nonventilatory effects and role in toxicity models. *Academ Emerg Med* 1996;3:1106-1112.

40. Kaufman B, Wright DC, Ballou WR, Monheit D: Protection against tetrodotoxin and saxitoxin intoxication by a cross-protective rabbit anti-tetrodotoxin antiserum. *Toxicon* 1991;29:581-587.

41. Chang FT, Bauer RM, Benton BJ, et al: 4-Aminopyridine antagonizes saxitoxin and tetrodotoxin induced cardiorespiratory depression. *Toxicon* 1996;34:671-690.

42. Sims JK, Ostman DC: Pufferfish poisoning: Emergency diagnosis and management of mild tetrodotoxication. *Ann Emerg Med* 1986;15:1094-1098.

43. Fukiya S, Matsumura K: Active and passive immunization for tetrodotoxin in mice. *Toxicon* 1992:30:1631-1634.

44. Matsumura K: A monoclonal antibody against tetrodotoxin that reacts to the active group for the toxicity. *Eur J Pharm* 1995;293;41-45.

45. Rivera VR, Poli MA, Bignami GS: Prophylaxis and treatment with a monoclonal antibody of tetrodotoxin poisoning in mice. *Toxicon* 1995:33:1231-1237.

46. Anonymous: 1965 Nobel Prize awards. Nobel Foundation http://www.nobel.se/chemistry/laureates/1965/index.html (accessed August 29, 2002).

47. Sato S, Kodama M, Ogata T, et al: Saxitoxin as a toxic principle of a freshwater puffer Tetradon fangi, in Thailand. *Toxicon* 1997;35:137-140.

48. Armstrong R: The blooming killer of the sea. Australian Institute of Marine Science. http://www.amis.gov.au/pages/about/communications/blooming-killer.htm (accessed August 28, 2002).

49. Kaufman B, Wright DC, Ballou WR, Monheit D: Protection against tetrodotoxin and saxitoxin intoxication by a cross-protective rabbit anti-tetrodotoxin antiserum. *Toxicon* 1991;29:581-587.

Radiation Emergencies

■ Introduction

Perhaps nothing in modern technology incites greater fear than the thought of a **radiation accident**. Whether the fear is of the effects of bombs, a silent death, or changes in unborn generations is quite immaterial. In reaction to this fear, the news media have sensationalized any damage, injury, or fatality that has resulted from a nuclear spill or accident. Fictional portrayals further fuel the unmitigated horror that is inspired by radiation accidents.

Strictly speaking, a radiologic accident refers to the release of radioactive substances or radiation, while an incident is an event with the potential for radioactive contamination. If things get out of hand, an incident may become an accident.

With the end of the Cold War, the risk of global thermonuclear war portrayed in fiction has passed, but terrorist events force a reconsideration of the consequences of radiation as a weapon of mass casualties. The risk of a crude nuclear weapon or a radiation dispersal weapon used against a civilian population has increased with the rise of major organizations devoted to terrorism. These organizations are not deterred by the thought of personal destruction, and, indeed, some may embrace it as a religious inevitability.

The atomic bomb is a weapon of mass destruction, while the radiation-enhanced weapon produces mass casualties without much destructive power. Destruction from a nuclear explosion is caused primarily by the blast and thermal results of the weapon. In addition to the injuries from the blast and thermal release of the explosion, there is an added complication of acute radiation exposure and chronic radiation exposure from the **fallout**.[1,2] It is thought that only 15% of the deaths from the bombing of Hiroshima and Nagasaki were caused by the radiation.[3]

Neither the emergency responder nor emergency physician have any significant experience in managing radiation-related emergencies. These same providers may suddenly have to care for hundreds or perhaps thousands of such casualties.

Nuclear power has had a superlative safety record, worldwide, when compared to chemical spills, fires in plants, coal mining disasters, or the accidents of any construction industry. To get some idea of the rarity of serious radiation injuries, a look at some statistics is in order. During the 32-year period from 1943 to 1975, 10,086 accidents in the nuclear-related industries were reported to the Atomic Energy Commission. Of these 10,086 accidents, 0.4% (41) were caused by radiation exposure. There were three fatalities. From 1945 to 1986, there were fewer than 1,000 persons worldwide involved in serious radiation accidents (in about 11,000 incidents), and, of these, about 500 people received medically significant doses of ionizing radiation, resulting in 50 fatalities.[4]

There have also been a few major power reactor spills or accidents with fatalities. Accidents occurred at Los Alamos in 1945 and 1946 and at the National Reactor Testing Station in Idaho in 1961. In England, in 1957, a fire occurred in the graphite-moderated reactor in Windsdale; this reactor fire was contained within the reactor and resulted in only a minimal release of radiation to the outside environment. In the United States, the damage to the Three Mile Island reactor systems that occured in 1979 is still being decontaminated. Again, there was minimal release of radioactive material to the outside environment, and absolutely no injuries were caused by the accident.[5]

Of course, this all changed on April 26, 1986, in the northern Ukraine town of Chernobyl, when at least 30 people died in history's worst nuclear accident.[6,7] Because of Soviet restrictions on reporting, the toll this accident took may never be known. The ill effects of this accident will be with us for years to come, as more than 100,000 people were exposed to high levels of radioactive fallout. The accident should serve as a warning to all that the power of the atom can cause damage far from the source when appropriate precautions are not taken. Sensationalists had a field day with this unmitigated disaster, yet other natural disasters have caused more fatalities or injuries (for example, Pompeii, the Johnstown flood, the San Francisco earthquake, the 1988 Armenian earthquake, and even the Bhopal chemical incident).

Unfortunately, little Russian data on the management of these casualties were reported in the emergency medicine literature, and few responders or providers received more than token briefings on how to manage a contaminated casualty.

Chernobyl does show that a major disruption of a nuclear power plant can release large quantities of radionuclides into the environment. It also shows that such a release causes the immense local and national disruption of essential services. Terrorists have noted this and have already demonstrated the ability to build and deploy radioactive dispersal devices. They have also plotted to destroy nuclear power plants to the same end.

The possibility of a radioactive spill or nuclear power plant accident is real, and all nearby medical facilities should be ready to manage such an accident. Hospitals and other medical care facilities near nuclear power plants are designated to handle the potential problems from such an accident and have prepared approved radiation accident protocols.[8] However, these well-prepared hospitals and their associated providers may not be involved in the management of a deliberate release of radiation by a terrorist or the mitigation of the effects of a crude nuclear weapon.

Other sources of radiation are far more prevalent than bombs or reactors.[9] The use of radioactive materials and radiation-producing equipment has infiltrated American industry at all levels. The most common radiation source is the familiar diagnostic x-ray unit in hospitals and physician's and dentist's offices. Radiation sources are also used in

INCIDENTS INVOLVING Radiation

Los Alamos

A laboratory in Los Alamos, New Mexico, was the site of the top secret World War II era Manhattan Project. The project, led by J. Robert Oppenheimer, was commissioned in 1943 to conduct research on radioactive materials for government use. The product of this research was, of course, the world's first atomic bomb. In 1945, at the Trinity Site at the Los Alamos lab, the first nuclear bomb was tested. Only a few weeks later, the United States dropped nuclear bombs on the Japanese cities of Hiroshima and Nagasaki. The activities at Los Alamos resulted in significant radiation contamination of the area.

Three Mile Island

In 1979, the nuclear power plant located on Three Mile Island, Pennsylvania, caused the most serious nuclear power accident in US history. On March 28 of that year, a series of malfunctions caused the plant's nuclear fuel to overheat. The fuel overheated to the point where the zirconium cladding (the tubes that hold nuclear fuel pellets) reacted with surrounding water and generated hydrogen. This hydrogen subsequently leaked into the reactor containment of the building. Radioactivity in the reactor's coolant increased dramatically, and there were resultant leaks in the coolant system. These leaks caused high radiation levels in other parts of the plant and small releases into the environment. Although no deaths were reported as a result of the accident, the accident resulted in a 10-year cleanup effort and caused the US Nuclear Regulatory Commission to make sweeping changes in how the commission regulated its licensees.

INCIDENTS INVOLVING Radiation

Chernobyl

The accident at the nuclear power plant located near the Ukraine town of Chernobyl was the worst nuclear power disaster in history. On April 26, 1986, two mechanical explosions destroyed the plant's reactor core and blew a hole in the roof of the building. It is estimated that over 100 million curies of radiation subsequently leaked into the atmosphere. Although 30 people were immediately killed by the blast, the event's long-term consequences have been devastating. One of the most significant environmental impacts was made by the radioactive material that settled in the top layers of the soil, which rendered hundreds of acres infertile and contaminated cows and, eventually, the human population. Tragically, the incidence of childhood thyroid cancer skyrocketed in the areas surrounding Chernobyl, and increases in a number of other cancers have been linked to the disaster.

thickness gauges and moisture gauges, and they are used in the sterilization process of medical supplies, food, and materials. Radioactive tracers and sources are used in pipelines and in the nondestructive testing of aircraft and machined parts. Radioactive tags are common in research in all fields of chemistry. In short, sources of radiation exposure may be much more widespread than usually realized by the emergency provider. Radioactive sources are NOT confined to weapons and reactor materials. Any of these devices may be used as the source for a radioactive dispersal weapon.

The transportation of **radioactive isotopes** may present the greatest nonterrorist risk of exposure for the emergency provider. These radioactive sources range from industrial and medical **isotopes** to spent fuel from reactors and, of course, nuclear weapons material. The substances should be clearly marked and appropriately packaged.

Fortunately, the greatest risks for accidents do not occur with the nuclear weapons material and related items. Military security and military nuclear accident and incident control (NAIC) teams are stationed throughout the United States. Two designated military Radiologic Advisory Medical teams are further available 24 hours a day to aid the NAIC teams, should they need additional medical help or consultation. The NAIC teams closely monitor the movement of nuclear weapons and weapons material because of the obvious terrorist threat with these items. They also respond rapidly to any accident involving aircraft or ships that carry nuclear weapons.

A civilian emergency department is more likely to be involved with industrial or medical radioactive sources than military sources or a military transportation accident. Such accidents may involve other trauma to the victim besides the effects of radiation. The most common medical scenario is a spill occurring within the hospital's own nuclear medicine department or resulting from the transportation of materials within the vicinity of the hospital's immediate response area.

The emergency management of radiation casualties depends upon the type of exposure and the amount of exposure. A person may be irradiated with x-rays or **gamma (γ) rays**, may have incorporated radioactive material into his body, or may be contaminated with radioactive material.

■ Radiation Physics

In order to concisely discuss the management of the radiation emergency, a short review of the physics of radioactivity and radioactive materials is needed. Various elements will be mentioned throughout this chapter; **Figure 14-1** shows the periodic table of elements for reference.

People are exposed to radiation every day. This radiation can be produced or occur naturally from the decay of the nu-

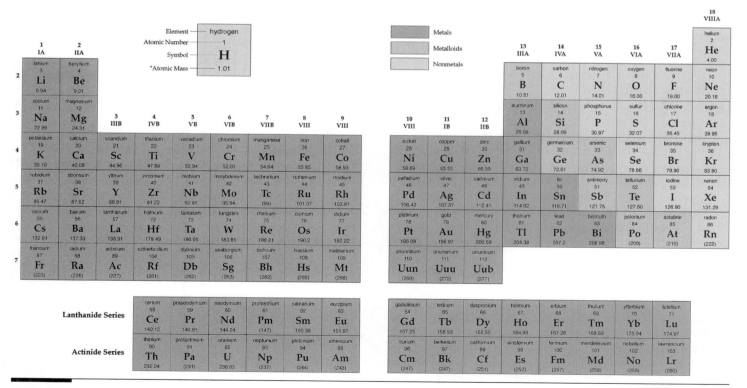

Figure 14-1 The periodic table of elements.

*Note: For radioactive elements, the mass number of an important isotope is shown in parenthesis; for thorium and uranium, the atomic mass of the naturally occurring radioisotopes is given.

cleus of an unstable isotope or from cosmic radiation. This residual radiation may be found in foods, soil, and water.

Artificially produced radiation may occur when an artificially produced unstable **radioisotope decays**, or when a stream of electrons, protons, or neutrons hits a target and causes a naturally occurring element to decay or to emit radiation. Sources could include diagnostic x-ray procedures, deliberate radiation of materials to produce radioactive isotopes, and even your television screen. Additional sources of exposure include nuclear medicine procedures (such as scans), fallout from prior weapons tests, and even residuals from prior nuclear reactor incidents.

Types of Radiation

The biological effects of the various forms of radiation are a function of the mass, charge, and energy of the particular type of radiation. There are two types of radiation: electromagnetic and particulate.

Electromagnetic Radiation

Electromagnetic radiation is energy. Electromagnetic radiation has no mass or charge. Electromagnetic radiation includes light, microwaves, infrared rays, ultraviolet rays, x-rays, and gamma rays.

Electromagnetic radiation is usually described as a low LET radiation. Linear Energy Transfer (LET) describes the rate at which radiation leaves its energy behind as it travels through matter. This means that electromagnetic radiation is much more penetrating than particle radiation. Exposure to an external source of low LET radiation creates a potential for significant biological damage deep within the body.

In a disaster scenario, gamma radiation would present a risk to rescuers as well as victims. Gamma and x-ray radiation is best shielded by very dense materials, such as lead, concrete, or steel.

Particulate Radiation

Alpha (α) particles are highly energetic and have a large mass. Because the mass of the alpha particle is so great, it is easily stopped by other matter. Alpha particles come from the decay of heavy elements such as radium, thorium, and uranium. Inside the body, alpha particles are quite dangerous. They undergo many interactions with surrounding tissues. These particles typically deposit all of their energy in a very small volume (high LET). An energy transfer of this magnitude within a cell will virtually guarantee the death of the cell. This means that alpha particles present a very serious hazard if they are deposited or incorporated into wounds, bone, or lungs.

Alpha particle radiation is a negligible hazard to patients, even if the alpha emitter is in direct contact with intact skin, because the alpha particle is unable to penetrate the keratin layer of the skin. Alpha radiation is not able to penetrate turnout gear, clothing, or a cover on a probe. Turnout gear and dry clothing can keep alpha emitters off of the skin. Respiratory protection is, however, of paramount importance, since the alpha emitter does damage only when within the body.

A variety of specific instruments have been designed to measure alpha radiation **(Figure 14-2)**. Special training in the use of these instruments is essential for making accurate measurements, because of the increased sensitivity of the

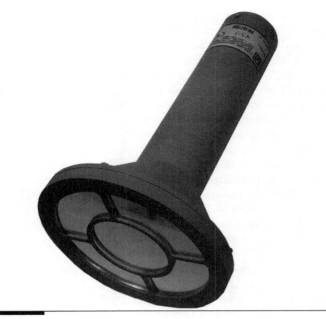

Figure 14-2 Alpha emitter detection device.

instruments. These instruments cannot detect alpha radiation through even a thin layer of water, blood, dust, paper, or other material, because alpha radiation cannot penetrate these substances.

A Geiger-Mueller survey meter cannot detect the presence of radioactive materials that produce alpha radiation unless the radioactive materials also produce beta or gamma radiation **(Figure 14-3)**.

In **Figure 14-4,** the black star shows the tracks made over a 48-hour period by alpha rays emitted from a radioactive particle of plutonium lodged in the lung tissue of an ape (the particle itself is invisible). In living lung tissue, if one of the cells adjacent to the particle is damaged in a certain way, it can become a cancer cell later on, spreading rapidly through the lung and causing almost certain death.

Beta (β) particles are often produced in nuclear reactors and **cyclotrons**. (A cyclotron is a particle accelerator in which the particles spiral inside two D-shaped, hollow, metal electrodes under the effect of a strong vertical magnetic field, gaining energy by a high-frequency voltage applied between these electrodes. The impact of the high-speed particles on a target can create new radioisotopes.) With its greater speed and smaller mass, the beta particle penetrates more deeply than the alpha particle. A beta particle represents a significant internal threat to the human body and only a minimal external threat. The small mass of the beta particle means that only a small amount of shielding is needed to protect from beta particles. In the laboratory, beta-emitting isotopes are common. High-energy electrons can also be emitted by electron microscopes and **particle accelerators**.

Radioisotopes find considerable use in the medical field both as the basis of a diagnostic technique and in the treatment of certain cancers. These radioisotopes are usually beta-emitting radioactive compounds. If a compound that emits beta particles is injected into a tumor, the beta particles will destroy the tumor. Because the beta particles only travel a short distance, little other tissue will be destroyed.

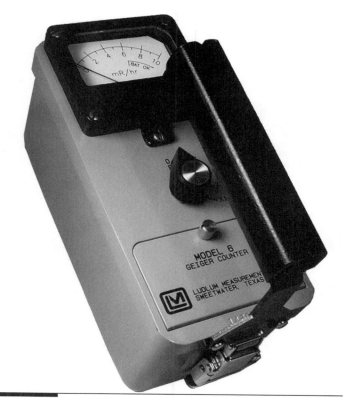

Figure 14-3 The most common type of radiation detector is a Geiger-Mueller tube, also called a Geiger counter.

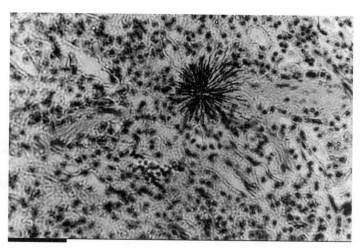

Figure 14-4 Emission tracks on photographic film resulting from alpha rays emitted from a radioactive particle of plutonium lodged in the lung tissue of an ape.

Iodine 131 (^{131}I) is used both to diagnose the activity of the thyroid and to treat a thyroid cancer. Cobalt 60 (^{60}Co), phosphorus 32, gallium 67, and cesium 137 (^{137}Cs) are used in the radiation treatment of many cancers. Sodium 24 is used for circulatory scans.

The greatest hazard to humans is from an internal contamination and the subsequent local irradiation from the particles. Beta radiation can also penetrate through to the germinal layer of the dermis and cause "beta burns" to the skin. The internal hazard is far greater than the external hazard, however. Beta radiation is a significant concern in fallout, but clothing and decontamination are generally adequate to protect both the staff and the patients from beta-particle hazards. Beta and gamma detection devices are shown in **Figure 14-5.**

Protons are the stripped nuclei of hydrogen atoms with a single positive charge. Although particle beam accelerators use protons, proton radiation is not a significant problem for emergency providers.

The **neutron** is a particle of the nucleus that has no charge. Neutrons are emitted by reactors, neutron beams, and some radioactive isotopes. The rate at which a **fission reaction** proceeds is regulated by controlling the number of neutrons available to interact. The atomic bomb produces an uncontrolled nuclear fission reaction and produces vast quantities of neutrons.

Neutron radiation is not commonly encountered, except during fission reactions. Either the detonation of a nuclear weapon or a criticality incident at a nuclear reactor or fuel-processing center will produce vast quantities of neutron radiation.

Unfortunately, if a sufficiently powerful slow neutron flux strikes the human body, many of the elements in the body such as sodium, chlorine, phosphorus, and gold fillings will become radioactive. This residual-induced radioactivity is proportional to the number of neutrons that hit the material and can be used to measure the dose of neutrons received. It is rarely significant enough to cause a danger to medical providers, because an active fission reaction is required to produce these neutrons.

Exposure to neutron radiation is quite concerning, because extensive biological damage occurs both from the neutrons and from the radioactive particles that are created as the neutrons impact other nuclei. This biological damage is considerably greater than equivalent amounts of beta or gamma radiation.

Neutrons have a relatively strong ability to penetrate and are difficult to stop. Moderate- to low-energy neutron radiation is shielded by materials with a high hydrogen content, such as water or polyethylene plastic. High-energy neutrons are better shielded by more dense materials, such as steel or lead. Often, a multi-layer shield will be used to first slow down fast neutrons, and then absorb the slow neutrons. **Figure 14-6** illustrates the materials that shield from various forms of radiation. **Table 14-1** lists the amounts of radiation that result from various types of exposures. **Table 14-2** lists recommended radiation exposure limits.

Half-Life

The **half-life** is the time required for a given amount of radioactive material to be reduced to one half of its original activity **(Figure 14-7).** The half-life for a given isotope is always the same; it does not depend on how many atoms you have or on how long they have been sitting around. The half-life values for radioisotopes vary widely. **Table 14-3** shows the half-lives for some common radioisotopes.

Biological Half-Life

The **biological half-life** is the time an organism takes to eliminate one half the amount of a compound or chemical. Thus, if a stable chemical compound were given to an individual and

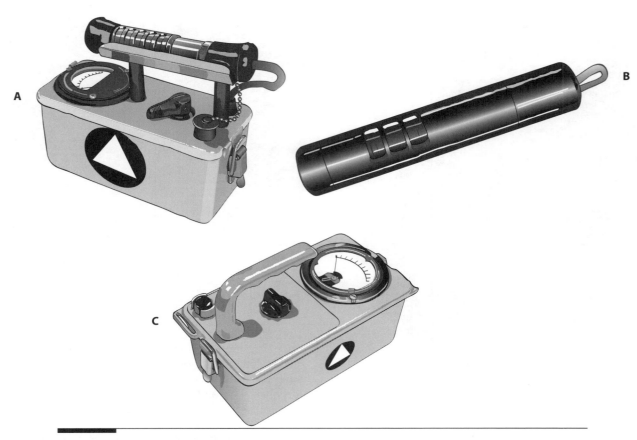

Figure 14-5 Beta and gamma detection devices. **A.** CD V-700 radiation instrument (civil defense). **B.** Close-up view of the probe from CD V-700 with the window open. **C.** CD V-715 radiation instrument.

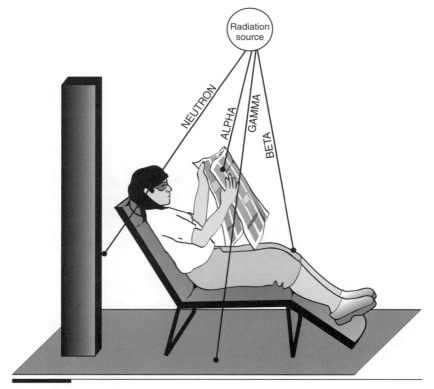

Figure 14-6 Alpha particles are stopped by paper. Beta particles can be stopped quite well by materials such as cloth. Gamma rays can be stopped by a thick sheet of lead or concrete. Neutron rays can be stopped by dense materials, such as steel or lead.

Table 14-1 Nominal Radiation Exposures

Radiation Source	Resulting Exposure
Natural and therapeutic exposures	
Living near normally functioning reactor	<1 mrem/yr
Watching color television	1 mrem/yr
New York to San Francisco flight	5 mrem
Chest x-ray	50 mrem
Natural background radiation (Denver)	150 mrem
Intravenous **pyelogram**	500 mrem
Pathologic exposures	
Acute lymphocytopenia	25 REM
Nausea and vomiting	100 REM
LD$_{50}$ (untreated human)	**450 REM**
LD$_{100}$ (100% death in humans)	**1,000 REM**
Acute CNS/cardiovascular syndrome (death within hours)	**5,000 REM**

Adapted from: Conklin JJ, Walker RI, eds. *Military Radiation.* Academic Press, Inc., New York, 1987, pp. 165–190.

Table 14-2 Recommended Exposure Limits

Exposure	Yearly Dose*
General public Occasional radiation worker Fertile women Minors	500 mrem
Emergency workers (whole body)	25,000 mrem (once in lifetime)
Lifesaving actions	100,000 mrem (once in lifetime)
Radiation worker: Whole body including gonads, lens of eye, and red bone marrow	5,000 mrem
Radiation worker: All other organs including thyroid	15,000 mrem
Radiation worker: Hands	75,000 (25,000 per quarter)
Radiation worker: Forearms	30,000 (10,000 per quarter)

*Please note that it is generally agreed that radiation exposure should be kept as low as reasonably achievable.

Adapted from: Anonymous: Document 22.6. Exposure to Radiation in an Emergency Lawrence Livermore National Laboratories Found athttp://www.llnl.gov/es_and_h/hsm/doc_22.06/doc22-06.pdf (Accessed July 20, 2003)

half of it were eliminated by the body (perhaps in urine) within 3 hours, the biological half-life would be 3 hours. The concept of biological half-life is equally applicable to chemicals such as pesticides and radioactive isotopes.

The **body burden** is used in reference to internally deposited radioactive material. The amount of a radioactive isotope that may be present in the body for a lifetime and pose no reasonable risk of illness is referred to as the maximum permissible body burden (MPBB). This quantity is different for each isotope. The amount of internally deposited isotope is usually expressed as a percentage of the MPBB that has been established for that isotope.

Effective Half-Life

The **effective half-life** incorporates both the radioactive and biological half-lives. It is used when health physicists calculate the dose received from an internal radiation source. To determine the effective half-life of a **radionuclide** in a human, one needs to know the radioactive half-life as well as the biological half-life of the radionuclide, as well as the half-lives of the compounds it forms.

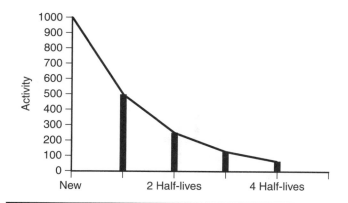

Figure 14-7 The half-life is the amount of time required for a material to be reduced by half.

Table 14-3 Half-lives for Some Common Radioisotopes

Radioisotope	Half-life
Barium 140	13 days
Carbon 14	5,730 years
Cesium 137	30 years
Hydrogen 3 (tritium)	12.3 years
Iodine 131	8 days
Iodine 125	60.1 days
Phosphorus 32	14.3 days
Phosphorus 33	25.3 days
Plutonium 238	85.3 years
Plutonium 239	24,000 years
Plutonium 240	6,500 years
Potassium 40	1.3 billion years
Strontium 90	29 years
Sulfur 35	87.6 days
Technecium 99	2 million years
Uranium 235	1.3 million years
Uranium 238	4.5 billion years

Measurement of Radiation

The amount of instantaneous radiation may be measured at the moment it strikes an object or a cumulative dose can be determined. Two different systems are used to measure these two types of units.

Flux Measurements

The classic radiation flux meter is the **Geiger-Mueller survey meter** or the scintillation counter, commonly called the Geiger counter. These devices measure the number of flashes or ionized sparks caused by the radiation per unit of time. They describe how much radiation would be absorbed if the flux stayed at the same level for the prescribed time period.

Hans Geiger was the first to see alpha particles and later invented the Geiger counter. A Geiger counter usually contains a metal tube with a thin metal wire along its middle. The space between the wire and the tube is sealed off and filled with a suitable gas, such as argon. The wire is then charged to about +1,000 volts relative to the tube.

An ion or electron penetrating the tube (or an electron knocked out of the wall of the tube by x-rays or gamma rays) will rip electrons off atoms in the gas. Because of the high positive voltage of the central wire, those electrons are then attracted to the wire. As they move to the wire, the electrons gain energy, collide with more atoms, and release more electrons, until the process snowballs into an avalanche, which produces an easily detectable pulse of current. With a suitable filling gas, the flow of electricity stops by itself, or else the electrical circuitry can help stop it.

The disadvantage of the Geiger counter is that this avalanche of electrons takes a certain amount of time, and the detector is unable to detect another particle or wave during this "dead time," while the avalanche occurs and the electronics reset.

Geiger counters alone do not discriminate between gamma, x, beta, or alpha rays. However, a feature found on some Geiger counters is an open window over the Geiger-Mueller tube. This allows for energy discrimination (that is, the determination of what type of radioactivity the unit is measuring) between gamma and x-rays that are strong enough to pass right through the housing of the Geiger counter and beta and alpha rays, which are too weak to pass through the housing, but can be read through the open window of the detector. **Survey meters** often convert the current pulses into audible clicks, producing the sound popularly associated with Geiger counters.

The **scintillation counter** works because the impact of radiation on a suitable material (which can be matched to the radiation) causes the emission of a minute flash of light, called a scintillation. The advantages of a scintillation counter are its efficiency, high precision, and high counting rate. Another advantage is the lower power requirements of the scintillation counter in comparison with the Geiger-Muller tube. This means that batteries last much longer in these devices.

Absorbed Radiation Measurements

The usual measurement of absorbed radiation is the **radiation absorbed dose (rad)**. It is the deposition of 100 **ergs** of energy per gram of material by the radiation. Another term often used is the roentgen (R), which is the deposition of 87 ergs of x-ray or gamma radiation per gram of air. For most purposes, the rad and the roentgen are equivalent.

Different types of radiation damage tissues in different ways, and the absorbed dose of radiation in rads does not always correlate with the apparent effects of the radiation on the tissues. This effect on the tissues may be correlated with the radiation that impinges on tissue, called the **roentgen equivalent in mammals (rem)**. The tissue effects of specific types of radiation are expressed as a **relative biological effectiveness (RBE)** times the measurement of absorbed radiation, the rad. RBEs vary from 1 for most x-rays, gamma rays, and beta emitters to 2 to 11 for neutrons and about 20 for alpha particles.[10]

When the RBE for neutrons is about 2, then 150 rad of neutron radiation is thought to be equivalent to 300 rad of gamma rays in effects on the tissue. Both would be expressed as a 300-rem dose. For most exposures, the millirem (mrem) is used.

Table 14-4 summarizes radiation measurement. **Table 14-5** lists the relative biological effectiveness for various types of radiation.

Dosimeters

The usual measuring device for absorbed doses of radiation is the **dosimeter**. The dosimeter provides a measurement of the total amount of radiation received by the dosimeter during the time measured, but it must be worn during exposure. The dosimeter will not measure the radiation received by a person if it is not worn by the person during the exposure. *The dosimeter may consist of a small film badge that increases in "fog" with absorbed radiation.* The density of the fog can be measured and correlated to known radiation doses for similar film held in a controlled environment.

Film badges provide a permanent record of the radiation exposure. Indeed, close examination of the film may provide evidence of contamination or of the direction of the exposure. Film badges suffer from fogging as a result of humidity and temperature. They are usually collected after only a month's wear (or a single exposure for an incident). The film must be processed at a laboratory before the dose can be determined.

Film badges are suitable for monitoring doses received from photon and beta radiations. They are ideal for workers who encounter x-ray fields.

Another type of dosimeter, a pencil dosimeter, uses the decay of an electrical charge from radiation-induced **ionization.** A movable filament is fixed to a hollow tube. An electrostatic charge is placed on the chamber wall and on the filament, causing the filament to be repelled toward the center of the tube. As the radiation causes the charge to decay, the filament falls toward the wall. The travel of the filament toward the wall is measured and is proportional to the amount of radiation. The reading from a pencil dosimeter is

Table 14-4 Radiation Measurement

Quantity	Unit	What Is Measured	Amount
Activity	Curie (Ci) Becquerel (Bq)	The number of disintegrations taking place per unit of time from 1 g of radium. In the International System of Units (SI), the becquerel (Bq) is the unit of radioactivity.	3.710 disintegrations per second 1 Bq = 1 disintegration per second (dps)
Exposure	Roentgen (R) Coulombs/ kilogram	Amount of charge produced in 1 kg of air by x-rays or gamma rays. The roentgen does not apply to alpha particles, beta particles, or neutrons. In the International System of Units (SI), coulomb/kilogram (C/kg) is the unit of exposure.	$1 R = 2.58 \times 10^{-4}$ C/kg
Absorbed dose	Rad (rad) Gray (Gy)	A rad is the amount of energy absorbed in 1 g of matter from radiation. In the International System of Units (SI), gray (Gy) is the unit of exposure. 20 rad of x-ray does not inflict the same damage to humans as 20 rad of alpha particles.	1 rad = 100 ergs/g (10 mJ/kg) 1 Gy = 100 rad
Dose equivalent	Rem Sievert (Sv)	Absorbed dose modified by the ability of the radiation to cause biological damage. In the International System of Units (SI), the sievert (Sv) is the unit of absolute biological damage. Rem is the biological damage unit.	rem = rad × RBE (see Table 14-5) 1 Sv = 100 rem

Table 14-5 Relative Biological Effectiveness

Radiation RBE (rem/rad)	Example: How many rads of protons will kill a person?
Alpha particles: 20 Neutrons: 10 (on average) Protons: 10 Beta particles: 1 Gamma rays: 1 X-rays: 1	Given: 600 rem is a fatal exposure. Given: The RBE for protons is 10. Given: rem = rad × RBE Therefore: 600 rem ÷ 10 rem/rad = 60 rad Answer: 60 rad of protons will kill a person.

immediately available so it can be used to minimize general exposure or in situations when a worker will be exposed to very high radiation fluxes. The pencil dosimeter is sensitive to impact and will give false readings if dropped. For this reason, film badges are often used in conjunction with the pencil dosimeter.

A third type of dosimeter, which is replacing both the pencil dosimeter and the radiation badge dosimeter, is the thermoluminescent dosimeter (TLD). This latest and most sophisticated entry into the field of dosimetry is a small chip made of lithium fluoride crystals. The principle behind

the TLD is that the lithium fluoride crystal gives off light in an amount proportional to the amount of radiation impinging upon it. When excited by radiation, some of the electrons are raised to a higher energy level and remain at that level until they are heated. The TLDs are inserted into badge holders containing filters to help determine the type and energy of the ionizing radiation to which the badge was exposed.

When the TLD chip is heated, the electrons return to the base state and release energy as light. A TLD reader heats and reads the subsequent light release in one operation. The electrons are then returned to their base state, and the TLD chip is ready to be used again. The reader is portable, and field measurements can be readily made. TLDs are sensitive, measuring as low as 10 mrem. They have a long shelf life and may be worn for as long as 3 months. In addition to these qualities, TLD materials are relatively unaffected by long-term storage or exposure to light, and they do not suffer serious effects from environments with high ambient temperature or humidity. The major drawback to the TLD system is that once a chip is read, the information is lost, and there is no permanent record of the person's exposure.

TLD badges are suitable for measuring doses from photon radiation and beta radiation. A TLD badge is ideal for monitoring workers who work with sealed or unsealed radioactive sources.

TLD extremity monitors are molded from translucent plastic and slide easily onto the finger of the wearer. They are worn under thin, preferably loose latex or vinyl gloves to

INHOSPITAL INFO

prevent contamination. They are capable of detecting low-energy beta radiation. These devices measure the radiation dose received by the extremities of a worker and are ideal for people who handle radioactive sources or solutions.

Biological Dosimetry

The effects of radiation upon animals and humans have been well documented as the result of our experiences following the bombing of Hiroshima and Nagasaki, infrequent radiation accidents, and especially the experience at Chernobyl. These biological effects form a crude **biodosimeter**.

An early and important clinical indicator of radiation damage is the lymphocyte count. As the absorbed radiation dose increases, the magnitude and rapidity of the lymphocytopenia increases. If the patient has fewer than 500 lymphocytes per cubic centimeter at 48 hours, the prognosis is poor. If the lymphocyte count is above 1,200 per cubic centimeter, the chances of survival are excellent. Lesser counts at 48 hours suggest more serious exposures.

Skin erythema, akin to a sunburn, also can act as a biodosimeter. The amount of erythema may be unreliable, because it varies substantially with the type of radiation. Erythema that develops within minutes to hours after exposure to gamma rays suggests serious exposure and possible systemic injury.

Gastrointestinal symptoms, such as nausea and vomiting, can also serve as indicators in biodosimetry. The severity of symptoms varies tremendously from person to person and is, therefore, not particularly useful. The timing of the symptoms is more useful. Early fever, diarrhea, decreasing level of consciousness, or hypotension are associated with extreme doses. The absence of gastrointestinal symptoms connotes a minimal exposure.

■ Management of Radiation Exposure

Notification

Although patients with radiation exposure or their coworkers may notify the EMS dispatcher, a company radiation physicist, or the hospital of all details, it is imperative that the hospital is given as much advance notice as possible. For most cases that are seen by EMS responders, the closest hospital has a well-developed radiation emergency plan. This plan, however, must be activated. The scene response crew must gather as much information as possible to ensure the proper and prompt notification of both the hospital and state authorities. The responsibility for the notification of state and federal authorities should be outlined for all hazardous materials response teams, hospitals, and nuclear laboratories.

An important point to note for all medical personnel is that if the agent is known, such as in a power plant, radioisotope treatment facility, or nuclear laboratory, the personnel working with the isotope often know more about the nature of the exposure than most emergency providers. Guidance given by these nuclear workers (even as patients) may well limit the spread of contaminants, decrease the absorption of radioisotopes, or limit the exposure for all concerned. This source of information and guidance must not be neglected.

Initial Response

The first question that the field emergency provider must answer is: *Is the exposure continuing?*

If the answer is yes, then the rate of exposure must be ascertained, and an appropriate tolerable exposure time for rescue workers must be calculated—BEFORE entry into the area of exposure. If the source is a ^{60}Co radiation therapy or sterilization machine, shielding the source stops further exposure for all. If the source is an x-ray machine, the removal of power stops the production of radiation. In all cases, do the following:

- Secure the safety of the scene for responders and bystanders alike.
- Limit further exposure to the hazardous substance.
- Provide lifesaving emergency care.
- Contain the spread of the hazardous substance.

Table 14-6 summarizes overall management of radiation exposure. If the source is diffuse from a terrorist event, then evacuation of the area is required. The scene should be secured, and walking victims should be corralled in a safe area. A controlled entrance to the scene should be established.

The emergency worker's first priority should be his or her own safety. If the radiation source is continuing, and the emergency worker becomes seriously exposed, he or she becomes a patient, not a rescuer.

After the exposure has ceased, or a tolerable time of exposure has been established, the next question that needs to be answered is: *Was the exposure irradiation or contamination (incorporation)?*

Radiation accidents can be best managed if the patients are separated into one of three categories:

1. Externally irradiated patients
2. Externally contaminated patients
3. Internally contaminated patients (potential incorporation)

The contaminated patient continues to pose a danger to the medical staff, because the contamination can be washed off, brushed off, or rubbed off onto the medical staff. Irradiated patients are not a danger to the staff. The internally contaminated patient may present no danger to medical staff or may have a lethal contamination.

Table 14-6 Overall Management of Radiation Exposure
• Treat conventional threats to life first.
• Manage fluid and electrolyte abnormalities as needed.
• Liberally use antiemetics for nausea and vomiting.
• Maintain infectious disease precautions; this is unnecessary in the field response, but should be considered soon after hospitalization of the patient.
• Consider antiviral prophylaxis; this is also unnecessary in the field, but necessary soon after hospitalization.
• Consider early consultation with appropriate specialties.

It is essential that the type and amount of the contaminating radioactivity is measured. If the source cannot be shielded or removed, then the allowable radiation exposure times must be calculated. The need to determine safe exposure times has prompted hospitals to designate a radiologist or radiotherapist as the chief physician when dealing with accidents from radioactive sources.

Facilities that include a radiation therapy unit are likely to have a medical health (radiation) physicist on staff, while all facilities with a Nuclear Regulatory Commission license must have a designated radiation control officer. Either of these two people are likely to be able to provide concrete advice about the management of radiation sources.

When the accident is purely from irradiation, the designation of a radiologist or nuclear medicine physician as the physician in charge may be appropriate. Unfortunately, beyond training, these physicians may have had little practical experience with the management of radioactive materials or calculations of absorbed radiation doses. Few radiologists understand the constraints and vagaries of the field environment. When blast, trauma, or burns are included, a radiologist may be an inappropriate physician to coordinate all activities. However, the emergency physician or general surgeon who is coordinating the management of the traumatized, contaminated patient would be well advised to solicit the help of those physicians experienced with the management of radiation sources.

Irradiation

Irradiation occurs with either x-rays, neutrons, gamma rays, or, in lesser amounts, beta particles. Penetrating radiation produces damage only in the portion of the body exposed. Most injuries and fatalities from radiation have been of this nature. Typically, the patient had been working and knows that he or she has been exposed to an x-ray source, a radiation sterilizing device, or a radiation source. The estimate of damage and the determination of treatment is likely to be a more difficult problem than the initial diagnosis or the nature of the injury.

There are occasional exceptions where the diagnosis is not obvious, however. Symptoms typical of flu, nausea, vomiting, skin burns or ulcerations, and bone marrow depression have been noted when a history of radiation exposure was not known or immediately suspected. This may be a very difficult differential diagnosis when the radiation exposure was days or weeks prior and the patient is completely unsuspecting of the event, as might occur in some terrorist scenarios.

It should be emphasized that an irradiated person has the equivalent of a burn. Just as a person with a thermal burn does not give off heat, an irradiated person does not give off radioactivity. Cells have been damaged or killed, but the person is not radioactive. The person does not glow in the dark. The irradiated person generally presents no danger to the medical staff.

The sole exception to this rule is a person's exposure to exceptionally high levels of neutron radiation. The neutron radiation can induce secondary radioactivity in such places as fillings and prosthetics. However, exposure to this level of neutron radiation is exceedingly rare, and the induced radiation is not a danger to the medical staff.

Protection From Irradiation

Protection of the medical personnel involved in a continuing irradiation accident revolves around three factors: duration, distance, and defenses (shielding).

Duration The duration of the exposure can be carefully monitored to ensure that each scene responder does not receive a dangerous irradiation. In this manner, the first responder may carry a piece of equipment into a hallway and then retreat. The next responder may carry the equipment farther into the building and retreat and so on. In this way, no single responder will receive a dangerous level of radiation, but if one responder were to perform the whole task, the yearly or lifetime limit for that responder could be exceeded.

Distance Radiation exposure decreases by the square of the distance from the radiation source. The inverse square law means that doubling the distance decreases the radiation to one fourth of the original intensity. Exposed personnel can move farther away from the area so that the inverse square law will afford protection.

Defenses Defenses, such as lead shielding, can be used by those who must enter an area to perform a technical task. These defenses may allow a surgeon to perform an amputation or a technician to lower a high-intensity source into a shielding well. Lead aprons and thyroid shields, which are commonly used during x-ray procedures, can offer significant protection. Protection from continuing radiation is listed in **Table 14-7**.

■ Mechanisms of Damage

Injury to living tissue results from the transfer of energy to atoms and molecules in the cellular structure of the tissue. The radiation can do the following:

- Produce **free radicals**
- Break chemical bonds
- Produce new chemical bonds
- Cross-link molecules
- Damage molecules that regulate vital cell processes (such as DNA, RNA, and proteins)

The cell can repair some cellular damage. At low radiation doses, such as that received from background radiation, the cellular damage is minor and readily repaired. At higher radiation levels, death of the individual cell will result. At extremely high radiation levels, many cells are killed, and cells cannot be replaced rapidly enough. This causes tissues to fail to function, and serious disease or death results.

Table 14-7 Protection From Continuing Radiation

- **Duration**
  Keep the duration of exposure to the lowest possible limits.
- **Distance**
  Doubling the distance between you and the radioactive source decreases exposure to one fourth of the original exposure.
- **Defenses**
  Shielding can markedly attenuate the radiation.

The alteration of cellular genetic material may cause no visible change in the cellular appearance, but it may cause a mutation that may or may not be passed to future generations of cells. This may cause **carcinogenesis** or nonspecific life-shortening. Depending on the type of cell affected, the mutation may be passed to offspring. This leads to an increased probability of abnormalities in offspring.

In general, the sensitivity of a tissue to radiation is proportional to the rate of proliferation of its cells and inversely proportional to the degree of cell differentiation. This means that a developing embryo is most sensitive to radiation during the early stages of development. (An embryo is more sensitive to radiation exposure during the first trimester than in later trimesters.)

As an illustration of cell sensitivity, **Table 14-8** lists tissues and organs from the least radiosensitive to the most radiosensitive. The systems of primary involvement are those with the tissues that have rapidly proliferating cells. The observed effects may occur rapidly with massive exposure to radiation or may occur 1 to 3 weeks after radiation exposure.

Acute Radiation Syndrome

The acute radiation syndrome describes a pattern of illness that results from whole body radiation. Large doses of penetrating radiation, irrespective of source, produce a predictable illness pattern. There are four stages to this illness: prodrome, latent stage, overt illness, and recovery or death. The severity and rapidity of progression through the stages parallels the dose of radiation received.

Prodrome

The prodrome phase is caused by immediately induced cell death and cellular dysfunction. Symptoms include nausea, vomiting, diarrhea, fatigue, and malaise. At higher doses of radiation exposure, the patient may develop prostration, fever, and respiratory distress. In some patients, hyperexcitability may occur.

Gastrointestinal prodrome symptoms generally resolve within 48 hours for patients with a survivable exposure. This may serve as a clinical biological dosimeter for survivable exposures.

Latent Stage

After the prodromal phase resolves, a period of relative wellness may occur in patients with significant exposure. This reflects the compensation of the body for immediate cellular dysfunction. At this point, the depletion of **precursor cells** and the death of high-turnover tissues, such as gut-lining cells, have not yet occurred.

The duration of the latent stage is inversely related to the total radiation dose. A higher exposure will produce a shorter latent period. With massive exposures and central nervous system failure, there may be no latent period at all.

Most patients in the latent phase may be treated as outpatients.

Overt Illness

When the short-lived cells are depleted and the failure of tissue regeneration occurs, the patient will quickly develop overt radiation illness. The **hematopoietic syndrome** occurs at the lowest radiation dose and will occur with all higher exposures. Overwhelming sepsis associated with neutropenia is a major cause of death in all significant radiation exposures.

Recovery or Death

Following the overt clinical illness, the patient either dies or recovers. Appropriate and intensive care markedly increases the percentage of survivors in moderate radiation exposures. In a terrorist or mass-casualty situation, only basic care may be available to the vast majority of patients.

Clinical Radiation Syndromes

Mild Exposure

Mild exposure is categorized as an exposure of less than 1 **gray** (Gy). The mild exposure patient (a patient with fewer than 125 rad of whole body exposure) will generally require only reassurance that there are no serious effects anticipated. White and red blood cell counts will be lowered in most people with over 25 rad exposure. Nausea will be a problem for about 5% to 10% of those exposed to over 50 rad, and this percentage increases with increasing amounts of exposure. The nausea and vomiting will usually last no longer than 48 hours. Ten percent of the exposed population will experience a transient hair loss after an exposure of 100 to 200 rad.

The lymphocytes are the most sensitive cells to the effects of radiation. Changes can be seen within a few hours after exposure. The lymphocyte count drops quickly to about 60% of the original circulating value and slowly recovers over the next 6 months.

The **neutrophils** drop to about 70% of their original value over the 45 days after exposure. The neutrophil count will slowly recover over the next few months. The

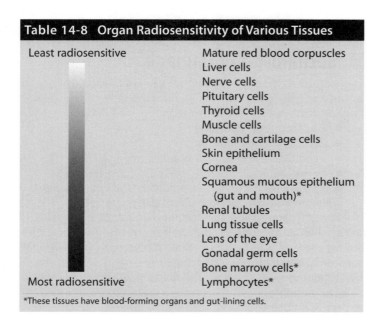

Table 14-8 Organ Radiosensitivity of Various Tissues	
Least radiosensitive	Mature red blood corpuscles
	Liver cells
	Nerve cells
	Pituitary cells
	Thyroid cells
	Muscle cells
	Bone and cartilage cells
	Skin epithelium
	Cornea
	Squamous mucous epithelium (gut and mouth)*
	Renal tubules
	Lung tissue cells
	Lens of the eye
	Gonadal germ cells
	Bone marrow cells*
Most radiosensitive	Lymphocytes*

*These tissues have blood-forming organs and gut-lining cells.

platelets also decrease to about 60% of the original circulating value. The nadir is noted at about 30 days after exposure. Despite these decreases, with only 100 R exposure, the patient does not develop any increase in infection or bleeding tendencies.

The patient should be advised that this dose may slightly increase the relative risk of developing cancer or leukemia. There is no known early preventative measure that will eliminate the slight increase in risk of the late effects (cancer and leukemia) for any significant exposure to radiation.

Males should be advised to employ a form of contraception for about 6 months following the exposure to avoid potential congenital malformations if conception were to occur during this period. After this period, precautions should not be needed. These measures are unnecessary for females, because eggs are not affected in the same way as sperm.

Intermediate Exposure: Bone Marrow Hematopoietic Syndrome

Intermediate exposure is an exposure of 1 to 4 Gy. Treatment is likely to be effective for this level of exposure. Exposure in the 100- to 400-rem range will cause symptoms of nausea, vomiting, and often diarrhea.

After an intermediate exposure, the bone marrow is suppressed, often completely, with later neutropenia, lymphopenia, and a decrease in platelets. The lymphocyte count may begin to fall as soon as 3 hours after an exposure. Hemorrhage from the thrombocytopenia may occur but more often infection supervenes.

Patients exposed to an intermediate dose of radiation will require medical observation and possibly active treatment. Without appropriate medical therapy, 5% to 50% of those exposed to 200 to 400 rad will die within 60 days. The time of greatest risk is during the bone marrow depression phase, which occurs 3 to 4 weeks after exposure. The problem, quite simply, is one of keeping the exposed patient alive for the 5 to 6 weeks until the bone marrow begins to recover.

At about 200 rad of acute exposure, the hematologic responses to radiation exposure are more profound. The lymphocyte count drops first and may fall to 40% of the original count within a few days. The neutrophil count also reaches a low of about 60% of the original level at about 45 days. There is a slight increase in the neutrophil count at about 2 to 3 days after exposure and about 2 weeks after exposure. The platelets continue to drop over the 30 days after exposure to about 30% of the original count. Despite the neutropenia, lymphocytopenia, and thrombocytopenia, there are usually no signs of bleeding or infections at the intermediate exposure level.

Therapeutic requirements for these patients fall into three categories:

1. **Control of infection:** Protect the patient from exogenous and nosocomial infections during the first 5 weeks. The use of strict isolation or "clean" room environments, use of appropriate antimicrobial drugs, and possible use of immune globulins are all indicated if available.

2. **Control of bleeding:** Initiate the use of blood, platelets, and blood products as needed to control bleeding diatheses. Of course, the patient should be protected from trauma.

3. **Supportive therapy:** Provide psychological support, rest, and counseling about the genetic and personal effects of the dose received. For the health physicist, radiologist, or radiation therapy technician who has just received a total lifetime exposure and must seek new work, this counseling cannot be emphasized enough. In addition, the patient may have concomitant poor wound healing and poor response to shock.

Just as the complex burn is best managed by a burn team, the complex course of a severely irradiated patient is best managed by a radiation injury team. The long-term care of these patients, quite appropriately, falls outside the province of the emergency provider. The emergency physician should consider early consultation with appropriate specialists in the management of these patients. Fortunately, there is a period of about 1 week available to arrange for special consultations and advice on the needed hospital services. During this time, the patient may be transferred to a radiation injury team facility that is staffed to provide the needed expertise, hematologic, oncologic, and laboratory services.

Growth factors G-CSF and GM-CSF may help preserve bone marrow function if there are regions where bone marrow still survives.

High-Level Exposure: Gastrointestinal Syndrome

Exposure of 4 to 8 Gy is considered to be a high-level exposure. Maximal lifesaving effort will be required for these patients. An exposure in the 400- to 1,000-rem range will produce both hematologic and gastrointestinal effects. An exposure of 500 rad of acute total body irradiation is nearly the LD_{50} for 60-day survival.

The early course of the patient's illness will be marked with severe and persistent nausea, diarrhea, and vomiting. Occasionally, gastrointestinal bleeding will be noted. Gut motility, fluid movement, and electrolyte balance are all affected by the gastrointestinal component. As the nausea abates, the profound hematologic effects become manifest.

After a high-level exposure, the marrow is completely suppressed, often with early neutropenia, lymphopenia, and thrombocytopenia. As always, the lymphocyte response occurs first, with a decrease to 20% of the normal occurring within the first few days. The biphasic neutrophil response, noted at 200 rad, again occurs, but it is much more exaggerated. All three blood component counts reach their lowest levels at about 4 weeks after exposure.

The previously outlined therapeutic requirements and concerns regarding infection and bleeding in the intermediately exposed patient are mandatory for patients with high-level exposures. The use of clean rooms or filtered laminar airflow rooms is also mandatory.

Treatment should include the careful management of fluid and electrolyte balances in the face of vomiting and diarrhea. The prevention of sepsis is paramount.

Heroic efforts to save a patient's life in suspected lethal or near lethal exposures (500 to 1,000 rad) might include the use of marrow transplantation during the first 10 days after exposure. This is about 2 weeks before the period of maximum bone marrow suppression is expected. Cross-circulation of a patient with another has also been proposed.

At 4 Gy exposure, 50% of all untreated patients will die. At 6 Gy exposure, all will succumb.

Very High-Level Exposure: Central Nervous System Syndrome

Very high-level exposure is considered to be an exposure that exceeds 10 Gy. In this event, death is probable. A constellation of immediate symptoms, including mental confusion, nausea, vomiting, diarrhea, and shock will be caused by exposures greater than 1,000 rad. Nausea and vomiting may occur within minutes.

The neutrophil count rises rapidly and then falls equally rapidly to fewer than 100 within 24 hours. Lymphocyte counts approach zero within 24 hours.

Such large doses of radiation may produce acute central nervous system and cardiovascular deterioration. Previously, it was thought that central nervous system effects accounted for most rapid deaths, but recent experience has shown that cardiovascular deterioration may also be rapid following these supralethal doses. The rapid neurologic and cardiovascular deterioration is the basis for the effectiveness of the so-called neutron bomb. A neutron bomb is a low-yield antipersonnel thermonuclear device specifically designed to produce maximum amounts of high-energy neutrons with little blast and fallout damage.[11]

At 1,000 rad of total body irradiation, the bone marrow is irreversibly damaged. The lymphocyte count falls to zero by 5 days after exposure. The neutrophil count falls to zero at about 10 days after exposure. The platelets become absent at about 15 days after exposure. Circulating red blood cells are not appreciably affected because of the long life span of a red blood cell.

There is no effective therapy at this exposure level. These surely terminal patients will require symptomatic therapy during what will probably be a short course (at most 2 to 10 days). Treatment will be supportive and palliative and includes sedation, antiemesis, and fluid replacement. Bone marrow transplant is an option. The maximal survivable radiation doses may be significantly higher with current therapy, and if there is even a remote chance of success, vigorous therapy should be administered. **Table 14-9** summarizes the symptoms caused by various levels of radiation exposure.

Local Exposures

Possibly, the most frequent type of irradiation accident seen in the emergency department is the local exposure of a hand in a high-level radiation field. These accidents often occur with gamma source x-ray cameras or sterilizing devices. Typically, a technician deliberately defeats the safety precautions (usually to service the machine), accidentally exposes himself or herself, and presents for therapy.

The amount and depth of damage are proportional to the level of exposure. Fortunately, only infrequently will a technician receive a total body irradiation in this manner. Because the gastrointestinal tract and the bone marrow are not irradiated, the patient does not develop the symptoms of whole body irradiation. Soft tissue exposed to radiation has far greater resistance than more rapidly reproducing tissues.

With a dose of fewer than 500 rem, the patient may have local erythema. There may be a slightly increased level of localized tumors as a late complication, but early complications are few.

With doses of about 2,500 rem, the patient may develop localized depilation, followed by a temporary but slowly healing ulcer. Skin atrophy, **telangiectasia**, and localized **vitiligo** may be late complications. At doses of greater than 5,000 rem to a localized area, ulcers are permanent, and a marked increase in neoplasms is noted. Doses greater than 50,000 rem cause great destruction in the path of the beam, with severe necrosis resulting.[12] Management of these lesions is frustrating, because deep vascular damage often precludes successful grafting.

Early treatment of these localized lesions should proceed as if the patient has incurred a skin burn. The patient should be dressed with a common burn ointment, such as silver sulfadiazine. Referral to a surgeon knowledgeable in the management of these patients may be accomplished at leisure. Dermal effects of localized exposure to radiation are summarized in **Table 14-10**.

Long-Term Effects

Long-term effects usually occur many years after acute or chronic radiation exposure and include:

1. **Tumor development:** Radiation in large amounts is an effective carcinogenic agent.

INHOSPITAL INFO

Table 14-9 Clinical Radiation Injury Classifications		
Classification	Exposure*	Symptoms
Mild exposure	Fewer than 125 rad	Minimal or no symptoms (may cause distant long-term effects)
Intermediate exposure	About 400 rad	Moderate to severe illness resulting from hematopoietic syndrome (probably nonlethal)
High-level exposure	About 400–600 rad	Severe illness resulting from gastrointestinal syndrome (may be lethal)
Very high-level exposure	About 600–1,500 rad	Quite lethal from 600 to 800 rad, surely lethal above 800 rad
Extreme exposure	Greater than 1,500 rad	Central nervous system syndrome (surely lethal)
*It must be emphasized that the approximate dose values may vary as much as 50% in individual patients.		

Table 14-10 Dermal Effects of Localized Exposure to Radiation

Dose	Early Effects	Late Effects
<500 rem	Erythema	None (may cause a slight increase in neoplasms)
>500 rem	Erythema depilation	Usually minimal increase in neoplasms
2,500 rem	Ulcerations	Local atrophy Telangiectasia
5,000 rem	Depilation	Altered pigmentations
>50,000 rem	Ulcerations	Chronic ulcerations Substantial carcinogenesis

Adatped from: Hopewell JW. The skin: its structure and response to ionizing radiation. *Int J Radiat Biol.* 1990;57:751-753.

2. **Sterility:** Temporary sterility can be induced at exposure levels of approximately 150 rem. Females are more often permanently affected than males.
3. **Cataracts:** Because of the high sensitivity of the lens of the eye, opaque areas of the lens develop after exposure levels of 200 to 600 rem.
4. **Life-shortening:** The aging process is increased. Nutrition to the cell appears to be impaired. The total cell number is decreased, and there is a modification of the composition of cellular material.
5. **Fetal damage:** The fetus is highly radiosensitive because of the rapid division of cells. No measurable fetal damage has been caused by exposures less than 1 rem.
6. **Chromosomal damage:** Detection of chromosomal damage requires many generations. An Oak Ridge study suggests that low intensity (1 to 10 rem/day) continuous exposures have only 10% to 25% of the mutagenic efficiency of acute exposures.[13,14]

The long-term effects of radiation exposure are important, but are beyond the scope of a book dedicated to emergency providers. Long-term follow-up varies greatly depending on the type of accident, the amounts of exposure or contamination encountered, and the nature of the isotopes involved in the accident.

Local areas of exposure should be closely watched for the appearance of viability and healing and the development of radiation burns. Areas of chemical or thermal burns that were also exposed to significant irradiation may show altered viability or poor healing. These symptoms take days to weeks to develop. Lymphocyte counts, platelet counts, and neutrophil counts should be performed on a daily basis.

Contamination

If the patient is radioactive, this may be a result of contamination or (rarely) induced activity from a neutron source. Induced radiation from neutron exposure does not produce any hazard to medical workers and serves mostly to aid in an estimation of the size of the dose received by the patient.

Perhaps the most important point for medical personnel to realize is that radioactive contamination is similar to a chemical burn. Until the radioactive or chemical contaminant is removed, it will continue to burn. If it is spread to a medical worker, it will burn the medical worker also. If it is a weak source of radiation, it will burn at a slower rate, just as weak solutions of chemicals will burn at slower rates than strong solutions.

In further comparison to a chemical burn, radioactive contamination may be external, may be ingested, or may be incorporated in a wound. The radiation and contamination exposure may also be complicated by other injuries, such as blast injuries or burns. When treating a chemical contamination, there is often no way of knowing when the chemical has finally been diluted or washed out. This is not true in radiation emergencies. When treating radiation contamination, the residual contamination can be measured with the appropriate instruments.

Protection From Contamination

When responding to emergencies involving contamination, ambulance and rescue personnel should don the appropriate protective gear for the scene. Filtration-type masks or self-contained breathing apparatus are minimal requirements for most scenes of radioactive contamination. Exposure to continuing high-level radiation should be managed as outlined previously, with limits to duration, increased distance, and appropriate defenses. A radiation biologist will usually determine these needs.

Protection of the environment of the ambulance may be a problem. It is unlikely that word of an accident will be received in such time and in such detail that all nonessential equipment can be removed from the ambulance and the interior can be covered with plastic or paper prior to arrival on the scene. Ambulances and ambulance personnel should be considered to be contaminated. Scene responders should not be released until both they and their vehicles are decontaminated and cleared by the radiation biophysicist. If the hazard area involves multiple casualties, the decontamination of a vehicle and crew will be at the joint discretion of the radiation biophysicist and the mass-casualty scene commander (usually a physician). A minor level of contamination may be tolerated in order to transport further patients, particularly those who may already be contaminated.

Medical and nursing staff should handle the patient with (at the least) masks, scrubs, gowns, and gloves to avoid exposure to themselves. Medical and nursing staff must be decontaminated after care of the patient, just as if a chemical agent were involved.

Medical attendants are permitted 5 R for the routine treatment and decontamination of patients. For emergency treatment, up to 25 R are permissible. This level of exposure will constitute a lifetime's exposure for a radiation physicist and will preclude work in that or a related field. For lifesaving treatment, up to 100 R are permitted in 1 year's time. Pregnancy should preclude participation in any voluntary radiation exposure.

Internal Contamination (Incorporation)

Internal contamination can occur by either ingestion or inhalation of radioactive compounds. Incorporation may also result from particles driven into the body by a blast effect. Although the incorporation of radioactive agents may be lethal to the patient, incorporated agents pose little risk to emergency providers. The sole exceptions to this are, of course, during the handling of bodily wastes and disposal of the fragments from wounds.

The seriousness of internal contamination is determined by the following:

1. The route of the contamination
2. The half-life of the isotope
3. The chemical nature of the isotope
4. The location of the isotope within the body
5. The level of exposure to the isotope
6. The specific therapy indicated for each radioactive isotope

The level of exposure must be assayed by the radiation physicist. This can be done by gastric washings, urinalysis, nasal smears, and, if available, whole body counters. The location of the isotope can be determined in the patient's body by a gamma camera assay, if, of course, the isotope emits gamma rays.

There are multiple agents that prevent the uptake or hasten the excretion of a radioisotope. The first few hours after the incorporation of a radionuclide may be crucial for effective treatment. A radiation physicist or physician who is experienced in nuclear medicine should be consulted in all cases of suspected incorporation of radioisotopes.

Increasing Excretion or Interrupting Absorption

Ipecac, charcoal, and magnesium citrate or sorbitol will all enhance excretion or interrupt gastrointestinal absorption. Metals, such as copper, iron, and plutonium, are generally better absorbed in an acid environment, such as the stomach. Neutralizing stomach acids with antacids may cause the formation of hydroxides or reduce the solubility of these metals.[15-17] Sorbitol, sodium alginate, or aluminum salts should be used for strontium ingestions.

Bronchoalveolar Lavage

Bronchoalveolar lavage may be used for inhaled contaminants, but it causes significant side effects and complications. It is customarily reserved for those who have far exceeded the maximum allowable body burden of the isotope.

Isotope Competition

Isotope competition can reduce the absorption of an isotope by providing an excess of a similar but nonradioactive form of the element. A familiar example would be the use of iodine salts to prevent the uptake of ^{131}I by the thyroid.

One of the most biologically important fission products released by reactor accidents is [131]I. If given within 1 hour of exposure to ^{131}I, 300 mg of stable iodine will reduce the uptake in the thyroid by about 90%.[18] The agent used in this technique is often called a blocking agent. This must be administered rapidly. There is little effect when potassium iodate is administered after 12 hours of exposure.

According to FDA recommendations, this prophylactic treatment should be initiated only when the estimated radiation exposure from radioactive iodine to the thyroid will be greater than 10 to 30 rem.[19] The administration of iodine can be preplanned, and the civilian population can self-administer the dose upon public health recommendations.[20] Note that this therapy is only good for exposure to [131]I.

There is some controversy about both public application of this therapy and the threshold of radiation for the administration of iodine. Blocking therapy with stable iodine was used in the wake of the Chernobyl accident with good effect.

Another blocking agent is used to prevent the uptake of strontium. Strontium behaves like calcium within the body. It is taken up by the bones and incorporated into the bony matrix. To prevent this, calcium can be administered to help displace the strontium and enhance excretion through the kidneys.

Isotope Dilution

A related technique is **isotopic dilution**, in which large quantities of a stable isotope are added in order to decrease the statistical probability of the incorporation of a specific atom of the radioactive form. The typical example is the use of ordinary water when faced with a radioactive dihydrogen (tritium) oxide incorporation. Caution should be taken by regularly monitoring the electrolytes during this treatment.

Sometimes, the dilution is accomplished with a completely different element that shares chemical properties with the radioactive isotope. Examples of this technique, called displacement therapy, are the use of calcium to block radioactive strontium uptake and the use of iodine to block radioactive technetium uptake.[21] Contact your department of nuclear medicine or radiologist regarding the specific agents used for the displacement of specific radioisotopes.

Chelating Agents

For some isotopes, specific heavy metal chelating agents will remove all isotopes of that type from the body **(Table 14-11)**. The prototype for this action is the medical use of deferoxamine to remove excess iron from the body. Radioactive iron can be removed in similar manner. Great care must be taken when using these chelating agents, because they do not discriminate between radioactive and nonradioactive elements. Massive and dangerous electrolyte disturbances may result from the use of these agents. Contact your department of nuclear medicine or a radiologist regarding the specific agents used and the appropriate doses for the chelation treatment of specific radioisotopes. The FDA has recently approved two new chelation agents: Ca-DTPA and Zn-DTPA suitable for treatment of incorporation of plutonium, americium, and curium.

Table 14-12 lists treatment for radiation exposures from various isotopes. If these various blocking or chelating agents are used in the first 1 to 3 hours after the ingestion, absorption can be reduced. In order to supply prompt treatment, the emergency department must have a well-defined plan, based on knowledge of the plant or lab operations, the radionuclides used, and the medications required. This may not be possible when a street accident or terrorist event is the cause of the exposure.

Table 14-11 Chelation Therapy for the Incorporation of Isotopes[22]

Isotope	Chelating Agent
Iron	Deferoxamine
Cesium	Prussian blue
Copper, gold, lead, mercury, and cobalt	Penicillamine
Rubidium	Chlorthalidone
Polonium	Dimercaprol (British anti-lewisite [BAL])
Cadmium, chromium, lead, and zinc	Calcium EDTA (ethylenediaminetetra-acetic acid)
Transuranic rare earths*	Zinc DPTA (diethylenetriaminepenta-acetic acid)

* Americium, californium, cerium, curium, lanthanum, plutonium, promethium, scandium, and yttrium.

Adapted from: Anonymous. Medical Management Of Radiological Casualties, ed 2. Armed Forces Radiobiology Research Institute. http://www.afrri.usuhs.mil/www/outreach/pdf/2edmmrchandbook.pdf (Accessed January 5, 2004).

After treatment, repeat assays of the isotopes, including both gamma camera and whole body counter assays, should be conducted to document the decontamination. The radiation physicist can then calculate the total absorbed radiation dose in order to determine whether a clinical radiation syndrome is likely.

Decontamination

The decontamination effort is started at the scene. If the patient's condition permits, the ambulance personnel should remove the patient's clothing and wash contaminated areas with soap and water. This action alone will remove the bulk of the surface contamination and will quickly decrease the risk of exposure to the medical staff. The effluent and clothing should be stored in plastic bags in order to ensure that the contamination does not spread. Removed clothing should be bagged, tagged with name and location, and marked radioactive as described subsequently, especially in a potential terrorist attack.

Decontamination should start, if medical status permits, with the cleansing of the areas of highest contamination first. Gentle washing is mandatory, as scrubbing and denuding skin will allow the entry of particles. Give special attention to skin folds, creases, hair, and body orifices. Remeasure the radioactivity levels after each washing and showering, and record the results.

Medical providers should ensure that decontamination does not take priority over lifesaving measures. The traumatized patient is more likely to die from the trauma than from the radioactive contamination. Providers, at all levels, should complete appropriate primary and secondary surveys, treating life threats as if there were no contamination. The sole exceptions to this might be invasive bodily procedures that could cause incorporation and mouth-to-mouth resuscitation that could expose the rescuer to the incorporation of radioactive materials.

A separate decontamination area within the hospital is essential. Walls and floors should be covered with plastic sheeting, and light switches should be protected with plastic. Entry and exit should be permited only at the discretion of a radiologist or radiation biophysicist who can check for radioactive contamination. If an installed decontamination shower with holding tank is not available, portable showers with large plastic holding tanks should be considered. All refuse water from the shower should be considered contaminated until cleared by a radiation biophysicist.

Table 14-12 Potential Treatment for Internal Contamination

Isotope	Route	Affected Area	Method of Treatment	Treatment	Dose
Iodine 131	Inhalation Ingestion Percutaneous absorption (small amount)	Thyroid	Block uptake by thyroid	SSKI (saturated solution of potassium iodide)	390 mg/day orally for 7 to 14 days
Cesium 137	Inhalation Ingestion	Whole body	Mobilization Decrease gastrointestinal uptake	Prussian blue (ferric ferrocyanide)	1 g in 100 to 200 mL of water orally three times daily for several days
Plutonium 239	Inhalation Absorption Wound incorporation	Bone Liver Lung	Chelation Increase excretion of the isotope	DPTA	1 g/day for 5 days
Hydrogen 3 (tritium)	Ingestion Inhalation Small amount by percutaneous absorption	Whole body	Dilution Increase excretion of the isotope	Water diuresis	3 to 4 L/day of water orally for 2 weeks
Strontium 90	Inhalation Ingestion	Bone	Displacement with calcium	Calcium	
Technetium 99	Inhalation Ingestion	Thyroid	Displacement with iodine	SSKI	390 mg/day orally for 7 to 14 days

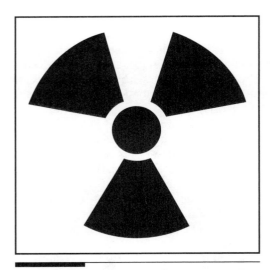

Figure 14-8 The international sign for radioactivity.

only verified uncontaminated supplies and personnel move from the "dirty" area to the clean area.

The patient's clothing and bedding should be removed and then put in plastic bags, if this has not previously been done. All jewelry and metal items should also be removed and placed in plastic bags. These plastic bags should be labeled "Radioactive material, **DO NOT DISCARD.**" Use of the international sign for radioactivity is appropriate **(Figure 14-8).**

Areas of contamination should be measured and recorded on an anatomic chart **(Figure 14-9).** A Lund and Browder burn chart is excellent for this recording. A second reading at the end of decontamination will verify the adequacy of the effort.

The use of specific agents for skin decontamination is determined by the properties of the contaminant, and this information should be made readily available to the health physicist. If there is no specific chemical or diluent that will remove, stabilize, or aid in dissolving the agent, then the use of detergent solution is indicated. Vigorous scrubbing should be avoided, because it tends to break down the skin barrier. Large amounts of water or other diluent is appropriate. Tepid water should be used rather than hot water, because hot water will open pores and allow internal contamination. Decontamination solutions that have been used successfully include soap and water; green soap and water; phosphate-based detergents, such as Tide or Cheer; chelating agents,

A single person, preferably a radiation physicist, should assume responsibility for ensuring that all personnel have and wear a dosimeter and ensure that the dosimeter readings are recorded. The same person should ensure that all nonessential personnel are excluded from the area and that

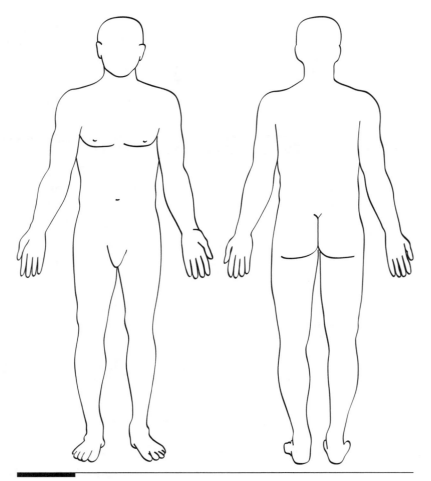

Figure 14-9 Sample radiation marking diagram.

such as EDTA and DPTA; potassium permanganate followed by sodium bisulfite; and titanium oxide.[23]

Surgical debridement and decontamination is best accomplished by a surgeon who has been trained in the treatment of radioactive wounds. Additional surgical staff may be needed if a patient has been contaminated with a very high-level source or if multiple patients have been injured. In extreme cases, the surgeon may operate from behind a lead shield while removing fragments.

Problem Areas in Decontamination

Wounds and body orifices are the first priority of decontamination efforts because of the potential for systemic absorption.

Wounds If a wound is involved, prepare and cover the wound with a self-adhering disposable surgical drape. The majority of skin decontamination should be removed with gentle, copious irrigation. Cleanse the surrounding areas until they are decontaminated. Remove the wound covering, and irrigate the wound with sterile water. Catch the irrigating fluid, and store it in a large, marked plastic container. Each step of the decontamination procedure should be monitored, and the extent and location of the contamination should be recorded. *Vigorous scrubbing for decontamination may damage the skin and allow absorption of skin contaminants.*

If a wound is grossly contaminated, both wet debridement as described above, and sharp surgical debridement may be indicated. Again, at each step of the decontamination process, the extent and location of contamination should be measured and recorded.

If contamination persists, further surgical debridement may be indicated. Do not mutilate to decontaminate without very good reason. Check with the radiation biophysicist about the nature and extent of the injury if the contamination was not removed, and use appropriate judgment.

Poor metabolic function and immunosuppression resulting from radiation may complicate the treatment of an otherwise simple injury. Injuries or burns that typically result in a 50% fatality rate with ordinary treatment may result in a rate as high as 90% for patients who have only 150 rem (1.5 Gy) of total body radiation.

Ears, Mouth, and Eyes Irrigate the contaminated area with saline or water and save the irrigating fluid for analysis. Be sure to get swabs of these areas before irrigation and save them in plastic bags for the use of the radiation biophysicist. Gastrointestinal absorption may be reduced with gastric lavage, emetics, and purgatives. Antacids containing aluminum oxide may cause radioactive metals to precipitate as insoluble hydroxides.

Hair Hair may retain some isotopes and should be cut in such cases. Do not shave the scalp if possible, as a skin injury may increase absorption and later incorporation into the body.

Inhalation About 50% of the contaminated material that is inhaled is returned to the pharynx by ciliary action in the trachea. This portion is often swallowed. Save all sputum for analysis. Lung lavage may be indicated, but it is often not used in the United States. The physician should consult the radiation biophysicist.

Measurements of the amount of contamination that has been removed and, most importantly, the amount that yet remains must be obtained. The radiation biophysicist will

need nasal and oral swabbings to estimate the amount of ingested contamination. Also, 24-hour urine and 72-hour fecal collections will prove helpful. All sputum, vomit, debrided tissue, particles and fragments, shaved hair, and exudates must be collected and saved separately. Extra samples of blood should be drawn for use by the radiation biophysicist in the estimation of exposure. Whole body radiation counts and radioiodide counts may be indicated.

When all patients have been decontaminated, the medical staff will need to be decontaminated themselves. All clothing, masks, booties, and linens should be bagged and labeled. Showers should be taken and fresh scrubs donned. A radiation biophysicist should monitor the medical staff and record any sites of radiation, ensuring that all is removed.

Finally, the suite, ambulances, litters, gurneys, and other equipment used must be decontaminated under strict control. All disposable materials will be discarded, whether used or unused, as contaminated waste. Severely contaminated equipment may need to be replaced. Any articles that are contaminated will be either decontaminated, stored for a length of time until the isotope decays, or disposed of as radioactive waste in accordance with federal regulations.

Laboratory Data

Laboratory data may provide clues to the extent of exposure, information on the nature of the radioactive agent, and the prognosis of the exposed person. Minimal laboratory tests should include the following:

- Complete blood count with platelets every 6 hours
- Urinalysis (Save all urine from the time of the accident.)
- Fecal analysis for affected radionuclide (Save all feces from the time of the accident.)
- Nasal swabs before blowing nose, washing face, or showering
- Patient's dosimeter reading, if any

Laboratory specimens should be handled as if they were radioactive until proven otherwise. Personal effects, such as jewelry and clothing, may be decontaminated and returned to the patient after approval of the radiation control officer. Never let the patient touch laboratory specimens or other objects until the patient has been decontaminated and verified to be free of residual contamination.

■ Threat Analysis

Nuclear Weapons

Two major scenarios describe the possibility of terrorists obtaining a nuclear weapon that is capable of impacting the United States. In the first, a stolen weapon is sold to terrorists, who then seek to smuggle it into the United States or within range of US overseas assets, such as an aircraft carrier. This could be a "suitcase nuke" that was originally designed for special forces troops to demolish bridges, railways, ammunition depots, or troop rally points. Both the United States and the Soviet Union produced a few hundred of these small nuclear weapons.

In 1997, former Soviet general Alexander Lebed announced that some of the Soviet portable weapons, as many as 100, were lost. Russian press reports noted that Chechen rebels stole nuclear weapons from a military base. In Miami, in 1997, ethnic Russians offered to sell a suitcase nuke to undercover US Customs agents. Terrorists may have already purchased such small nuclear weapons and may only be waiting for the opportune moment to smuggle them into the United States. Furthermore, because the Russians have lost much of the control and loyalty of their military forces, terrorists may have already purchased a full-size nuclear weapon from former military sites.

The second scenario involves a terrorist group building its own nuclear weapon using smuggled material. The International Atomic Energy Agency has documented at least 18 cases of weapons-grade nuclear smuggling since 1993. About a dozen countries possess this kind of material. The largest amount sits in Russian weapons facilities and laboratories, and the accounting of this material is slipshod and inaccurate. The Russians themselves admit that they do not know how much they have.

Most authorities feel that a terrorist group could produce a nuclear weapon without assistance from a state-sponsored nuclear weapons program. However, acquiring and enriching uranium or creating plutonium in a nuclear reactor is an expensive and difficult process that requires both substantial equipment and sophisticated techniques. Many authorities feel that the technical challenges inherent in building an atomic bomb preclude terrorists from building a functioning atomic bomb, even if they were to obtain the fission-grade materials. Unfortunately, the theory on which the atomic bomb is based is quite well documented, and the construction of a gun-type weapon is not a complex task. Although the yield of this weapon would be "only" the size of Hiroshima or Nagasaki, building this weapon is an entirely achievable task for dozens of nuclear physicists.

The detonation of even a crude nuclear weapon in an American city would cause tens of thousands of casualties. Most casualties would be caused by the blast and thermal effects of the weapon. This is the ideal terrorist weapon and has been sought by both terrorists and nations alike. This is truly a weapon of both mass destruction and mass casualties.

Blast

The extremely rapid heating of the air by the nuclear reaction of a nuclear weapon creates an explosion. Indeed, the explosion of a nuclear weapon is often measured with the equivalent amount of tons of TNT that would create a similar sized explosion.

As the rapidly expanding gas cloud moves outward, it creates a shock or blast wave, followed by a blast of wind. The shock wave and the blast of wind produce the same injuries associated with a conventional explosive device. The effect of the atomic weapon, however, is much, much greater, and the range of injury outwards from the point of the explosion (ground zero) is also much greater. The blast winds from a nuclear explosion can reach over 250 km/h. The magnitude of the blast wave associated with a nuclear weapon is the major reason why these weapons deserve the title *weapons of mass destruction* (Figure 14-10).

Thermal Injuries Although the blast injuries and destruction associated with a nuclear weapon are fearsome, the greatest numbers of casualties and fatalities are produced by

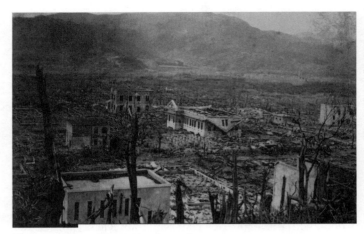

Figure 14-10 Hiroshima after the explosion.

the thermal burns caused by the nuclear explosion. The nuclear reaction releases vast quantities of thermal energy, which travel both through the air and in the shock wave.

Although the thermal radiation occurs over a very short duration, it is quite intense. The radiant energy is absorbed by any surface exposed to the nuclear explosion. For exposed human skin, this causes burns. For any combustible surfaces, it may cause ignition or incineration. A 1-kton nuclear weapon will result in a 50% mortality rate, caused by burns, of exposed persons within 500 meters of the point of explosion.

Because the majority of these burns are caused by radiant energy, protection is quite easy. The burns only occur on the surfaces exposed to the radiant energy. Any wall or opaque object will absorb the radiant energy before it strikes the human. Even white or light-colored clothing will reflect much of the radiant energy.

If the victim looks at the explosion, the retina can be permanently damaged. Eyes may also be damaged by the thermal burn.

Primary Radiation Injuries If one considers the consequences of a 1-kton yield, then the following would occur within 1 minute around the point of ground zero:

1. The blast would cause 50% casualties at a distance of approximately 400 to 500 m.
2. Thermal radiation (burns) would cause casualties within the same distance as the blast effects.
3. Nuclear radiation pulse (that is, gamma and neutron radiation) would cause 50% casualties within approximately 0.5 km.
4. The radioactive fallout could produce very high exposure rates within up to 0.8 km, depending on wind and weather conditions.

Obviously, larger weapons will have larger effects (Table 14-13).

Fallout

There are over 300 different fission byproducts that result from a typical fission reaction. Many of these isotopes have widely varying half-lives, from fractions of a second to thousands of years. The principle decay is through beta and gamma ray emission.

About 60 grams of these fission products are formed per kiloton of bomb yield. The estimated activity of these radioisotopes is about 1.1 to 10^{21} Bq or the equivalent of 30 million kg of radium.[24] Much of this intense activity rapidly decays with the short-lived half-life isotopes **(Figure 14-11)**.

In a nuclear explosion, excess plutonium or uranium or both are scattered about by the force of the explosion and add to the fallout. The plutonium or uranium dispersed during the explosion decays through its usual pathway. The alpha particles produced are of importance if ingested or inhaled.

An additional effect discovered early in the course of the development of nuclear weapons is the transformation of dust and debris into potentially lethal toxins. The intense neutron bombardment occurring during fission leads to neutron capture in rocks, dust, and even air. The rocks, dust, and air then acquire their own radioactivity.

These transmuted materials, decay products, and leftover fission materials are vaporized and then sucked up by

Table 14-13 **Effects of Various Blast Sizes**			
Blast Energy	Blast Injury Effect	Initial Radiation	Burns
1 Mton	4.5–5.0 km	2.2–2.5 km	14–15 km
100 kton	2.0–2.5 km	1.7–1.9 km	5–6 km
10 kton	1 km	1 km	1 km
1 kton	0.5 km	0.5 km	0.5 km

Adapted from: Glasstone, Samuel and Dolan, Philip J., *The Effects of Nuclear Weapons (third edition)* http://www.cddc.vt.edu/host/atomic/nukeffect. U.S. Government Printing Office, 1977. (Accessed 12 July, 2005)

the fireball into the atmosphere. This plume of small particles is carried by the wind and subsequently falls onto the surrounding area. Some are carried into the stratosphere and are scattered worldwide. This collection of radioactive debris is termed fallout **(Figure 14-12)**.

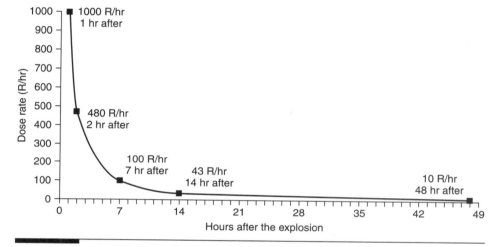

Figure 14-11 Decay ratio.

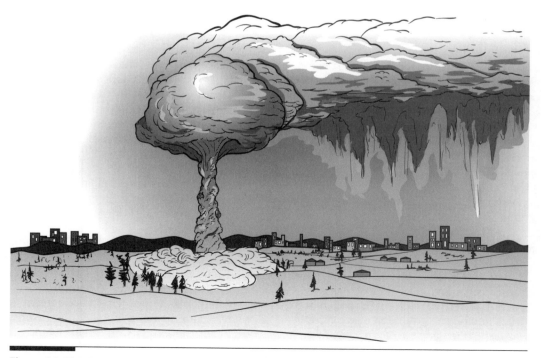

Figure 14-12 Fallout.

It was also realized that another method of creating such toxins is a direct result of the nuclear reactors. When the fission materials are consumed in the nuclear reaction, the resulting storm of neutrons transmutes the other components of the reactor fuel rod and all of the surrounding structures into radioactive isotopes. Although this material is not useful, it is extremely radioactive—indeed, much more so than simple fallout.

Although the blast effects and thermal effects of the nuclear explosion are far more important and produce more casualties than the radioactivity, most people are more fearful of the radioactivity.

Reactor Accidents and Sabotage

Most people are aware of the reactor accidents of Three Mile Island and Chernobyl. The accident at Chernobyl was caused when approximately eight safety systems were bypassed. The explosion resulted in the meltdown of the core and the destruction of the roof of the containment vessel. The explosion and subsequent release of radioactivity caused widespread contamination of vast areas of land. This accident caused the deaths of 28 individuals from acute radiation injury, and 237 people were treated for acute radiation syndrome.

In the Western world, the probability of terrorism involving a reactor is low. This is because of the high security surrounding reactors and the redundant safety systems incorporated into the reactor design. There is extensive shielding around a reactor; therefore, a significant amount of explosives would be required to breach this containment. Before reaching the containment vessel, the terrorists must also traverse armed security guards and exclusion fences. This is a low probability event.

There is some evidence that terrorists have contemplated crashing an aircraft into a nuclear reactor or the fuel storage pits. This could be more damaging than most cases of internal sabotage of the reactor.

Radiation Dispersal Weapons

The fear of radiation-related casualties has led to the development of a crude weapon of terror—the **radiation dispersal weapon** (RDW, or dirty bomb). In this device, an explosion or sprayer is used to disperse a radioactive mixture onto a populated area. The material becomes dangerous to anyone nearby and requires expensive and extensive cleanup efforts. Some people will become ill or even die from the radiation exposure. The majority of people who are exposed will only develop problems years after the exposure. The effects and costs of this kind of weapon can be easily illustrated by the examination of several accidents in which radioactive materials were scattered among an unsuspecting public.

The first major obscured radiation accident occurred in 1982 in Juarez, Mexico. In this accident, a radioactive source of about 400 Ci of ^{60}Co within a radiotherapy unit was stolen from a warehouse and dismantled. The radioactive core of 6,000 pellets of ^{60}Co was exposed and cut up. The pellets were spilled in a pickup truck and on the ground in a junkyard.[25]

The machine was dismantled and sold for scrap to a steel company. Some of the cobalt pellets, together with other scrap metal, were recycled into construction reinforcing rods. The cleanup started when a pickup truck carrying these reinforcing rods was found to be quite radioactive when it tried to drive through detectors in the Los Alamos Laboratory.

During the two months between the theft and the detection, many people had been exposed to large doses of radiation. The Juarez incident has been downplayed by the Mexican authorities and has received little publicity.

The resulting exposures sickened hundreds and killed 1.[26] About 4,000 persons were exposed, including 5 who received doses ranging from 300 rem (3 Sv) to 700 rem (7 Sv). Four Mexican workers in the junkyard received very large whole-body doses and 2 others were severely burned on the hands and feet. Seventy-five more people received doses ranging from 25 rem (0.25 Sv) to 300 rem (3 Sv), while another 720 received doses ranging from 0.5 rem (5 mSv) to 25 rem (0.25 Sv). Six thousand tons of reinforcement bars were contaminated, of which 950 tons were imported into the United States. Eight hundred and fourteen houses were demolished because these contaminated steel bars were used in their construction.

A similar episode occurred in 1987 in Goiana, Brazil, after two junk collectors broke into an abandoned building and found a gamma-ray radiotherapy unit.[27,28] They removed the head of the unit and took out the capsule containing about 20 g of radioactive ^{137}Cs, which had an emission activity of 1,400 Ci. The capsule was forced open and the powdered compound was scattered. Indeed, the luminescent blue powder was rubbed into the body by several people, including children. The first symptoms of radiation poisoning were felt within days. The victims sought help in local pharmacies and hospitals and were treated as if they had an infectious disease.

The nature of the illnesses was finally diagnosed over 2 weeks after the exposure occurred. Out of 111,800 people who required testing, 249 were found to be contaminated. In spite of decontamination, 5 people died, and 1 required the amputation of a limb. Forty-nine patients required hospitalization, and 21 of these required intensive care.

To decontaminate the area, 125,000 drums and 1,470 boxes were filled with contaminated clothing, furniture, dirt, and other materials. Eighty-five houses were demolished. The medical response and cleanup phases took several months to complete. In this case, there was both an exposure and a contamination problem.

The RDW has a tremendous terror effect, because the thought of exposure to a radioactive source is, bluntly, terrifying to most people. The accidents in Mexico and Brazil are illustrative of the probable course of an actual RDW exposure and the subsequent cleanup efforts. A recurring trend is that almost a month elapses between the exposure and the realization by authorities that there is a radiologic emergency at hand.[29]

The lethality of an RDW is dependent on a number of factors, including the type of radioactive material used, the wind and weather conditions, and the speed at which the target area is evacuated. A small bomb would likely kill nobody, but it would receive maximum media exposure and render an area uninhabitable for an extended period of time. Whatever the lethality, the RDW would create panic.

Manufacturing an RDW is both simple and inexpensive. Clearly it is an easier task than trying to create a nuclear bomb.

In one scenario, an expended fuel rod is cut or ground up and simply released into an air-conditioning vent, along a subway course, or from the top of a tall building in the wind. Any sort of aerosol- or liquid-dispersing device that could disperse radioactive material into air, water, or food would do. The exposure could be external or internal and could cause immediate and long-term health effects. This method sacrifices the person who carries and dumps the pail of radioactive powder in front of the fan. The terrorist who comes that close to a significant radiation source will shortly become a martyr.

This method has one singular advantage. There is no loud bang to alert authorities to a potential problem. Hours or even weeks after exposure, casualties may show up in emergency departments as the first clue to the release. If alpha emitter agents are chosen, the populace and area may be well contaminated before the authorities realize that there is a problem.

In another, more popular scenario, the nuclear waste is packed around an explosive device. When detonated, the radioactive waste is dispersed. If the detonation occurs at the top of a skyscraper, the radioactive waste is widely dispersed. A ground-level explosive device would cause much less dispersal.

The size of the RDW could be as small as a hand grenade or briefcase bomb or as large as a truck bomb. The packaging could be a crate or a cylinder, such as a water heater. Because these RDW's are totally unsophisticated, anyone can build and deliver this type of weapon. The waste material could range from radioactive slurry from fuel rod production to parts of reactor linings.

Fortunately, the devil is in the details. To be effective, there must be a substantial dispersal of a fairly "hot" agent. For maximum dispersal, the material must be ground to a fine powder or dissolved in an appropriate solvent. This requires substantial risks or sacrifices by the organization that grinds up the agents.

The more radioactive the material, the greater the chance of discovery as a result of escaped radiation, and the more danger to those carrying the material and preparing the material for the RDW. The very high dose that would be received while assembling the source with the explosive, packaging it, and then transporting it to the target location would be a major impediment. A lethal and—most importantly—rapidly incapacitating dose from the concentrated and unshielded source is likely.

Three other problems confront the would-be terrorist wanting to build and employ an RDW.

- The kinds of extremely radioactive materials ideal for these RDWs have short half-lives. This means that the terrorist must use the bomb material soon after procuring it.
- An RDW with a highly radioactive casing would literally be hot. The highly radioactive isotopes give off a substantial amount of heat—enough to fuel thermal generators in space probes.
- Substantial amounts of shielding would be required to prevent detection—as much as 4,500 kg of lead shielding. This is a lot of mass to move.

Nonetheless, at least one group of terrorists has already constructed an RDW, so the threat has substantial credibility. In 1995, Chechen rebels left a container of ^{137}Cs in a popular Moscow park. To lend credibility to their threat of possessing such a weapon, a Chechen commander, Shamil Basayen, publicly announced where the bomb was buried. Russian bomb disposal experts removed the bomb.[30]

Abdullah al Mujahiwar was arrested on May 8, 2002, in Chicago's O'Hare International Airport. With him were purportedly documents that outlined an RDW. The Bush administration appears to suspect that Osama bin Laden's Al Qaeda network has already obtained such radioactive materials as strontium 90 (^{90}Sr) and ^{137}Cs.

Customs officers in 2000 in Uzbekistan found 10 lead-lined containers in a truck after their radiation detectors went wild.[31,32] The Iranian driver apparently was carrying ^{90}Sr to Pakistan with false papers. Quetta, Pakistan, was his purported destination. Quetta is the major crossing point into southern Afghanistan, which has been known to harbor terrorists.

According to UN reports, Iraq tested a 1-ton radiologic dispersal weapon in 1987. They apparently abandoned the project because the radiation levels were not deadly enough.

■ Summary

As noted, most medical providers feel that they will never be faced with the possibility of a serious radiation incident. Our increasing use and transportation of radioisotopes puts all emergency departments in jeopardy of being involved in a nuclear spill.

The present ability of terrorists to use either stolen nuclear weapons, improvised nuclear weapons, or RDWs should be considered a real threat in every town. Even if the town is not the target of such a nuclear device, there is a significant possibility that refugees from an exposed target area may bring contamination to the outlying areas. The town may also become contaminated by the fallout plume of a detonated nuclear device.

The most likely threat is a radiologic dispersal weapon. These are technologically feasible weapons to manufacture and can be constructed with materials already available to terrorists. The procurement of nuclear wastes on the black market has probably already occurred, and explosives are already in the terrorists' hands. Considering that at least one nation experimented with RDWs several years ago, it is likely that the design is available to terrorists today. Premade devices may also be available on the black market from this and other state sources.

Statements from public and protected sources suggest that the use of nuclear weapons is a substantial threat at this time. The author feels that the risk is high, and the author's confidence in the sources is high. Recent efforts by the administration to find manufacturing facilities for such devices indicate that the authorities also support this analysis and conclusion.

A medical facility's established radiation emergency protocol should be updated by a manager or physician director on a yearly basis. Personnel may receive training on the management of a radiation accident upon initial orientation in some hospital and emergency services. Unfortunately, what is not used is lost, and training on radiation emergencies is no exception. All emergency providers should receive initial and annual training in the management of radioactive accident victims.

■ Resources

US Department of Energy
REACTS daytime phone: (423) 576-3131
REACTS 24-hour phone: (423) 481-1000 (for emergency use)

Regional coordinating offices for radiologic assistance
Brookhaven Area Operations Office   516-282-2200
Upton, NY 11973
Responsible for Connecticut, Delaware, Maine, Maryland,
   Massachusetts, New Hampshire, New York, New Jersey,
   Pennsylvania, Rhode Island, Vermont, Puerto Rico, and the
   Virgin Islands

Oak Ridge Operations Office   615-576-1005
PO Box E, Oak Ridge, TN 37830
Responsible for Arkansas, Kentucky, Louisiana, Mississippi,
   Missouri, Tennessee, Virginia, and West Virginia

Savannah River Operations Office   803-726-3333
PO Box A, Aiken, SC 29801
Responsible for Alabama, Georgia, Florida, North Carolina, South
   Carolina, and the Canal Zone

Albuquerque Operations Office   505-844-4667
PO Box 5400 Albuquerque, NM 87185
Responsible for Arizona, Kansas, New Mexico, Oklahoma, and Texas

Chicago Operations Office   312-972-4800 or 312-972-5731
9800 South Cass Ave, Argonne, IL 60439
Responsible for Illinois, Indiana, Iowa, Michigan, Minnesota,
   Nebraska, North Dakota, South Dakota, Ohio, and Wisconsin

Idaho Operations Office   208-526-1515
785 DOE Pl, Idaho Falls, ID 83402
Responsible for Colorado, Idaho, Montana, Utah, and Wyoming

San Francisco Operations Office   415-273-4237
1301 Clay St, MS 700-N, Oakland, CA 94612
Responsible for California, Hawaii, and Nevada

Richland Operations Office   509-373-3800
PO Box 550, Richland, WA 99352
Responsible for Alaska, Oregon, and Washington

■ References

1. Glasstone S, Dolan PJ: *The Effects of Nuclear Weapons,* ed 3. Washington, DC, US Department of Defense, 1977.
2. Walker RI, Cerveny TJ: *Medical Consequences of Nuclear Warfare.* Falls Church, VA, Office of the Surgeon General, 1989.
3. *Medical Effects of Ionizing Radiation Course.* Uniformed Services University for the Health Sciences, Bethesda, MD.
4. Federal Emergency Management Agency: *Course for Radiological Monitors.* Washington, DC,US Government Printing Office, 1979.
5. Fabrikant JI: The effects of the accident at Three Mile Island on the mental health and behavioral responses of the general population and nuclear workers. *Health Phys* 1983;45:579-586.
6. Anonymous: Chernobyl Accident, http://www.uic.com.au/nip22.htm (Accessed July 12, 2005).
7. Geiger HJ: The accident at Chernobyl and the medical response. *JAMA* 1986;256:609-612.
8. Bores RJ: The scope of nuclear regulatory commission requirements for arrangements for medical services for contaminated injured individuals. *Bull NY Acad Med* 1983;59:956-961.
9. Stasiak RS, Stewart CE, Redwine RH: Symptoms and treatment of radiation exposure. *Emerg Med Serv* 1986;15:21-26.
10. Casarett AP: *Radiation Biology.* Englewood Cliffs, NJ, Prentice Hall, 1968.
11. Taylor TB: Third generation nuclear weapons. *Sci Amer* 1987;256:30-39.
12. Anonymous: *Basic Radiation Protection Criteria.* Bethesda, MD, National Council on Radiation Protection and Measurements (Report No 39), 1971.
13. Littlefield LG, Joiner EE, Colyer SP, Frome EL: Radioprotective chemicals as tools for studying mechanisms of radiation-induced chromosome damage in human lymphocytes, in *Chromosomal Alterations: Origin and Significance* (G. Obe and A.T. Natarajan, eds. with contributions by F. Adlkofer et al.). New York, Springer-Verlag, pp. 132–139, 1994.
14. Wing S, Shy CM, Wood JL, Wolf S, Cragle DL, Frome EL: Mortality among workers at Oak Ridge National Library. Evidence of radiation effects in follow-up through 1984. *JAMA* 1991;265:1397–1402.
15. Baxter DW, Sullivan MF: Gastrointestinal absorption and retention of plutonium chelates. *Health Phys* 1972;22:785.
16. Tompsett SL: Factors influencing the absorption of iron and copper from the alimentary tract. *Biochem J* 1940;34:961.
17. Jacobs AG, Rhodes DK, Peters H, et al: Gastric acidity and iron absorption. *Brit J Haemat* 1966;12:728.
18. Ramden D, Passant FH, Peabody CO, Speight RG: Radioiodine uptakes in the thyroid studies of the blocking and subsequent recovery of the gland following the administration of stable iodine. *Health Phys* 1967;13:633.
19. Saenger EL: Radiation accidents. *Ann Emerg Med* 1986;15:1061-1066.
20. Fowinkle EW, Sell SH, Wolle RH: Predistribution of potassium iodide: The Tennessee experience. *Pub Health Rep* 1983;96:123-126.
21. Lincoln TA: Importance of initial management of persons internally contaminated with radionucleides. *Am Ind Hygiene Assoc J* 1976;16-21.
22. Anonymous: *Management of Persons Accidentally Contaminated with Radionucleides.* Washington, DC, National Council on Radiation Protection and Measurements (Report No 65), 1980.
23. Saenger EL: Radiation accidents. *Ann Emerg Med* 1986;15:1061-1066.
24. Nuclear weapon radiation effects. Federation of American Scientists, http://www.fas.org/nuke/intro/nuke/radiation.htm (accessed November 3, 2002).
25. Bunce N, Hunt J: The Mexican radiation accident. The University of Guelph, 1984, http://helios.physics.uoguelph.ca/summer/scor/articles/scor24.htm (accessed November 4, 2002).
26. Marshall E: Juarez: An unprecedented radiation accident. *Science* 1984;223:1152-1154.
27. Zylbersztajn A: Not to commemorate, but to remember: 10 years since the Goiania nuclear accident. *Int Nwsltr Phys Educ* 1997;35:1.
28. Ortiz P, Friedrich V, Wheatly J, Oresegun M: Lost and found dangers: Orphan radiation sources raise global concerns. *IAEA Bulletin* 1999;41:18-21.
29. Lloyd D, Clark M: Editorial: Déjà vu again. *Radiological Protection Bulletin* 2000;220.
30. AFIO weekly intelligence notes. Association of Former Intelligence Officers, April 28, 2000, http://www.afio.com/sections/wins/2000/2000-17.html (accessed November 2, 2002).
31. West J: Atomic haul raises fears of bin Laden terror bomb. April 23, 2000.
32. AFIO weekly intelligence notes. Association of Former Intelligence Officers, April 28, 2000, http://www.afio.com/sections/wins/2000/2000-17.html (accessed November 2, 2002).

Electronic Terrorism and Directed Energy Weapons

Coauthored with M. Kathleen Stewart MSCIS, MSLA

■ Introduction

The list of weapons available to terrorists ranges from passenger jets to atomic devices and includes all of the chemical and biological weapons developed over the last hundred years. To this list must be added the growing threat of widespread damage to domestic electronic systems from weapons of cyber- and electronic terrorism. These cyber- and electronic terrorist weapons could also be characterized as weapons of mass disruption.

This chapter will review the basic principles and attributes of the technology of electronic weapons and cyber terrorism as they may affect the EMS system. It should be stressed that this chapter is not exhaustive and is intended only to illustrate how the technology base of the world and EMS in particular is vulnerable to a variety of attacks.

■ Terrorism, Computers, and the Internet

Every machine connected to the Internet is potentially a printing press, a broadcasting station, and a place of assembly. The astute observer should note that a majority of the 33 organizations deemed foreign terrorist organizations by the US Department of State have a formal Web presence on the Internet.[1] With the advent of the Internet, the terrorist group can disseminate its information, undiluted by the media and untouched by government sensors. It should come as no surprise, then, that these same organizations have used the Internet to spread gospel, instructions, propaganda, and plans for both devices and attacks.

Unfortunately, actual terrorist use of computers, networks, information architectures, and the Internet has been largely ignored in favor of a headline-grabbing cyber attack or act of cyberterrorism. The reality of our weaknesses and our vulnerabilities is both more chilling and far more reassuring.

Cyberterrorism has no clear-cut, widely accepted definition. The pejorative connotation of terrorism has been wrongly applied to computer abuse. For example, an e-mail list that the authors subscribe to on terrorism routinely reports cases of child pornography as incidents of terrorism. Child pornography is certainly criminal and certainly perverted, but it is hardly an act of terrorism. The term *terrorism* is defined in one public law as premeditated, politically motivated violence perpetrated against noncombatant targets by subnational groups or clandestine agents, usually intended to influence an audience.[2]

How Vulnerable Are We to a Cyber Attack or Electronic Attack?

We are easy prey for two reasons: First, the growing technological sophistication of terrorists includes, not only weapons of mass destruction and casualties, but a growing use of computers. Secondly, our own economic and technological systems have an increasing vulnerability to carefully timed attacks as we increase our dependence on computers.

The entire critical infrastructure of the United States, including electrical power, telecommunications, health care, transportation, water, and the Internet, is quite vulnerable to a cyberattack. Control systems, communication systems, and dispatch systems are now connected to the Internet and are, thus, potentially open to intrusion. This does not include the possible effects that a cyber attack could have on finance or national defense. Three major avenues of attack that could affect EMS operations are the viral attack, the denial of service attack, and the electromagnetic pulse attack.

■ Viruses and Worms

Malignant computer programs are often called **viruses**, because they share some of the traits of biological viruses. Unlike a cell, the biological virus has no way to reproduce by itself and requires a functioning host cell. Similarly, the computer virus requires a functioning "host" machine in order to replicate, and will only work with the proper host. Furthermore, the computer virus passes from computer to computer, just as a biological virus passes from person to person.

There are other similarities. A virus is a fragment of DNA inside a protective jacket. A computer virus must piggyback on top of another program, document, or e-mail in order to get into the computer. It often must disguise itself from antiviral software with a surrounding innocuous package, like its biological counterpart.

People create computer viruses. A person must write the code for the virus, and then test it to make sure that it functions as intended and spreads as designed.

A computer that has an active copy of a virus on its hard drive is considered **infected**. The way that the virus is activated depends on the design (coding) of the virus. Some viruses become active if the user simply opens an infected document. Others require specific actions of the user.

Traditional computer viruses were first noted in the 1980s. During that decade, the use of computers spread from large centralized locations to small businesses and homes as a result of the availability of small personal computers—the advent of the PC. The first viruses were Trojan horse viruses.

A **Trojan horse** is simply a malignant computer program that claims to do something (often to perform as a game or a utility) but actually does something else instead—such as erase your disk. A Trojan horse program has no way to replicate automatically.

Another early virus was the **boot sector virus**. The boot sector is a small program that initializes the computer and the process of loading the operating system—"booting"

it into the memory. By putting code in the boot sector, the virus guarantees that it will be loaded into memory immediately and will be able to run whenever the computer is on. A boot sector virus will infect the boot sector of any floppy disk that is inserted into an infected machine. Boot sector viruses are seldom seen anymore, because the manufacturers of operating systems and antivirus software protect the boot sector; most users boot from a hard drive; and programs are most often loaded from CDs, which are less susceptible to boot sector modifications.

Once the virus is active on the computer, it can copy itself to files, disks, and programs as they are used by the computer (whether they are accessed automatically or by the computer user). The big difference between a computer virus and other programs is that the computer virus is specifically designed to make a copy of itself. When the viral programs are executed, the virus examines the hard drives to see if there is a susceptible program on the disk. When such a program is found, the virus modifies it by adding the viral code to the program or replacing the program or file with its own code. When this is accomplished, the virus has effectively reproduced itself so that two or more programs are infected. Every time the user runs any infected program, the virus has another chance to reproduce by attaching to other programs, and the cycle continues. This replication often occurs without the knowledge of the computer user (sometimes the programs infected are system programs that the user does not control).

Attachments that come as program files, such as Microsoft Word files (.DOC), Microsoft Excel spreadsheets (.XLS), and images (.GIF and .JPG), can contain viral attachments. A file with an extension such as EXE, COM, or VBS is executable and can deliver a viral program that can do any level of damage to a computer. Many viruses disguise themselves by doubling the file name extension (for example, STUFF.GIF.VBS).

A virus often contains a **payload,** or additional action that the virus will carry out besides replicating itself. Payloads vary from the trivially annoying to the destructive. Some nondestructive and nontrivial payloads include logging programs that record every keystroke typed in, programs that automatically send e-mails to every address in the computer, and programs that open portals for strangers to examine and use your computer. If the payload is well designed, the user may not even be aware that the computer is infected.

Previous attacks have already illustrated the ability of a program to acquire both data and passwords and then e-mail this information to an individual. Public machines, nonsecure business or official machines, and some secure systems can be used as remote intelligence gathering devices. Locating the offending program is often difficult, because many of the key-logging programs are titled or disguised as necessary system files or folders.

A **worm** is simply a virus that has the ability to copy itself from machine to machine. A copy of the worm looks around and infects other machines with the same security defect through any available computer network. Using the networks and the Internet, worms can infect other machines incredibly quickly.

INCIDENTS IN Electronic Terrorism

Juju Jiang

For more than a year, unbeknownst to people who used Internet terminals at Kinko's stores in New York, Juju Jiang was recording what they typed, paying particular attention to their passwords. Jiang had secretly installed, in multiple Kinko's stores, software that logs individual keystrokes. He captured more than 450 user names and passwords, and used them to access and open bank accounts online.[3]

Modern computer viruses can be found in programs available on floppy disks, CDs, and DVDs. They can also be hidden in multiple kinds of e-mail attachments and in material that is downloaded from the Web. Why is this important for EMS? What possible harm could come from a virus that is spread by e-mail other than to disrupt the e-mail? Some answers to these questions become apparent after reviewing recent viruses and worms.

One of the most recent destructive viruses and worms is **Code Red** (now with multiple variants), which first appeared in July 2001 and ultimately affected over 300,000 computers in the United States. This worm exploited a hole in Microsoft's IIS Web servers. Authorities still do not know where this worm originated or who the writer was.

The worm was activated based on dates. From days 1 to 19 of the month, the worm would propagate; from days 20 to 27, it would launch a denial of service attack against a particular site; and from day 27 to the end of the month, the worm would "sleep" in the computer.[4] Some variants have opened covert access ports (back doors) in operating systems that allow other intrusions.

The concept of the covert access port is important. These covert sites of entry allow a malignant programmer access and even control of programs running on the affected computer. The access may be gained with a virus by contaminating programs that are part of the "remote help" services in some operating systems, or the access port may be built into a program by the designer or a programmer (either disgruntled or operating under instructions).

Although Microsoft provided a patch for Code Red, many system administrators did not obtain or apply the patch to their systems. These unprotected computers remain vulnerable to this virus.

The newer intrusions may have a more malignant purpose. During the summer of 2001, the coordinator for the Website run by the city of Mountain View, California, noticed a suspicious pattern of intrusions. During an FBI investigation, it was found that several other US cities had had the same intruders. These probes originated from the Middle East and southern Asia. The invaders were looking up information regarding the cities' utilities, government offices, and emergency systems.

This information took on new importance after several computers were seized from Al Qaeda operatives after the September 11, 2001 attacks. Officials discovered a broad pattern of surveillance of US infrastructure on these computers.[5]

The Nimda worm appeared 1 week after the September 11 terrorist attacks and attacked the financial sector. A more intelligent worm, Nimda could replicate itself in several ways: by infecting e-mail programs, copying itself onto the computer servers, or infecting users who downloaded infected pages from the infected Web servers. Nimda affected millions of computers and brought the Internet to a crawl. Nimda replicated itself much faster than the Code Red worm and caused billions of dollars in damage.[6]

The Slammer worm or Sapphire worm, as it is also known, surfaced January 25, 2003 (Super Bowl weekend). The Slammer exploited a vulnerability in the servers that deliver Web pages to users. It was the fastest cyberattack in history. The number of Slammer infections doubled every 8.5 seconds and the Slammer did over 90% of its damage in the first 10 minutes of its release. Slammer incapacitated parts of the Internet in Korea and Japan, disrupted the phone service in Finland, and markedly slowed airline reservation systems, credit card networks, and ATM machines in the United States.[7]

Slammer could have been much more destructive had it been properly programmed. A new, improved Slammer could do much more damage. It could even affect phone and other trunked communication systems (including some radio links) for a city or larger region of the country.

Although control systems are unlikely to be directly damaged by an Internet virus like Slammer, the denial of service to control points for water distribution systems, railroad switch points, power grids, chemical plants, and telephone systems may cause widespread nondestructive failures. After the mapping of access points described previously, terrorists may well have targeted specific weak spots for harassment.

Implications

Any of the modern viruses and worms could be redesigned to destroy, or at least severely cripple, the 9-1-1 system here in the United States. They could also cripple or destroy electrical power systems, transportation systems, telecommunications systems, water supply systems, and perhaps our defense systems.

What Can You Do to Help?

One of the best things you can do is install a good virus protection program on your computers and update your virus protection frequently, not just occasionally. Set up a schedule for operating system updates and run a virus scan. If a virus is found, eliminate it.

Each virus is tailored for a specific operating system. If you are running a variation of Microsoft Windows (Windows 98, 2000, or XP, for example), then a virus tailored for Unix will not affect your computer. Likewise, if you use Linux, a Windows virus will not affect your computer. Some viruses are built to exploit known weaknesses in popular programs. If you do not run Microsoft Outlook as your e-mail program, then viruses that affect Outlook will not trouble you.

- Have the virus protection set to scan a document before it is opened.
- Do not open any file sent to you unless you were expecting that file from someone you know and trust. If you do, the file will execute as soon as it is open, and if it contains a harmful or destructive virus or worm, you will infect your system and anyone else you may e-mail.
- Never "double-click" on an attachment that arrives in e-mail unless you are specifically expecting that (and only that) attachment. As noted previously, attachments may be executable, even if you think that you are simply opening a picture.
- Do not use macros in Microsoft application programs unless they come from a known source. Macros are common vehicles for introducing viruses into Microsoft systems.
- Make sure that your administrator has a solid backup plan that can restore your operating system and essential programs in an emergency. Make sure that he or she keeps these backup copies readily available and updated to reflect the most recent operating system and program updates.
- Those working with essential operating systems, such as dispatch centers, should have an expert evaluate their computers for the presence of covert back doors that allow other intrusions.
- Those working with essential operating systems should require that known uninfected working copies of all necessary software be immediately available should a disruption occur. Trained personnel who are able to revive the computer system should be on duty and in-house 24 hours a day for just this type of problem.

Perhaps the most important action is to report any suspicious e-mail or unusual computer activity to the person in charge, the system administrator, or other designated person. Establish an on-call point-of-contact to your Internet service providers and appropriate law enforcement officials should you discover a launching of a cyberattack by either someone in your organization or an external operator. Remember that the Mountain View, California, attacks were discovered by astute and observant local operators.

■ Denial of Service Attack

A **denial of service (DoS)** attack is not a virus but a method hackers use to prevent or deny legitimate users access to computers or servers. The loss of service may be as simple as the inability of a particular network service to use e-mail, or the loss of all network connectivity and services for every computer attached to the Internet in any way.

The most common kind of DoS attack is simply to send more traffic to a network address than the programmers who planned its data buffers anticipated. The attacker may be aware that the target system has a weakness that can be exploited, or the attacker may simply try the attack, not knowing if it will work.

For a good example, imagine a terrorist creates a program that calls 9-1-1. The 9-1-1 operator answers the telephone, but learns that it is a prank call. If the program repeats this task continuously, it prevents legitimate customers from using 9-1-1, because the telephone line is busy. This is a denial of service, and it is analogous to a DoS attack.

Many DoS attack tools are also capable of executing a **distributed DoS (DDoS)** attack. For example, imagine that the terrorist secretly plants his or her program onto many computers on the Internet. This would create a bigger impact, because there would be more computers calling the 9-1-1 operators. It would also be more difficult to locate the attacker, because the program would not run from the attacker's computer; the attacker would only control the computer that originally had the program secretly installed.

In the worst case, a DoS attack can force an Internet-connected site to cease operation. If this were a critical control system, the organization would lose the use of the control function. A DoS attack can also destroy programming and files in a computer system. However, a DoS attack is a type of security breach to a computer system that does not usually result in the theft of information or other security loss. Although usually intentional and malicious, a DoS attack can sometimes happen accidentally.

How Can Antivirus Software Help Against DoS?

Using a virus, the DoS attack tools can be secretly installed onto a large number of innocent computer systems. Systems that unknowingly have DoS attack tools installed are called **zombie** agents or **drones**. These zombie systems can be centrally managed by a hacker to initiate DoS attacks at targeted computers. Zombies are not the victims of the DoS attack, but they are used to perform the actual attack.

Antivirus software detects viruses that can inject the DoS agents, but it does not detect the DoS attacks. By extracting a pattern or a signature from known zombie agents, antivirus products can detect malevolent software on the compromised system. Antivirus software may also detect when a hacker is secretly installing zombie agents.

It is difficult to trace the origin of the request packets in a DoS attack, especially if it is a distributed DoS attack. It is impossible to prevent all DoS attacks, but there are precautions server administrators can take to decrease the risk of being compromised by a DoS attack. These precautions are beyond the scope of this chapter. However, by keeping your antivirus software up to date and using good computing practices as listed previously, you can keep your system from becoming a zombie and aiding a DoS attack.

■ Attacks Against the Power Supply

Brute Force Attacks

Attacks against the power supply are a method of sabotage that precedes World War II. The US military has long recognized the critical importance of power supplies to an industrialized country. Significant strategic bombing targets in

New York City

On a hot, humid afternoon in August 2003, millions of people in the northeastern United States and parts of southern Canada experienced what has been called the most widespread power outage in North American history. Starting at approximately 4:00 PM eastern standard time, power went out from parts of Connecticut, New York, and New Jersey, all the way west to Michigan and north to Ontario. The outages caused severe disruptions in the communications, transit, and economic systems in the affected areas. With the tragic events of September 11, 2001 still fresh in the minds of many North Americans, many initially feared that the power outage was the result of terrorism. However, government officials quickly ruled out terrorist acts as the cause.

World War II were dams (for hydroelectric power), generator plants, and power distribution systems.

The United States has become more dependent on electrical power for EMS operations, EMS communications, and multiple services and diagnostic devices within the hospitals. If a command and control system has no electricity, it is simply wire, metal, and plastic, not a functioning system. One only has to examine the consequences of accidental power supply disruptions to graphically illustrate this point.

Although emergency power supplies exist for each of the critical systems such as hospitals, EMS communications, police and fire communications and dispatching, and high-rise elevator systems, the usual duration of emergency power is about 24 hours. Shortly after this, the emergency power supplies will run out of fuel, backup generators will exceed maximum safe continuous operating times, or emergency battery supplies will be exhausted.

Attacks against the power supply system may be combined with other attacks to increase disruption. The attacks may be as simple as a person-portable bomb placed against a critically located transformer or as complex as deliberate sabotage or attack on a nuclear power plant. The latter is, of course, feared because of the possibility of radiation release, which is covered in Chapter 14.

In the 1991 Gulf War, cruise missiles with "soft bombs" were extensively employed in Iraq. These soft bombs sprayed conductive graphite wire and metal shards over open-air transformer switching yards that connected power stations to the electrical distribution grid. When the graphite threads fell onto the electrical wires of the switching stations, they would short out the power lines and send surges of electricity through the power grid.

The idea for these soft bombs apparently grew out of a training accident in southern California. Military aircraft were dropping "chaff"—hundreds of metallic strips used to confuse enemy radar. An airplane released its chaff near a power switching station and many of the strips fell onto a power switching station, blacking out a large area of Orange County, California.[8] These bombs have been used in Iraq, Kosovo, and Serbia.

This technique of power supply disruption has been experienced by many sponsors of terrorism. There is no question that this lesson has been learned by those who teach terrorism. There should be no question that this will be a target of future terrorists. Improvisational devices, such as aluminum coated Mylar strips and metallic kite wires, may be used to effect this kind of disruption.

■ Electromagnetic Pulse Devices

When detonated, an electromagnetic pulse (EMP) weapon (also known as an E-bomb) generates a pulse of energy capable of short-circuiting a wide range of electronic equipment, including computers, radios, and public utility power supplies **(Figure 15-1)**.

First described in 1870 by Heinrich Hertz, the EMP effect was again noted after early experiments with nuclear weapons. When the nuclear weapon explodes, it also produces a brief EMP (measured in nanoseconds) that radiates away from the bomb like a shock wave.

This very short pulse of electromagnetic energy can produce short-lived transient voltages, measured in thousands of volts, on exposed electrical conductors, such as wires, electronic chips, and the conductive tracks on printed circuit boards. These transient voltages can destroy or "wound" the electronic circuitry within a device. A wounded device may still function, but its reliability may be seriously impaired. It may keep working intermittently, which could be more disturbing than a complete breakdown.

The EMP device is only effective in a finite area around the device. The calculation of electromagnetic field strength at a given radius for a given device is not difficult. Determining the probability of an "electronic kill" is much more difficult. A large device may destroy all communications and semiconductor devices for several miles in a swath extending in all directions from the weapon.

The lethality of an EMP devise to electronic equipment is determined by the power generated and by the characteristics of the pulse. The shorter pulse waveforms, such as microwaves, are far more effective against electronic equipment and are more difficult to protect against. A short pulse is more dangerous, because it produces greater power for a given amount of weapon energy and can produce a broader frequency spectrum. The broad frequency spectrum improves the coupling of energy into the targeted devices.

Equipment with an antenna, designed to conduct power in or out of the device, is particularly vulnerable to EMPs. This is often called **front door coupling**. The power flow from the EMP weapon is readily able to enter the system and cause damage through the antenna and connections. The best energy transfer occurs when the wavelength of the pulse is close to the wavelength of the antenna or a multiple of the antenna's length. UHF and VHF radio receivers, televisions, and cell phones are all vulnerable to the effects of EMP through front door coupling.

Today, most receivers use computer controlled frequency synthesizers. Many of them advertise this fact by dis-

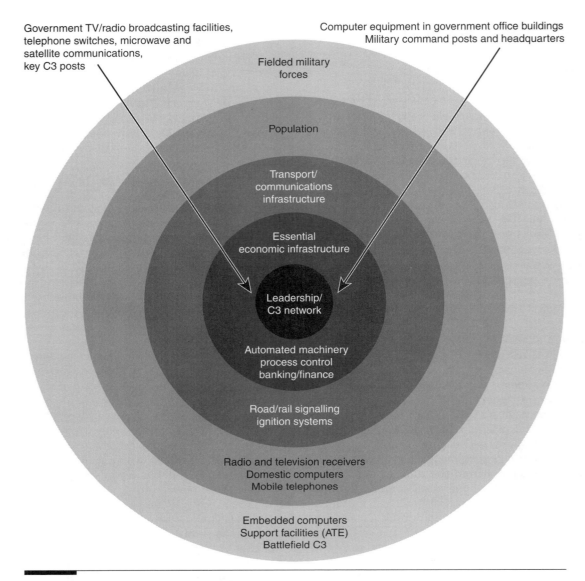

Government TV/radio broadcasting facilities, telephone switches, microwave and satellite communications, key C3 posts

Computer equipment in government office buildings
Military command posts and headquarters

Fielded military forces

Population

Transport/communications infrastructure

Essential economic infrastructure

Leadership/C3 network

Automated machinery process control banking/finance

Road/rail signalling ignition systems

Radio and television receivers
Domestic computers
Mobile telephones

Embedded computers
Support facilities (ATE)
Battlefield C3

Figure 15-1 Warden's "five rings" strategic air attack model in the context of electromagnetically vulnerable target sets. (John Warden III is the author of Operation Thunder, the strategic bombing plan used in 1991 in the Gulf War.)

playing words like *PLL, synthesized,* or *quartz* on their front panels or in the advertising literature. These computer controlled synthesizers offer tremendous advantages to the operation of a receiver. Not only do they enable receivers to have the same stability as the quartz reference, but they also enable many other facilities to be introduced, because they can easily be controlled by a microprocessor. This enables facilities such as multiple memories, keypad frequency entry, scanning, and much more to be incorporated into the set.

Back door coupling occurs when the electromagnetic field from the weapon produces a large transient current in the wiring infrastructure that connects to the device. This can include telephone lines, networking cables, and power lines. For a car's computer, the spark plug wires, the connecting wires from the sensors to the computer, and the power wires from battery and alternator to the computer are sufficient means for the pulse to enter the car's computer.

Anyone who lives in a lightning-prone area of the country is familiar with a much milder EMP associated with a lightning strike to the local power grid that can destroy computers, televisions, and phones. These lightning-derived pulses are longer and buffered by circuits in the power grid designed to mute the electromagnetic spike. This surge down the power grid is equivalent to back door coupling.

The deployment of the weapon causing this effect is easy, because at least a few of the connecting wires will be properly oriented to absorb some of the electromagnetic energy. Electrical equipment, consumer electronic goods, computers, and communication equipment will be extensively damaged by back door coupling.

There are four basic types of EMP weapons: nuclear weapons, propellant driven magnetohydrodynamic generators, explosively pumped flux compression generators, and high-power microwave generators (based on virtual cathode ray oscillator or viractor technology).

Nuclear Weapons

The EMP effect was first observed and associated with nuclear weapons in 1962, when a 1.4-megaton nuclear weapon was detonated 400 km above the mid-Pacific ocean. The pulse from this explosion destroyed radios and satellite equipment, and the ionization effects of the bomb blocked high-frequency radio communications for 30 minutes. This EMP incident resulted in power system failures as far away as Hawaii.

A high-altitude nuclear detonation produces an immediate flux of gamma rays from the nuclear reactions within the device. These photons in turn produce high-energy free electrons by Compton scattering at altitudes between (roughly) 20 and 40 km. These electrons are then trapped in the Earth's magnetic field, giving rise to an oscillating electric current. This current is asymmetric in general and produces the EMP. Because the electrons are trapped essentially simultaneously, a very large electromagnetic source radiates coherently.

The pulse can easily span continent-sized areas, and this radiation can affect systems on land, sea, and air. A large device detonated at 400 to 500 km over Kansas would affect all of the continental United States. The signal from such an event extends to the visual horizon as seen from the burst point.

At lower levels, the effects of a nuclear weapon's detonation on electronics are somewhat different. Source region electromagnetic pulse (SREMP) is produced by low-altitude nuclear bursts. A vertical electron current is formed by the asymmetric deposition of electrons in the atmosphere and in the ground from the nuclear explosion, and the formation and decay of this current emits a pulse of electromagnetic radiation. A low-altitude explosion produces an asymmetric pulse, because some electrons emitted downward are trapped in the Earth's surface, while others, moving upward and outward, can travel long distances in the atmosphere, producing ionization and charge separation.

Within the source region, peak electric fields greater than 10^5 V/m and peak magnetic fields greater than 4,000 A/m can exist. These pulse amplitudes are much larger than those from high-altitude nuclear explosions or from lightning strikes and pose a considerable threat to all civilian computer systems and much of the electronic equipment in the affected region. The ground provides a return path for electrons at the outer part of the deposition region toward the burst point. Positive ions, which travel shorter distances than electrons and at lower velocities, remain behind and recombine with the electrons returning through the ground. Thus, strong magnetic fields are also produced in the region of ground zero.

When the nuclear detonation occurs near to the ground, the SREMP target may not be located in the electromagnetic far field, but may instead lie within the electromagnetic induction region. As a result, the region where the greatest damage can be produced is from about 3 to 8 km from ground zero. In this same region, structures housing electrical equipment are also likely to be severely damaged by blast and shock.

Magnetohydrodynamic Generators

The technology of explosive and propellant driven magnetohydrodynamic (MHD) generators is not well discussed in the open-source literature. MHD generator technology has been extensively explored by the former Soviet Union. It has not yet been used in a weapon system.

The major advantage of MHD generators is their lack of moving parts and their compactness. The major research effort of the Russians was focused on the potential of the MHD generator as a compact source of electrical energy, rather than as a weapon system.

Flux Compression Generators

To generate a seriously powerful one-off pulse, old-fashioned explosives are perhaps the best energy source. The energy stored in a kiloton or two of TNT can be turned into a huge pulse of microwaves by using a device called a flux compressor. This device uses the energy of an explosion to cram a current and its magnetic field into an ever-smaller volume. Sending this pulse into an antenna creates a deadly burst of radiowaves and microwaves.

Simplicity is one of the flux compressor's big attractions for military strategists and terrorists alike. These flux compression generator (FCG) EMP devices are highly portable and can even be operated from a distance.

The device consists of a cylindrical copper tube filled with a fast, high-energy explosive, surrounded by a helical coil of heavy copper wire, which has a horn antenna attached at the far end (**Figure 15-2**). A capacitor is discharged into the coil to produce an initial magnetic field just before the explosives are detonated.

Setting off the detonator triggers the explosive, sending the explosion hurtling along the tube at almost 5,400 m/sec. A structural jacket of a nonmagnetic material contains the coil as the explosion progresses. Before the explosive pressure wave begins to shatter the device, the blast flares out the inner metal tube. The distorted metal makes contact with the coil, causing a short circuit that diverts the current—and the magnetic field it generates—into the undisturbed coil ahead of it. As the explosion proceeds down the tube, the magnetic field is squeezed into a smaller and smaller volume. Compressing the magnetic field this way creates a huge rise in current in the coil ahead of the explosion, building a mega-amp pulse just 500 picoseconds wide. Finally, just before the whole weapon is destroyed in the blast, the current pulse flows into the antenna, which radiates its electromagnetic energy outwards. The whole process is over in less than a tenth of a millisecond, but in that tenth of a millisecond, a terawatt of power is generated and radiated.

A small FCG can be used to start the current in a larger device. In this case, the current pulse flows into a larger coil just before the explosives in the large device are detonated, repeating the process above on a huge scale. At its peak, a large FCG device may produce tens of terawatts of power, or more than a thousand lightning strikes.

Weapons that utilize this technique produce most of the power in the frequencies below 1 MHz, making it difficult to focus the energy. Detonating the EMP in the air or near the

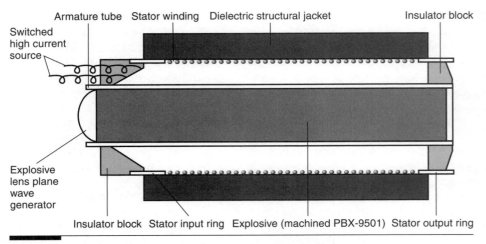

Figure 15-2 Theoretical construction details of a FCG EMP generator.

top floors of a skyscraper maximizes the effects of the weapon.

These weapons are quite inexpensive and simple. The electronics and explosives, although not usually available at your local electronics parts emporium, are much easier to procure than any type of nuclear materials. Any nation or large terrorist group that has the engineering drawings and specifications for these weapons could easily produce them for as little as $2,000 apiece.[9] Considering that both Russia and China, major players in this field, are struggling under economic difficulties, the proliferation of these devices is very real.

High-Power Microwave Generators

High-power microwave (HPM) sources have been under investigation for several years as potential weapons for a variety of combat, sabotage, and terrorist applications. Because of classification restrictions, details of this work are relatively unknown outside of the military community and its contractors. Sometimes these weapons are also called high-energy radio frequency weapons.

The most straightforward HPM weapon is a viractor (virtual cathode-ray oscillator) attached to a large capacitor bank to provide a current spike through it. Other devices that could be used to produce HPMs include the magnetron (a device present in every microwave oven), the klystron, and the reflex triode.

The basic viractor produces a very powerful electron beam that is aimed against a mesh anode within a tube. Many electrons will pass through the anode and form a bubble of space charge—the virtual cathode—behind the anode. If the virtual cathode is placed in a tuned resonant cavity, very high-power microwaves can be generated. The viractor is a small, mechanically simple, and robust device that is capable of producing a very powerful pulse of radiation from 170 kW to over 40 GW in microwave frequencies. The duration of the output pulse is limited by the melting of the anode **(Figure 15-3)**.

The viractor is particularly important, because the output can be focused and has the ability to couple into equipment through ventilation holes in shielding, gaps between

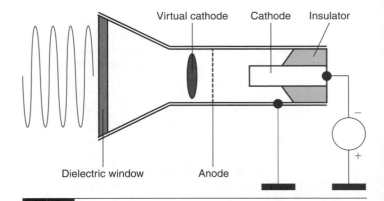

Figure 15-3 Viractor.

shielding panels, and poorly shielded interfaces. A key point to recognize is the insidious nature of HPM. Because of the gigahertz-band frequencies (4 to 20 GHz) involved, HPM has the capability to penetrate through the antenna, but also through minute shielding leaks throughout the equipment.

There are various reports that a small portable version of this could be used by the police to stop cars by burning out their engine-control computers.[10] Other reports speculate that criminals have used these devices to destroy security electronics in banks or warehouses, prior to robbing them.

Implications

EMP and HPM weapons pose a significant threat against electronic equipment that is susceptible to damage by transient power surges. The EMP weapon is a weapon of mass destruction that is particularly tuned to the weaknesses of a modern, computer-reliant city. The conventional EMP and HMP weapons can disable nonshielded electronic devices within the effective range of the weapon. (Most military-grade radios and electronic equipment are designed to resist some levels of EMP, but civilian equipment is not adequately shielded for this type of attack.)

Commercial computer equipment circuits are particularly susceptible to EMP (even circuits that are contained in ignition systems in cars and trucks and those that operate traffic lights). These circuits are often made of high-density metal oxide semiconductor (MOS) devices, which are very sensitive to exposure to high-voltage transients. Very little energy is required to permanently destroy a MOS device.

Computers used in data processing systems, communications systems, displays, and industrial control applications, including road and rail signaling and those imbedded in vehicles, cardiac monitors, digital engine controls, electronic flight controls, and signal processors (found in many types of modern radio equipment) are all vulnerable to the effects of EMP through back door coupling. Computer networks are particularly susceptible, because the hundreds of feet of cabling connecting their workstations can act as an efficient radiowave receiving antenna.

The electronic control module of modern cars and most trucks is a computer. The 1970 EPA requirements for reduced emissions was the driving force that prompted the shift to electronically controlled engines and the introduction of computers into almost all vehicles. These computers are found in all modern fire trucks and ambulances—whether diesel or gasoline powered. The computer system tells the engine when to feed fuel and air to the cylinders. It also gives and receives signals to and from engine sensors to find the best fuel economy.

US federal laws regarding computer engine controls in vehicles started with the requirement of an oxygen sensor in 1982. The first was the IM-240 federal regulation. The IM-240 federal regulation has since been enhanced from the original OBD (on-board diagnostics) regulation to the current OBD-II federal regulation (which is applicable for 2003 US vehicles as well as vehicles around the world as mandated by European OBD). These mandatory on-board computers would be disabled by an EMP and the vehicle would no longer run.

Because of the universal reliance on electronics in the United States, EMP weapons could cripple an EMS system that is dependent on computers, computer networks, and electronic communications systems. This damage from the burnout or overload of the electronic circuits would extend far beyond the area directly affected by the blast and radiation of a nuclear weapon.

In such an attack, civilian airliners may be lost. In short, pilots will lose communication, navigation aids, landing lights, and, in some cases, even the ability to control the aircraft after electronic fly-by-wire circuits are destroyed by a massive EMP. The pilot's instrumentation may display incorrect readings, and displays may blank out at critical times. It is unknown whether the nation's air traffic control system has been "hardened" against EMP.[11] The extent of the risk to Federal Aviation Administration systems from EMP is probably (and appropriately) classified.

Although the initial design is technologically difficult, EMP technology can be harnessed by those who have only basic engineering and technical skills. EMP weapons can be built with materials that are available to governments and terrorists alike. Fully developed, ready-to-deploy weapons may be available to clandestine markets at any time. Reports state that at least one country, India, has built such a weapon "for peaceful purposes." Because the United States has actually deployed such a weapon, it is quite possible that the design is available to terrorist nations today. (The United States deployed an EMP weapon in Operation Desert Storm that was designed to mimic the flash of electricity from a nuclear bomb.)

Future advances may provide the compactness needed to weaponize the capability in a bomb or missile warhead. Currently, the effective radius of the weapon is not as great as nuclear EMP effects. Open-source literature indicates that effective radii of "hundreds of meters or more" are possible.

■ Implications and Protective Measures

It is difficult to protect against an EMP without purchasing military-grade communications equipment. It should also be noted that electromagnetic weapons can be sneaky. The perpetrators don't have to destroy every electronic device in sight. Instead, they can hit just hard enough to make electronics crash. The military calls this a soft kill—the damage is done without the victim ever knowing it.

Criminals may have already used microwave weapons, according to Bob Gardner, who chairs the Electromagnetic Noise and Interference Commission of the International Union of Radio Science in Ghent, Belgium.[12] Reports from Russia suggest that these devices have been used to disable bank security systems and to disrupt police communications. Another report suggests a London bank may also have been attacked in this way. Although these incidents are hard to prove, they are perfectly plausible. "If you're asking whether it's technologically reasonable that someone could do something like this," says Gardner, "then the answer is yes."[13]

Some anti-EMP measures that EMS providers can take are as follows:

1. The only reliable protection against EMP emitters is accomplished by completely encasing susceptible equipment in a heavy-gauge metal shielding or surrounding it with a special metal screening—the Faraday cage **(Figure 15-4)**. A Faraday cage can be made from fine metal mesh. This cage is connected to a ground and completely encloses the items it protects. If any power cables, data cables, or antennae penetrate the cage, the protection may be worthless. Keep all equipment in the cage disconnected from batteries and other power supplies.

2. Maintain a supply of spare radio, monitor, and engine ignition spare parts. Keep the spare parts in a Faraday cage. Smaller pieces of equipment can be placed in empty, metal military ammunition containers or similar tightly sealed metal boxes.

3. Use one system at a time during a threat period. Disconnect other systems from power and antennas and keep them in the Faraday cage.

4. If your vehicle ignition fails, disconnect the negative battery terminal, wait 2 minutes, reconnect the terminal, and attempt to restart the vehicle. Some computerized ignition systems on late-model cars might possibly be reset in this way.

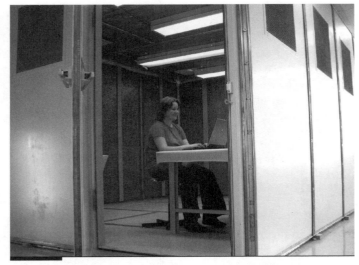

Figure 15-4 Faraday cage with computer inside. During operation, the door is closed. The Faraday cage is ineffective when the door is open.

Equipment that has been shielded or hardened against electromagnetic discharges may withstand higher electromagnetic fields. Radios and other equipment that use vacuum tube technology will be spared, as these circuits are not damaged by EMP.

There is no doubt that system hardening is a must to avoid damage to any part of the electromagnetic equipment; however, hardening has its limitations. New equipment may be hardened by design. Older equipment may be impossible to harden.

Because the development and deployment of EMP weapons is at an early stage, no one really knows what the total effect is going to be. Only with retrospective data or the release of military data compiled during the development of the weapons can we effectively plan preparedness for these weapons.

■ Directed Energy Weapons

Directed energy weapons include microwave radiation emitters, particle beam generators, and lasers. Directed energy weapons rely on electromagnetic waves or subatomic particles that impact at or near the speed of light. Several of these weapons have already been tested in combat and may be available to terrorists in the very near future.

Lasers

In 1954, the maser (microwave amplification by stimulated emission of radiation) was invented by Charles Townes and Arthur Schawlow. Using ammonia and microwave radiation, they created the maser well before theorizing the laser (light amplification by stimulated emission of radiation) in 1958. The technology of the maser is very similar to the laser, but it does not use a visible light. Gordon Gould was the first person to use the word *laser* in 1957.

There is good reason to believe that Gordon Gould made the first light laser. (He holds patent numbers 4,053,845 and 4,704,583 for optically pumped laser amplifiers; these are

light amplifiers that employ collisions to produce a population inversion laser.) Following his work on the Manhattan project, Gould was a doctoral student at Columbia University under Charles Townes, the inventor of the maser. Gordon Gould was first inspired to build his optical laser in 1958. In 1960, while working as a section head at Hughes Research Laboratories, Theodore Maiman created the ruby laser, which is considered by some to be the first successful optical or light laser.

Laser Background

There are multiple techniques for producing a laser, including the use of gas, crystals, or semiconducting diodes. All of these techniques have a similar basic construction.

You can see all of the components of laser construction in **Figure 15-5,** which illustrates how a simple **ruby laser** works. The laser consists of a flash tube (like those found on cameras), a ruby rod, and two mirrors (one half-silvered). The ruby rod is the lasing medium, and the flash tube pumps the laser.

The following occurs to form laser light with the ruby laser **(Figure 15-6)**:

1. The flash tube (pump) fires and injects light into the ruby rod. The light excites atoms in the ruby.
2. Some of these atoms emit photons.
3. Some of these photons are emitted in a direction parallel to the ruby rod's axis, so they bounce back and forth between the mirrors. As these photons bounce back and forth through the crystal, they stimulate emission in other atoms.
4. When enough photons are emitted, the light will pass through the half-silvered mirror. This will be monochromatic, single-phase, collimated light— laser light.

Laser light has special qualities **(Figure 15-7)**:

■ The light released is monochromatic, meaning it contains one specific wavelength of light or one specific color. The wavelength of light is determined by the amount of energy released when the electron

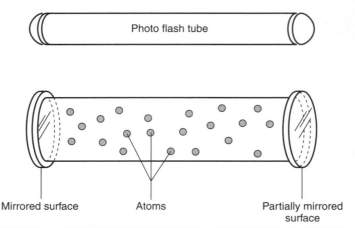

Figure 15-5 A ruby laser consists of a flash tube, a ruby rod, and two mirrors.

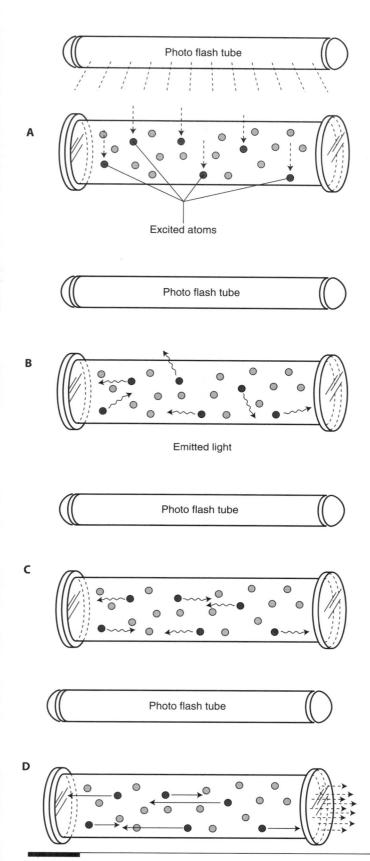

Figure 15-6 **A.** The flash tube fires and injects light into the ruby rod. The light excites atoms in the ruby. **B.** Some of these atoms emit photons. **C.** Some photons are emitted and bounce off the mirrors. **D.** Light passes through the half-silvered mirror, forming a laser.

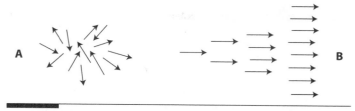

Figure 15-7 A. Irregular nature of normal light, for example, from a light bulb. **B.** Coherent nature of laser light.

drops to a lower orbit. This wavelength depends on the material of the laser and the method by which it was stimulated to emit light.

- The light released is coherent, meaning it is "organized"—each photon moves in step with the others. (The waves of the electromagnetic radiation are in phase in both space and time.) This means that all of the photons have wave fronts that launch in unison.
- The light is very directional. A laser light has a very tight beam and is very strong and concentrated. A lightbulb, on the other hand, releases light in many directions, and the light is very weak and diffuse.
- The design of the laser device makes the beam parallel.
- Finally, laser light does not disperse over long distances because of this parallel nature (collimation) of the laser beam.

In 1990, the International Red Cross developed a useful classification of lasers that have been developed for use on the battlefield or in industrial settings. The material that the laser is made of determines the frequency and, to some extent, the available power. All lasers are classified by the manufacturer and labeled with the appropriate warning labels. The following criteria are used to classify lasers:

1. **Wavelength** is considered for all lasers. If the laser is designed to emit multiple wavelengths, the classification is based on the most hazardous wavelength.
2. For continuous wave or repetitively pulsed lasers, the **average power** output (in watts) and **limiting exposure time** inherent in the design are considered.
3. For pulsed lasers, the **total energy per pulse** (in joules), **pulse duration**, **pulse repetition frequency**, and **emergent beam radiant exposure** are considered.

Tables 15-1 and **15-2** list two different classifications of lasers. **Table 15-3** lists types of lasers.

Immediately after the development of the first functional laser, the military (and hence terrorist) potential of the laser was apparent. Modern pulsed lasers can reach energy levels of up to millions of watts in a fraction of a second **(Figure 15-8)**.

Eye Injuries

The eye is the part of the body that is most vulnerable to laser hazards. Eye damage can occur at much lower power levels than the level that affects the skin. This damage may be either

Table 15-1 Laser Classification

Class 1 Lasers	Lasers that are not hazardous for continuous viewing or are designed in such a way that human access to laser radiation is prevented. These consist of low-power lasers (up to 0.4 μW) or higher power embedded lasers. There may be a more hazardous laser embedded in the enclosure of a class 1 product, but no harmful radiation can escape from the enclosure (eg, laser printers).
Class 2 Visible Lasers (400 to 700 nm)	Lasers emitting visible light which, because of normal human aversion responses, do not normally present a hazard, but would if viewed directly for extended periods of time (like many conventional light sources). Laser pointers fit in this classification.
Class 2a Visible Lasers (400 to 700 nm)	Lasers emitting visible light that is not intended for viewing, and under normal operating conditions would not produce an injury to the eye if viewed directly for less than 1,000 seconds (eg, bar code scanners).
Class 3a	Lasers that normally would not cause injury to the eye if viewed momentarily, but would present a hazard if viewed using collecting optics (fiberoptics loupe or telescope). Many military targeting lasers would fit in this class. These lasers have power ranging from 1 to 5 mW and are considered a "marginal eye hazard."
Class 3b	Lasers that present an eye and skin hazard if viewed directly. This includes both intrabeam viewing and specular reflections. Class 3b lasers do not produce a hazardous diffuse reflection except when viewed at close proximity. Class 3b lasers have power ratings from 5 to 500 mW and are considered "significant eye hazards."
Class 4 Lasers	Lasers that present an eye hazard from direct, specular, and diffuse reflections. Class 4 lasers are dangerous to both skin and eyes. In addition, such lasers may be fire hazards.

Adapted from: http://web.princeton.edu/sites/ehs/laserguide/sec2.htm; Laser safety at http://web.princeton.edu/sites/ehs/laserguide/sec2.htm; Laser safety background at http://www.femto.sims.nrc.ca/LaserSafety/lsafety7.htm; The Royal School of Artillery at www.atra.mod.uk/atra/rsabst/pdf/G-Electro-Optics/G02-SAFE.pdf. Accessed March 22, 2004.

Table 15-2 International Committee of the Red Cross Battlefield Laser Classification[14]

Category A Lasers	Systems not designed primarily for antipersonnel use, but which under battlefield conditions may present an ocular hazard.
Subcategory A1	Range finders, target designators, laser target markers, optical radar systems (LIDAR). Most laser range finders are NOT eye-safe.
Subcategory A2	Sighting, training, simulation, and other small, portable systems. An example of a subcategory A2 system is the day/night laser sight clipped to the barrel of a pistol, where the light spot shows the place of bullet impact.
Category B	Antisensor systems. These systems are designed to find, block, or destroy enemy optical viewing, scanning, ranging, guiding, and communications systems. The risk of injury to the unprotected eye from a category B system is extremely high. Examples of US category B systems are the Stingray, Dazer, and Cobra.
Category C	Antipersonnel systems. Antipersonnel systems are specifically designed to harm the individual—in this case, to injure the eyes. Most information about these systems is classified. An exception that shows the nature of the category is the British Navy's Laser Dazzle Sight (LDS). This system was employed on British naval vessels and was used in the Falklands War in 1982. It is important to realize that the energy and wavelength capable of dazzling the eye at 5 km may blind at 1 km. The Chinese 33-kg ZM-87 portable laser disturber is marketed on the international market as a weapon against both soldiers and sensors. The target market for the Chinese ZM-87 is the Third World.
Category D	Antimaterial systems. The tactical laser and the American Space Defense Initiative weapons are examples of such systems. These systems do not just cause eye injury; they may kill.
Category E	Nonlaser intense light systems. These systems include searchlights, aircraft landing lights, and strobe lights. These systems may cause damage to eyes or skin from the intensity of the light at close ranges.

temporary or permanent, depending on the wavelength and the power of the laser. Because the eye is more sensitive and the pupil is larger during darkness, laser weapons have a greater effect at night than during the day. Generally, eye injuries are far more serious than injuries to the skin.

Laser weapons concentrate intense light and heat upon a target. Depending on the power of the laser, this light can burn out optical devices or permanently blind those who operate them. If the person is using a see-through optical device such as binoculars, the beam strength is magnified and greater injury to the eye can result. Even modestly powered lasers can temporarily blind an unprotected person looking through a telescope. Higher power lasers can be used to destroy objects in flight or on the ground.

The human eye is a complex optical system. It is designed to transmit, focus, and detect light. Light passes into the front portion of the eye through the cornea. The light that enters is focused on a spot in the back of the eye (the retina). There it forms an image on cells that are specifically designed to detect light.

The cornea is the outermost, transparent layer of the eye. The cornea can withstand dust, sand, and other envi-

Table 15-3 Types of Lasers*

The following table gives details of a selection of the most important lasing materials and corresponding types of laser. The list of potential applications is far from complete.
The shaded rows represent the effective wavelength of solitary colored lasers. A white row means that many colors are found.

	Wavelength	Power	Operating Mode	Applications
Semiconductor diode lasers				
Single diodes	Infrared to visible	1 mW–100 mW	Continuous and pulsed modes	Optoelectronics: DVD, CD, etc.
Diode laser bars	Infrared to visible	Up to 100 W	Continuous and pulsed modes	Pumping light source for solid-state lasers
Solid-state lasers				
Nd:YAG laser	1.06 μm Near infrared	1 W–3 kW	Continuous and pulsed modes	Materials processing, measurementation, medicine
Ruby laser	Red	Several MW	Pulsed mode	Measurementation, pulse holography
Gas lasers				
CO_2 laser	10.6 μm Farr infrared	1 W–40 kW (100 MW in pulsed mode)	Continuous and pulsed modes	Materials processing, medicine, isotope separation
Excimer laser	193 nm, 248 nm, 308 nm (and others)	1 kW–100 MW	Pulsed mode 10 ns–100 ns	Micro-machining, laser chemistry, medicine
HeNe laser	632.8 nm (most prominent)	1 mW–1 W	Continuous mode	Measurementation, holography
Argon ion laser	515 458 nm (several)	1 mW–150 W	Continuous and pulsed modes	Printing technology, pumping laser for dye laser stimulation, medicine
Dye laser	Continuous between infrared and ultraviolet (different dyes)	1 mw–1 W	Continuous and pulsed modes	Measurementation, spectroscopy, medicine

Adapted from: Fraunhofer ILT-Laser-Tutorial.htm, accessed August 18, 2003.

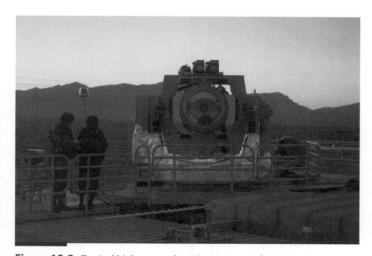

Figure 15-8 Tactical high-energy laser (static mount for testing).

ronmental hazards. The corneal cells grow quite rapidly and replace themselves within about 48 hours. This means that mild injuries to the cornea heal rapidly.

The aqueous humor is a thick liquid between the cornea and the lens. The water in the aqueous humor absorbs heat, so that it protects the internal parts of the eye from thermal radiation.

The lens of the eye is a flexible tissue that changes shape to focus light on the back of the eye. When the lens changes shape, it allows the eye to focus on both near and far objects.

The iris controls the amount of light that enters the eye. The iris is the pigmented part of the eye that adjusts to light intensity by contracting or dilating. The change in the iris size adjusts the size of the pupil, which controls the amount of light that enters the eye.

The retina is the light-sensitive area at the back of the eye. The retina contains two types of photoreceptor cells: rods and cones. These cells convert the optical image on the retina into electric signals. The optic nerve carries these electric signals to the brain.

The fovea is the most sensitive, central portion of the retina. It is the area of the retina that is responsible for detailed vision. When the fovea is destroyed by a laser beam (or any other means), the person is rendered legally blind, because detailed vision is lost.

The vitreous humor is a colorless gel that fills the area between the iris and the retina. The vitreous humor does not replace itself if it leaks out of the eye, so a perforation that results in a vitreous humor leak can cause permanent blindness.

Laser-induced eye injuries occur with a severity that depends on the exposure dose and the location of the expo-

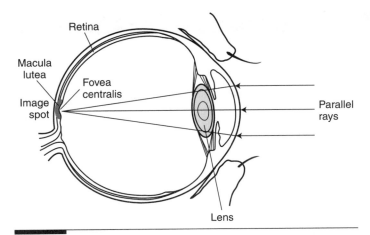

Figure 15-9 The effects of a laser beam are magnified by the optics of the eye.

sure within the eye. The exposure dose to the eye tissue depends on the nature of the laser beam and the atmosphere that it traverses. The nature of the laser beam includes the pulse energy, the pulse duration, and the wavelength of the laser. The atmosphere that it traverses also affects the energy delivered by the laser; factors include the range, the water content of the atmosphere, atmospheric turbulence, and pollution.

The light intensity of the image formed on the retina is 100,000 times greater than the light intensity received at the front of the eye. It is this considerable optical gain that creates an eye hazard when a laser beam enters the eye (**Figure 15-9**). When a person is exposed to laser light, the person can become temporarily blinded (dazzling), become blinded for a prolonged time (photolysis), or suffer permanent changes in visual function from retinal lesions or hemorrhages.

The potential for eye injuries is increased when lasers are used in open, uncontrolled environments. Complaints of disruption of vision or visual performance by laser glare from laser aiming devices, entertainment lasers at concerts, or outdoor laser displays are becoming more common. These laser exposures have temporarily blinded commercial pilots of both helicopters and fixed-wing aircraft.[15,16]

Treatment There is no currently accepted treatment for laser or light-induced eye injuries. A laser eye injury can worsen with time, so anyone with a suspected laser eye injury should be evaluated promptly and then again at regular intervals. The patient with a laser eye injury may experience sharp eye pain, sudden loss of vision, streaky or spotty vision, or disorientation. The damage to the eye tissue may vary with the wavelength of the laser.

Wavelengths of various types of lasers are listed in **Table 15-4.** This table is far from complete as new lasers are developed almost daily. The shading of the row roughly shows the location on the spectrum of the laser's wavelength. **Figure 15-10** shows the spectrum of light and where different types of light fall in terms of wavelength.

Far-infrared radiation, which ranges from 3,000 nm to 1 mm, is absorbed primarily by the cornea (**Figure 15-11**). A high-energy laser pulse may severely burn or perforate the cornea. Severe burns or perforations should not be patched,

Table 15-4 Laser Wavelengths*

Lasing Medium	Laser Type	Wavelength
FAR INFRARED		
CO$_2$	Gas	10,600 nm
NEAR INFRARED		
HeNe	Gas	1,152 nm
Argon	Gas-Ion	1,090 nm
Nd:YAG	Solid State	1,064 nm
InGaAs	Semiconductor	980 nm
Krypton	Gas-Ion	799.3 nm
Cr:LiSAF	Solid State	780-1,060 nm
GaAs/GaAlAs	Semiconductor	780-905 nm
Krypton	Gas-Ion	752.5 nm
Ti:Sapphire	Solid State	700-1,000 nm
VISIBLE LIGHT		
Ruby	Solid State	694 nm
Krypton	Gas-Ion	676.4 nm
InGaAlP	Semiconductor	635-660 nm
HeNe	Gas	633 nm
Ruby	Solid State	628 nm
HeNe	Gas	612 nm
HeNe	Gas	594 nm
Cu	Metal vapor	578 nm
Krypton	Gas-Ion	568.2 nm
HeNe	Gas	543 nm
DPSS	Semiconductor	532 nm
Krypton	Gas-Ion	530.9 nm
Argon	Gas-Ion	514.5 nm
Cu	Metal vapor	511 nm
Argon	Gas-Ion	457.9 nm Several others
HeCd	Gas-Ion	442 nm
N2+	Gas	428 nm
Krypton	Gas-Ion	416 nm
NEAR ULTRAVIOLET		
XeF	Gas (excimer)	351 nm (UV-A)
N2	Gas	337 nm (UV-A)
XeCl	Gas (excimer)	308 nm (UV-B)
FAR ULTRAVIOLET		
KrF	Gas (excimer)	248 nm (UV-C)
Argon SHG	Gas-Ion/BBO crystal	229 nm (UV-C)
KrCl	Gas (excimer)	222 nm (UV-C)
ArF	Gas (excimer)	193 nm (UV-C)

Adapted from: http://www.lexellaser.com/techinfo_wavelengths.htm, accessed March 22, 2004.

<UV   IR>

400   450   500   550   600   650   700   750

*Visible light portion of spectrum shown.

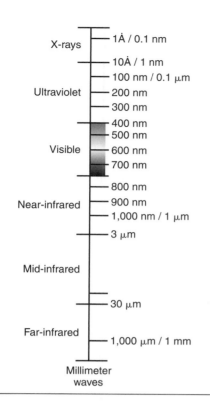

Figure 15-10: The optical spectrum. Laser light is nonionizing and comprises a range that includes ultraviolet (100 to 400 nm), visible (400 to 700 nm), and infrared light (700 nm to 1mm).

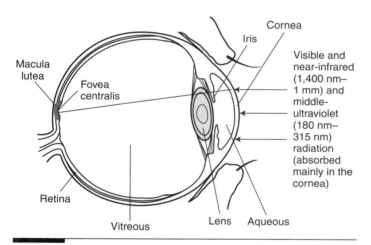

Figure 15-11 Wavelengths that damage the cornea.

and the eye should be protected to ensure that the vitreous humor does not leak out. Minor laser burns to the cornea may be treated with an eye patch and appropriate eye antibiotics.

Some infrared radiation from IR-A wavelengths, which range from 700 to 1,400 nm, and IR-B wavelengths, which range from 1,400 to 3,000 nm, is absorbed by the lens.

Radiation from visible and IR-A wavelengths (400 to 1,400 nm) is the most hazardous and is transmitted by the optical components of the eye. It eventually reaches the retina, where most of the radiation is absorbed in the retinal pigment epithelium and in the choroid, which is a dark

brown layer with exceptionally large blood vessels and a high blood-flow rate. Laser burns to the retina do not require an eye patch. Indeed, an eye patch may reduce the person's remaining vision. Damage to the retina or hemorrhaging from retinal damage can cause a complete loss of vision.

A person who sees large dark spots at or near the center of his or her vision, has a large floating object in the eye, or who has an accumulation of blood in the eye should be promptly evacuated to a hospital with ophthalmologic support. Hemorrhage into the eye should be treated by positioning the patient in a head-up position, to allow the blood to settle into the lower part of the eye. **Color plates 15-1, 15-2, and 15-3** depict laser eye injuries.

Skin Burns

The risk of skin injury is greater than the risk of eye injury by a laser because we have a lot more skin tissue than eye tissue. However, skin injuries from lasers are much less serious than eye injuries. This is partly because skin injuries do not often produce the dire consequences of eye injuries and partly because the eye concentrates the laser's beam as described previously.

Skin injuries from lasers primarily fall into two categories: thermal injury (burns) from acute exposure to high-power laser beams and photochemical injury from chronic exposure to scattered ultraviolet laser radiation.

- **Thermal injury** can result from direct contact with the beam or the specular reflections of a laser. These injuries (although painful) are usually not serious and are normally easy to prevent through proper beam management and hazard awareness.
- **Photochemical injury** may occur over time from ultraviolet exposure to the direct beam, the specular reflections, or even the diffuse reflections of a laser. The effect can be the equivalent of a minor or severe sunburn. Prolonged exposure may promote the formation of skin cancer. Proper protective eyewear and clothing may be necessary to control ultraviolet exposure to the skin and eyes.

Skin injuries usually only affect the external dead layer of the epidermis. Even if the injury penetrates the skin, the damage will heal readily. Laser-induced skin damage is most pronounced from far-infrared wavelengths such as those produced by carbon dioxide lasers. Skin damage can also be caused by visible or near-infrared wavelengths, but this requires higher laser intensity than for far-infrared wavelengths. (The skin reflects most visible and near-infrared wavelengths and absorbs UV-B and UV-C wavelengths). With enough power and duration, a laser beam of any wavelength in the optical spectrum can penetrate the skin and cause deep internal injury.

The pain from thermal injury to the skin by most targeting lasers is enough to alert a victim to move out of the beam path. Unfortunately, a number of high-power and visible lasers and infrared lasers are now used in industry. These are capable of producing significant skin burns in less than a second.

Threat

The laser is the only directed energy weapon that is currently fielded by both the United States and other military forces. In many cases, the laser is not intended as a weapon per se, but rather as a targeting device for another weapon, such as a missile or a "smart" bomb. The properties of the laser are particularly suited for this purpose. The militaries of many nations developed lasers for use as range finders and target designators. When the range of the laser was found to be too low, a higher powered laser was developed to illuminate the target.

There is a potential problem with many such military laser devices—they can easily cause retinal injury in the eyes of anybody who looks into the beam, even at a distance of many miles. This rapidly became an advantage when the military realized that the laser could be used to actively disable personnel by blinding or dazzling them. By 1985, the British Navy had developed an unclassified weapon that was fitted aboard ships to blind oncoming enemy pilots at ranges of up to 3 miles.

Many thousands of target-designation and distance-ranging lasers have been manufactured and sent out with troops of multiple countries. As such, they may find their way into the hands of terrorists and be employed against US civilians. Other civilian lasers can be easily adapted to similar purposes.

Indeed, muggers in England have used simple laser pointers to blind victims before robbing them.[17] There have been many anecdotal reports of eye pain and headaches lasting for several weeks following brief ocular exposures to laser pointer beams.[18] (This is difficult to understand, because lasting pain is not a common consequence of laser treatment for diabetes, for which a considerable amount of laser energy is delivered to the retina.)[19,20]

Lasers have already been used by terrorists in an attempt to blind helicopter pilots. It would be no great stretch for a terrorist to mount a relatively powerful laser on a truck or within a car and attempt to blind pilots who are landing at a commercial airport.[21] Likewise, simple lasers may be used to destroy the vision of law enforcement personnel responding to a terrorist attack.

It is unlikely that a class 3b or class 4 laser will be employed by terrorists, but it is, of course, possible. The EMS provider at all levels should be prepared to treat eye injuries from class 2 and class 3a lasers, as these injuries occur rarely in civilian life without terrorists.

Protection

There is no foolproof countermeasure for a blinding laser. Each of the following protective efforts will hinder the ability to see and to carry out activities requiring sight.

Avoidance

Laser radiation does not travel through opaque objects. Any opaque cover will provide protection against all but military class 4 lasers. Avoid looking directly at any laser beam or its reflection, if at all possible. Reflections off of shiny surfaces may cause damage despite forward cover.

Patching

Wearing an eye patch on one eye offers partial protection from blinding lasers. Unfortunately, it also deprives the wearer of depth perception and peripheral vision. Patching only prevents blinding in the patched eye.

Filter

The present method of protection from the laser threat is quite simple: Build a pair of protective sunglasses that reflect the laser light but let other wavelengths through, so the wearer can see. These helmet visors or goggles prevent laser radiation from damaging the wearer's eyes. This works well if the laser threat has been previously identified and is limited to one or two wavelengths.

As always, thorough research by a terrorist would reveal what protective equipment is currently available for military, law enforcement, and EMS providers. With this information, the terrorist could choose a wavelength from which there is no protection. In addition, the level of attenuation provided by visors at present is only adequate against laser powers used at present and may not be adequate against higher-power Soviet, Chinese, North Korean, or Pakistani lasers, should these be used as antipersonnel weapons.

It is expected that a tunable (frequency agile) laser threat will also develop soon. The technical approach used to protect against fixed-frequency lasers cannot be applied to protection from the agile threat or even to the protection from a larger number of fixed-frequency threats. As more band rejection filters are built into a sandwich, transmissivity of the visor at other wavelengths decreases also, making it unusable at night and limiting its utility in the daytime.

It must be stressed that to be effective, laser protective goggles and glasses must be on before exposure to the laser, and must have the appropriate frequency rejection characteristics for the laser used. This presents a difficult problem for law enforcement and EMS providers who may be faced with any of these lasers as a terrorist threat.

■ Microwave Radiation Emitters

Microwave radiation emitters were also covered in the previous section on EMP weapons. The effects on equipment were covered in that section.

Long-term exposure to HPMs can produce both physical and psychological effects in humans and include sensations of warmth, headaches, generalized fatigue, weakness, and dizziness. The effect depends on the power output of the weapon and the distance from the generator to the person.

■ Particle Beam Generators

A particle beam is a directed flow of atomic or subatomic particles. These high-energy particles, when concentrated into a beam, can melt or fracture metals and plastics. They also generate x-rays at the point of impact. These weapons are in development stages only and are quite unlikely to be found in the hands of terrorists. **Table 15-5** summarizes the effects of commonly used lasers.

Table 15-5 Summary of Effects of Commonly Used Lasers

Laser Type	Wavelength (nm)	Bioeffect Process	Skin	Cornea	Lens	Retina
				Tissue Effected		
CO_2	10,600	Thermal	X	Thermal corneal injuries		
HFl	2,700	Thermal	X	Thermal corneal injuries		
Erbium-YAG	1,540	Thermal	X	Thermal corneal injuries	Glassblower's cataracts	
Nd:YAG [a]	1,330	Thermal	X	Thermal corneal injuries	Glassblower's cataracts	Retinal damage
Nd:YAG	1,060	Thermal	X			Retinal damage
Gas (diode)	780–840	Thermal	[b]			Retinal damage
He-Ne	633	Thermal	[b]			Retinal damage
Ar	488–514	Thermal/Photochemical	X			Retinal damage[c]
XeFl	351	Photochemical	X	Photokeratitis (welder's flash)		Retinal damage
XeCl	308	Photochemical	X	Photokeratitis (welder's flash)		

Adapted from: http://web.princeton.edu/sites/ehs/laserguide/sec2.htm; Laser safety at http://web.princeton.edu/sites/ehs/laserguide/sec2.htm; Laser safety background at http://www.femto.sims.nrc.ca/LaserSafety/lsafety7.htm; The Royal School of Artillery at www.atra.mod.uk/atra/rsabst/pdf/G-Electro-Optics/G02-SAFE.pdf. Accessed March 22, 2004.

[a] Wavelengths of 13,300 nm (very far-infrared spectrum) or more are common in some Nd:YAG lasers and have demonstrated simultaneous cornea/lens/retina effects in biological research studies.
[b] Power levels of these lasers are not normally sufficient to be considered a significant skin hazard.
[c] Photochemical effects dominate for long-term exposures to the retina (exposure times of more than 10 seconds).

Visible and near-infrared wavelengths are particularly hazardous since they are readily transmitted through ocular media and are focused to a spot on the retina 10–20 μm in diameter. Thus the intensity of such light at the retina will be on the order of 105 times greater than at the cornea. Self-focusing of femtosecond pulses within the eye can further enhance retinal intensities. Hence, retinal damage thresholds are several orders of magnitude lower than those for corneas.

■ References

1. Conway M: Reality bytes: Cyberterrorism and terrorist 'use' of the internet. *First Monday,* http://www.firstmonday.dk/issues/issue7_11/conway/ (Accessed July 4, 2003).
2. Title 22, US Code, § 2656f(d)2.
3. Jesdanun A: Cybercafes pose security problems. CBSNews.com. http://www.cbsnews.com/stories/2003/07/22/tech/main564568.shtml (Accessed March 20, 2004.)
4. Cyber war! The warnings? "Frontline." PBS, April 24, 2003 http://www.pbs.org/wgbh/pages/frontline/shows/cyberwar/warnings/ (Accessed April 28, 2003).
5. Cyber war! Introduction. "Frontline." PBS, April 24, 2003 http://www.pbs.org/wgbh/pages/frontline/shows/cyberwar/etc/synopsis.html (Accessed April 28, 2003).
6. Cyber war! Introduction, "Frontline." PBS, April 24, 2003 http://www.pbs.org/wgbh/pages/frontline/shows/cyberwar/etc/synopsis.html (Accessed April 28, 2003).
7. Cyber war! Introduction, "Frontline." PBS, April 24, 2003 http://www.pbs.org/wgbh/pages/frontline/shows/cyberwar/etc/synopsis.html (Accessed April 28, 2003).
8. Saltus, R: Blackout led to weapon that darkened Serbia. *Boston Globe,* May 4, 1999:A27.
9. Izakovic (NI): Conventional electromagnetic pulse warheads. Deepspace4, http://www.deepspace4.com/pages/science/mp/empwarheads.htm (Accessed March 26, 2003).
10. Amos D: Police chase psychology. *ABCNews.com,* http://abcnews.go.com/onair/CloserLook/wnt000713_CL_policechase_feature.html (Accessed April 15, 2003).
11. Rogers K: Are electromagnetic pulses terrorists' next weapon of choice? *Las Vegas Review-Journal,* September 1, 2001, http://www.globalsecurity.org/org/news/2001/010930-attack04.htm (Accessed March 26, 2003).
12. Sample I: Just a normal town . . . *New Scientist,* http://www.newscientist.com/nl/0701/end.html (Accessed August 17, 2003).
13. Sample I: Just a normal town . . . *New Scientist,* http://www.newscientist.com/nl/0701/end.html (Accessed August 17, 2003).
14. Doswald-Beck L (ed): *Blinding Weapons: Report of the Meeting of Experts Convened by the International Committee of the Red Cross on Battlefield Laser Weapons, 1989–1991.* Geneva, Switzerland, International Committee of the Red Cross, 1993.
15. Kurtzweil P: Investigators' reports: Laser light shows nixed until fixed. US Food and Drug Administration, http://www.fda.gov/fdac/departs/496_irs.html (Accessed August 21, 2003).
16. Coleman, J: Assembly panel approves laser pointer bill. *Las Vegas News,* May 08, 1999, http://www.lvrj.com/cgi-bin/printable.cgi?/lvrj_home/1999/May-08-Sat-1999/news/11141492.html (Accessed August 21, 2003).

17. Anonymous: Killer pens. *Newsweek,* November 24, 1997:8.
18. Seeley D: *Laser point causes eye injuries?* Orlando, FL, Laser Institute of America, 1997.
19. Mainster MA, Sliney DH, Marshal J, et al: But is it really light damage? *Ophthal* 1997;104:179-190.
20. Yolton RL, Citek K, Schmeisser E, et al: Laser pointers: Toys, nuisances, or significant eye hazards? http://www.opt.pacificu.edu/journal/Articles/archives/laserpaper.html (Accessed August 20, 2003).
21. Anonymous: Russian ship's laser caused eye injury, Navy officer says. http://www.aeronautics.ru/nws002/ap036.htm (Accessed August 21, 2003).

Personal Protection and Decontamination

■ Introduction

Until very recently, emergency providers have been woefully negligent about both infection precautions and hazardous materials management. Every medical provider who works in an emergency department or with an EMS agency must understand that an accident involving hazardous materials places the lives of the rescuers, the victims, the emergency staff, and the surrounding community in jeopardy. When either chemical or radioactive agents are involved, there will likely be more casualties among the police, fire, and rescue personnel than among the original accident victims.[1] The addition of an intention of terrorism markedly increases the likely number of casualties among the public and the response teams.

This chapter will present simple guidelines to prevent contamination and explain expedient methods for the decontamination of field casualties and providers. It is not intended to replace specific guidelines for a particular agent, but rather to give an overall approach that is applicable to all casualties. EMS providers and physicians are reminded that exposures to some substances mandate self-contained, airtight protective overgarments with completely self-contained breathing equipment. Fortunately, these exposures are rare, and shipments of these substances are usually quite well controlled.

Goals of Decontamination

The necessity and principles of decontamination are well known to all medical providers. One form of decontamination, antiseptic technique, is used daily throughout the world. The surgical scrub decontaminates both patient and provider; the scrub clothes, drapes, and sheets provide a containment vessel, and antiseptics act as neutralizing solutions. Indeed, the reproductive abilities of viruses and bacteria add a magnitude to biological decontamination that the radiation physicist or chemical engineer will never know. The incident in Bhopal killed 2,500, and Chernobyl contaminated tens of thousands, but smallpox devastated the native population of the Americas and the Sandwich and Polynesian islands.[2] The Black Death killed nearly one third of the population of Europe.

There are conflicting purposes and goals in decontamination:

- **Prevention of personal contamination**
  This is a significant goal that is important during decontamination. The contaminated rescuer rapidly becomes a casualty, and, as such, not only becomes useless as a care provider, but becomes a burden to his or her own rescue team. Remember, dead rescuers rescue nobody.

- **Prevention of contamination of the responders' equipment and workplace**
  Assuming that you are already in personal protective gear, this goal often takes lower priority than tasks that are pressing at the moment, but mismanagement of this decontamination task may expose both patients and health care providers to lethal chemical exposure and render the emergency department unusable for an indefinite time period. With some chemicals, emergency department contamination may make exposed emergency equipment, such as monitors and defibrillators, unsalvageable. Contamination with these chemicals may require the closure of the emergency department until such time as the space can be decontaminated or rebuilt.

- **Patient care**
  Removal of contamination will decrease the absorption of chemicals by the patient and lessen the seriousness of the toxic illness. It also removes the risk of cross-contamination with other patients.

  The balance between the protection of the staff and the provision of emergency medical care to a patient is complex and requires mature judgment. Immediate life-threatening illness should generally be cared for before complete decontamination is accomplished. This must be balanced against the precepts of the preceding two goals. Again, if the patient is cared for by an unprotected rescuer who subsequently becomes a casualty, there is no net benefit.

  This consideration must also be balanced against the needs of the many. If there are multiple casualties, the rescuer should not waste time or material on unsalvageable patients, but should concentrate on the most salvageable of the patients in order to benefit the most people with the least expenditure of time. This is standard triage for mass-casualty situations.

- **Protection of the environment**
  Protection of the environment is of secondary importance to personal protection and patient care. The US Environmental Protection Agency (EPA) will find no fault with a large-scale decontamination operation that is initially unable to control chemical runoff. The EPA liability increases as the scene becomes more manageable and the duration of the response becomes longer. Once the initial impact of the incident has been mitigated or additional aid has arrived, the incident commander MUST start to properly contain any hazardous materials.

- **Satisfaction of legal requirements**
  There are also legal requirements. Occupational Safety and Health Administration (OSHA) requirements, as described in Regulation 29 CFR 1910.120q, require staff safety and response training in all workplaces where exposure to dangerous chemicals could reasonably be expected to occur. Because EMS and emergency departments are logical recipients of chemical casualties, they fall under this regulation. For an unknown substance, OSHA strongly recommends Level B protection (or better Level A), as described elsewhere in this text.

■ Identification

Vital to all decontamination and containment procedures is the identification of the offending substance. In industrial cases, this is a trivial problem. Simply asking the foreman or manager at the plant what the plant is using or making may provide the answer (often in greater detail than other resources that are readily available). In transportation accidents, identification may be equally simple. The fumes of anhydrous ammonia or chlorine are quite easy to identify. The bill of lading or manifest may describe the contents in detail. The shipper or the consignee may know the contents well. Usually, the manifest and other data are available on the vehicle or with the driver. The vehicle may also bear an appropriate placard. The problems start when these documents are lost, missing, or destroyed, and the vehicle has no placard or an inappropriate placard.

In a military attack, identification is often easy, because the intelligence officer has a very good idea what the opposition is capable of making and how they are able to disseminate it. This leads to a fairly short list of possible substances. Unfortunately, the soldier must assume that the enemy has an ongoing research and development team that is actively looking for new substances that are not detected by current technology, are not repelled by current protective garments, or are not susceptible to current antidotes. An example of this strategy is the use of mustard gas in World War I, which penetrated the then-current masks and clothing designed for phosgene and chlorine. Similar avenues of research led the Russians to the Novichok agents, which are suspected to be impervious to current antidotes for nerve agents.

When dealing with terrorism, the identification of the offending substance may be quite difficult. Indeed, the terrorist may use the shock value of employing an obscure chemical with an equally obscure antidote that, when mixed with another chemical, renders the antidote useless. The terrorist may have access to state-sponsored military research, as outlined previously. The terrorist may also set secondary or auxiliary explosive devices to kill or maim the rescuers. Likewise, the terrorist may scatter **caltrops** or similar devices to rend protective suits. Although the soldier expects such complications, the civilian is unaccustomed to multiple threat avenues.

In rare cases, the substance must be identified by a laboratory. This identification will rarely arrive in time to be useful for field or EMS decontamination procedures.

■ Field Decontamination Operations

The Decon Team

Table 16-1 shows the components and organization of a decontamination team.

Decon Team Leader

All members of a decontamination (decon) team report to the decon team leader or incident commander. This individual is responsible for all decisions relating to the management of the decontamination operation. The decon team leader should be formally trained as an incident commander and should also be trained up to the level of his or her responders (operations or technician level). The decon team leader must handle the flow of information, analyze the hazard, and decide what type of personal protective equipment (PPE) is required for the responders. He or she must decide how and when to call in additional aid, and when to initiate and terminate the decontamination operation. In some cases, a safety officer will work closely with the decon team leader. When a safety officer has not been assigned, the team leader must oversee the health and safety of all the decon team members. The decon team leader must constantly analyze and reanalyze the overall situation for safety issues.

Operations Team

The operations members are the personnel who will actually perform the decontamination of casualties. Team members must be trained to the operations level or technician level. To operate in the hot or warm zone, they must don no less than Level B PPE with some form of self-contained breathing apparatus (SCBA) or supplied air respirator (SAR). The operations team must be medically prescreened before donning PPE, and then evaluated again after doffing PPE. Members work in pairs of two, with two backup members in full PPE on standby. Team member responsibilities include the operation of decontamination equipment, the decontamination of patients, the decontamination of self and partner, the direction of the flow of patients in transition, and the predecontamination treatment of patients (if necessary).

Suit Support Staff

The primary goal of suit support is to assist the operations team members in the following tasks: taking pre-entry vital signs, donning or doffing PPE, ensuring hydration, and monitoring overall medical well-being. Although the suit support staff operates in the cold zone, they should also be trained to the operations level and must don Level C PPE with splash protection and a full-face air purification device. As a collateral responsibility, suit support staff will assist with the flow of decontaminated patients and prepare backup operations teams for entry.

Equipment Support Staff

The equipment support members may operate in both the warm and cold zones. Their responsibilities include erecting, operating, servicing, and disassembling decontamina-

Table 16-1 The Decon Team

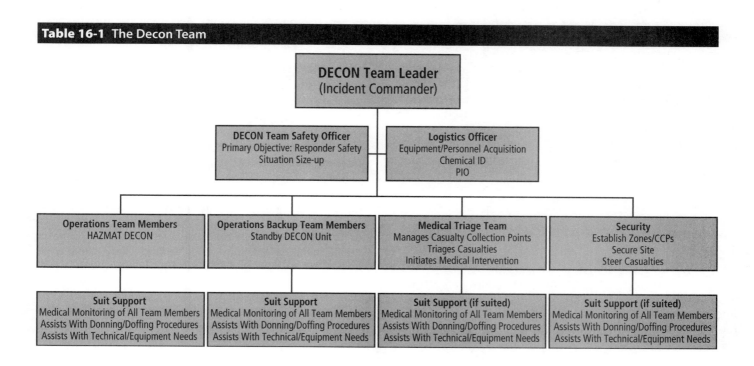

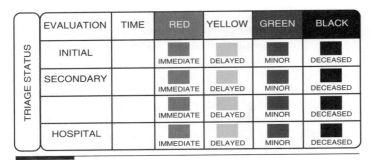

TRIAGE STATUS	EVALUATION	TIME	RED	YELLOW	GREEN	BLACK
	INITIAL		IMMEDIATE	DELAYED	MINOR	DECEASED
	SECONDARY		IMMEDIATE	DELAYED	MINOR	DECEASED
			IMMEDIATE	DELAYED	MINOR	DECEASED
	HOSPITAL		IMMEDIATE	DELAYED	MINOR	DECEASED

Figure 16-1 Symbols for triage categories.

tion showers and apparatus; securing a water supply for the showers; servicing breathing apparatus; and operating water containment and pumping equipment. The level of training, as well as PPE, will vary for these personnel. Those operating in the warm zone should have a minimum of operations level training and must wear Level B PPE with SCBA or SAR. Those in the cold zone may not require operations knowledge, but should have some form of awareness training, and they may require Level C PPE with NBC filtered masks.

Triage Staff

The triage team's responsibility is to manage the flow of casualties from the decontamination area to the established treatment and casualty collection sectors **(Figure 16-1)**. This individual or group of individuals must have emergency medical credentials. The best candidates for this job are emergency department triage RNs (for hospital decontamination), paramedics (if any are available), or EMTs. Physicians and physician assistants are not encouraged to assist with triage because of their lack of familiarity with the mass-casualty triage system, and simply because their expertise is best used in treating casualties, not directing their flow. Triage is a stressful task, and team members should be selected for their decisiveness and ability to perform rapid triage under pressure. They must resist the urge to treat patients, as that would greatly degrade their ability to direct casualty flow. By virtue of the fact that they are assessing decontaminated patients, there is no need for PPE. This is predicated on the assumption that a perimeter and security has been established to prevent contaminated victims from bypassing the decontamination area. If there is porous security, then it is recommended that these individuals don Level C PPE with an NBC filtered mask. This precaution will afford the team member the ability to redirect any contaminated casualty that has slipped by, without much risk of contamination.

Treatment Staff

Members of the treatment staff receive patients at the casualty collection point. The casualty collection point should be located in close proximity to the triage area. Patients should be segregated from each other based on the triage group that they have been assigned. This helps to concentrate re-

sources on those who require aggressive management. The treatment staff is made up of medical professionals who are familiar with the effects caused by chemical agents and the appropriate antidote administration for all age groups.

Security Staff

This often overlooked assignment is a key to a successful decontamination effort. Hospital decontamination operations are predicated upon the staff's ability to control the flow of patients into the facility. Without adequate security, the hospital may find critical areas compromised and contaminated. Tasks performed by security staff include directing the peaceful and organized flow of patients throughout the decontamination process, preventing access to areas by unauthorized persons, and posting caution markers and tape. By virtue of the job description, security staff must operate in both warm and cold zones. Their level of PPE should reflect the area in which they are operating.

Decontamination Operation Considerations
Prevention of Contamination

The very best method of decontamination is to prevent the contamination before it occurs. This can be accomplished by minimizing contact with potentially hazardous substances. When there is a spill of unknown substances at the scene of an accident, *assume that it is dangerous*. Medical providers should not walk through areas of obvious contamination and should not touch objects that are potentially contaminated.

Disposable outer garments and disposable equipment may prevent the spread of contaminants and, therefore, should be both carried and used. Monitoring and sampling instruments should be protected by plastic bags or sheaths. Monitor leads should be brought through the neck of the bag and taped. (Sampling ports may be cut in the bags where needed.)

Site Selection and Management:
Location, Location, Location

Is the site appropriate? Nearby streams and ponds make sites environmentally unsuitable for agents that persist. Hospitals generally make poor decontamination sites, because of the added risks to other patients. Hospital incident commanders must consider runoff, the flow and direction of patients, surge capacity, and the well-being of noncontaminated patients and staff. Numerous hospitals have field decontamination facilities located within feet of their entrance or in line with the ambulance bay. This type of poor planning does not take into account spillage, vapor lines, or the expansion of the decontamination area by splash.

When a suitable decontamination site has been established, a decontamination station is constructed. This decontamination station should be clearly marked, and all firefighters, police, rescue workers, and cleanup technicians should be aware of the site.

Logistics

Before beginning decontamination, the officer in charge should decide how much decontamination is necessary and how much decontamination can be accomplished at the scene of the accident. The following questions need to be answered:

- *Are existing resources available to decontaminate both personnel and equipment? If they are not readily available, how long will it take to make them available?* Decontamination at hospitals or fire stations will complicate the problem and may contaminate multiple areas and vehicles.
- *Can the decontamination be safely accomplished with the equipment on hand?* Dilution is difficult to use as a decontamination technique when the temperature is −20°F!
- *Can equipment be decontaminated?* The toxicity of some agents may make equipment unsafe or unusable. Disposal may be the only safe method of handling some agents. If the county only owns one ambulance, contamination could be a major problem.

Scene Decontamination Officer

The decontamination officer's responsibilities, duties, and authority should be clearly outlined in disaster plans. An appropriately trained medical triage officer should have joint authority, so that truly life-threatening injuries are not neglected. The decontamination officer and medical triage officer should be responsible to the incident commander.

The decontamination officer, medical triage officer, and incident commander should confer with specialists, such as chemical engineers, toxicologists, nuclear physicians, and physicists, as needed to determine which decontamination methods will be used, how much decontamination is required, and how much decontamination can be completed at the scene. Patients with life-threatening emergencies may have to be treated at higher levels of contamination. The receiving hospital must be forewarned and be able to handle decontamination and emergency treatment simultaneously.

Transport Vehicles

Although ambulances are traditionally used for the transport of casualties, this is a poor idea for contaminated victims. Ambulances are exceedingly difficult to decontaminate, filled with expensive gear, and carry very few patients. Multiple radioactive material incidents have proven the inadequacies of ambulances in contamination situations.

Although helicopter ambulances can move patients rapidly, they are more expensive than land ambulances and are even more difficult to decontaminate. Moving equipment to a scene by air may be allowable, if the landing site is carefully selected and does not endanger others. Moving contaminated patients by air transport is an exceedingly poor idea. A pilot, unaccustomed to wearing protective gear, may not be able to safely pilot the vehicle. An unprotected pilot, overcome by contaminants, endangers himself or herself, the crew, the patients, and those on the ground.

Pickup trucks are far better vehicles to transport contaminated patients than ambulances. They have steel beds, carry large numbers of patients, and are relatively easy to decontaminate. In the worst outcome, a pickup truck is far easier to replace than an ambulance. Four-wheel drive trucks provide added mobility in inclement weather and rough terrain. Plain-body vans, SUVs, or delivery vans (bread vans) provide acceptable substitutes in cases of inclement weather.

Decontamination Techniques

The specific techniques required to adequately decontaminate an object will depend upon the nature of the object, the contaminant, the weather, and the tools and equipment available. Likewise, the size and complexity of the decontamination station will depend upon the physical and chemical properties of the contaminant, the potential for exposure and location of that exposure to the workers, the availability of equipment, and the weather. Simply, spilled ammonia from an overturned railroad tank car will require a different level of protection than a spilled 60-mL beaker of medical radioiodine solution.

Physical Removal

The most common technique to dispose of a contaminant is to physically remove it. Physical removal is simple, effective, and requires few specialized tools. Physical methods of removal include brushing, scraping, wiping, diluting, absorbing, and vacuuming. In special situations, the area may be cleaned by pressurized streams of water, steam, or sand. Some liquids may evaporate or may be vaporized.

Chemical Removal

Chemical removal involves the neutralization or dissolution of the substance with another chemical. It is more complex than physical removal, because it requires an understanding of the chemical structure and reactions of the offending agent. Chemical removal techniques include neutralizing the substance, dissolving the substance, and reducing the adhesion of the substance with surfactants. Remember that the chemicals used to dissolve the substance may also dissolve or alter protective clothing.

Isolation or Disposal

It may not be possible or practical to decontaminate some equipment or clothing. This is most often true with radioactive agents and some chemical agents. Special areas for the storage of these items will be designated by decontamination officers in conjunction with state and federal officials.

Chemical Decontamination

Generally, all skin exposures should be initially treated with irrigation with large volumes of water at low pressure for more than 30 minutes. Only after exposure to metallic sodium, lithium, and potassium should this not be done immediately. In these cases, the metallic fragments should be expeditiously removed. Specific antidotes to skin exposure do not generally exist, and providers should not waste time looking for such antidotes.

The following guidelines may be helpful when medical providers are faced with an unknown hazardous material. The solutions are designed to chemically destroy the agents and not merely remove them. The components that formulate these solutions may be prepackaged and stored for long periods of time in an appropriately sized receptacle (in which a person may "just add water"). In all cases of suspected chemical contaminations, the medical provider should irrigate the contaminated area with large volumes of water at low pressure while awaiting these solutions.

Decontamination Solution A Decontamination solution A contains 5% sodium bicarbonate and 5% trisodium phosphate. These chemicals are available in most hardware stores and chemical supply houses. Mix 4 lb of sodium bicarbonate and 4 lb of commercial grade trisodium phosphate in 10 gallons of water to obtain the proper concentrations.

Decontamination solution A may be used on intact skin, followed by copious irrigation. Do not use solution A on open wounds, mucous membranes, or eyes. Generally, these areas are best treated with copious irrigation with large volumes of water at low pressure for long durations.

Decontamination solution A may be used for the following:

- Inorganic acids
- Acidic caustic wastes
- Metal processing wastes
- Solvents and organic compounds, such as chloroform
- Trichloroethylene and toluene
- Plastic wastes and polychlorinated biphenyls (PCBs)
- Biological contamination

Decontamination Solution B Decontamination solution B is a concentrated solution of bleach (sodium hypochlorite). A 10% solution may be made by mixing 8 lb of anhydrous calcium hypochlorite powder with 10 gallons of water. Anhydrous calcium hypochlorite powder is commonly known as HTH and is available from swimming pool supply houses. HTH should always be stored in plastic containers.

Decontamination solution B may be used for the following:

- Heavy metals, such as lead, mercury, or cadmium
- Pesticides, chlorinated phenols, dioxin, and PCBs
- Cyanide
- Ammonia
- Inorganic wastes
- Organic wastes
- Biological contamination

Decontamination solution B may be used on intact skin after it is diluted with water in a 50:50 ratio. An equally good alternative for use on skin is household strength hypochlorite bleach solution. Follow the use of either solution with irrigation with water. Do not use solution B on open wounds, mucous membranes, or eyes. Household bleach may be used on mucous membranes and sparingly on open wounds.

Rinse Solution (Decontamination Solution C) A general purpose rinse solution suitable for use with all of the chemical decontamination solutions is a 5% solution of trisodium phosphate. To prepare the rinse solution, add 4 lb of trisodium phosphate to 10 gallons of water.

Rinse solution is an effective decontaminant for the following:

- Solvents and organic compounds
- PCBs
- Oily wastes not suspected to be contaminated with pesticides

Following a rinse with this solution, equipment may be rinsed again with water. Decontamination solution C may be used on intact skin and should be flushed off with water. Do not use solution C on open wounds, mucous membranes, or eyes.

Alkali Decontamination Solution (Decontamination Solution D) The decontamination solutions listed above are not effective with strong alkali contaminating agents. A dilute solution of hydrochloric acid may be made by mixing 1 pt of concentrated hydrochloric acid in 10 gallons of water.

Decontamination solution D is suitable for the following:

- Inorganic bases
- Alkalies
- Alkali caustic wastes

All skin, eyes, or mucous membranes exposed to any of these alkaline agents should be treated with copious irrigation with water. Irrigation should involve large volumes, low pressures, and long durations.

Biological Decontamination

Biological decontamination has abruptly changed from an issue taught and largely ignored to a critical step as a result of the rise of AIDS-related diseases and the experience with anthrax in Florida and Washington. The principles have been taught to medical providers since Semmelweis and are applicable to EVERY contagious disease. Note that the hysteria of AIDS has not been supported by an increase in AIDS transmission to medical providers, other than through high-risk activities such as illicit drug use.

These principles are widely promulgated and known by medical providers at all levels. Specific guidelines on the decontamination of personnel, equipment, and ambulances are available from the CDC in Atlanta, Georgia. If an unknown agent is thought to have some bacterial or viral component, decontamination solution B—sodium hypochlorite—will ensure that no viable organisms remain.

Level 1 Decontamination Level 1 decontamination is required if there is a possibility of contamination, but it has not been proven. It is appropriate for victims in the area of a chemical spill or release. The victim should show no signs or symptoms of chemical exposure. If hospital emergency personnel handle a possibly contaminated victim, this is the minimum level of decontamination required.

Procedure: All clothing should be removed, bagged, and labeled. (Depending on the incident, these items may be used as evidence by law enforcement personnel.) The removal of clothing and shoes will remove as much as 90% of the contaminants. The patient should then be washed with a fog spray or shower (if available) for 1 minute. If possible, the runoff water should be retained for later evaluation and proper disposal. (It should be noted that water is suitable decontamination for many toxic materials. There are two in particular for which water decontamination may not be suitable: Vx and mustard. Likewise, water will not decontaminate spore forming organisms such as anthrax.)

Level 2 Decontamination Level 2 decontamination is required if contamination is known, but there are no signs or symptoms of exposure.

Procedure: All clothing should be removed, bagged, and labeled. Remove the respirator last (if applicable). The victim should then be moved away from the contaminated clothing. The patient should be washed in a holding basin with a fog spray or shower (if available) for 1 minute. If possible, the runoff water should be retained for later evaluation and proper disposal. Following this, the patient should be thoroughly showered with soap and water.

Level 3 Decontamination Level 3 decontamination is required if the patient is symptomatic. This may include skin irritation, chemical burns, or respiratory symptoms.

Procedure: All clothing should be removed, bagged, and labeled. Remove the respirator last (if applicable). The victim should then be moved away from the contaminated clothing. The patient should be washed in a holding basin with a fog spray or shower (if available) for 1 minute. If possible, the runoff water should be retained for later evaluation and proper disposal.

Continue to flush all areas that are known to be contaminated or that are irritated with water for 15 minutes. This may require a decision whether to transport the victim to the hospital at this point, or to continue to decontaminate at the scene. The toxicity of the chemical, the availability of decontamination showers at the hospital, the distance or time of transport, the types of other injuries, and the available protection for the EMS personnel are all factors in this decision. Following irrigation, the patient should be thoroughly showered with soap and water.

Provider Decontamination

Responders and hospital personnel that are involved with decontamination procedures should receive the same level of decontamination as the patient. If there is no protective equipment available to responders, then the victims should be instructed how to decontaminate themselves if possible. This may be appropriate for an alert and awake victim of a spill, but it is grossly inappropriate for a patient with significant additional injuries.

Emergency Department Decontamination

In the emergency department, there will hopefully be no continuous exposure to the noxious agent. A discontinuous exposure is possible as a result of inadequate field contamination. This is most likely to occur with the first few casualties, before the field teams recognize the contamination threat. Because the hospital medical teams are also unaware of the contamination threat and wear no protection, the contaminating agent may be spread rapidly and widely within the hospital.[3] Emergency department staff should all be aware of this potential and be empowered to seal a room, a

suite, or even the entire emergency department until appropriate identification and decontamination can be instituted.

Setup

Upon receiving notification, the hospital should activate the internal plan that is appropriate for the suspected contaminant. Depending upon the number of estimated casualties, the emergency physician should make a decision whether to initiate a limited or a full response. Appropriate ancillary help should be summoned prior to the arrival of the victims. There is no need to act hastily, unless a patient has sustained life-threatening injuries. Remember that some chemicals or radioactive materials are so difficult to decontaminate that monitors, defibrillators, and other quite expensive equipment may need to be discarded. It is always preferable to minimize the spread of contaminants than to explain the losses afterward.

The emergency staff has three primary missions when dealing with these potentially contaminated patients. The process of decontamination must address each of these missions in detail:

1. Prevent damage to themselves.
2. Prevent contamination of the workplace, thereby reducing the threat to themselves, their colleagues, and their patients.
3. Decontaminate and treat the patient(s).

Decontamination

Although patient care may be delayed slightly, it is simpler and safer for all involved if the patient is decontaminated at the incident scene. Decontamination should occur prior to contact or transport by EMS personnel. This will minimize the level of risk to the EMS personnel who may not be properly protected against contamination. Ambulances may not be properly ventilated to keep contamination from patient attendants, and patient compartments provide close quarters, further increasing attendants' susceptibility to exposure. Unfortunately, history shows that the *vast majority* of casualties will not be transported by EMS and may arrive in the emergency department contaminated.

If patients are not decontaminated before care is initiated, contamination may spread via blood pressure cuffs, stretcher pads and straps, immobilization devices, or oxygen and suction units. Some of this equipment is not easily decontaminated, and personnel may not even be aware that it has become contaminated. Transporting contaminated patients may allow the spread of contamination from the emergency scene to the ambulance and to the hospital.

Chemical-specific decontamination should be performed when the chemical is positively identified and the chemical-specific decontamination procedures are known and can be implemented. It is critical for responders to interface with plant or company personnel to attempt to obtain this information. **CHEMTREC** or other sources of technical information can be contacted (see the resources section at the end of this chapter). Be sure to follow the specified decontamination procedures.

Otherwise, **field decontamination** must be performed. The following three levels of field decontamination

INHOSPITAL INFO

are simple procedures that can be accomplished by almost any emergency response organization.

Preplanning

Decontamination principles, equipment, and techniques remain unchanged from field to hospital setting. In theory, it should be easier to preplan for decontamination in the hospital environment than in the field setting; however, the reality is that preplanning tends to take lower priority in the face of day-to-day urgent matters. Hospital decontamination plans that have not been practiced are often found to be completely unworkable when needed. With the frequency of hazardous materials transport, literally any hospital in the country could receive contaminated victims at any time.

Receiving Committee

A reception area should be set up and considered to be an exclusion zone. Appropriate decontamination areas and procedures as discussed previously are necessary for this area. Incoming ambulances and other transportation vehicles should be clearly identified as either contaminated or decontaminated, and separate entry areas should be provided for each.

Ideally, this decontamination and reception area should be outside. If this is not possible because of space or weather constraints, decontamination will have to occur within the hospital. The receiving area should be carefully chosen with this eventuality in mind. A controlled indoor environment is essential. All nonessential and nondisposable equipment should be removed.

The receiving committee should be outfitted with protective garments. The level of this protection must depend upon the nature of the contamination. Minimal protection includes a respirator, a multi-layer Tyvek suit, and nitrile gloves and boots. Only after a responsible survey officer has examined the patient and ensured that residual contamination does not place unprotected personnel in jeopardy should protection be doffed. It is always easier (and safer) to prevent contamination than it is to decontaminate.

All incoming patients should be considered potentially contaminated, despite the best assurances of the field decontamination officer. These patients should be scanned for any signs of contaminants. This is quite easy for radioactive or odiferous materials, but may be exceptionally difficult for slower-acting, concentrated contaminants. If there is any doubt, the patient should be completely decontaminated again.

The incoming contaminated patient requires thorough decontamination with the same materials and principles previously discussed. It should be assumed that a patient who has bypassed decontamination has a potentially life-threatening injury. The difficult question that must be answered by a competent and well-trained triage officer is: *Does this patient need treatment or decontamination first?* As noted earlier, the balance between the protection of the staff and the provision of emergency medical care to a patient is complex and requires mature judgment. In all cases, simply removing clothing and washing the patient markedly reduces the decontamination burden for other medical providers. In selected cases, simultaneous decontamination and lifesaving care may be provided.

Resuscitation

Rarely, lifesaving procedures will be necessary for patients who remain contaminated. It is anticipated that these casualties will be contaminated with toxins other than nerve agents, which are extremely lethal. (The military axiom is, "If you arrive alive, you will survive!")

Wherever possible, bare rooms with ventilation ports plugged should be used for resuscitation. An appropriate resuscitation room should be set aside in the disaster plan for this contingency. This room must allow easy access to the outside, with a corridor that can be both protected and decontaminated. An adjacent area must be available for decontamination of the medical personnel. Ideally, the waste drainage from the room should be routed to a separate holding tank.

All equipment should be removed from the resuscitation room, and only that equipment needed for the operation or procedure should be passed into the room. All articles and equipment that enter or remain in the exclusion zone should be considered both expendable and expended. Suction should be provided by portable units to eliminate the contamination of wall suction tubing throughout the hospital. Portable electrical junction boxes eliminate the decontamination of wall sockets.

Plastic sheeting on walls and floors will aid the decontamination process after the disaster response is over. This sheeting should be stocked with the disaster equipment, together with sufficient gaffer's tape to secure it to walls and floors. The emergency department should practice building this "containment vessel" from sheeting during every practice disaster, so that the operation proceeds smoothly and quickly.

The surgeon, emergency physician, or other provider, together with scrub nurses, should wear protective garments that will withstand the contaminant for at least twice the expected duration of the procedure (generally Level B). (This allows a margin for additional procedures or for clumsiness because of the garments.) The surgeon should practice handling tools and instruments while wearing these garments prior to an actual disaster, because tactile skills will be changed by the protective garments.

All contaminated objects should be bagged and labeled. These objects should be stored in a separate waste container for each patient. Wherever possible, these articles should be handled with tongs or other remote handling equipment. Remember that all articles may end up as evidence in a crime laboratory.

■ Personal Protective Equipment

The use of PPE to protect the airways, skin, and eyes is an indispensable component for the emergency department that receives chemically contaminated patients. Ideally, each and every patient that presents to the emergency department will be completely decontaminated prior to arrival onto hospital property. However, this prehospital decontamination is unlikely. There are multiple reasons for this, including self-referral; bystander transport; transport by ill-equipped or ill-trained emergency service providers, firefighters, or police officers; and contaminated patients triaged as critical because of injuries and rushed to medical care. The medical provider must assume that decontamination has not occurred, and, hence, personal protection is needed.

The EPA has outlined detailed combinations of respirators and chemical protective attire that may be used in certain hazardous environments. These grades of protection are classified as Levels A, B, C, and D. All emergency personnel who enter the contaminated zone or who have direct contact with contaminated victims will require PPE. Rescue workers entering a contaminated area require a greater level of protection than medical personnel providing care to contaminated or potentially contaminated patients.

Level A

Level A equipment provides the greatest degree of protection and consists of an encapsulated, vapor-impermeable, and chemical-resistant garment; double-layer chemical-resistant gloves and boots; and a positive-pressure SCBA **(Figure 16-2).** Airtight seals should be in place between the suit and the inner layer of hand, face, and foot protection. Level A protection usually is required only of those working in areas of very high concentrations of toxic agents.

Level A suits and equipment will protect against most military and industrial compounds. Many municipal and corporate hazardous materials response teams in the United States have some Level A capabilities.

Level B

Level B equipment consists of a positive-pressure SCBA, a chemical-resistant suit, and chemical-resistant gloves and boots **(Figure 16-3).** Airtight seals on the face, hands, and feet are unnecessary. Level B protection is used when full respiratory protection is required, but skin exposure presents less danger. Many hazardous materials response teams outfit their decontamination squads with Level B protection.

Level C

Level C equipment is required when concentrations of the toxic agent are expected to be much lower, and little likelihood of skin exposure exists. Generally speaking, Level C protection should be used when the chemical hazard is known, the concentration is low, and the ambient oxygen concentration is normal. This is the usual situation for medical decontamination outside the emergency department. Level C protection consists of a full-face air purification device, such as a canister mask, a nonencapsulating chemical-resistant suit, and chemical-resistant gloves and boots **(Figure 16-4).** For the medical decontamination of chemically

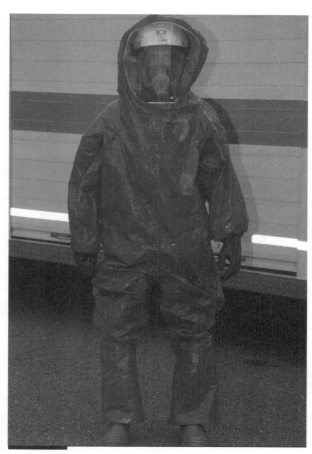

Figure 16-2 Level A protective gear, designed for use in areas contaminated with nerve gas.

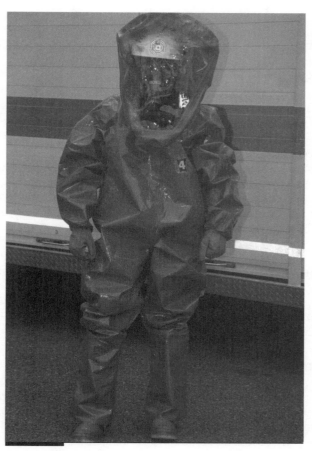

Figure 16-3 Level B protection.

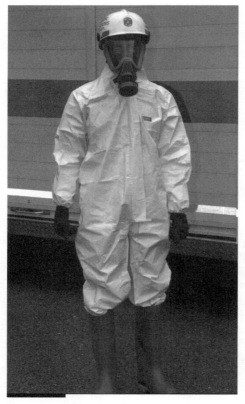

Figure 16-4 Level C protection.

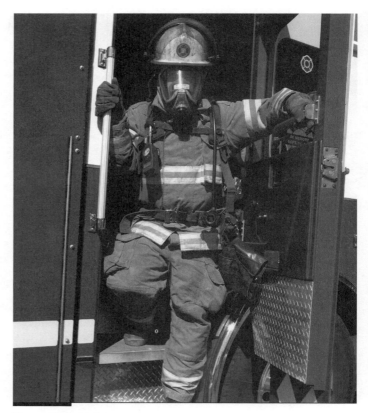

Figure 16-5 Firefighter turnout gear.

contaminated patients, inexpensive disposable chemical-resistant multi-layer polymer suits are available that correspond to Level C protection.

Technically, full military MOPP gear is equivalent to Level C protection, because complete splash protection, impermeable garments, and SCBA or SAR are not included.

Level D

Level D equipment consists of standard work clothes and no respiratory protection. The usual Level D protection prescribed includes a long sleeve shirt and long pants, so scrubs do not even qualify as Level D protection. Level D is used only when there is no danger of chemical exposure.

Special purpose decontamination squads should have appropriate garments with them or readily available at all times. Decontamination officers should review the available types and compare protection times with the types of agents most commonly found in the community. *Remember that no garment is impermeable forever.* Level D protection is sometimes mixed with Level A protection.

Firefighter Turnout Gear

Turnout gear is designed to shed embers and water **(Figure 16-5).** It will provide protection for the medical provider for a short period. (Approximately 30 minutes when combined with SCBA. This may be enough time to affect a rescue of living patients through a possibly contaminated area.) It is difficult to decontaminate, and may need to be discarded after contamination. It should not be considered as worthwhile protection from a chemical weapon hazard, because it is categorized as Level D protection.

Tyvek Suits

Many types of special purpose protective garments are available that provide more protection than Tyvek does. However, Tyvek is relatively inexpensive and readily available. It will provide short-term protection from small quantities of most materials. For medical professionals who are not involved in gross decontamination and cleanup, this level of protection will usually suffice. It is not suitable for the decontamination of the patient who has been exposed to nerve agents or vesicle-forming agents as part of a terrorist attack. Quite simply, the protection from splashes and spills that Tyvek provides is not adequate when one considers the consequences of the penetration of this barrier, which is merely Level D protection with some additional liquid-splash barrier protection.

Note that several special-purpose garments that have been classified as Level B or even Level A protection may have Tyvek as one of the layers of protection. This is not the same as having Tyvek as the ONLY protection. Because no one material can protect against all chemicals, multiple layers are used to combine the resistant qualities of each.

Gloves

Glove material is an important consideration, because the practitioner's hands make the most contact with the patient. Unfortunately, there is no one glove material that can provide adequate protection against all chemicals. Many authorities recommend multiple gloves of multiple materials, but this is bulky and decreases the practitioner's ability to feel a pulse or use tools.

Thin, flexible, nitrile gloves permit manual dexterity and offer significant resistance to chemical contamination. They cost only a fraction more than similar rubber gloves. Because medical providers must often touch casualties before decontamination is complete, they should use this protection. Both short (regular) and gauntlet-length gloves should be provided.

Latex gloves allow chemical agents to pass through so quickly that they are effectively useless, even if doubled or tripled gloves are worn.

Nitrile Boots

As with nitrile gloves, nitrile boots offer significant resistance to chemical contamination. Because the medical decontamination provider will step in water and contaminants, overboots are essential.

Face Protection

Either full-face protection masks (preferred) or eye protection goggles should be available for all medical personnel. These may be built into the SCBA or respirator.

Respirators and Breathing Systems

Respirators and breathing systems can be designed to supply air under positive pressure, or to require the operator to inhale forcibly (negative pressure). Because the contamination of hazardous materials face masks would be best prevented by positive air pressure, OSHA has banned the use of all negative-pressure devices in environments that are immediately hazardous to life and health. This ban applies when working with ANY nerve agent at ANY concentration. This includes all military style protective masks.

Self-Contained Breathing Apparatus

The best breathing system is a **self-contained breathing apparatus** or SCBA system **(Figure 16-6)**. If you have ever seen a firefighter wearing a full-face mask with an air tank

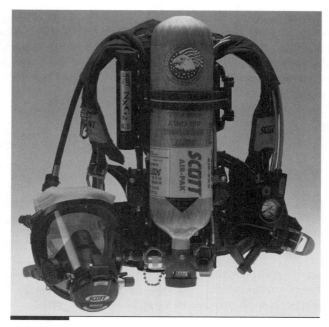

Figure 16-6 Self-contained breathing apparatus.

on his or her back, then you have seen an SCBA system. The air tank contains high-pressure purified air and works exactly like the tank used by a scuba diver. The tank provides constant positive pressure to the face mask. A SCBA provides the best protection against chemical hazards, but has the following problems:

- The tanks are heavy and bulky.
- The tanks contain only 30 or 60 minutes of air.
- The tanks have to be refilled using special equipment.
- SCBA systems are expensive.

The compressed-air reservoir limits the duration of the use of the suit, because the entire air supply must be carried on the user's back. Spare cylinders must be stocked in a ratio of about 4 cylinders to each mask unit in order to ensure a continuous supply in more remote areas.

For firefighting and scene response and decontamination, an SCBA system makes a lot of sense. The smoke is thick, dangerous, and contains an unknown mix of poisonous gases. The fire may consume most or all of the oxygen in the air. The fire engine or hazardous materials response van can carry extra tanks or refilling equipment, and a firefighter spends a limited time in the burning building or contaminated environment. For civilians in a decontamination area or for soldiers on the battlefield, however, an SCBA system is unworkable because of the limited air time available.

SCBA requires substantial training to use safely. It is also quite expensive, both for original purchase and upkeep. All members of the decontamination squad who enter the exclusion areas should have their own SCBA.

Supplied Air Respirators

Supplied air respirators, or SARs, provide an uncontaminated source of air through an external supply. That air supply can be provided by a hose that runs from a pump or supply canister located outside the contaminated zone.

A hose-fed breathing apparatus provides supplemental oxygen or purified air to an encapsulated worker from a central supply point. It is not suitable for those who are working in the hot zone, because of the potential for the entanglement of the hoses or the need for excessively long hose lines. Hoses provide much longer duration, but they may become tangled, break, or rupture, and they may be too short to effectively separate the air supply from the hazards. Two types of masks are available for the SAR: a valve actuated air supply and a continuous flowing air supply.

A hose-fed breathing apparatus may be most useful for decontamination work, where motion and exposure are both decreased. It is suitable for those members of a decontamination team who will be quite close to the hospital.

The major problems of the SAR are as follows:

- If the hose kinks, the air is cut off.
- If the air supply becomes contaminated, so does the user.
- If the hose is too short, it will not reach the area where help is needed.

These problems can be temporarily solved by a "rescue" SCBA worn together with the SAR. This rescue bottle allows 10 or 15 minutes of additional air to allow the member to escape the environment, even if the hose is broken or kinked.

Powered Air Purifying Respirator

Another type of supplied air respirator, the **powered air purifying respirator**, uses the same sort of filter cartridge found in an air purifying respirator. However, instead of placing the filter directly on the mask and requiring the user's lungs to suck air through it, the filter attaches to a battery-operated canister. The canister uses a fan to push air through the filter, and then the purified air runs through a hose to the mask. The advantage is that the air coming into the mask has positive pressure. Any leak in the mask causes purified air from the canister to escape, rather than allowing contaminated air from the environment to enter. Obviously, positive pressure creates a much safer system, but it has two disadvantages:

- If the batteries die, so does the user.
- The constant airflow through the filter means that the filter does not last as long.

The SAR may be the only option for infants and children, because their small faces make masks difficult to fit reliably.

A valve actuated air supply is much more efficient than the continuous flow type. The fit of either type of mask is much less critical than with a cartridge respirator, because air is supplied to the user under pressure and leakage will be away from the airway.

Cartridge Respirators

Cartridge respirators are the typical military style gas masks often seen in the media. The term *gas mask* is now controversial, and authors seem to avoid the common term. Although many authors have coined complex terms for this device, including air purifying respirator, protective respirator, negative-pressure canister filter protective masks, and cartridge respiratory protective devices, the operating principles of the gas mask remain unchanged from its pre–World War I origins. Even the origin of the mask itself is shrouded in controversy. Generally, it is credited to Mr. Garrett A. Morgan and a 1912 patent for a Morgan Safety Hood and Smoke Protector.[4]

Cartridge respirators are inexpensive, portable, and easy to use and store. A cartridge respirator functions by filtering the air through a special sorbent material that binds the chemical vapors.

There are three different filtration tasks that the filter of a gas mask may perform:

- Particle filtration
- Chemical adsorption
- Chemical neutralization

Particle filtration is the simplest of the three tasks. In a gas mask designed to guard against a biological threat, very fine particulate filtration is useful. This is called high-efficiency particulate protection or HEPA. A bacteria or spore might have a minimum size of 1 m. Most HEPA particulate filters remove particle sizes as small as 0.3 m. Any particulate filter eventually clogs, and breathing becomes more difficult.

Chemical adsorption requires a different approach, because chemical weapons are most often dispersed as mists or vapors that are largely immune to particulate filtration. The most common approach with any organic chemical (whether it is paint or a nerve toxin like sarin) is to adsorb it to activated charcoal.

Activated charcoal is charcoal that has been treated with oxygen to open up millions of tiny pores within the structure of the charcoal. The use of special manufacturing techniques results in highly porous charcoals that have surface areas of 300 to 2,000 sq m/g. The huge surface area of activated charcoal gives it countless bonding sites. Activated charcoal is good at trapping carbon-based impurities (organic chemicals), as well as chemicals like chlorine. When these chemicals pass next to the carbon surface, they attach to the surface and become trapped. This means that an activated-charcoal filter will remove certain impurities while ignoring others. Many other chemicals are not attracted to carbon at all, so they pass right through. It also means that, once all of the bonding sites are filled, an activated-charcoal filter stops working.

Chemical neutralization is the third technique used within the gas mask. For example, during chlorine gas attacks in World War I, masks were made that contained chemicals that react with and neutralize chlorine and phosgene. Certain low-molecular chemical warfare agents, such as hydrogen cyanide and cyanogen chloride, are poorly adsorbed by activated charcoal. In order to also protect against these agents, modern military masks are augmented by impregnating the charcoal with metallic salts of copper, chromium, and sometimes silver. Further impregnation with organic substances that augment protection against nerve agents are also used, the most common additive being triethylenediamine.

For industrial respirators, there are a variety of filters available that are specific for the chemical that must be eliminated. These often contain a neutralization agent to afford better protection against a specific chemical. The different filters are color coded by NIOSH standards.

The cartridge may be chosen for general purpose or for the specific agent that is identified. A wide variety of filters is available that protect against special chemicals or combinations of chemicals. Different cartridges must be used to protect from nerve gases, organic vapors, acid gases, chlorine, ammonia, and methylamine. The general purpose cartridges will often have a markedly shorter effective protection life span than the specific agent cartridges. Multiple filter sets should be carried that will protect against commonly encountered hazards in the area.

Cartridge respirators have a finite lifetime during use. If the concentration of the agent is high or the time that the cartridge is used is lengthy, then the chemicals will saturate the sorbent material or use up the reactive agents. When this happens, the respirator starts to deliver contaminated air to the user. The typical military filter provides protection against at least 10 (but probably up to 100) attacks before chemical warfare agents start to leak through the filter elements.

If the protective mask is used in a noncontaminated atmosphere the filter will gradually become ineffective as it absorbs moisture and pollution from the air. Long-term use or unsuitable storage may degrade the protective ability against some chemical warfare agents. As mentioned, when the HEPA portion of the filter element is saturated with particulates, it becomes increasingly difficult to draw in another

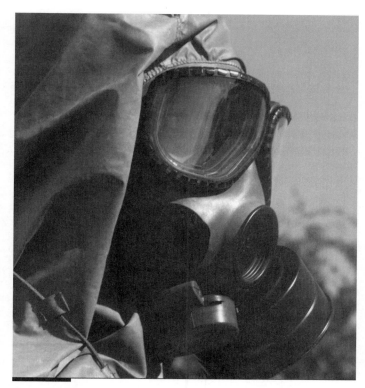

Figure 16-7 M40 military canister style protective mask (modern issued protective mask in the US military).

breath. These factors limit the use of cartridge respirators to short-term use or to low concentrations of chemicals in the air. Because all filters have a finite duration of protection, spare filters of each type selected should be readily available.

The user provides the power to draw his or her breath through the canister and filter the air. This negative pressure can also draw contaminated air through the edges of a poorly fitting mask. A moderate amount of respiratory work is involved when inhaling across the pressure resistance of the filter cartridge. As noted earlier, negative pressure masks are *not* approved by OSHA, despite use by the military.

Cartridge respirators must be fitted to the user with an airtight seal **(Figure 16-7)**. The major problem with any air purifying respirator is that any leak in the mask renders the protection ineffective. The leak could come from a poor fit between the mask and the user's face, or from a crack or hole somewhere on the mask. Facial hair will also destroy this seal and render the mask useless.

Although masks may be found that only cover the nose and the mouth, the user must still have eye protection with goggles. There is little sense to using a half-face mask for decontamination work.

■ Responder Health and Safety

Preentry and Postentry Medical Examination

A brief physical examination is *mandatory* for all operations responders and those donning Level B or C PPE. The well-being of all responders should be monitored irrespective of the level of PPE; however, donning Level A and B PPE places re-

sponders at a higher risk for illness and injury. A minimum of vital signs and a brief subjective interview should be performed before donning and immediately after doffing PPE. The exam should assess for the following criteria:

Physical Examination
- Blood pressure should not be greater than 150/90 mm Hg
- Pulse should not be greater than 110 beats/min
- Respiration should not be greater than 24 breaths/min
- Temperature should not be greater than 99.2°F
- Lung sounds should be bilateral, equal, and clear, with good expansion

Subjective Interview Questions
Are you experiencing any of the following?
- Chest pains
- Dizziness or light-headedness
- Difficulty breathing or shortness of breath
- Palpitations
- Nausea
- Fear or anxiety that is disproportionate to the magnitude of the incident (Remember, hazardous materials responders are a select group of individuals, who may feel greater than normal pressure to perform. They often suppress their fears and anxieties in order to get the job done. Although danger is part of the job, a high degree of anxiety may adversely affect a member's performance, and place that member and his or her partner in danger.)

Anyone who does not meet the criteria above should be excluded from the operation. However, stress and anxiety can alter many of the examination benchmarks. A certain degree of common sense and discretion should be exercised when assessing responders. For example, was a responder excluded because he or she ran two blocks with equipment to the suit support area and, as a result, is now tachycardic? In this case, the responder who is excluded because of the pulse criterion should be advised to find someplace to relax for some time and come back when he or she has calmed down a bit.

■ Problems Caused by Protective Gear

Patient Evaluation
Vital Signs

It has been well established that obtaining reliable vital signs is difficult to impossible when either the examiner or the patient is wearing protective garments.[5-7] Adequate monitoring of the patient's condition may require that the patient's protective garments be breached. Of course, vital signs are easy to obtain and treatment easy to provide when protective garments have been removed. However, once this occurs, the patient is exposed to further contamination. A major consideration is the determination of a safe time to remove the patient's protective garments.[8]

Pulse

It is indeed difficult to measure a normal pulse when a patient is wearing protective garments, particularly when the examiner is also gloved. When the patient is hypotensive, in protective garments, and in transit, this may become an exercise in futility. Direct contact of the examiner's fingers to the patient's skin will eliminate many of these problems, but at a cost of the exposure of both patient and examiner to the agents that prompted the use of garments in the first place.

Pulses may be remotely measured by a **piezoelectric crystal plethysmograph** attached to a finger. An alternative may be the use of infrared light emitting **diodes** and receivers, such as are used in pulse oximeters. Both of these methods require the exposure of the casualty, at least of the finger. If there are only a few people in protective garments, it may be possible to wire the patient with earlobe pulse oximeter probes prior to donning protective garments. This will be an unlikely scenario in most field operations, unfortunately.

Doppler flow devices are quite efficient at detecting flow, but they require direct contact with naked, gel-covered skin. This mandates exposure of the casualty. Doppler flow devices will allow a very accurate determination of systolic blood pressures.

Oxygenation

Oxygen saturation is easily measured with pulse oximeters, which are available from a wide variety of manufacturers, and is the best guide to the state of perfusion. The provider may also note cyanosis under protective garments, but it is much more difficult if the patient is wearing a protective mask or SCBA. The respiratory status provides only indirect evidence of oxygenation, which can be markedly changed by some chemical agents.

Respiration

The patient's respiratory rate can be measured by a cogent and attentive observer, even when both the patient and the observer are in protective garments. If the trained observer has to attend to multiple casualties, this measurement is discontinuous. Lay helpers can be rapidly taught to assess depth and rate of respirations in static victims, but subtle nuances will be missed. When the victim is being transported, such lay observers may be unable to adequately evaluate the patient.

Transthoracic impedance devices, such as used for premature infants, are available and quite reliable. However, they are relatively expensive and require a breach of the protective garments to apply. Diaphoretic patients may rapidly shed the electrodes, necessitating multiple exposures of the patient in order to reapply electrodes.

■ Responder Stresses Caused by Protective Gear

Protective Garments

Not only are protective garments annoying, they result in serious decrements of performance.

Irritation

As any first-year resident or scrub nurse in training realizes, the moment that protective garments are donned, the itches start, sneezes begin, snuffles commence, and the latrine starts to issue a summons. Whether motivated by fear or by heat, sweating starts, and there is no way to keep it from running into the eyes. These irritations all add to distraction. When job performance is critical, distraction may result in an increase in accidental injuries, breaches in protection, and a decrease in performance.

Anxiety

As soon as the provider realizes there is a threat, anxiety will cause psychological casualties. These psychological casualties may constitute a major problem for the incident scene commander, because the medical services will have to treat not only casualties from the support and evacuation units, but from their own ranks. These casualties may not be overt and may only suffer major decrements in performance.

A major relief to stress is socialization and communication with friends and colleagues. When one is wearing protective gear, normal facial expressions are unreadable even at a close distance. Voices are changed, and clarity and timbre are lost during transmission through masks and face pieces. Eye contact may also be lost. Body contact becomes difficult and muffled by the protective garments. This loss of socialization and communication heightens the anxiety.

The process of decontamination itself may cause an increase in anxiety. Unless decontamination is complete, the clean areas will rapidly become dirty. This will produce substantial amounts of distrust and anxiety about the thoroughness of the decontamination. An anxious, hungry, hot, dehydrated, exhausted squad member who is forced to go through the decontamination station "yet another time" is a fused and primed explosive device. Obsessive and compulsive decontamination squads must be tempered by leaders with compassion and understanding about the job stress of the field member.

Respiratory Effort

Until one has abundant experience with either a respirator or SCBA, the increased effort of respirations becomes an annoyance. If the activity requires substantial physical exertion, then the increased work of breathing will cause a decrease in performance. Because difficulty in breathing is an early sign of poisoning by some chemical agents, the increased work of breathing may provoke anxiety about the integrity of the protective garments.

Heat Load

The use of saunas and total body occlusive wraps and other conditions of high humidity and heat stress will increase the incidence of heat stroke. A black or dark brown, totally sealed, protective suit will easily qualify as a sauna on a hot day. The inability of a person in full protective garments to lose heat by radiation, convection, or evaporation is well documented.[9-11] If a casualty results from this high heat load, it may be impossible to differentiate the early effects of a nerve agent from that of exertional heat stroke. Lesser heat loads may lead to a decrease in attention span and performance, resulting in accidental injuries. The medical team must constantly monitor the team members for such signs of heat stress.

Dehydration

Drinking is possible with only a few of the protective mask designs, and then only from specially designed containers.[12] Even when one has all the right equipment, drinking is difficult to accomplish without practice with the assembled equipment. Inadequate amounts of water may be consumed during the use of this equipment, especially when one considers the increased water loss caused by heat load. Dehydration becomes a distinct possibility. Even modest dehydration will produce a marked decrease in both physical and mental abilities.

Use and Condition of the Garment

Damaged or improperly donned protective clothing will allow the entry of contaminants and set the stage for potentially disastrous results. At the very least, decontamination will be more difficult.

Improper protective garments will afford little or no protection. Chemicals may rapidly permeate through and into incompatible garments and respirator filters.

■ Summary

The next pages summarize the protective equipment needed for a decontamination operation and the steps of a field decontamination.

■ Equipment

This equipment list will provide MINIMAL protection to the emergency squad responding to an accident or to the hospital receiving casualties from such an accident. It is not designed or intended to replace specific guidelines for known agents.

Containment Equipment
Pools and Buckets

A child's rigid sided or inflatable wading pool provides an ideal sump to contain contaminated wash water and decontamination solutions. These wading pools may be purchased in quantity and stored until needed, with little chance of degradation. Of course, specific supplies for the EMS trade are available, but these are usually several orders of magnitude more expensive that the substitutes.

Plastic Bags

Bags of all available sizes should be available for preserving samples and disposing of contaminated materials. Small sizes may be used for valuables and specimens, while large sizes may be used for contaminated clothing and equipment. Clear zip-front body bags will minimize contamination to both the transport personnel and the transport vehicle.

Plastic Sheeting

Plastic sheeting may be used to cover nonessential and nonmovable equipment. Ventilation ducts may be sealed with duct tape and plastic sheeting. "Safe" corridors may be marked with plastic sheeting. It is almost impossible to have enough of this material during an actual incident.

Plastic tarps may be used to further contain spills, to provide privacy for decontamination operations, and to serve as tool or equipment dumps. They may be purchased in a variety of sizes and weights.

Engineer's Tape or Police Marker Tape

Engineer's tape comes in 100-ft rolls of bright colors and may be used to mark out exclusion zones and decontamination stations. Police or special purpose marker tape is somewhat more expensive and serves the same purpose. Marker cones are also useful.

Saw Horses

Saw horses or military litter stands may be used to provide an elevated and level surface to work on patients. Both military litters and backboards can be placed on the stands. Elevation of the litters allows the triage and treatment teams to work with much less fatigue.

Cleaning Supplies
Clothing and Hair Removal Supplies

The following should be kept on hand for clothing and hair removal:

- 2 pairs of paramedic scissors
- Hair clippers
- Disposable combs and brushes

Bleach, Detergent, and PEG

The well-equipped emergency department has at least one bottle of bleach and a box of phosphate-containing Tide or similar detergent. If possible, access should be arranged to a 55-gallon drum of polyethylene glycol solution (PEG-400). For some situations, stripping paint may be appropriate.

Contaminated Storage Supplies

The following should be kept on hand for storing contaminated items:

- 6 small steel drums (5-gallon size)
- 8 waste-disposal pails
- 25 half-gallon polyethylene plastic bottles
- 50 to 100 polyethylene bags (10-gallon size)
- 50 1-quart ice cream containers

Kitty Litter or Similar Absorbent Material

This material will allow spills of contaminants to be absorbed and then cleaned up easily.

Sponges and Soft Brushes

Abundant disposable brushes, cloths, and sponges should be stored. These may be used for cleaning victims or equipment. Do not forget some sort of remote handling tongs and cotton-tipped applicators for the removal of items.

Surgical Equipment

Remember that all equipment within the decontamination area must be considered disposable!

- Suction machine (manual or electric)
- Anesthesia dispensing equipment
- Oxygen tanks
- Surgical lamps

INHOSPITAL INFO

- Surgical drapes and towels
- Surgical instruments for minor surgery
- Instrument carts
- 2 tracheotomy trays
- 2 cut-down trays
- Physical examination equipment
- Nasal-irrigation sets
- Syringes and needles for administering medication and obtaining blood samples
- 2 or 3 disposable suture sets should be available for the removal of particulate contamination
- Normal saline for irrigation
- Bulb syringes

Medications

- Appropriate irrigating solutions
- Emergency drug trays
- Ophthalmic ointments
- Phenylephrine 0.25% nasal spray

Sample Equipment

- Cotton swabs
- Blood drawing equipment
- Blood collection containers
- Urine collection containers
- Sputum collection containers

Clerical Supplies

- Marking tags and labels
- Approximately 200 large envelopes for wallets, documents, keys, etc.
- Pens and pencils
- Triage tags
- Clipboard
- Magic markers
- Masking or gaffer's tape (This tape can be used to secure bags or markers to items. It may also be used to mark containers.)
- 1 tape recorder and 12 cassettes
- Polaroid camera, flash-bulbs, and film. Alternatively, a digital camera with abundant memory or multiple memory cards.
- 2 emergency logs

Water

This may be more difficult to provide and control than anticipated. Showers and decontamination scrubbings consume frightfully large amounts of water. Check with the fire department and arrange for a water resupply prior to an incident. Both hot and cold running water are desirable (and, in some climates, absolutely necessary). Additional supplies of cool potable water are needed for hot climates.

Garden hose and a portable showerhead may allow you to bring the shower to the critical patient, rather than move the patient to the shower. Fifty feet or more of garden hose is recommended. Fire units may charge a small line with a fog nozzle for the same purpose.

■ Nine-Step Field Decontamination Plan

The following nine steps summarize the decontamination process.

Step 1: Entry

A specified entry point allows the control of contaminated personnel. A tool drop within the contaminated area ensures that any tools, which may be needed by other personnel at the accident site, are left in the "dirty" place. This will keep the tools available for replacements or for those who only need to decontaminate enough to safely change the SCBA units.

Step 2: Gross Cleaning

In this step, as much solid, liquid, or gas as possible is removed from contaminated personnel. When working with high-risk agents, everyone who is working at step 2 should be wearing SCBA and have a level of protection equal to or better than the person being decontaminated. These step 2 workers will also have to be completely decontaminated when their job is done.

Step 3: SCBA and Respirator Servicing

At this point, additional SCBA equipment must be made available. For high-risk hazardous materials, the entire SCBA must be changed. For lower-risk agents, air bottle or filter changes may be appropriate. Clean units are handed from the clean side of the decontamination station, and dirty units are left in the contaminated area for cleaning and resupply.

Step 4: Protective Clothing Removal

Protective clothing should be removed and isolated at step 4. It may be necessary to dispose of protective clothing, rather than attempt detoxification. Abundant supplies of protective garments are needed for replacement workers in these cases.

Step 5: Personal Clothing Removal

In the management of extremely hazardous materials, the complete removal of personal clothing is required. This may include undergarments and personal effects, such as watches and jewelry.

Step 6: Body Washing

Again, in the management of extremely hazardous materials, showers and body washing are required. Heated overhead showers are much better than cold water hose lines. Sumps or tubs may be used to control water runoff.

The decontamination officer should ensure that the wash is complete, including behind and in the ears. Soap and water will usually suffice for these areas. In extreme cases, hair clipping may be necessary. Shaving may increase the absorption of agents, so it should be avoided. Contact lenses should be removed, and the eyes should be irrigated to remove contaminants.

When materials do not present an extreme hazard, the shower area may be set up at a fire station, gym, or school. Prior arrangements with the owners are essential.

Step 7: Dry and Redress

Towels and clean replacement clothes must be provided. Disposable coveralls, surgical scrubs, and hospital slippers are inexpensive and easy to obtain.

Step 8: Medical Evaluation

After decontamination is complete, the decontaminated personnel should be evaluated by medical providers. A log should be maintained of each and every person who was in the hot zone. Vital signs should be taken on every person.

Any open wounds or skin breaks should be noted by the medical personnel. Even if these are not new injuries, they should be cleansed and properly evaluated for the presence of contaminants. Physicians who are trained in the management of the agent involved should be consulted for advice regarding these wounds.

Step 9: Observation, Medical Treatment, and Debriefing

Special decontamination may be required for personnel who may have inhaled an agent, sustained a contaminated wound, or handled an agent that readily penetrates intact skin. At this point, further observation may be necessary for personnel who have been exposed to chemicals with late effects. These personnel should be transported to an emergency department for further medical evaluation and therapy.

All personnel should be debriefed by a recorder, noting the duration of exposure, protection used, and any special features of the accident. This information may be quite useful for both medical and administrative investigations regarding casualties.

■ Resources

See this book's Website for contact information for the following organizations.

CHEMTREC

Chemical Manufacturers Association's Chemical Transportation Emergency Center (CHEMTREC) is available for emergency assistance 24 hours per day. This single resource will aid in contacting all other agencies and correlating available data for protection and decontamination hazards. CHEMTREC cannot provide adequate medical help for physicians treating contaminated patients.

Oil and Hazardous Materials Technical Assistance Data Service

The Oil and Hazardous Materials Technical Assistance Data Service (OHM-TADS) will provide help about petroleum and derivatives through physical characteristics. OHM-TADS can be contacted through CHEMTREC.

The Chlorine Emergency Plan

Chlorine manufacturers' Chlorine Emergency Plan (CHLOREP) can be contacted through CHEMTREC.

These resources emphasize safety, containment, decontamination, and cleanup. They are weak on medical care. Because of this, the responsibility for care of the patient continues to rest with the treating physician.

■ Suggested Additional Reading

- Hazardous Materials Incident Response Operations (Unit 3), in *US Environmental Protection Agency Training Manual*. US Environmental Protection Agency, (not available for public distribution).
- *Hazardous Materials Emergency Response Guidebook*. Department of Transportation (DOT publication 5800.3).

■ References

1. Heully F, Gruninger M: Collective intoxication caused by the explosion of a mustard gas shell. *Annales de Medicine Legale* 1956;36:195-204.
2. Lorin HG, Kulling PEJ: The Bhopal tragedy: What has Swedish disaster medicine planning learned from it? *J Emerg Med* 1986;4:311-316.
3. Okumura T, Takasu N, Ishimatsu S, et al: Report on 640 victims of the Tokyo subway sarin attack. *Ann Emerg Med* 1996;28:129-135.
4. Bellis M: Garrett Morgan gas mask patent. *What you need to know About* Web site. http://inventors.about.com/library/inventors/blgas_mask2.htm (accessed April 2, 2002).
5. Burgin WW, Gehring LM, Bell TL: A chemical field resuscitation device. *Mil Med* 1982;147:873-874.
6. Bennion SD: Designing of NBC protective gear to allow for adequate first aid. *Mil Med* 1982;147:960-962.
7. Hodson PB: Assessment of casualties in a chemical environment. *J R Army Med Corps* 1985;131:116-117.
8. Gaston B: Casualty decontamination during amphibious assault. *Navy Med* 1988;7:8-9.
9. Stephenson LA, Kolka MA, Allan AE, Santee WR: Heat exchange during encapsulation in a chemical warfare agent protective patient wrap in four hot environments. *Aviat Space Env Med* 1988;59;345-351.
10. Nishi Y, Gonzalez RR, Gagge AP: Prediction of equivalent environments by energy exchange and assessments of physiological strain and discomfort. *Israel J Med Sci* 1976;12:808-861.
11. Stewart C: *Environmental Emergencies*. Baltimore, MD, Williams and Wilkins, 1989.
12. Cadigan FC: Battleshock: The chemical dimension. *J R Army Med Corps* 1982;128:89-92.

CHAPTER

17 Summary and Conclusions

■ Threat

In attempting to evaluate agents that can be used to cause mass casualties, the question, *What can cause a maximum credible event?* is often posed. A maximum credible event is an event that could cause a large loss of life, in addition to the disruption, panic, and overwhelming use of civilian health care resources. Experts state that for an agent to be considered capable of causing a maximum credible event, it should be highly lethal, inexpensively and easily produced, stable in aerosol form, and able to be dispersed.

As was evident with the anthrax-contaminated letters sent to individual targets in the media and Congress in late 2001, this may not be the appropriate question when considering a terrorist event. A terrorist is in the business of seeding terror. If a miniscule amount of a lethal agent achieves widespread media attention, then the terrorist has adequately performed the job. If the event changes the behavior of the police, media, and public alike, then the terrorist has achieved his or her objectives.

Perhaps a better question is, *What agents are credible as terrorist weapons?* Subcategories of this question include:

- Which agents are easily manufactured?
  - Which agents are readily available, particularly in the countries that sponsor terrorism or their close allies?
  - Which agents could be adapted, stolen, or genetically engineered?
- Which agents would cause significant morbidity or mortality?
  - Which agents would cause significant casualties that require significant health care resources?
- Which agents would strike fear into the hearts of the public?
  - Which agents have had substantial media exposure?
  - Which agents have a high lethality?
  - Which agents cause a high morbidity?
  - Which agents have a high communicability?

Despite mass infusions of federal cash into the fields of chemical and biological warfare and terrorism, we are still not prepared. Our experience with biological terrorism in the public mail has certainly shown that there is little or no ability to anticipate a chemical or biological attack, little or no ability to detect one if it occurs, and little ability to manage the consequences if attacked.[1] Quite simply, the United States is unprepared to deal with a biological or chemical attack.[2]

There are multifactorial reasons for this unpreparedness in the United States. Areas that need improvement are listed in the next sections.

Availability

Biological warfare agents can be easily procured from the environment, clinical specimens, universities, and biological supply houses.[3] In 1995, the Aum Shinrikyo cult, famous for its use of sarin gas, was found to possess biological weapons including anthrax, botulism, and Q fever. Plague is endemic in Colorado prairie dogs, and anthrax can be found in North Dakota and South Dakota.

Common fermentation techniques used for producing antibiotics, toxoid vaccines, and some beverages can be used to grow large quantities of biological agents. Viral agents are an order of magnitude more difficult, but well within the training of a PhD in microbiology. The argument that bioweapons must be state-sponsored ignores much historical precedent.[4]

Chemical weapon availability has already been discussed in detail in this text. There is no question that terrorists can obtain sufficient materials to build small quantities of several common agents. Chemical agents can also be manufactured in small quantities in a warehouse or small manufacturing plant. Large quantities of ready-made agents can be stolen by hijacking trucks or tank cars.

Detection

Intelligence and the detection of biological agents is most often retrospective. When a suitable facility can be contained in the space of a large garage, intelligence services have great difficulty finding clandestine production facilities for biological agents. Biological agents are likely to be delivered covertly, and sick individuals may be the initial indication that an attack has occurred. If the agent is delivered properly, then a large number of casualties may result during a short period of time. In the midst of treating all of the casualties, emergency services must not only provide effective care, but protect themselves.

Currently available detection equipment can identify four biological agents. The improved version of this equipment, to be fielded in the near future, will be able to detect at least eight, although the exact number has not been released. There are dozens of agents that could be used as biological weapons. Our current systems that identify four or eight agents essentially serve as an obvious warning to terrorists to avoid these agents and use another agent that evades detection. This is analogous to the development of the Novichok agents in response to our current nerve agent detection equipment.

Biological agents are easily shipped from place to place, and detection during transport is nearly impossible. As noted, most of these agents are uncontrolled and can be found endemically throughout the world. Obtaining a culture is not nearly as expensive or conspicuous as obtaining nuclear material. Processing and refining a culture requires equipment that is considered suitable for a well-equipped hospital laboratory or research facility and thus is easily ordered and diverted. The fact that Saddam Hussein bought his original anthrax cultures from a mail-order house in the United States and had them shipped by a commercial overnight carrier is an example of the ease with which materials can be obtained.[5] Anthrax is a listed and watched bacterium and has been for many years.

The detection of biological agents is an intense interest of the military research and development communities. The principle difficulty in detecting a biological weapon aerosol is differentiating it from the background organic matter. Because these devices detect the agent after dispersal, there will be a huge body of exposed victims. The devices use a specific characteristic of the microbe or toxin for detection and are quite specific to those agents that are detectable. It is absurdly easy to visualize the release of an agent that is not on the highest threat list and hence not detected by the employed detectors. This may be as simple as using a virulent derivative of monkeypox instead of smallpox.

Some limited battlefield detection devices exist, but these are totally unusable in the majority of US cities. They may be helpful for a special event, such as the Olympics, where crowds are moderately constrained and threats are quite high. Current equipment includes the Biological Integrated Detection System—a truck mounted unit that samples air in search of selected agents. The Long Range Biological Standoff Detection System employs an infrared laser to detect aerosol clouds at up to 30-km distance. The Short Range Biological Standoff Detection System uses ultraviolet and laser-induced fluorescence to detect biological aerosols at distances of up to 5 km. These two latter systems provide some early warning and can cue other detection efforts.

An alternative threat is the infected pawn sacrifice. In this case, a volunteer becomes deliberately infected and goes into a crowded area to touch and infect as many others as possible. This would be an effective way to disseminate smallpox, because the patient could well be ambulatory during the early skin lesion phase of the infection.

Again, the biowarfare threat may not be directed toward humans. Livestock and crops are strategic targets and vulnerable to attack. It is not inconceivable that a Muslim terrorist would attempt to destroy all pork and pork products in the United States. Although not a killing blow for the United States as a whole, such a plague would certainly hinder the US economy. The detection of this plague would be very difficult prior to symptoms in a substantial number of affected animals.

Planning

Most planning for emergency response to terrorism has been concerned with overt attacks, such as bombings or chemical agent attacks. These attacks elicit immediate response from emergency responders, such as fire, police, and EMS personnel. To a varying degree, hospitals, EMS providers, and city, county, and state officials have paid only lip service to the idea that bioterrorism presents a clear and present danger. One only has to poll emergency physicians, paramedics, and police officers in any major city to find out that the response plans to an event in which multiple patients with similar symptoms present within a short time have not been disseminated to the responders who will be implementing them "on the ground."

Training

In order to diagnose these agents, the health care professional must be astute and suspicious regarding the possible use of biological weapons. Emergency physicians must be aware of symptoms and epidemiologic patterns that may indicate a biological attack; yet, they have never been taught these techniques. Understanding the behavior, pathogenesis, modes of transmission, means of diagnosis, and available treatment options may be as easy as reading from a chart, or may be quite difficult if an altered and weaponized agent is used.

Emergency services, police, and even hospitals must purchase equipment and train employees for work in protective gear that yet has only been found in the military and specialized fire department squads **(Figure 17-1)**. Following the release of sarin in the Tokyo subway system in 1995, 10% of the prehospital responders experienced symptoms of nerve agent poisoning as a result of exposure to victims and the contaminated environment.[6] As many as 46% of the hospital staff that cared for the victims also became symptomatic because they handled the victims. Emergency services must realize that they are significant targets and conduct their routine operations accordingly.

Attack victims may not present as ambulance patients, and the EMS providers may not be involved in the early care of these victims. Following the release of sarin in the Tokyo subway system in 1995, less than 10% of victims arrived at the hospital by ambulance. The rest arrived on foot, by taxi, or by private car. It is unlikely that the pattern of arrival will be any different with a biological agent. Indeed, with the slower onset of symptoms, one can expect that more patients will present without EMS involvement.

Timely Response

A biological agent is slow moving and may well be covert. The use of most germ agents will involve a delay between the exposure and the onset of illness—the incubation period. Only a short window of opportunity will exist between the time that the first cases are identified and the second wave of the population starts to become ill. During that brief period, public health officials must verify that the attack has occurred, identify the specific organism or organisms used, and start mitigation and prevention with quarantine and mass vaccination or prophylactic treatment.

Even if an astute emergency physician notes that an unusual number of patients have a certain disease and contacts the CDC for help, the crisis is recognized immediately as a biowarfare attack, and help is dispatched immediately, the lag time may be unwieldy. Remember that with some of the agents that have been identified, there is an incubation period of up to 20 days from the time of dissemination of the agent before the first symptoms occur. The patient may be quite infective during latter parts of this incubation period. The secondary contacts may be untraceable. (Just imagine a single patient infected with smallpox sitting in a busy waiting room in a metropolitan emergency department for 4 to 6 hours before being seen and having the condition diagnosed as smallpox.)

If an attack occurs in a targeted city, such as Los Angeles, New York, San Francisco, Denver, Chicago, or Washington, we can presume that plans have been made and supplies have been stockpiled.[7] The response time for these cities can be measured in hours from the first notification or recognition of a problem.

Given absolute best case scenario response times after notification, it will take at least 2 to 3 hours for a qualified team of local predesignated physicians and prehospital providers to assemble, draw gear, and convene in the response area. It will take another few hours to assess the situation, draw appropriate clinical samples, and formulate an idea of what illness or toxin was employed. When local teams are unavailable, incapacitated, or delayed by events, such as panic or simultaneous attacks with other devices or agents, the on-scene response time grows rapidly.

During this time, others would be exposed and potential carriers may leave the city bound for other destinations. When casualties exceed the available medical resources, then additional resources must be identified and assembled, after which the resources must be transported to the casualties, or the casualties must be transported to the resources. This could take days or weeks. If news services broadcast any warning, one can expect a panic-stricken response that may cause gridlock on the roads and further complicate any response team's travels to the area.

If the attack occurs in a nontargeted city, such as Kansas City, then there is far less likelihood of adequate prepositioned stocks of protective garments, antibiotics, vaccines, and supplies. Qualified medical providers will not only have to bring their own protective garments, but may have to provide all other supplies at the scene. This response will be measured in tens of hours rather than hours.

Prophylaxis

There is no question that there are not enough emergency providers who have received enough immunizations to care for the population in the event of an attack against a US city.

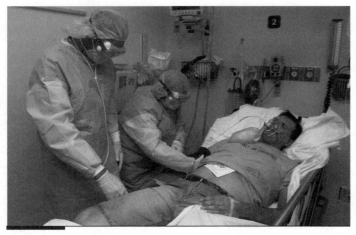

Figure 17-1 Training with protective gear is needed in order to properly prepare for a terrorist attack.

There is also no question that the providers will be at the highest risk of exposure if active agents are employed. Because it is unlikely that we will know the agent in advance, it is unlikely that advanced protection is possible.

Federal officials often note that antibiotics have been stockpiled and vaccines have been developed for many of the possible terrorist agents. A simple look at one of the most common agents, smallpox, will quickly verify that the United States simply does not have enough vaccine to immunize the bulk of any one large city. If a coordinated attack on two or more cities were mounted, then current stocks would be woefully inadequate. This does not even include the vast problems associated with the dispersal of the vaccine to all who need it.

Furthermore, in the case of anthrax, it has been noted that the most common prophylactic antibiotics used are contraindicated in children (quinolones and tetracyclines).[8] Because these contraindications are widely promulgated, the response of parents and medical community might be problematic if these antibiotics were dispensed to the pediatric population.

Finally, the stockpiled antibiotics and vaccines may be worthless. Biowarfare specialist Ken Alibek described multiresistant strains of *Yersinia pestis* and aggressive strains of anthrax that were developed by BioPreparat in the former Soviet Union.[9] There is further indication that BioPreparat developers were working on a chimeric virus with the lethal potential of both smallpox and the Ebola virus.

Politics and Jurisdictional Control

When given the choice of where to spend defense money, it is easier to put it into real and visible tools such as guns, battleships, and troops. Bluntly speaking, cruise missiles are easier to sell to a congressional committee than protective garments in Tulsa.

Another debatable issue that affects preparedness is one of control. When a biowar incident occurs, who will be in charge?[10,11] Will it be local fire, police, or emergency services personnel? Will it be medical authorities from state, county, or local departments of health?

Certainly these questions have not been adequately answered, and control issues are always best answered in advance of the incident, rather than during the emergency. Any governor, city manager, or mayor should consider these factors and establish a firm grasp of who is to be in charge and why they are to be in charge before an emergency happens. These questions have all been answered for conventional hazardous materials operations, explosives, and conventional terrorist actions, yet much posturing and politicking occurred during such events as the World Trade Center bombing and the Oklahoma City bombing. In the Atlanta 1996 Olympics, thousands of man-hours of planning were devoted to establishing who was to be in charge (and why) in the event of multiple kinds of terrorism. Because that planning was already accomplished, the basic outline should be applicable for every city and should be made available and modified as required.

This thought has not escaped the federal government. President Clinton signed Executive Order 12938 on No-

vember 14, 1994. This order declared a national emergency because of the unusual and extraordinary threat that the proliferation of weapons of mass destruction poses to the national security, foreign interest, and economy of the United States. Following the sarin gas attack in Japan and the Oklahoma City bombing, President Clinton signed Presidential Decision Directive 39, which addresses how the United States should deal with the prospect of terrorist use of weapons of mass destruction. In this document, consequence management of weapons of mass destruction attacks rests with the Federal Emergency Management Agency (FEMA) for domestic incidents. The preparations include site surveys, assessments of local hospitals' abilities to treat victims, and an accounting of the size, condition, and locations of local stocks of various antidotes. The Congress followed this with Public Law 104-201, the Defense Against Weapons of Mass Destruction Act.

Theoretically, the FBI has leading responsibility for crisis response. This arm of the US Department of Justice is not responsible for medical care. Will the FBI attempt to assume control of the scene to preserve evidence? The FBI's record of cooperation with medical providers in a biological incident is unknown. It will be essential that the FBI share its threat assessment with the emergency providers who will be treating the patients.

Considering the role of FEMA, established by Presidential Decision Directive 39, it remains to be seen how the FBI and FEMA will interact. Will FEMA attempt to usurp control of the incident? FEMA has no experience in chemical or biological terrorism.

President Bush addressed some of these problems with the creation of the US Department of Homeland Security in 2002. This coalesces many disparate federal agencies and theoretically makes them more responsive. Because (at the time of publication) the Department of Homeland Security has no experience, track record, or established organization, its ability to coordinate and participate is completely unknown. Likewise, its ability or willingness to work with the local and state authorities has yet to be determined. (There is no criticism intended in these statements, just simply the acknowledgment that the new federal administration is untested.)

Will martial law be declared and render the military in control of a city? Even if martial law is declared, it will be impossible to implement without calling out the National Guard or transporting in the standing military. This too, will take tens of hours and will allow terrorists and carriers to escape. Based on responses to natural disasters, such as floods and hurricanes, a minimum response time of 36 hours seems to be an appropriate estimate.

Responsibility is also not an easy consideration. Although the US Department of Defense has the greatest capability in biological defense, the responsibility for dealing with the effects of bioweapons falls into multiple venues, including many federal, state, and local city governments and ultimately the civilian medical community.[12] Many of these organizations are completely unprepared to deal effectively with this problem.[13] Will the responsible authorities be medical experts from the CDC or even military specialists from one of the biowar development centers at Dugway or Fort Detrick? Where do these experts fit in?

Finally, will civil liberties be suspended? If so, for how long, and who will decide? Our constitution guarantees freedom of assembly, guards against unreasonable search and seizure, and upholds significant guards against the limitation of travel within the states. For some biological agents, quarantine is a logical method of decreasing the possibility of spread. Likewise, the seizure and destruction of contaminated articles, vehicles, and even houses may be required. Decisions that fall within the realm of national security are usually made by federal officials. Decisions about quarantines are usually reserved for local officials. Recent exercises have not answered these questions.[14-16]

Impact

An agent could be disseminated in a shopping mall, airport, subway, or sports arena and infect or contaminate tens of thousands of people who subsequently travel to thousands of destinations. With agents that take days for first symptoms to appear and are infective before the symptoms appear, mitigation and control of the infection may be close to impossible. Chemical agents act much more quickly and are likely to require less mitigation.

The effects of a terrorist attack are potentially catastrophic. In a paper by researchers at the CDC, the projected economic impact alone ranged from $477 million per 100,000 people exposed to brucellosis to $26.2 billion if anthrax were used.[17] Over 30,000 deaths were predicted if anthrax were used as the biological agent. The paper consistently used the lowest possible costs for all factors that affected costs, *including the virulence of the disease*. It is clear that this would not be the case in an actual disaster of this magnitude. The costs of both preparedness and intervention were not low. Even so, the authors concluded that the reduction in preventable losses through preparedness and intervention have a significantly greater impact than reductions in the probability of an attack through intelligence gathering and related activities.

The authors also noted that the best possible measures to decrease both costs and deaths were those that would enhance the rapidity of the response to an attack. "These measures would include developing and maintaining laboratory capabilities for both clinical diagnostic testing and environmental sampling, developing and maintaining drug stockpiles, and *developing and practicing response plans at the local level.*"[18]

When examining past epidemics for any clues about the potential of man-made epidemics, lay authors often look at the Black Death in Europe in the 1300s. They cite knowledge of public health, cleanliness, microbiology, and antibiotics as evidence that this kind of plague will not happen again from biological agents. Unfortunately, the devastation of a noncurable disease that is rapidly spread and causes significant casualties would not be prevented by these factors.

Other authorities look at the multiplicity of anthrax threats involving letter bombs or other small-scale dissemination of anthrax. As was shown in Sverdlovsk in 1979, point dissemination of a noncontagious agent (even in relatively large quantities) will affect only a limited area and a relatively small population.[19]

Additional Problems

There are risks in overestimating the possibility of domestic terrorism as well. These downside perils have received scant attention. The dangers include the following:

1. The increased media presence about possible threats may increase the terrorists' inclination to try certain agents.
   a. An increase in media coverage makes terror a likely outcome of the dissemination of these agents—even when the release is on a small scale.
   b. Media can illuminate the weaknesses of the country so that a terrorist can more effectively mount a successful terror operation.
   c. The media magnify strategically minor problems into countrywide incidents. Only a foolish strategic planner would fail to note the massive operation mounted to capture two snipers in Baltimore and Washington and the immense amount of media coverage expended during this operation. Thousands of citizens were paralyzed by the actions of only two terrorists.
2. The media (and the government) can falsely reassure the public about levels of preparation and the ability to mitigate disaster. This false assurance of capability often ignores the reality of logistics.
   a. Carefully staged exercises are simply not the same as the real thing.
   b. The surge capacity of hospitals and the numbers of intensive care unit beds are quite limited. Stockpiling drugs does not ensure that there are qualified physicians and nurses to properly administer these drugs, and stockpiling ventilators does not ensure that there are technicians qualified to use, monitor, and even repair these devices.
   c. Disaster medical assistance teams are equipped to treat about 300 to 400 patients per day, with a response time of about 4 to 6 hours in best case planning. Aum Shinrikyo caused about 5,000 patients to seek care within a 4-hour period.
   d. The chemical and biological agents that the terrorist employs may not be the ones for which the US government has prepared. Classic examples are dusty mustard, Novichok agents, and carbamate-based nerve agents.
   e. The Joint Commission on Accreditation of Healthcare Organizations certification implies that a hospital has paperwork that supports a disaster plan and an ability to handle disaster-related casualties. Having the paperwork in place does not mean that the hospital has actually prepared to handle excessive numbers of chemical casualties.

3. The undermining of US civil liberties in the name of enhanced security is quite likely and is probably happening today, but this does not necessarily result in adequate security.
   a. "Politically correct" screening ignores the undisputed fact that the vast majority of terrorists have been males between the ages of 15 and 40. Searching white-haired grandmothers is only window-dressing security.
   b. Confiscation of tweezers, nail clippers, and tiny Swiss Army knives is also window dressing. Pencils, pens, and belts make equally good weapons and are ignored. Hair spray cans or metered dose inhalers can be reloaded with chemical or biological agents and constitute a far greater threat.
4. The focus on large-scale attacks may be a mistake.
   a. As noted previously, small-scale attacks are much more likely than a large-scale attack with military agents.
   b. The guiding assumption is that small-scale events are an included contingency within the preparations for a high-end mass-casualty attack. This may not optimize state and local response capabilities of dealing with the much more probable simultaneous small-scale threats.

The Future

There is no question that the well-funded supranational terrorist can afford to purchase the equipment to build biological weapons or that the equipment will be sold when ordered. Unfortunately, with the downfall of communism and the resulting economic problems in the former Soviet Union, BioPreparat employees have lost their jobs. There is no question that some of these former Soviet researchers, production engineers, and munitions design engineers have sought employment elsewhere. There is equally no question that some of the new employers are not on friendly terms with the United States.

Likewise, vast stores of biological weapons (including anthrax, smallpox, plague, and other organisms) were scattered throughout the Soviet Union. Because that country has had difficulties with control of nuclear weapons and nuclear weapons components and materials since the downfall of communism, it is a sure bet that the former Soviet Union no longer retains control of all of these biological weapons stocks. Where these agents have been dispersed is sheer conjecture. Like Russia's nuclear materials, Russia's biological warfare technology may be vulnerable to leakage to third parties through either theft or outright sale.

In the Gulf War in 1991, the threat that Iraq would use biological warfare was a major concern for all coalition forces, and extensive preparations were made for this threat. Iraq conducted research and development work on anthrax, botulinum toxins, clostridial toxins, wheat smut, ricin, and aflatoxins. Field trials were conducted with botulinum toxin and aflatoxin. Anthrax release was simulated with *Bacillus subtilis* (as the United States did in the 1950s). Weapons delivery systems, including rockets, bombs, and spray tanks were tested. In all, Iraq produced nearly 20,000 L of botulinum toxin, nearly 9,000 L of concentrated anthrax, and over 2,000 L of aflatoxin and had munitions loaded to deliver these agents.[20]

Although these agents were the justification for the invasion of Iraq, the agents have not been found, despite nearly two years of occupation by US-led forces. Idle speculation would lead to the belief that the agents do not exist. Since there is abundant evidence that they were deployed in at least two conflicts, the appropriate question might be, where did they go?

Unclassified information from CIA and Defense Nuclear Agency documents indicate that numerous rogue states such as Iran, Libya, and North Korea have or are pursuing biological weapons programs.[21]

The alleged use of biological weapons has been and will continue to be controversial. Proof of use is much easier to document after nuclear or chemical weapons have been employed than after most biological agents have been employed. Biological warfare does not require a plague with thousands of deaths to be effective. If enough critical positions were vacant because of people acquiring upper respiratory infections or diarrhea, defenses could be substantially degraded. A potato famine, such as Ireland experienced, will destroy a country's economy without a single overt casualty.

To complicate matters, some biological weapons may be developed to destroy crops or livestock. It is also likely that in the future, biological weapons may be produced that can do the following:
- Damage military equipment
- Degrade the plastics used in aircraft or computers
- Render fuels useless
- Destroy rubber in tires and equipment

Nature's Biowarfare

Mother Nature has delivered several pandemics that have simulated the effects of a full-blown biological warfare attack. The most often talked about is plague or the Black Death in the 1300s. As noted previously, bubonic plague caused over 25 million deaths. Much of this lethality would be mitigated by modern medical care and pharmacology, provided it was not overwhelmed.

A significant model of what might happen after a viral bioweapon release is found in the influenza pandemic of 1918 and 1919. This pandemic happened during well-recorded history, and good accounts of the desperation and damage it wreaked on the United States are available.[22] The influenza pandemic of 1918 and 1919 killed more people than World War I. Influenza rapidly spread, made almost half of the world's population ill, and killed between 21 and 40 million people. It has been cited as the most devastating epidemic in recorded world history. More people died of influenza in a single year than in 4 years of the Black Death bubonic plague from 1347 to 1351.[23]

The influenza of 1918 and 1919 was a global disaster. This pandemic was not curable by the medical technology of 1918 (nor is it curable by today's technology). All medical care in the United States was overwhelmed. Society was unable to contain the infection, as the spread of influenza was aided by ship, railroad, and the mass migrations of both civilians and military personnel during World War I. Acute illness caused critical personnel shortages in sanitation, law enforcement, postal delivery, food delivery, transportation, and health care. Enough physicians were killed that medical students were graduated early, and dentists relicensed as physicians for the duration.

Inundated with patients, hospitals turned away people for lack of space and personnel. This was despite makeshift patient accommodations in halls, offices, porches, school gymnasiums, armories, and even tents (even during late fall). Basic supplies, such as linens, bedpans, and gowns, were difficult to obtain. Customers desperate for any hope of protection or relief emptied pharmacy shelves of over-the-counter remedies.

Bodies piled up as the massive deaths of the epidemic ensued. Besides the lack of health care workers and medical supplies, there was a shortage of coffins, morticians, and gravediggers.[24,25] Indeed, cities were so short of coffins that Washington, DC, seized a trainload of coffins en route to Pittsburgh. Many patients were buried in mass graves. Public gatherings were suspended, retail hours were curtailed, and churches were closed. The conditions in 1918 and 1919 were not so far removed from the Black Death in the era of the bubonic plague of the Middle Ages.

At the time of this writing, severe acute respiratory syndrome (SARS) has been diagnosed in multiple cities. As noted with influenza, this acute illness has caused significant morbidity and mortality among physicians and EMS providers who cared for the initial casualties. The WHO has declared that (for now) SARS is contained. Because upper respiratory illnesses have a seasonal cycle, this may or may not be accurate in the months and years to come.

■ Summary

It is said that if you do not study history, you are doomed to repeat it. Certainly, the likelihood of chemical and biological weapons being used against the United States is greater than at any other point in our history. Awareness of this threat and the appropriate education of our medical care providers, public health officials, law enforcement personnel, and leaders are crucial.

Compared to conventional, chemical, and nuclear weapon threats, biological weapons are unique in their ability to cause disruption and panic. Imagine the chaos if an agent similar to the influenza of 1918 and 1919 were deliberately spread throughout the United States. We still don't have the ability to produce a vaccine rapidly enough to protect the entire population of the United States in any reasonable time frame. It takes 6 months from the identification of a strain to produce a live attenuated virus vaccine. This prohibits the production of vaccine in time to protect the first wave of illness of any viral agent.

Our hospitals already have acute shortages of staff, beds, and equipment as a result of a harsh fiscal climate. In many parts of the country, emergency departments routinely have 4- to 8-hour waits for current patient loads. The health care system was barely able to cope with the nominal up-

swing in patient load during the 1999 and 2000 flu season. There is simply no reason to think that it will be able to cope with a deliberately engendered pandemic.

One must also look at the panic that accompanies such a pandemic. One may expect panic that would make people fight for supposed protective agents, flee for supposedly safe locales, or even just try to protect family and loved ones. Panic and the threat of death would suborn the already decimated law enforcement services and make martial law inevitable. Think about how difficult it would be to enforce quarantine for smallpox in Los Angeles, for example, with multiple ways to get out of the city, including both land and sea. With current news reporting, this panic would be spread by news media on a real-time basis.

It looks sufficient to stockpile various antibiotics and vaccines, but it really takes a while to detect the diseases that would respond to these treatments. Most physicians will fail to consider bioterrorism until they have several cases of a certain disease in their emergency department on their shift. If the disease causes common initial symptoms, such as fever, sniffles, and a sore throat, and occurs in the winter, they will not consider it until many patients start to arrive. This may be 5 to 10 days after the initial exposure and the now-exposed medical providers will be part of the second wave of casualties. Some of the new casualties will be lethally sick, and some will be simply extremely scared. The patients with the usual illnesses will continue to need emergency care, but they may be far sicker because of a mild infection on top of their already fragile health.

Unlike the typical focal disaster, the bioterrorist pandemic may well be widespread, with many geographic areas affected simultaneously. Thus, every community will have to be self-prepared, rather than pooling resources from several contiguous counties or relying on state personnel for help.

If bioterrorism-associated illness is especially severe (in the magnitude of the 1918 and 1919 flu epidemic, for example), local health services could easily and rapidly become overwhelmed. Supplies of intensive care unit beds, ventilators, and other critical-care equipment may prove to be inadequate. Shortages of antiviral agents and antibiotics for treatment of secondary infections may also result. There may be an increased demand for ancillary or nontraditional treatment centers, and certainly there will be an increased demand for mortuary and funeral services.

If you normally see 100 patients per day in your emergency department, think about how you would respond to 1,000 patients or more in a day. Do not just consider the problem of personally examining all of these patients, consider the logistics involved in simply providing bandages for them, caring for them, feeding them, and keeping life support going for a significant percentage of them. Remember that you cannot plan on significant external help for a minimum of 24 hours after the need is declared. It really does take a while to load crates, transport them, and unload them at the site.

Moreover, unlike natural disasters, demands on medical care in each community from a massive biological weapon release may last 6 to 8 weeks until the first wave of infection is complete. Unlike the typical disaster, essential community servants themselves (such as medical care personnel, police officers, firefighters, ambulance drivers, and other First Responders) will be just as likely—or even more likely (because of increased exposure)—to be affected by an influenza or other pandemic than the general public.

In order to ensure responsible biowarfare planning, a hospital administrator should consider staffing for 10 times (or more) the rated bed capacity of the hospital. This includes deciding where the extra cots, blankets, gloves, and gowns are going to come from and how they will be transported to the hospital. The administrator must also decide how he or she is going to staff the hospital when 25% of the staff (including physicians, nurses, registration clerks, cooks, lab technicians, bottle washers, security personnel, and janitors) are casualties and 50% of the staff is panicked and wants to stay home.

We should include in our plans the concept that leaders are mortal too. The designated leader may be one of the first casualties of the event, and the plan must include this possibility. Responsible biowarfare exercises should begin by declaring 10% of all "players" dead just before the exercise starts, and another 2% to 3% should be eliminated with each passing "day" of the exercise until the mitigation stage. This requires a random distribution, and all leadership positions should be included in the lottery. We will certainly find casualties among our leadership positions in both the medical and governmental communities. We cannot ignore these consequences if this nightmare becomes reality, and we must be certain that subordinates can carry out the appropriate plans in the harsh landscape of a pandemic.

■ References

1. Simon JD: Biological terrorism: Preparing to meet the threat. *JAMA* 1997;278:428-430.
2. Harris R, Paxman J: *A Higher Form of Killing.* New York, NY, Wang and Hill, 1982, pp 75-81.
3. Osterholm MT: The medical impact of a bioterrorist attack. *Postgrad Med* 1999;106:121-130.
4. O'Toole T, Inglesby TV: Facing the biological weapons threat. *Lancet* 2000;356:1128-1129.
5. Harris R, Paxman J: *A Higher Form of Killing.* New York, NY, Wang and Hill, 1982, pp 75-81.
6. Okumura T, Suzuki K, Fukuda A, et al: The Tokyo subway sarin attack: Disaster management, Part I: Community response. *Acad Emerg Med* 1998;5:613-617.
7. Shapiro RL, Hatheway C, Becher J, et al: Botulism surveillance and emergency response. *JAMA* 1997;162:156-161.
8. Chemical-biological terrorism and its impact on children: A subject review. *Pediatrics* 2000;105:662-670.
9. Alibek K: *Biohazard.* New York, NY, Random House, 1999.
10. Cole TB: When a bioweapon strikes, who will be in charge? *JAMA* 2000;284:944-948.
11. Vastag B: Experts urge bioterrorism readiness. *JAMA* 2001;285:30-32.
12. Fidler DP: The malevolent use of microbes and the rule of law: Legal challenges presented by bioterrorism. *Clin Infect Dis* 2001;33:686-689.
13. Inglesby TV, Grossman R, O'Toole T: A plague on your city: Observations from TOPOFF. *Clin Infec Dis* 2001;32:436-445.
14. Fidler DP: The malevolent use of microbes and the rule of law: Legal challenges presented by bioterrorism. *Clin Infect Dis* 2001;33:686-689.
15. O'Toole T, Inglesby T: Shining light on dark water. Johns Hopkins Center for Civilian BioDefense. http://www.hopkins-biodefense.org/lessons.html (accessed October 10, 2001).
16. Inglesby TV, Grossman R, O'Toole T: A plague on your city: Observations from TOPOFF. *Clin Infec Dis* 2001;32:436-445.
17. Kaufmann AF, Meltzer MI, Schmid GP: The economic impact of a bioterrorist attack: Are prevention and post-attack intervention programs justifiable? *Emerg Infect Dis* 1997;3:83-94.
18. Kaufmann AF, Meltzer MI, Schmid GP: The economic impact of a bioterrorist attack: Are prevention and post-attack intervention programs justifiable? *Emerg Infect Dis* 1997;3:83-94.
19. Walker DH, Yampolska O, Grinberg LM: Death at Sverdlovsk: What we have learned. *Am J Pathol* 1994;144:1135-1141.
20. Jarrett DG: *Medical Management of Biologic Casualties Handbook.* Frederick, MD, US Army Medical Research Institute for Infectious Diseases, 2001.
21. Horrock N: The new terror fear: Biological weapons. *US News and World Report,* May 12, 1997. http://static.highbeam.com/u/usnewsampworldreport/may121997/thenewterrorfearbiologicalweapons/index.html (accessed April 1, 2004).
22. Schoch-Spana M: Implications of pandemic influenza for bioterrorism response. *Clin Infect Dis* 2000;31:1409-1413.
23. Billings M The influenza pandemic of 1918. http://www.stanford.edu/group/virus/uda/ (accessed October 3, 2001).
24. On the eve of peace in WWI influenza cast shadow of death. *Deseret News,* http://www.desnews.com/cen/hst/01260133.htm (accessed March 4, 2003).
25. Knox R: Scientists check 1918 killer flu's genes and issue a warning similarly virulent strain could hit again. *Boston Globe,* March 21, 1997, http://www.boston.com/tools/archives/ (accessed April 1, 2004).

A-230 A Soviet nerve agent similar to V-gas.

A-232 A Soviet nerve agent similar to V-gas; this agent was not formally approved.

A-234 A Soviet V-series nerve agent.

Abattoir A building that houses facilities to slaughter animals; to dress, cut, and inspect meats; and to refrigerate, cure, and manufacture meat byproducts.

Abattoir fever A synonym for Q fever. Caused by *Rickettsia burnetii*.

Abelikov anthrax A form of weapons-grade anthrax developed by Ken Alibek (Kanatjan Alibekov) that is said to be four times more deadly than natural anthrax.

AC NATO military designator for hydrogen cyanide (HCN). CAS Number 74-90-8.

Acalculous cholecystitis An infection/inflammation of the gallbladder that occurs in the absence of gallstones.

Accomodation Adaptation of the eye for distance viewing, resulting in pupil constriction or dilation.

Acetylcholine A compound that causes muscles to contract, found in various organs and tissues of the body. Broken down rapidly by the enzyme cholinesterase. Often abbreviated as Ach.

Acetylcholinesterase An enzyme that stops the action of acetylcholine by separating it into acetic acid and choline. Nerve agents combine with acetylcholinesterase to prevent it from inactivating acetylcholine. Acetylcholinesterase values in serum and red blood cells confirm nerve gas poisoning. Often abbreviated as AchE.

ACTH Adrenocorticotropic hormone.

Active topical skin protectant A topical skin cream developed by the U.S. Army to protect the skin from nerve agents and vesicants.

Acute chemical pneumonitis Acute inflammation of the lungs (pneumonitis) caused by inhalation of chemicals.

Adamsite The common name for DM, also known as *nausea gas,* DM is the NATO military designator for the vomit agent having the chemical name diphenylaminochloroarsine (or phenarsazine chloride). Causes the rapid onset of rhinorrhea and lacrimation symptoms as well as headache, nausea, and severe vomiting. CAS Number 578-94-9.

Aerosol A fine mist or spray containing minute particles.

AFB₁ Aflatoxin B_1

AFB₂ Aflatoxin B_2

AFIP Acronym for the *Armed Forces Institute of Pathology*.

African swine fever The virus that causes hog cholera. May be employed as a biological weapon.

Agent 15 The NATO military designator for an incapacitating agent allegedly produced by the Iraqis. Thought to be chemically related to BZ.

Agent L Another name for Lewisite (dichloro (2-chlorovinyl) arsine), which is a potent vesicant agent. CAS Number 541-25-3.

Agent Q A variant of mustard that has the chemical name 1,2-bis-(2-chloroethylthio) ethane. Also known as sesquimustard. It is a potent vesicant agent that is often used with mustard. CAS Number 3563-36-8.

Agent T A variant of mustard that has the chemical name bis-(2-chloroethylthio ethyl) ether. It is a potent vesicant agent that is often used with mustard. CAS Number 693-07-2.

Agglomeration The process whereby moist sticky particles collide due to the air turbulence and adhere to each other.

Aging Dealkylation of acetylcholinesterase that has been phosphorylated by a nerve gas. Reactivation is impossible once the dealkylation of phosphorylated AChE occurs. Once aging occurs, new AChE must be synthesized.

Air hunger The feeling of not being able to catch your breath; often used as a synonym for *dyspnea.*

Al Hakam An Iraqi biological production facility on the Tigris River, 60 kilometers southwest of Baghdad. According to UN inspectors, the Iraqis produced bacillus anthracis weapons there.

Alimentary toxic aleukia A condition that occurs when humans ingest mycotoxins, usually from contaminated grains. Begins with burning sensations in the mouth, throat, esophagus, and stomach; continues with vomiting, diarrhea, and gastric cramps; and finally progresses to severe leukopenia (a drop in white blood cell count). *See also* Yellow rain.

Alkyl An organic functional group that contains carbon and hydrogen atoms arranged in a chain. Has the general formula C_nH_{2n+1}. Examples include methyl, CH_{3*}, which is derived from methane, and butyl, C_2H_5, which is derived from butane.

Alkylation reactions Alkylation is the organic reaction in which an alkyl group replaces a hydrogen atom in an organic compound.

Allergic contact dermatitis A skin rash caused by an allergic reaction to a substance applied to the skin. A classic example is the reaction to oils in poison ivy (*Rhus* species).

Alpha-bromophenylacetonitrile A highly irritating agent similar to CN, but that is much more toxic. It is no longer used routinely. It is also called bromobenzylcyanide or CA. It has been replaced by CN and CS. CAS Number 16532-79-9.

Alpha particles (also *α-particles* or *α-radiation*) Alpha particles are heavy and slow and do not pass through intact skin. The radiation hazard from alpha emitters occurs if they are ingested or absorbed into open wounds.

Alphaviruses A genus in the family Togaviridae. Includes the Eastern, Western, and Venezuelan equine encephalitis viruses. Alphaviruses cause fever, rash, myalgia/arthralgia, and lymphadenopathy syndromes (eg, Chikungunya haemorrhagic fever, O'Nyong-nyong, Mayaro, Ross River, and Sindbis viruses) and encephalitis (eg, Semliki Forest encephalitis).

Amyl nitrite A yellowish oily volatile liquid having the formula $C_5H_{11}NO_2$. It is used as a heart stimulant and a vasodilator. Inhalation of its vapor produces instant flushing of the face.

Analogues A structural derivative of a parent compound that often differs from the parent compound by a single element or chemical chain. It is also a methemoglobin-forming compound that has treatment effects in cyanide intoxication.

Animal venom Toxins obtained from cobras and other snakes, scorpions, wasps, shellfish, etc.

Anthrax A blood-poisoning, spore-forming disease of cattle and sheep caused by *Bacillus anthracis*. Develops in humans if they inhale, ingest, or have skin contact with the spores. The pulmonary form of anthrax can be lethal. Symptoms include fever, malaise, fatigue, coughing, and mild chest discomfort followed by severe respiratory distress. *See also* Woolsorter's disease.

Antibiotic A compound that kills or slows the growth of bacteria. Antibiotics are one class of antimicrobials, a larger group that also includes antiviral, antifungal, and antiparasitic drugs.

Antibody Proteins produced by an organism's immune system to recognize and destroy foreign substances.

Anticholinergic A substance that inhibits the ability of nerve fibers to liberate acetylcholine at a synapse when a nerve impulse arrives.

Anticholinesterase A substance that inhibits the action of the enzyme cholinesterase.

Antigen Any substance that stimulates an immune response by the body. The immune system recognizes such substances as being foreign and produces antibodies to fight them.

Anxiolytics A class of drugs that reduce anxiety.

Aplasia Failure of a tissue or organ to develop.

Apnea The cessation of respiration.

Apoptosis Programmed cell death signaled by the nuclei in normally functioning cells when the age of the cell or its condition dictates. It may be triggered by some viruses.

Arsine The most toxic form of arsenic; it causes hemolysis and kidney failure in humans. The NATO military designator for arsine is SA. CAS Number 7784-42-1.

Arthralgia Ache or pain in the joints. Arthritis is arthralgia with inflammation in the joint.

Arthropod Any invertebrate possessing jointed limbs and a segmented exoskeleton. Belonging to the phylum Arthropoda, the group includes crustaceans, arachnids (eg, spiders, scorpions, and mites), myriapods (eg, millipedes and centipedes), and insects. Used in this text to describe vectors of biological warfare agents.

Aspergillus flavus A fungi that produces the toxin aflatoxin, which causes cancer.

Assay A quantitative or qualitative evaluation, or test, of a substance. Frequently used to describe tests that determine the presence or concentration of infectious agents, antibodies, etc.

Asymptomatic Without symptoms.

Ataxia An inability to coordinate voluntary muscle movements, resulting in unsteady movements and staggering gait.

ATNAA (Antidote Treatment Nerve Agent Auto-Injector) An auto-injected antidote to a nerve agent.

ATP Adenosine 5' triphosphate.

Atropine An anticholinergic agent that is a first-line therapy for emergency treatment of anticholinesterase agents. Reverses the muscarinic effects of nerve agent poisoning, such as bronchospasm, excessive respiratory secretions, and intestinal hypermotility. Note that unopposed action of atropine in high doses produces effects similar to BZ.

Atropine sulfate An alkaloid derived from species of belladonna and related plants or produced synthetically. It is an anticholinergic and antispasmodic drug that can be used to relax smooth muscles, relieve the tremor and rigidity of Parkinsonism, and increase the heart rate by blocking the action of the Vagus nerve. Atropine sulfate is the sulfated form of the alkaloid.

aTSP An acronym for *active topical skin protectant*.

Aum Shinrikyo A religion based on mixed Buddhist and Hindu beliefs that orginated in Japan. It gained international notoriety in 1995 when a group of followers carried out a poison gas attack on the Tokyo subways on the orders of its founder, Shoko Asahara. The group also investigated several biological weapons.

Australia Group An informal group of nations which aims to allow exporting or transshipping countries to minimize the risk of assisting chemical and biological weapon (CBW) proliferation.

Autoclaving A device that exposes items to high-pressure steam in order to decontaminate materials or render them sterile.

Avian influenza virus Pathogen that affects poultry. Similar viruses have caused several severe epidemics of influenza when they cross species barriers and infect humans.

BA An obsolete lacrimator agent. Its chemical name is 1-bromo-2-propanone. Was used as a harassing agent in World War I. BA is the NATO military designator for bromacetone. CAS Number 598-31-2.

Bacillary dysentery A form of dysentery caused by *Shigella dysenteriae*.

Bacillus anthracis The bacteria that causes anthrax. Humans can be affected when they inhale, ingest, or have skin contact with the spores. The pulmonary form can be lethal. Symptoms include fever, malaise, fatigue, coughing, and mild chest discomfort followed by severe respiratory distress.

Back door coupling Occurs when the electromagnetic field from an EMP weapon produces a large transient current in the wiring infrastructure that connects to a targeted device. The resulting electrical surge damages or destroys circuits within the device.

Bacteria Single-celled microorganisms that reproduces by binary fission. These organisms reproduce rapidly. Some can form spores (encysted variants) when environmental conditions are harsh.

BAL British Anti-Lewisite, also called 2,3 dimercaptopropanol. It is an antidote for Lewisite. CAS Number 59-52-9.

Balkan grippe A synonym for Q fever. It is caused by *Rickettsia burnetii*.

Balkan influenza A synonym for Q fever. It is caused by *Rickettsia burnetii*.

Bananabunchy top virus A pathogenic plant virus.

Bartonella quintana A bacteria that causes trench fever, which was a significant problem during World War I. It is a rickettsial disease. Also called *Rochalimaea quintana*.

Batrachotoxin A poison derived from a South American toad.

BDS Acronym for *British Biological Detection System*. The system uses luciferase, an enzyme produced by fireflies, to detect ATP (adenosine triphosphate), which is present in all living cells, as an indicator of biological weapons. This system was deployed during the first Gulf War.

Belladonna A plant-derived poison with atropine-like effects. It is similar to BZ in its effects.

Beta-adrenergic agonists A type of drug that stimulates the adrenergic nerves directly by mimicking the action of norepinephrine through beta receptor sites. Adrenergic stimulants (agonists) may have three modes of action: direct interaction with specific receptors (examples are epinephrine and phenylephrine); indirect action by stimulating release of neurotransmitters; or a mixed action involving both of the above (examples are phenylpropanolamine and ephedrine).

Beta particles (also *β-particles* or *β-radiation*) A historical term used in early descriptions of radioactivity to describe a charged particle emitted from a nucleus during radioactive decay. Its mass is 1/1837 that of a proton. The radiation hazard from beta particles is greatest if they are ingested. Strontium-90 (^{90}Sr) is an example of a material that emits beta particles.

Bhopal The location of an incident in 1984 which was the worst industrial disaster in the history of the world. It was caused by the accidental release of 40 metric tons of methyl isocyanate (MIC) from a Union Carbide India, Limited (UCIL) pesticide plant located in the heart of the city of Bhopal in the Indian state of Madhya Pradesh. The MIC leak killed thousands outright and injured anywhere from 150,000 to 600,000 others, at least 15,000 of whom died later from their injuries.

BIDS Acronym for the U.S. Army's *Biological Integrated Detection System*, a system that samples the air for evidence of biological weapons.

Bilateral perihilar fluffy infiltrate Fluid that accumulates in the alveolar (airspace) compartment or the interstitial compartment of both lungs (bilateral) around the root of the pulmonary vessels (the hilum). It increases the lungs' density and cancels the contrast between vessels and lung boundaries; these structures disappear and air bronchograms are created.

Binary munitions Chemical warfare munitions that are activated by the combination of two (or more) chemicals, either in flight or shortly before launch of the munition. Some documents identify these weapons by the codes VX-2, GD-2, or GB-2. *See also* DF.

Biodosimeter A biological or biochemical indicator of the effects of exposure, such as a change in blood chemistry or blood count. A highly accurate biological dosimeter has yet to be found.

Biological agent A living organism, including viruses and infected materials derived from them, produced for biological warfare against plants, animals, or human beings. These agents cannot be readily detected by our physical senses. There are about 60 different known biological agents.

Biological half-life The time an organism takes to eliminate one half the amount of a compound or chemical from the body.

Biological weapons Microorganisms, including bacteria, viruses, fungi, rickettsiae, and protozoa, or their products (ie, toxins) that can be used to incapacitate an opponent via acts of biological warfare. Tend to be more lethal than toxic chemical materials, but less lethal than nuclear weapons (10 grams of anthrax are said to have the same lethality as 1,000 kilograms of Sarin, under optimal dispersion conditions). The active agents are biologically produced toxins or pathogenic infectious organisms. Exposure to such organisms or their toxins often leads to death after an incubation period of a few days.

Biopreparat The Soviet Union biological weapons program. This secret program involved 35,000 workers, including 9,000 scientists working at laboratories at 47 sites across the former Soviet Union.

Bioregulators A new class of weapons that can damage the nervous system, alter moods, trigger psychological changes, and even kill. Cannot be traced by pathologists.

Biosafety cabinets (BSCs) The primary means of containment for working with infectious microorganisms. *See also* Biosafety level.

Biosafety level Specific combinations of work practices, safety equipment, and facilities that are designed to minimize the exposure of workers and the environment to infectious agents. Level 1 applies to agents that do not ordinarily cause human disease. Level 2 is appropriate for agents that can cause human disease, but whose potential for transmission is limited. Level 3 applies to agents that may be transmitted by the respiratory route and that may cause serious infection. Level 4 is used for the diagnosis of exotic agents that pose a high risk of life-threatening disease that can be transmitted by the aerosol route and for which there is no vaccine or therapy.

BiPAP Acronym for *Bi-level Positive Airway Pressure*.

Biphasic disease A disease that occurs with two phases separated by a feeling of apparent wellness.

Black plague (Black death) A highly contagious disease caused by the bacteria *Pasturella pestis*. Its three forms: pneumonic, septic, and bubonic. All forms can be quite contagious. Normally carried by rodents and transmitted by fleas, this disease caused millions of deaths in the 13th and 14th centuries.

Blackpox The disease that would result from a genetic combination of Ebola and smallpox.

Blepharospasm A spasm of the eyelid muscle resulting in closure of the eye.

Blister agent A chemical warfare agent that produces local irritation and damage to the skin and mucous membranes, pain and injury to the eyes, reddening and blistering of the skin, and damage to the respiratory tract when inhaled. Include mustards (HD and HN), arsenicals (L), and mustard and Lewisite mixtures (HL).

Blood agent An antiquated term that refers to a chemical warfare agent that is inhaled and absorbed into the blood. Most are tissue toxins. Examples are AC and CK.

Blood urea nitrogen (BUN) A measure of the amount of urea, a waste product of protein metabolism, in the blood. Urea is formed by the liver and carried by the blood to the kidneys for excretion.

Body burden Refers to the industrial chemical residue each of us has in our bodies. These chemical residues, also called the *chemical body burden*, can be detected in blood, urine, and breast milk. In this text, it is used in reference to internally deposited radioactive material.

Boot sector virus A computer virus that acts on the first few sectors of a disk. Because the operating system is "booted" from these sectors, the virus affects the entire operating system.

Botulinum toxin The toxin that causes botulism. The toxin is produced by the bacteria *Clostridium botulinum*. It is among the most potent toxins known. Also known as *Botulinum neurotoxin* and commonly refered to as *botox*. The NATO military designator is X.

Brill-Zinsser disease Recrudescence of epidemic typhus years after the initial attack. The agent that causes epidemic typhus (*Rickettsia prowazekii*) remains viable for many years. When host defenses are down, it reactivates, causing recurrent typhus. Named for the physician Nathan Brill and the bacteriologist Hans Zinsser.

British Anti-Lewisite (BAL) An effective antidote developed by the British that reverses the toxic symptoms of Lewisite. Its chemical name is 2,3 dimercaptopropanolol.

Bromoacetone The NATO military designator for the obsolete lacrimator agent BA CAS 598–31–2.

Bromobenzylcyanide A highly irritating agent similar to CN, but much more toxic. No longer in use. Also called alpha-bromophenylacetonitrile. The NATO military designator is CA. CAS Number 16532-79-9.

Bronchiectasis Persistent and progressive dilation of bronchi or bronchioles as a consequence of inflammatory diseases, chemical action, obstruction, or congenital abnormality. Symptoms include foul breath odor, paroxysmal coughing, and production of purulent sputum.

Bronchoalveolar lavage A diagnostic and therapeutic procedure conducted by placing a small fiber-optic scope into the lung of a patient and injecting sterile water (saline) into the lung and removing the fluid. The sterile solution removed contains secretions, cells, and protein from the lower respiratory tract.

Bronchorrhea Excessive discharge of mucus from the lungs.

Bronchoscopy A procedure in which an instrument is passed into the airway to look at the lung structures and/or obtain specimens.

Brucellosis An infectious disease, also called *undulant fever*, caused by bacteria of the genus *Brucella*. These bacteria are primarily passed among animals and cause disease in many different vertebrates. In humans, can cause a range of symptoms that are similar to the flu and may include fever, sweats, headaches, back pains, and physical weakness.

BTX An often used abbreviation for botulinium toxin. *See* Botulinum toxin.

Bubo A tender, enlarged, inflamed lymph node, particularly in the upper chest, clavicle, or groin areas.

Bulbar paralysis Paralysis of the muscles of the lips, tongue, mouth, pharynx, and larynx due to involvement of the motor nuclei of the lower brain stem (the bulbar area).

Bullae Large blisters.

Burkholderia mallei The causative agent of glanders, developed as a biological weapon by the United States and other countries.

Butyl A hydrocarbon radical, C_4H_9, that has the structure of butane and a valence of 1. The name is derived from *butyric acid*, a four-carbon carboxylic acid found in rancid butter.

BW Acronym for *biological warfare*.

BWC Acronym for the 1972 *Biological Weapons Convention*.

BZ NATO military designator for 3-quinuclidinylbenzilate, a delayed-onset (1 to 4 hours after exposure) incapacitation agent. It is a glycolate anticholinergic compound related to atropine, scopolamine, and hyoscyamine. CAS Number 6581-06-2.

C*t or C•t Concentration multiplied by time, also called the *concentration-time product*. A measure of the agent's concentration in the air multiplied by the time of the exposure. For most inhalation agents, the C•t associated with a biological effect is fairly constant.

CA The NATO military designator for a highly irritating agent similar to CN, but much more toxic. No longer used by civilian law enforcement. Also called *bromobenzylcyanide*. CAS Number 16532-79-9.

Calmatives Calming or relaxing agents; also called *anxiolytics*.

CANA An acronym for *Convulsant Antidote for Nerve Agents*. The military name for an injector loaded with diazepam.

Carbamates A class of toxic pesticides with the general formula R_1R_2-N-C(O)-O-R_3 that resemble the organophosphorus nerve agents. Carbamates are derived from carbamic acid and are used in industry, agriculture, and households.

Carbonic dichloride Synonym for *phosgene*. CAS Number 75-44-5.

Carbuncle Synonym for *boil*. Painful swellings of the skin caused by a deep bacterial skin infection.

Carcinogenic A substance that causes or tends to cause cancer.

Carcinogenesis The process by which normal cells are transformed into cancer cells.

Cardiac Pertaining to the heart.

Cardiomegaly Enlargement of the heart.

Cardiovascular Pertaining to the heart and vessels.

Carrier A person or animal that harbors a specific infectious agent without having visible symptoms of the disease. Acts as a potential source of infection.

Cartridge respirators Protective masks that use a filter cartridge to protect the wearer from inhalants. The typical military "gas mask" is a cartridge respirator.

CAS Acronym for the *Chemical Abstracts Service*.

Case-fatality ratio or proportion The ratio of the number of cases of a disease that end in death and the total number of cases of the disease. Usually expressed as a percentage.

Case-to-infection ratio or proportion The ratio of the number of cases of a disease compared to the number of infections with the agent that causes the disease. Usually expressed as a percentage.

Castor bean A bean produced by the plant *Ricinus communis* from with castor bean oil and ricin are derived.

Casualty An individual rendered incapable of performing normal tasks by a disease. Includes both those who are temporarily incapacitated and those who have died.

Cathartics Medications designed to induce a bowel movement. Often used to relieve long-term constipation.

CBDCOM Acronym for the U.S. *Chemical and Biological Defense Command*.

CBIRF Acronym for the U.S. *Marine Chemical Biological Incident Response Force*. A rapid-response team that deals with chemical and biological warfare threats.

CCK Abbreviation for *cholecystokinin*.

CCEP Acronym for *Comprehensive Clinical Evaluation Program*.

CDC Acronym for the *Centers for Disease Control and Prevention*.

Cerebral edema The presence of abnormally large amounts of fluid in the brain. Swelling of the substance of the brain.

CG The NATO military designator for phosgene. A colorless chemical agent designed to cause pulmonary damage and asphyxia that is heavier than air. Has caused more war casualties than any other war gas and was also used quite extensively in World War I. Also called *carbonic dichloride*. CAS Number is 75-44-5.

CHe Shorthand for cholinesterase.

Chemical adsorption Adhesion of the molecules of liquids, gases, and dissolved substances to the surfaces of solids.

Chemical Agent Monitor (CAM) A handheld, soldier-operated device that is used to monitor chemical warfare agent contamination on individuals and equipment.

Chemical neutralization Inactivation of a chemical by a chemical process.

Chemical pneumonitis Pneumonia caused by inhalation of a chemical.

Chemical warfare All aspects of military operations involving the employment of lethal and incapacitating munitions/agents and the warning and protective measures associated with such offensive operations.

Chemical warfare agent A chemical substance used in military operations to kill, seriously injure, or incapacitate humans (or animals) through its toxicological effects. Subcategorized by the military into nerve agents, incapacitating agents, blister agents (vesicants), lung damaging (pulmonary or choking) agents, blood agents, and vomiting agents.

Chikungunya virus A biological agent that is a positive-sense, single-stranded RNA virus. Family: *Togaviridae*, Genus: *Alphavirus*. Sudden severe headache, chills, fever, joint and muscle pain are the commonest symptoms.

Chlamydia pneumonia Pneumonia caused by bacteria of the genus *Chlamydia*.

Chlorine A common nonmetallic halogen having the chemical symbol Cl. Best known as a heavy, yellow, irritating toxic gas. It is a bleaching agent and disinfectant. In nature it occurs only as a salt (eg, as in sea water). CAS Number 7782-50-5.

2-Chloro-1-phenylethanone Chemical name for the lacrimator agent CN. CAS Number 532-27-4.

Chloroacetone A commonly available compound that was used as an irritant in the early days of World War I. CAS 78-95-5.

Chloroamide Synonym for *chloramine*. A chlorine compound that reacts with mustard. A component of SERPACWA.

Chloropicrin A heavy colorless insoluble liquid compound that causes tears and vomiting. Used as pesticide and as tear gas.

Choking agents Another name for pulmonary agents that damage the lung by inhalation. *See also* Pulmonary agents.

Cholera The diarrheal disease caused by the bacteria *Vibrio comma*. Causes profuse diarrhea (also called *rice water diarrhea*). Has been used as a biological agent to incapacitate humans.

Cholinergic Effects produced on the parasympathetic nervous system, similar to those produced by ACh.

Chronic carrier case. *See* Carrier.

CIA Acronym for *Central Intelligence Agency*.

Cidofovir A drug treatment for the cytomegalovirus, a type of herpesvirus. Proposed as a treatment for other viral infections. Use of cidofovir would be administered under an Investigational New Drug (IND) protocol. Trade name is Vistide, and it was formerly known as HPMPC.

Ciliary body A thin vascular (blood-vessel-filled) middle layer of the eye that is situated between the sclera (the white of the eye) and the retina (the nerve layer that lines the back of the eye, senses light, and creates impulses that travel through the optic nerve to the brain).

CK The NATO military designator for cyanogen chloride, a blood agent. CAS Number 506-77-4.

Clark I A vomit agent. Also called DA or diphenylchloroarsine. CAS Number 712-48-1.

Clark II A vomit agent. Also called DC or diphenylcyanoarsine. CAS Number 23525-22-6.

Clostridium botulinum The bacteria that produces the botulinum toxin. Causes botulism, or food poisoning. Botulinum toxin has been found with non-state actors such as the Japanese Aum Shinrikyo sect.

Clostridium perfringens The biological agent that causes gas gangrene.

Clostridium perfringens **toxin** A series of toxins produced by the *Clostridium perfringens* (gas gangrene) bacteria. The epsilon toxin is thought to have possible use as a biological agent.

Clostridium tetani The biological agent that causes tetanus.

CN Chloroacetophenone CN (1-chloroacetophenone) is the NATO military designation for the standard tear gas used by local law enforcement agencies. Synonyms are *phenacyl chloride, chloromethyl phenyl ketone,* and *2-chloro-1-phenylethanone.* CAS Number 532-27-4.

CNB The NATO military designation for a solution of chloroacetophenone in benzene and carbon tetrachloride. *See also* CN.

CNC The NATO military designation for a solution of chloroacetophenone in chloroform. *See also* CN.

CNS The NATO military designator for chloracetophenone combined with chloropicrin (pulmonary and lacrimator) and chloroform (tearing agent). *See also* CN and Chloropicrin.

Coccidioides immitis The fungus that causes coccidioidomycosis.

Code Red An extremely destructive computer worm that first appeared in July 2001 and ultimately affected over 300,000 computers in the United States. The worm exploited a hole in Microsoft's IIS Web server.

Command detonated The remote detonation of an explosive or munition.

Compound 19 The secret Russian biological weapons facility at Sverdlovsk.

Compound W The NATO military code name for ricin.

Concomitant Existing or occurring simultaneously. Therapeutic regiments employing more than one agent at the same time are often described as *concomitant therapies.*

Confluent Joining or running together. Often used to describe a rash. Lesions that are confluent join each other.

Congo-Crimean hemorrhagic fever virus A biological agent that causes hemorrhagic fever.

Conjunctival infection Redness (due to increased vascularity) of the conjunctiva. Often seen with irritation of the eye due to the effects of chemical agent.

Containment capability The ability to limit damage due to failure of a component or device. Often used in biological warfare discussions to mean the ability of the medical/public health systems to limit the spread of a biological warfare agent.

Convalescence Gradual healing (through rest) after sickness or injury.

Convention on the Prohibition of the Development, Production, and Stockpiling of Bacteriological and Toxin Weapons A 1972 treaty that prohibits the development, possession, and storage of biological weapons and the development of systems to develop these weapons. The shortened name of the treaty is the Biological Weapons Convention or BWC.

Corpus one A containment facility at the Russian biowarfare center in Oblensk.

Corynebacterium diphtheriae The causative agent for diphtheria.

Coxiella burnetii The biological agent found with the Japanese Aum sect.

CR The NATO military designator for dibenoxazephine. A lacrimator agent developed in Great Britain in 1962 as an alternative to CS and CN. CR is much more potent than CS. CAS Number 257-07-8.

Cranial nerve dysfunction Malfunction of the cranial nerves.

Creatinine A waste substance produced by the muscles when they are used or broken down. The name creatinine is also given to a blood test that measures the blood level of creatinine.

CS NATO military designator for a variant of tear gas having the chemical name o-chlorobenzylidene malononitrile. This is the standard military tear gas. About 10 times as strong as CN. CAS Number 2698-41-1.

CSIS Acronym for *Canadian Security Intelligence Service.*

Curare A toxic alkaloid found in certain tropical South American trees that is a powerful relaxant for striated muscles. Used by South American Indians as an arrow poison.

Cutaneous Relating to or existing on or affecting the skin (ie, *cutaneous nerves,* a *cutaneous infection*).

CW Acronym for *chemical weapons* or *chemical warfare.*

CWC Acronym for the *Chemical Weapons Convention.*

CX NATO military designator for phosgene oxime. Although not a blister agent, it is treated as one by the military. It is more correctly referred to as an urticant. CAS Number 1794-86-1.

Cyanide A highly toxic chemical agent that attacks the circulatory system. A cyanide is any chemical compound that contains the group CN^-, with the carbon atom triple bonded to the nitrogen atom. Two cyanide ions can bond to each other via their carbon atoms, forming the gas cyanogen (NC-CN). CAS Number 74-90-8.

Cyanogen chloride A cyanide compound (NATO designator CK) used as a chemical warfare agent. Its effects are similar to those of sycanide. CAS Number 506-77-4.

Cyclohexyl sarin A variant of sarin with a cyclohexyl ring. This is a G-series nerve agent with chemical name o-cyclohexyl-methylfluorophosphonate. The NATO designator is GF. CAS Number 329-99-7.

Cycloplegic A drug that paralyses the ciliary muscle, making it impossible to focus on near objects.

Cyclotron A particle accelerator in which the particles spiral inside two D-shaped, hollow, metal electrodes under the effect of a strong vertical magnetic field, gaining energy by a high-frequency voltage applied between these electrodes.

Cytotoxin A toxin that kills tissues.

DA NATO military designator for diphenylchloroarsine, a vomit gas. Has the formula $(C_6H_5)_2AsCl$. Causes rapid onset of both respiratory and skin irritation combined with nausea. Although it is an arsine, it acts more as an irritant than as a blood agent in usual concentrations. Also called Clark I.

DANC Acronym for *decontaminating agent, non-corrosive*. Also known as RH-195, this compound was developed by the DuPont Company. It is a whitish powder that liberates chlorine more slowly than ordinary bleaching material and therefore is more stable in storage.

DARPA Acronym for the U.S. *Defense Advanced Research Projects Agency*.

DAS Diacetoxyscipenol.

DC Military designator for the vomit agent having the chemical name diphenylcyanoarsine. It is an irritating agent that causes rapid onset of rhinorrhea and lacrimation symptoms associated with headache, nausea, and severe vomiting. Also called Clark II. CAS Number 23525-22-6.

DDT Dichloro-diphenyl-trichloroethane.

Debride To remove dead or dying tissue.

Decontaminating protective skin cream (DPSC) Protective skin cream under development by the U.S. Army as the replacement for SERPACWA. The goal is for the cream to actively destroy some chemical agents.

Decontamination The process of removing and destroying a harmful substance.

DEET Common name for N,N-diethyl-m-toluamide, the active ingredient in the most widely used insect repellent applied to the skin.

Denatured Changed in nature or natural quality.

Dengue fever virus A biological agent that has been investigated for its suitability for biological warfare by the U.S. military.

Dengue hemorrhagic fever, Dengue shock syndrome Severe manifestations of dengue fever.

Denial of service (DoS) A method hackers use to prevent or deny legitimate users access to computers or servers by calling/accessing a server so often and so rapidly that the service becomes overwhelmed.

Deoxynivalenol Also known as DON or vomitoxin, deoxynivalenol is one of about 150 related compounds known as the trichothecenes that are formed by a number of species of *Fusarium* and some other fungi.

Dermal Pertaining to the skin. Often used as synonym for *cutaneous*.

Descending flaccid paralysis A paralysis that starts from the head and works toward the feet (descending) with limp (flaccid) muscles.

Desquamation Loss of the outer layer of the skin.

Deuterophoma tracheiphilia A synonym for *Phoma tracheipl. hila*. A pathogenic plant fungus.

DF The NATO military designator for methylphosphonyldifluoride. Can be combined with isopropyl alcohol to form GB (Sarin). CAS Number 676-99-3.

DFP Abbreviation for *diisopropyl fluorophosphate*, a weak organophosphate nerve agent also known as agent PF3.

Diabetes insipidus A rare disorder, resulting in excessive thirst and excessive passage of very dilute urine, due to a hormone deficiency in the pituitary gland, which is situated at the base of the brain. Results from decreased production of the antidiuretic hormone vasopressin, which normally prevents the kidney from producing too much urine.

Diathesis A medical term meaning "predisposition" or "tendency."

Diatomaceous earth A nontoxic substance made up from crushed fossils of freshwater organisms and marine life. Diatomaceous earth has a high porosity because it is made of microscopically small coffinlike hollow particles. The U.S. Center for Disease Control recommends its use to clean up toxic spills.

Dibenoxazephine Usually referred to by the NATO designator CR, dibenoxazephine is a lacrimator agent developed in Great Britain in 1962 as an alternative to CS and CN. Much more potent than CS. CAS Number 257-07-8.

Dicobalt-EDTA Also known as KELOCYANOR; it is an antidote for acute cyanide poisoning. It chelates the cyanide ion and renders it inactive. CAS Number 36499-65-7.

Diffuse interstitial infiltrates Fluid accumulated in the alveolar (airspace) compartment or the interstitial compartment of the lung, and occurring throughout the lung. It increases lung density and cancels the contrast between vessels and lung boundaries; these structures disappear and air bronchograms are created.

2,3-Dimercaptopropanol Also known as British Anti-Lewisite. An antidote for Lewisite that is effective if used rapidly after exposure. CAS Number 59-52-9.

4-Dimethylaminophenol A cyanide antidote noted for its fast action that works by formation of methemoglobin, which subsequently combines with cyanide and deactivates it. Also called 4-DMAP.

Diodes Diodes allow electricity to flow in only one direction. Diodes are the electrical version of a valve, and early diodes were actually called valves. During an EMP, semiconductor diodes may be destroyed or damaged.

Diphenylchloroarsine A vomit agent having the formula $(C_6H_5)_2AsCl$. The NATO military designator is DA. It causes very rapid onset of both respiratory and skin irritation combined with severe nausea. CAS Number 712-48-1.

Diphenylcyanoarsine A vomit agent having the military designator DC. It is an irritating agent that causes the rapid onset of rhinorrhea and lacrimation symptoms associated with headache, nausea, and severe vomiting.

Diphosgene A lung irritant that is only slightly irritating to the eyes. Like phosgene, its effects are often delayed. Its chemical name is trichloromethylchloroformate, and it has the formula $ClCO_2CCl_3$. The NATO designation is DP. CAS Number 503-38-8.

Diphoterine An active eye and skin decontamination solution that has been tested and safely used for eye and skin splashes with a wide variety of irritant and corrosive chemical compounds.

Diplopia Seeing double.

Disease A condition whereby the body or a part of the body is interfered with or damaged. In a person with an infectious disease, the infectious agent that has entered the body causes it to function abnormally in some way. The type of abnormal functioning that occurs is the disease.

Distribution The act of dispersing or the condition of being dispersed; diffusion.

DMSO Dimethyl sulfoxide. This substance enhances penetration of intact skin by some chemical warfare agents.

DNA Acronym for *deoxyribonucleic acid.*

Dopant Impurities added to semiconductors. One of the main reasons that semiconductors are useful in electronics is that their electronic properties can be greatly altered in a controllable way by adding small amounts of impurities.

Doppler flow devices A meter with a probe sensor that measures blood flow in a blood vessel. The device transmits high-frequency soundwaves (640 kHz or more) that travel into the blood. Sound is reflected back to the sensor from solids or bubbles in the blood. If the blood is in motion, the echoes return at an altered frequency proportionate to flow velocity. This may be translated to a sound or to a flow speed, depending on the device.

Dosimeter An instrument that measures and indicates the amount of x-rays or radiation absorbed in a given period.

Doxycycline A type of tetracycline antibiotic that often is used to treat rickettsial and chlamydial diseases.

DP The military designator for diphosgene. A choking gas quite similar to phosgene in its effects. However, it is a liquid and more persistent than phosgene. Breaks down into chloroform and phosgene. CAS Number 503-38-8.

DTIC Acronym for *Defense Technical Information Center.*

Dusty mustard A mustard mixed with silica powder to make both detection and decontamination more difficult.

EA2192 A toxic byproduct from the hydrolysis of VX. During a basic hydrolysis of VX, up to 10 percent of the agent is converted to diisopropylaminoethyl methylphosphonothioic acid (EA2192). This byproduct is a major reason not to use water in decontamination of VX.

Eastern equine encephalitis virus A viral agent that causes encephalitis. Eastern equine encephalitis virus is a member of the Togaviridae family and is closely related to Western and Venezuelan equine encephalitis viruses.

Ebola A hemorrhagic fever, similar to Marburg, that is produced by a virus. Caused by infection with the Ebola virus, which is named after a river in the Democratic Republic of the Congo (formerly Zaire) in Africa, where it was first recognized. The virus is one of two members of a family of RNA viruses called the Filoviridae. Three of the four identified subtypes have caused disease in humans: Ebola-Zaire, Ebola-Sudan, and Ebola-Ivory Coast. The fourth, Ebola-Reston, has caused disease in nonhuman primates, but not in humans.

Ebolapox A genetic combination of Ebola virus and smallpox virus that is said to have been developed by the Russian Biopreparat weapons experts. These Russian bioweapons researchers may have created a recombinant Ebola-Smallpox, grafting a DNA copy of the disease-causing parts of Ebola into smallpox, thereby combining the hemorrhages caused by Ebola with the high contagion of smallpox. Also called *blackpox.*

ECt$_{50}$ Time-concentration product of an inhalation agent that will produce a specific biologic effect in 50 percent of a group. This roughly corresponds to the ED$_{50}$ for an absorbed agent.

ED Also known as *ethyldichloroarsine*, this compound produces a vapor that is harmful only after extended exposure. However, the liquid form causes blisters upon less than 1 minute of exposure. It is a vesicant.

ED$_{50}$ The dose of an agent that will cause a specific biologic effect in 50 percent of a group. *See also* LD$_{50}$.

EEG An electroencephalogram.

Effective half-life A concept that incorporates both radioactive and biological half-lives. It is used when health physicists calculate the dose received from an internal radiation source.

Ekaterinburg The alternate name for the Russian city of Sverdlovsk where anthrax was accidentally released in 1979.

Electromagnetic radiation Waves produced by the motion of electrically charged particles. These waves are called *electromagnetic radiation* because they radiate from electrically charged particles. They travel through empty space as well as through air and other substances.

Electroplating The process of putting a metallic coating on a metal or other conducting surface by using an electric current. It is used to improve the appearance of materials, for protection against corrosion, and to make plates for printing.

ELISA (enzyme-linked-immunosorbent serologic assay) A technique that relies on an enzymatic conversion reaction. It is used to detect the presence of specific substances, such as enzymes, viruses, antibodies, or bacteria.

Empiric That which is derived from experiment and observation rather than theory.

EMS Acronym for *Emergency Medical Services.*

Encephalopathy A general term describing brain dysfunction. Examples include encephalitis, meningitis, seizures, and head trauma.

Endemic A disease that is widespread in a given population.

Endemic typhus Disease caused by *Rickettsia prowazekii*. Characterized by fever, aches, headaches, weakness and pain, followed by stupor, delirium, and death (about 30 percent mortality). Spread by lice.

Endospore Any spore that is produced within an organism (usually a bacterium). Its primary function is to ensure the survival of a bacterium through periods of environmental stress. They are resistant to dessication, temperature extremes, starvation, ultraviolet and gamma radiation, and chemical disinfectants.

Endothelial The layer of thin, flat cells that line the interior surface of blood vessels, forming an interface between circulating blood and the vessel wall. These cells line the entire circulatory system, from the heart to the smallest capillary.

Endotheline A natural substance discovered in 1988 in Japan that causes blood vessel constriction. Because it is so easy to synthesize, it is considered to be one of the biggest threats to the conventions against chemical and biological weapons.

Endotoxin A component of the cell wall of all gram-negative bacteria that produces fever and shock. Effective both when the bacteria are alive and when they are killed, lysed, and their products released into the systemic circulation.

Enkephalin Either of two molecules found in the human brain that have pain-killing properties.

Enteritis necroticans Enteritis with necrosis of the intestinal wall caused by *Clostridium* species.

Enterohemorrhagic *Escherichia coli* 0157 A biological agent that produces a toxin causing serious diarrhea.

Enzootic A disease that is present constantly in the animal community, but that only manifests itself in a small number of cases.

Enzyme Any of the numerous complex proteins that are produced by living cells that catalyze specific biochemical reactions at body temperature.

Epidemic The occurrence of cases of an illness in a community or region that is in excess of the number of cases normally expected for that disease in that area at that time.

Epizootic An outbreak or epidemic of disease in animal populations.

Erg A metric unit of energy (dyne-cm). A joule is 100,000,000 ergs.

Erythema Redness and warming of the skin, typically due to inflammation caused by trauma or infection.

Erythema multiforme A skin disease characterized by papular (small, solid, usually conic elevation of the skin) or vesicular lesions (blisters) and reddening or discoloration of the skin, often in concentric zones about the lesion. Associated with many infections, collagen diseases, drug sensitivities, allergies, and pregnancy.

Erythema nodosum An inflammatory disorder that is characterized by tender, red nodules under the skin.

Erythrocyte A mature red blood cell that contains hemoglobin, which transports oxygen to tissues. It is a biconcave disc that lacks a nucleus.

Eschar A dry scab formed on the skin following a burn or cauterization of the skin.

Ethyl bromoacetate An irritant used in World War I by the French. One of the first chemical warfare agents. CAS Number 105-36-2.

Ethylene A flammable, colorless, gaseous alkene that is obtained from petroleum and natural gas. Used in the manufacture of a variety of different chemicals.

Exotoxin Toxic proteins secreted by bacteria, usually gram-positive ones.

Expectant In triage, those who have mortal injuries but who have not yet died.

Extrapyramidal syndromes The extrapyramidal system of the nervous system is part of the basal gangli and influences motor control through the pyramidal pathways. When the extrapyramidal system is disturbed (often as a side effect of chemicals such as BZ, benzodiazepines, phenothiazines, and haloperidol), motor control is affected. These neurologic effects include tremors, dystonia, and chorea.

Eyelid edema Swelling of the eyelids.

Faget's sign When a person exhibits a slow pulse and an elevated temperature. Often seen in yellow fever.

Fallout The precipitation of radioactive particulate matter from a nuclear weapon explosion to Earth from clouds. This term also applies to the particulate matter itself.

Fasciculations A small, local involuntary muscle contraction (twitching) visible under the skin that arises from the spontaneous discharge of a bundle of skeletal muscle fibers. May be caused by nerve agents.

Field decontamination Refers to the protection of patients and health care workers from continued exposure to chemical agents at a site.

Filovirus A virus belonging to the family Filoviridae, which is in the order Mononegavirales. They are single-stranded negative-sense RNA viruses that target primates. There are two genera: the Ebola viruses (Ebolavirus, with four species) and the Marburg virus (Marburgvirus). *See also* Ebola and Marburg.

Fission reaction An event in which a single nucleus of an element of high atomic weight (such as uranium) absorbs a neutron. Some nuclei become unstable and emit a nuclear particle or radiation, whereas others split into two nuclei and perhaps several additional neutrons. Used in atomic weapons or power generation, these are chain reactions in which the unstable nuclei split and release several neutrons, which in turn trigger additional fissions. When chain reactions occur in nuclear fission weapons ("atomic bombs"), all of the fissions and energy release occurs in an extremely short time and the energy release is uncontrolled.

Flavaviruses Linear, single-stranded RNA viruses. Yellow fever and dengue hemorrhagic fever are the most virulent flavaviruses. Other flavaviruses are St. Louis encephalitis and West Nile Virus.

Flea-borne typhus Synonym for *murine typhus,* which is caused by *Rickettsia typhi.*

Fluorescein staining A test that uses an orange dye (fluorescein) and a cobalt blue light to detect foreign bodies in the eye or damage to the corneal surface.

Fluoroquinolones A class of antibiotics derived from nalidixic acid. Cipro™ is a fluoroquinolone that is often used in the treatment of anthrax.

FM The NATO military designation for titanium tetrachloride, which is a noxious smoke.

Focal cutaneous necrosis Small spots (foci) of necrotic or dead skin and underlying tissues.

Focal hepatocellular necrosis Small areas of necrosis in the liver.

Foliant The Russian name for the program that developed the novichok agents.

Fomite Any inanimate object via which pathogenic organisms may be transferred but that does not support their growth.

Francisella tularensis The causative agent of tularemia, or infectious rabbit fever. Used by Japan in the World War II. Developed into a biological weapon by the U.S. military, but stocks were destroyed in 1972. Also called *Pasteurella tularensis.*

Free radicals Typically, stable molecules containing pairs of electrons. Free radicals can be created by radiation and chemical reactions. When a chemical reaction breaks the bonds that hold paired electrons together, free radicals are produced.

Front door coupling A term used to describe the effects of an electromagnetic pulse on equipment with an antenna designed to conduct power in or out of the device. This equipment would be particularly vulnerable to EMPs.

FS The NATO military designation for fuming sulfuric acid and chlorosulfonic acid, which is a choking agent.

G agents The first series of nerve agents; these agents were produced by Germany (hence the G) during and before World War II.

GA NATO designator for Tabun, which has the chemical name ethyl N,N-dimethyl-phosphoroamidocyanidate.

GAO Acronym for the U.S. *General Accounting Office.*

Gas chromatography (GC) The process whereby a very small amount of a liquid mixture is injected into a chromatograph and vaporized in a hot injection chamber. It is then swept by a stream of inert carrier gas through a heated column that contains a stationary, high-boiling liquid. As the mixture travels through the column, its components go back and forth at different rates between the gas phase and dissolution in the high-boiling liquid, separating into pure components. Just before each compound exits the instrument, it passes through a detector. When the detector "sees" a compound, it sends an electronic message to the recorder, which responds by printing a peak on a piece of paper.

Gastritis Inflammation of the stomach lining.

Gastrointestinal Pertaining to the stomach and intestines.

GB NATO military designator for Sarin.

GB-2 NATO military designator Sarin in binary form.

GC Medical shorthand for *gonococcus,* which is the causative agent for gonorrhea in humans. It is also an acronym for *gas chromatograph.*

GD NATO designator for Soman, which has the chemical name pinacolyl methyl methylphosphonofluoridic acid 1, 2,2-trimethylpropyl ester.

GD-2 NATO military designator for Soman in binary form.

GE Ethyl methylethyl phosphonofluoridate.

GE-2 GE in binary form.

Geiger-Mueller survey meter A type of radiation detector. Contains a gas and has a positively charged wire running down its center. A high voltage on the wire causes the charged particles to crash into atoms of the gas at high speeds that produce multiple ionizations from a single photon or charged particle. The wire attracts all the resultant electrons and the tube wall attracts all the ions. An electric pulse is generated that can be processed to deflect the meter's needle and to produce an audible click.

Genetically engineered organisms Bacteria or viruses treated in specific ways that could affect the genetic structure of specific human cells or increase lethality of an otherwise standard microbiologic agent.

Genetically modified microorganisms Organisms that have been genetically modified. In the case of weapons, these genetic elements that contain nucleic acid sequences associated with pathogenicity.

Geneva Protocol of 1925 The 1925 Geneva Protocol for the Prohibition of the Use in War of Asphyxiating, Poisonous, or Other Gases and Bacteriological Methods of Warfare was the first major treaty that prohibited the use of biological weapons.

Genitourinary Pertaining to the genitals and urinary tract.

GF NATO military designator for a G-series nerve agent having the chemical name o-cyclohexyl-methylfluorophosphonate. Also called *cyclohexyl sarin.* CAS Number 329-99-7.

Glanders A contagious bacterial disease that causes pneumonia and inflammation in horses and other equines. Has been weaponized by several countries.

Glucose-6-phosphate dehydrogenase deficiency Glucose-6-phosphatase dehydrogenase (G-6-PD) deficiency is the most common disease-producing enzymopathy in humans. The disease is highly polymorphic, with more than 300 reported variants. The *G6PD* enzyme catalyzes the oxidation of glucose-6-phosphate to 6-phosphogluconate while concomitantly reducing the oxidized form of nicotinamide adenine dinucleotide phosphate ($NADP^+$) to nicotinamide adenine dinucleotide phosphate (NADPH).

GosNIIOKhT The Russian State Scientific Research Institute of Organic Chemistry and Technology.

Granulation The formation of small rounded masses of tissue in wounds that are composed of inflammatory cells, capillaries, and fibroblasts.

gray SI unit for an absorbed dose. One gray is equal to an absorbed dose of 1 joule per kilogram (100 rads).

Greek Fire Invented by the Byzantines during the seventh century, this burning mixture floated on water and was used in naval engagements.

GS A fabricated G-agent created for disinformation by U.S. intelligence services to deceive Soviet chemical warfare experts.

Guanarito virus The etiologic agent of Venezuelan hemorrhagic fever (VHF). Guanarito virus is antigenically related to the Junin, Machupo, and Lassa viruses.

GV Dimethyl-dimethylamino-ethyl phosphoramidofluoridate.

H NATO military designator for H-series blister agents, which include Levinstein (Sulfur) mustards (H), distilled mustard (HD), nitrogen mustards (HN-1, HN-2, HN-3), and mustard-Lewisite mixture (HL).

Hagedorn oximes (H-oximes) A subset of conventional oximes, also called bispyridinium oximes, that includes agents such as HI-6, HGG-12, and HGG-42. Similar in action to the familiar 2-PAM. *See also* Pralidoxime.

Half-life The length of time it takes for a radioactive substance to lose half of its radioactivity from decay. At the end of one half-life, only 50 percent of the original radionuclide remains.

Hantaan virus A viral biological agent that produces a rapidly fatal pneumonia.

Hantavirus pulmonary syndrome (HPS) A recently identified hantavirus that can affect the lungs, causing a rapid viral pneumonia. The virus was originally called Muerto Canyon virus—later changed to Sin Nombre virus (SNV).

Hantaviruses A group of viruses found in wild rodents. Although they do not produce disease in their rodent hosts, hantaviruses can cause illness in humans. First isolated in the laboratory from striped field mice captured near Korea's Hantaan River.

HC NATO military designator for a concealing smoke mixture composed of granulated aluminum, zinc oxide, and hexachloroethane.

H/CC3 Mustard/CC3; a Hungarian version of the mustard blister agent.

HCN Chemical formula for hydrogen cyanide.

HD NATO military designator for distilled mustard, a blister agent.

Hematemesis Bloody vomit.

Hematochezia Bloody diarrhea.

Hematocrit The percent of whole blood that is composed of red blood cells. It is a measure of both the number and size of the red blood cells.

Hematological effects Effects pertaining to the blood and lymphatic system.

Hematopoietic Pertaining to the formation of blood or blood cells.

Hematopoietic syndrome One of the four effects of whole body radiation exposure, characterized by white blood cell, lymphocyte, and platelet deficiencies, resulting in immunodeficiency, complications from infection, bleeding, anemia, and impaired wound healing.

Hematuria The presence of blood in the urine; often a symptom of urinary tract disease.

Hemoconcentration Concentration of the blood, usually as a result of dehydration. Often results in a very high hematocrit.

Hemoglobinuria Presence of hemoglobin, usually from blood, in the urine. However, a positive test for hemoglobin in the urine may also be caused by the breakdown of muscle tissue because myoglobinuria reacts with the same tests as hemoglobin.

Hemolysis Breakdown of red blood cells and the subsequent release of hemoglobin.

Hemoptysis The expectoration (spitting) of blood or bloodstained sputum.

Hemorrhagic diathesis A condition in which clotting factors are altered, platelets are changed, or blood vessels are damaged so that the patient is more susceptible to bleeding.

Hemorrhagic fever with renal symptoms (HRFS) A disease caused by hantaviruses. The disease occurs mainly in Asia and the Balkans, where it is caused by the Hantaan virus. In Europe, the Puumula virus causes HRFS. The Seoul virus causes a milder form of HRFS throughout the world.

Hemorrhagic smallpox. *See Blackpox.*

Hendra virus A member of the Paramyxoviridae family, this virus was first isolated in 1994 from specimens obtained during an outbreak of respiratory and neurologic disease in horses and humans in Hendra, a suburb of Brisbane, Australia.

Hepatic necrosis Destruction or death of the liver. One of the effects of hepatitis.

Hepatitis Inflammation of the liver. May be caused by infection (viruses) or chemicals (such as alcohol or chloroform).

Hepatomegaly Enlargement of the liver.

HF Hafnium. Also, Hydrogen fluoride, a very toxic gas used in glass etching and production of integrated circuits.

HGG-12 An H oxime that may have some positive antidotal effects for Soman exposure. *See also* Hagedorn oxime.

HGG-42 An H oxime that may have some positive antidotal effects for Soman exposure. *See also* Hagedorn oxime.

HI-6 A subset of conventional oximes are the bispyridinium oximes, or H oximes (*H* for Hagedorn). These include agents such as HI-6, HGG-12, and HGG-42. H oximes have shown promise in reactivating aged enzymes after GD exposure. *See also pralidoxime.*

Histoplasma capsulatum The fungus that causes histoplasmosis.

HIV. *See* Human immunodeficiency virus (HIV).

HL NATO military designator for mustard and Lewisite mixture. *See also* Blister agent.

HN NATO military designator for nitrogen mustard. There are three varieties of nitrogen mustard HN1, HN2, and HN3. *See also* Blister agent.

H/PD The NATO military designator for a combination of mustard and phenyldichlorarsine (blister agent) that has both rapid and delayed effects.

Host An organism in which a parasite lives and by which it is nourished.

H-oximes. *See* Hagedorn oximes.

HT The NATO military designator for thickened mustard. *See also* Blister agent.

HT-2 Hydrolyzed T-2. *See also* T-2.

Human immunodeficiency virus (HIV) The virus that causes AIDS (Acquired Immunodeficiency Syndrome). Usually transmitted via blood or sexual contact.

Hun Stoffe (also Hun Stuff) A synonym for *mustard gas*. The military designator of *H* for mustard stems from this name.

Hydrocephalus A condition in which there is an overproduction, obstructed circulation or impaired absorption of CSF resulting in abnormal accumulation of fluid within the cerebral ventricles and/or subarachnoid spaces. There is dilation of the ventricles, depressed brain tissue, increased intracranial pressure and consequent neurological disturbances.

Hydrocyanic acid A synonym for *cyanide*.

Hydrogen cyanide The chemical name for the simplest cyanide compound. The NATO designation is AC.

Hydrogen sulfide A colorless gas with an offensive stench that smells like rotten eggs; however, the gas paralyzes the sense of smell rapidly. Considered a broad-spectrum poison, meaning that it can poison several different systems in the body, in particular the nervous system. Its toxicity is comparable to that of hydrogen cyanide.

Hydrolysis A chemical reaction in which water reacts with a compound to produce other compounds. The reaction involves the splitting of a bond and the addition of the hydrogen cation and the hydroxide anion from the water.

Hydroxycobalamin Also known as Vitamin B12a. Hydroxycobalamin readily binds body stores of cyanide. Used as a cyanide antidote throughout Europe.

Hyperalimentation A procedure in which nutrients and vitamins are given to a person in liquid form through a vein.

Hyperbaric oxygenation High-pressure oxygen provided via a pressure chamber. It is an antidote for several poisons, including cyanide.

Hyperemia Congestion with or engorgement of blood in a part of the body.

Hyperesthesia An increased sensitivity, particularly to touch.

Hypermotility Excessive movement; especially excessive motility of the gastrointestinal tract.

Hyperpnea Deep and rapid respiration that occurs normally after exercise or abnormally with fever or various disorders.

Hyperreflexia Reflexes that are stronger than normal.

Hypoalbuminemia Low blood serum albumin concentration.

Hyponatremia Low blood serum sodium concentration.

Hypopyon The presence of pus cells in the anterior chamber of the eye.

Hypovolemia A condition of abnormally low intravascular volume and decreased volume of the circulating plasma in the body. This can be due to blood loss or dehydration.

ICAM An improved version of the chemical agent monitor CAM.

ICD Acronym for *international classification of diseases*.

ICt$_{50}$ Time-concentration product of an inhalation agent that will incapacitate 50 percent of a group. This roughly corresponds to the ID$_{50}$ for an absorbed agent. *See also* ID$_{50}$.

ID$_{50}$ Dose of an incapacitating agent that will incapacitate 50 percent of a group. The lower the ID$_{50}$, the more potent the agent. *See also* LD$_{50}$.

IDLH Acronym for *immediately dangerous to life and health*.

IgG One of many antibodies present in blood serum. Usually indicative of a recent or remote infection. Most prevalent about three weeks after an infection begins.

IgM One of many antibodies present in blood serum. Usually indicative of an acute infection.

II NATO code name for rice blast, which is caused by *Pyricularia grisea*.

Immunity The ability of an organism to resist disease.

Immunohistochemistry A type of assay in which specific antigens are made visible by the use of fluorescent dye or enzyme markers.

IMPA Isoprophyl methylphosphonic acid.

Incapacitating agent A chemical warfare agent that produces a temporary disabling condition (physiological or psychological) that persists for hours to days after exposure has ceased.

Incendiary agents Agents and chemicals used to start fires.

Incubation period The time between the exposure to a biological agent and the appearance of the first clinical symptoms. Although there are no symptoms, the organism may be causing substantial damage during this period.

Infection The entry of an infectious agent in the body of a person or animal. In an apparent, "manifest," infection, the infected person appears to be sick. The organism enters the body, increases in number, and causes damage to the host in the process.

Infiltrate Usually refers to fluid in the lung. In addition to increasing the lung density, the infiltrate cancels the contrast between vessels and lung boundaries, and these structures disappear. Air filled bronchi, normally invisible, will be contrasted by infiltrate creating air bronchograms.

Influenza The flu, a viral infection of the respiratory tract, comes in three variants: A, B, and C. Type A influenza caused the Spanish flu in 1918, killing 20 million people in a few months, twice as many as in four years of war.

Inguinal lymph nodes The lymph nodes located in the groin (inguinal region).

Interferent A substance that, when present with a chemical warfare agent at or above the minimum detectable level, causes a false negative when otherwise a true positive would have resulted.

Interferon A protein that is produced by cells when they are invaded by viruses. The protein is then released into the bloodstream or intercellular fluid to induce healthy cells to manufacture an enzyme that counters the infection. There are three distinct types of interferon—alpha, beta, and gamma.

Interstitial fluid losses Fluid movement into the area between the tissues and blood vessels (the interstitial areas).

IOM Acronym for the U.S. *Institute of Medicine*.

Ionization The condition of being dissociated into ions. Ionization may be caused by heat, radiation, chemical reaction, or electrical discharge.

IPE Acronym for *individual protective equipment.*

Iritis Inflammation of the iris of the eye.

Irradiation Exposure to penetrating radiation. Occurs when all or part of the body is exposed to radiation from an unshielded source. *External irradiation does not make a person radioactive.*

Isocyanates A group of low-molecular-weight aromatic and aliphatic compounds containing the isocyanate group (-NCO). Isocyanates are powerful irritants to the mucous membranes of the eyes and the gastrointestinal and respiratory tracts. Symptoms include excessive tear secretion, dry throat, dry cough, chest pains, and difficulty in breathing.

Isotope competition Reducing the absorption of an isotope by providing an excess of a similar but nonradioactive form of the element.

Isotopic dilution The provision of large quantities of a stable isotope to decrease the statistical probability of the incorporation of a specific atom of the radioactive form.

Japanese B encephalitis virus A biological agent that causes brain membrane inflammation.

Johnston Atoll A United States open-air biological and chemical weapons testing and storage facility in the Pacific Ocean that is located about 1,000 kilometers southwest of Hawaii.

JSCMAD Acronym for the U.S. *Joint Service Chemical Miniature Agent Detector*, which is a small chemical weapons detector for battlefield use.

Junin virus The virus that causes Argentinian hemorrhagic fever. The Junin virus is a New World arenavirus. The virus is carried by rodents, especially mice of the genus *Callomys*.

Kampstoff LOST A synonym for *mustard gas.*

Kelocyanor The trade name for dicobalt EDTA, Kelocyanor is an antidote for acute cyanide poisoning that acts by formation of methemoglobin.

Ketosis The presence of abnormally high levels of acidic substances called ketones in the blood. The normal body fuel is glucose. Ketones are produced when there is not enough glucose in the bloodstream, and the body has to use fat for energy.

L NATO military designator for Lewisite, a blister agent having the chemical name dichloro-(2-chlorovinyl)arsine.

Lacrimal glands The tear glands.

Lacrimation The act of forming tears.

Lacrimator agents Also known as tear gas, these agents are used extensively by law enforcement agencies and the military. Lacrimator agents are irritating to the eyes and mucous membranes.

Laryngeal Relating to or situated in the larynx.

Laryngeal edema Edema around the larynx.

Lassa fever A viral hemorrhagic fever. A very contagious disease originating from Nigeria. It is a potential biological agent. The virus, a member of the virus family Arenaviridae, is a single-stranded RNA virus and is zoonotic, or animal-borne.

Lateral rectus (LR) Muscle that moves the eye away from the nose.

Lavage Washing out by flushing with water.

LCL$_0$ The lowest reported lethal concentration.

LCM Lymphocytic choriomeningitis.

LCt$_{50}$ The time-concentration product of an inhalation agent that will kill 50 percent of a group. Note that the lower the LCt$_{50}$, the more potent the agent. This roughly corresponds to the LD$_{50}$ for an absorbed agent. *See also* LD$_{50}$.

LD$_{50}$ The absorbed dose of an agent that will kill 50 percent of a group. Note that the lower the LD$_{50}$, the more potent the agent. *See also* LCt$_{50}$.

LDL$_0$ The lowest reported lethal dose.

Legionella pneumophila The organism that causes Legionnaires' disease. Has the potential to be used as a biological agent.

Legionnaire's disease An acute respiratory infection caused by the bacterium *Legionella pneumophila*, which can cause a broad spectrum of disease, from mild cough and fever to serious pneumonia. Discovered when 200 members of the American Legion became seriously ill during a conference in a U.S. hotel in 1976.

LET Acronym for the *lidocaine, epinephrine*, and *tetracaine* solution for topical anesthesia.

Leukocytosis An increase in the total number of white blood cells (WBCs) from any cause.

Leukopenia A reduction in the circulating white blood cell count to <4,000/μL. Predisposes the body to infections of all kinds and lowers the immune response.

Levinstein process A chemical process for the production of mustard. Consists of bubbling dry ethylene through sulfur monochloride, allowing the mixture to settle, and (usually) distilling the remaining material.

Lewisite A blister-forming agent similar to mustard. Following World War II, was considered obsolete by the major powers because of the discovery that 2,3-dimercapto-propanol ("British anti-Lewisite") was an inexpensive and effective antidote to Lewisite exposure. Penetrates ordinary clothing and even rubber. Chemically, Lewisite is dichloro-2-chlorovinyl arsine, $ClCHCHAsCl_2$. CAS Number 541-25-3.

Lewisite shock The result of protein and plasma leakage from the capillaries with subsequent hemoconcentration and hypotension after exposure to large amounts of Lewisite.

LOST A synonym for *mustard gas*.

LSD Acronym for *lysergic acid diethylamide,* a synthetic hallucinogenic (psychedelic) compound. Has been tested as an incapacitating agent.

Lymphadenopathy A swelling of the lymph nodes in any part of the body.

Lymphocytic choriomeningitis virus (LCMV) A single-stranded RNA virus that belongs to the Arenaviridae family. Other members of this family include Lassa virus and the Tacaribe group. LCMV produces a febrile, self-limited, biphasic disease, called lymphocytic choriomeningitis (LCM), which often is complicated by aseptic meningitis.

Lymphoid tissues The lymph nodes, in conjunction with the spleen, tonsils, adenoids, and Peyer patches, are highly organized centers of immune cells that filter antigens and circulating bacteria from the extracellular fluid.

Lymphopenia An abnormally low number of lymphocytes in the blood.

M18 Chemical Agent Detector Kit A portable, expendable kit that can be used for surface and vapor analyses. Designed primarily for detecting dangerous concentrations of vapors, aerosols, and liquid droplets of chemical agents. Can sample for unknown agents.

M19 Sampling and Analyzing Kit The M19 kit is a portable, expendable kit that can be used to identify chemical agents, perform preliminary processing of unidentifiable chemical or biological warfare agent samples, and delineate contaminated areas.

M256A1 Chemical Agent Detector Kit Consists of a carrying case, a booklet of M8 paper, 12 disposable sampler-detectors individually sealed in a plastic laminated foil envelope, and a set of instruction cards attached by a lanyard to the plastic carrying case. *See* M8 paper.

M291 kit A skin decontamination kit.

M687 An American 155-mm binary sarin chemical weapon artillery shell.

M8 paper A chemical detector and agent identifier that is designed to detect the presence and identity of chemical agents producing agent-specific color changes. When activated by chemical agents, the detector may appear to be polka dotted. The user compares the color of the dots with the colors marked on front to determine the identity of the specific agent. Differs from the M9 chemical detector in that it allows partial identification of the agent by color.

M9 paper A chemical detection paper that is placed on personnel and equipment to identify the presence of liquid chemical agent aerosols. Contains a suspension of an agent-sensitive red indicator dye in a paper matrix. It will detect and turn pink, red, reddish-brown, and red-purple when exposed to liquid nerve agents and blister agents.

Maceration Softening of the tissues after death (of either the body or the tissue) by autolysis.

Machupo virus The causative agent of Bolivian hemorrhagic fever (BHF), a viral hemorrhagic fever known to be endemic only in Bolivia. First described in 1959, it caused outbreaks in small communities in eastern Bolivia throughout the 1960s. The Machupo virus is a member of the family Arenaviridae and is maintained in populations of the rodent Calomys. *Genus callosus*.

Macules The simplest dermatological lesion. It is flat and can only be seen, not felt. Maculae are nonpalpable erythematous or purpuric spots of irregular shape and size. They are often confluent.

Malignant smallpox A form of smallpox. The rash is confluent, and lesions are soft and velvety, more macular than popular, and do not become pustular. The skin is fine-grained, reddish, and in some cases there are hemorrhages under the skin. The malignant form is frequently fatal.

Marburg virus A hemorrhagic viral fever caused by a filovirus similar to Ebola.

Mark I A military kit containing atropine and 2-PAM that can be administered to victims of a nerve agent attack. The commercial name is the AtroPen Auto-Injector & Pralidoxime Chloride Injector.

Mass spectrograph (MS) A device used to separate electrically charged particles by mass.

MD The NATO military designator for methyldichloroarsine, a blister/vesicant agent. CAS Number 593-89-5.

Medial rectus (MR) Muscle that moves the eye toward the nose.

Medial rectus paresis Paralysis of the muscles that move the eye, often seen with botox poisoning.

Melioidosis A disease produced by *Burkholderia* bacteria, which are gram-negative rods.

Meningoencephalitis An inflammatory process involving the brain (encephalitis) and meninges (meningitis). It is most often caused by pathogenic organisms that invade the central nervous system and occasionally by toxins, autoimmune disorders, and other conditions.

Menometrorrhagia Excessive uterine bleeding, both at the usual time of menstrual periods and at other irregular intervals. May also be called *metrorrhagia*.

Methemoglobin A type of hemoglobin that is not capable of carrying oxygen and delivering it to tissues. Because hemoglobin is the key carrier of oxygen in the blood, replacement by methemoglobin can cause cyanosis (a slate gray-blueness) of the skin. A small amount of methemoglobin is normally present in blood.

Methemoglobinemia Methemoglobin in the blood stream.

mg/m³ Milligrams per cubic meter.

mg-min/m³ Milligrams per minute exposure per cubic meter.

MHD Magneto-hydrodynamic generators.

Microorganisms Bacteria, viruses, rickettsiae, fungi, and protozoa.

Miosis Contraction of the pupil. The opposite of mydriasis.

Mission Oriented Protective Posture (MOPP) A flexible system used to direct the wearing of chemical protective garments and mask to balance mission requirements with the chemical warfare agent threat. MOPP gear consists of the following items: chemical suit, overboots, butyl rubber gloves, and protective mask with hood.

MLD₅₀ Median lethal dosage for 50 percent of the population.

Mnemonic A word-based memory aid that can aid in the memorization of information.

MOD The British Ministry of Defense.

Monkey pox virus A biological agent quite similar to smallpox that may be genetically engineered to produce a disease similar to smallpox.

MOPP Acronym for *Mission Oriented Protective Posture.*

Moribund In a dying state; at the point of death.

Murine typhus A form of typhus caused by *Rickettsia typhi*. It is characterized by the gradual onset of fever, aches, severe headaches, weakness, dry cough, and generalized pains. Transmitted by fleas or lice, the natural hosts are rats and mice. Synonyms include *flea-borne typhus fever, endemic typhus fever,* and *urban typhus.*

Murray Valley encephalitis virus A biological agent that causes inflammation of brain tissue.

Muscarinic receptors Receptors found in the parasympathetic nervous system. These receptors regulate cardiac contractions, gut motility, and bronchial constriction. The muscarinic receptors in exocrine glands stimulate salivation, lacrimation, and gastric acid secretion.

Mustard A prototype blister agent that has two basic forms: nitrogen mustard and sulfur mustard. Nitrogen mustard has been produced in three forms: HN1 bis-(2-chloroethyl), ethylamine; HN2 bis-(2-chloroethyl), methylamine; and HN3 tris-(2-chloroethyl), amine. Sulfur mustard is bis-(2-chloroethyl), sulfide.

MVD Acronym for *Ministerstvo Vnutrennikh Del,* the Russian Ministry of Internal Affairs.

Myalgia Pain in a muscle or a group of muscles.

Myasthenia gravis The most common disorder of neuromuscular transmission. In myasthenia gravis, the postsynaptic membrane is distorted. The concentration of acetylcholine receptors is reduced, and antibodies are attached to the membrane. Acetylcholine is released normally, but has less effect on the post-synaptic membrane.

Mycoplasma An infection is caused by *Mycoplasma pneumoniae,* a microscopic organism related to bacteria. The most common mycoplasmic infection is upper respiratory infection or pneumonia.

Mydriasis Reflex pupillary dilation as a muscle pulls the iris outward; occurs in response to a decrease in light or the presence of certain drugs.

Myelitis An inflammation of the spinal cord. Symptoms can include headache; loss of function, as though the spinal cord has been cut; tingling; pain; loss of feeling; and loss of bladder control.

Myocarditis An inflammation of the heart, usually caused by a virus or bacteria.

Myofibrils Cylindrical organelles found within muscle cells that are composed of thin filaments of actin and thick filaments of myosin.

Mutagenic An agent capable of inducing cell mutation.

N Abbreviation for *normal,* which is equivalents per liter, as applied to concentration.

NAAK Acronym for *nerve agent antidote kit.*

NATO Acronym for *North Atlantic Treaty Organization.*

Negative pressure isolation facility A room that has an interior pressure lower than atmospheric pressure. Organisms spread by respiratory means such as cough will be unable to escape to the outside world because the negative pressure means that air flow is always *into* the room.

Nephrotoxicity The activity of a chemical that causes damage to the kidney.

Nerve agents The most toxic chemical warfare agent. Absorbed into the body through breathing, by injection, or by absorption through the skin. Affect the nervous and the respiratory systems and various body functions. Include the G series and V series chemical warfare agents.

Neuropathy Inflammation of or damage to neurons (nerves).

Neutron The particle in the atomic nucleus that has a mass of 1 and a charge of 0. Penetrating particles found in the nucleus of the atom that are removed through nuclear fusion or fission.

Neutropenia Leukopenia in which the decrease is primarily in the number of neutrophils (the chief phagocytic leukocyte).

Neutrophil The chief phagocytic leukocyte. Stains with either basic or acid dyes.

New World arenaviruses Ambistranded RNA viruses that are divided into two groups based on whether the virus is found in the Eastern Hemisphere or the New World (Western Hemisphere). Include the Junin virus, the Machupo virus, the Guanarito virus, the Sabia virus, the Tacaribe virus, Whitewater arroyo virus, the Tamiami virus, and the Amapari virus.

Nicotinic Nerve endings that respond to acetylcholine are divided into muscarinic and nicotinic receptors. The nicotinic receptors are of fast onset, short duration, and almost always are excitatory in nature.

NIH Acronym for the *National Institutes of Health.*

NIOSH Acronym for the *National Institute of Occupational Safety and Health.*

Nitriles Any of a class of organic compounds containing the cyano radical –CN. Are nonreactive and do not allow passage of many chemical agents.

Nitrogen LOST A synonym for *nitrogen mustard gas*.

NO Nitrogen oxide. This compound is intensely irritating to the lungs.

Nonlethal chemical agents Agents designed to subdue or incapacitate a person, rather than kill them. Examples include calmatives, tear gas, vomit gas, and BZ.

Nonpersistant A chemical that is designed to either dissipate quickly (such as cyanide) or that can be easily destroyed by environmental factors such as sunlight. A nonpersistent agent does not stay around long.

Normal cardiac shadow The shadow of the heart on a chest x-ray.

North American Whitewater Arroyo Virus One of the New World arenaviruses. Found in California.

Nosocomial infection An infection occurring in a patient that is acquired at a hospital or other healthcare facility. Commonly called a *cross infection.*

Novichok# A binary form of Substance 33 (V-gas) developed by the former Soviet Union. Has no established name, but is often called novichok#.

Novichok 5 The first Soviet binary agent. Derived from the unitary nerve agent A-232 (also called V-gas). Estimated to be 5 to 8 times more effective than VX.

Novichok 7 A binary agent with similar volatility to Soman. Estimated to be 10 times more effective than Soman.

Novichok agents A type of binary nerve agent purported by Russian chemist Vil Mirzayanov to be developed in the late 1980s and early 1990s by the former Soviet Union, made of chemicals not controlled by the Chemical Weapons Convention, and more potent than VX. He was subsequently arrested by the Russian Security Service for disclosing state secrets. The status of this research is unknown. Novichok is Russian slang for "newcomer."

NRC Acronym for the *Nuclear Regulatory Commission* or the *National Research Council.*

NU The NATO military designator for Venezuelan equine encephalitis (VEE).

Nuclear incident Any occurrence or series of occurrences having the same origin that causes nuclear damage or that creates a grave and imminent threat of causing such damage.

Nystagmus Involuntary movements of the eyeballs; the presence or absence of nystagmus is used to diagnose a variety of neurological and visual disorders.

Oblensk A Russian biowarfare facilty.

OC Concentrated liquid extract from the cayenne pepper plant.

Ocular Pertaining to the eye.

Old World arenaviruses Arenaviruses are ambistranded RNA viruses that are divided into two groups based on whether the virus is found in the Eastern Hemisphere or the New World (Western Hemisphere). Include the lym-phocytic choriomeningitis virus, the Lassa virus, the Mopeia virus, the Mobala virus, and the Ippy virus.

Oleum A mixture of sulfuric acid and sulfur trioxide. Also, fuming sulfuric acid.

Oliguria Production of an abnormally small amount of urine.

Omsk hemorrhagic fever virus A flavivirus that causes a hemorrhagic viral fever. It is in the same family as the virus that causes dengue fever.

Omutninsk A Russian biowarfare facility.

ONR Acronym for the *Office of Naval Research* of the U.S. Navy.

OPA Isoprophyl amine.

Opacification The process of becoming cloudy or opaque.

Orchitis Inflammation of the testicle.

Organophosphorus chemicals Organic compounds that contain phosphorus as an integral part of the molecule.

Orthopox The family of viruses that includes vaccinia, variola, cowpox, monkeypox, camelpox, molluscum contagiosum, and ORF. Poxviruses are very large rectangular viruses with a complex internal structure.

OU The NATO military designator for Q fever.

Outgassing The loss of substance by evaporation or sublimation. Usually applied to a contaminant that affects others around the patient.

***p*-Aminoheptanoylphenone (PAPP)** A methemoglobin-forming compound that has treatment effects in cyanide intoxication.

***p*-Aminooctanoylphenone (PAOP)** A methemoglobin-forming compound that has treatment effects in cyanide intoxication.

***p*-Aminopropiophenone (PAHP)** A methemoglobin-forming compound that has treatment effects in cyanide intoxication.

PAC Acronym for the *Presidential Advisory Committee.*

Palsies Another term for paralysis.

2-PAM Also called pralidoxime chloride, the U.S. Army uses this oxime to reactivate acetylcholinesterase. (*See also* H oxime.)

Pandemic An epidemic occurring worldwide or over a very wide area that crosses international boundaries and usually affects a large number of people. *See also* Epidemic.

Papules Small (less than 1 centimeter) circumscribed, elevated skin lesions that are pointed, flat topped, dome shaped, smooth, or eroded.

Paralytic cobra toxin A toxin reputedly developed by the Russians whereby recombinant DNA techniques were used to induce cobra venom production in bacteria.

Parenteral That which is not done in or through the digestive system. Can refer to blood being drawn from the venous system, a drug being introduced into a vein, or injection of medications through the skin or into the muscle.

Parotitis Inflammation of the parotid gland (and other salivary gland).

Particle accelerator Apparatus that speeds a particle, such as an electron, to near the speed of light in order to collide the particle with an atom. The resultant collisions can form new or artificial radioactive isotopes and elements.

Pasteurella tularensis Causative agent of tularemia, or infectious rabbit fever. Used by Japan in World War II. Developed into a biological weapon by the U.S. military, but stocks were destroyed in 1972. The organism is also called *Francisella tularensis*.

Pathogen A pathogen is an organism that is able to evade the normal defenses of the host and cause an infection.

Pathogenicity The quality of being a pathogen, a measure of how easily an organism infects a host.

Payload The part of a missile or torpedo that carries an explosive charge.

PB Pyridostigmine bromide, a pretreatment compound for nerve agents. Acts as an antidote-enhancing compound.

PCR Acronym for *polymerase chain reaction. See also* RT-PCR.

PD NATO military designator for phenodichloroarsine, which is a variant of Lewisite. Very irritating to the eyes and mucous membranes and causes rapid blister formation if exposed to the skin. Although classed as a blister agent, it also acts as a vomiting compound.

PEG Polyethlene glycol.

Perfluroroisobutylene (PIFB) A compound that results from the combustion of Teflon™ and other similar plastics. It is intensely irritating to the lungs and has a latent period of 1 to 4 hours. Although not a "formal" war gas, it was developed as a chemical weapon by the former USSR. Its chemical name is 1,1,3,3,3- Pentafluoro-2-(trifluoromethyl)-1-propene. CAS Number 382-21-8.

Peripheral neuropathy A condition resulting from nerve damage that usually affects the feet and legs, causing pain, numbness, or a tingling. Also called *somatic neuropathy* or *distal sensory polyneuropathy*.

Petechia A minute red or purple spot on the surface of the skin as the result of tiny hemorrhages of blood vessels in the skin (as in typhoid fever).

PF3 Diisopropyl fluorophosphates, also known as DFP. It is a weak organophosphate nerve agent.

PFAPE Perfluoroalkylpolyether. An ingredient in the barrier cream SERPACWA.

PG NATO military designator for staphylococcal enterotoxin B, which was part of the U.S. biological weapons stockpile until 1978.

pH Measurement of acidity or alkalinity. The pH scale goes from 0 to 14, with 7 as the neutral point. A pH lower than 7 is acidic; a pH above 7 is alkaline.

Phenodichloroarsine A variant of Lewisite, this compound is very irritating to the eyes and mucous membranes. It causes rapid blister formation if exposed to the skin. NATO military designator is PD. CAS Number 696-28-6.

Phosgene A colorless gas that is heavier than air. It is a chemical agent designed to cause pulmonary damage and asphyxia. The NATO military designator for this agent is CG. CAS Number 75-44-5.

Phosgene oxime (CX) Also known as dichloroformoxime, this compound is a powerful irritant that produces immediate reactions varying from a mild irritation to severe local pain. Classified either as an urticariant or a blister agent. CAS Number 1794-86-1.

Photophobia Intolerance to light.

Piezoelectric crystal plethysmograph A pressure-sensitive piezoelectric crystal that generates its own voltage when pressed. When strapped against the skin, this device easily picks up pulses and generates voltages up to 200 mV with each pulse waveform.

Pinacolyl alcohol An aliphatic alcohol with the chemical name 3,3-dimethyl-2-butanol. Important ingredient in binary weapons in which Soman, GD, is formed at the time of use.

Pinacolyl methylphosphonyl fluoride The chemical name for Soman, GD. CAS Number 96-64-0.

Plague A highly contagious disease caused by *Pasturella pestis*. Has pneumonic, septic, and bubonic forms. Normally carried by rodents and transmitted by fleas. A defecting Soviet scientist, Vladimir Pasechnik told British and U.S. intelligence that Soviet scientists had developed a genetically engineered multi-drug-resistant strain of pneumonic plague.

Pleuritic chest pain Chest pain that increases with respiration.

Pneumorickettsiosis Synonym for Q fever, which is caused by *Rickettsia burnetii*. Has been investigated as a potential biological weapon.

Polymer-fume fever A fever caused by heavy exposure to pyrolysis products of polytetrafluoroethylene (PTFE, trade names Fluon, Teflon, Halon). Symptoms are usually flu-like illness with chest tightness and mild cough. Occurs when PTFE is heated above 300°C.

Porcine enterovirus type 9 Causative agent of swine vesicular disease. It has been investigated as a biological weapon.

Positive end expiratory pressure (PEEP) Ventilation method whereby airway pressure is maintained above atmospheric pressure at the end of exhalation by means of a mechanical impedance within the circuit. The purpose of PEEP is to increase the volume of gas remaining in the lungs at the end of expiration in order to decrease the shunting of blood through the lungs and improve gas exchange.

Positive pressure breathing (PPB) Inhalation of respiratory gases that are under a small constant positive pressure relative to ambient pressure, which forces air into the lungs. *See also* Positive End Expiratory Pressure (PEEP).

Powassan (POW) virus A member of the family Flaviviridae. It is an enveloped, single-stranded RNA virus. Although in the same family as St. Louis encephalitis virus and West Nile Virus, the POW virus is ecologically very different. Disease, when it occurs, takes the form of infection and inflammation of the brain (encephalitis and meningitis). Most infections do not result in disease.

Powered air-purifying respirator (PAPR) A device that uses a blower to force ambient air through air-purifying elements to the mask.

PPB Acronym for *positive pressure breathing*.

PPE Acronym for *personal protective equipment*.

Ppm Parts per million.

Pralidoxime (2-PAM) Currently used by the U.S. Army to reactivate cholinesterase.

Precursor cells Cells that form other cells through natural processes.

Precursor chemicals Chemicals that are commonly used in the manufacture of chemical warfare agents. May also refer to chemicals that are part of a binary chemical weapons system.

Prepositioned medical supplies Stocks of drugs, bandages, and other medical supplies that are preloaded into containers and stored in warehouses. These stocks may be rapidly deployed in case of a disaster.

Prerenal azotemia Elevation of blood urea nitrogen caused by effects other than kidney failure or disease.

Probenecid Lowers uric acid levels by increasing the amount of uric acid passed in the urine. Helps to dissolve tophi and prevent uric acid deposits in joints. Also used to increase the concentration (blood level) of antibiotics, because it competes for elimination of these antibiotics in the urine.

Prodrome Stage of infection in which the patient has nonspecific symptoms, such as headache, lethargy, or fever. It is the period before the development of a specific symptom complex that is suggestive of the classic infection. The patient may be quite contagious during this stage.

Progressive vaccinia A severe complication of smallpox vaccination that occurs because of an immune defect in the vaccinated individual or in a susceptible contact person. The primary vaccination site does not heal, but rather expands with extensive necrosis, eventually covering large portions of body with extensive destruction of normal tissue. Sometimes called *vaccinia necrosum, vaccinia gangrenosa,* or *disseminated vaccinia.*

Proteinuria Protein in the urine.

Proton A component of an atomic nucleus with a mass of 1 and a charge of +1. The nucleus of a hydrogen atom. A H^+ ion.

Pruritus The medical term for itching. It is a common manifestation of dermatologic diseases, including xerotic eczema, atopic dermatitis, and allergic contact dermatitis.

Prussic acid A synonym for *cyanide.*

PS Chloropicrin, an infrequently used lacrimator agent. CAS Number 76-06-2.

Psittacosis Also called *parrot fever,* caused by *Chlamydia psittaci,* a mycoplasma. This mycoplasma has been developed as an incapacitating agent.

Ptosis Drooping of the eyelids due to weakness of the muscles responsible for keeping the eyelids open.

Puccinia gramisis secalis Rye stem rust. Pathogenic plant fungus developed as a biological weapon by the United States for destroying rye harvest. Existing stocks were destroyed in 1972.

Puccinia gramisis tritici Wheat stem rust. Pathogenic plant fungus developed as a biological weapon by the United States for destroying wheat and barley harvest. Existing stocks were destroyed in 1972.

Pulmonary Pertaining to the respiratory system.

Pulmonary agent Agents that damage the lung by inhalation. They may or may not have a latent period. Examples of pulmonary agents are phosgene and chlorine. These may also be referred to as *choking agents.*

Pupura Bleeding from the skin. May be in the form of black and blue patches of varying sizes (*ecchymoses*) or pinhead-sized spots (*petechiae*), or both.

Pyricularia oryzea A plant disease, also called *rice blast.* This fungus causes "plague" in rice crops. It was developed by the U.S. military. Existing stocks were destroyed in 1972.

Pyridostigmine bromide A chemical that blocks the nerve-signal-regulating enzyme *acetylcholinesterase* (AChE).

QB3 Common abbreviation for *quinuclidinyl benzilate,* which is an incapacitating agent. Also known as *BZ.* CAS Number 6581-06-2.

Q-fever Also called *Query fever, Balkan influenza, Balkan grippe, abattoir fever,* or *pneumorickettsiosis.* This fever is caused by *Coxiella burnetii.*

QL The NATO designator for the liquid precursor used with sulfur to form VX. Its chemical formula is o-ethyl o-2-diisopropylaminoethyl methylphosphonite. CAS Number 57856-11-8.

Quality factor (Q). *See* RBE.

3-Quinuclidinylbenzilate A glycolate anticholinergic compound related to atropine, scopolamine, and hyoscyamine. Its NATO military designator is BZ. It is a delayed onset (1 to 4 hours after exposure) incapacitation agent. CAS Number 6581-06-2.

Radiation absorbed dose (rad) A quantity that expresses the amount of energy that ionizing radiation imparts to a given mass of matter. It is defined as a dose of 100 ergs of energy per gram of matter. The SI unit for absorbed dose is the gray (Gy), which is defined as a dose of one joule per kilogram. Because one joule equals 10^7 ergs, and since one kilogram equals 1,000 grams, 1 Gray equals 100 rads.

Radiation accident An accident involving facilities or activities from which a release of radioactive material occurs or is likely to occur and that has resulted or may result in an international transboundary release that could be of radiological safety significance for another state.

Radiation dispersal weapon Any device that causes the purposeful dissemination of radioactive material without a nuclear detonation; a dirty bomb.

Radioactive isotope A natural or artificially created isotope of a chemical element having an unstable nucleus that decays, emitting alpha, beta, or gamma rays until stability is reached. The stable end product is a nonradioactive isotope of another element (ie, radium-226 decays to lead-206). Also called a *radionuclide* or *radioisotope.*

RBC Acronym for *red blood cell.*

RBE Acronym for *relative biological effectiveness.*

Rebirth Island A Russian weapons testing facility in the Aral Sea used for open-air testing of biological weapons.

Red phosphorus (RP) A compound formed by heating white phosphorus to 250°C or by exposing white phosphorus to sunlight. It is not poisonous and is not as dangerous as white phosphorus, although frictional heating is enough to change it back to white phosphorus.

Relative biological effectiveness (RBE) The dose of a reference radiation, usually x-rays, required to produce the same biological effect as was seen with a test dose, D_T, of another radiation.

Reservoir Any person, animal, arthropod, plant, soil, or substance in which an infective agent normally lives and multiplies. The infectious agent primarily depends on the reservoir for its survival.

Reticuloendothelial system (RES) A part of the generalized immune system that consists of phagocytic cells, primarily monocytes and macrophages, located in reticular connective tissue. These cells accumulate in the lymph nodes and the spleen. The Kupffer cells of the liver and tissue histiocytes are also part of the RES.

Retrosternal Behind the sternum.

Reversible hemolytic anemia Breakdown of blood cells (hemolysis) that reverses over time or with treatment.

Rhinitis An inflammation of the nose.

Rhinorrhea Watery mucus discharge from the nose (as in the common cold).

Ribavirin An antiviral drug used in the treatment of respiratory syncytial virus infection and hepatitis C. Has been proposed as a potential treatment for several viruses that have been investigated for use as biological weapons. The chemical formula is 1-beta-D-ribofuranosyl-1,2,4-triazole-3-carboxamide.

Rice blast A plant disease is caused by *Pyricularia oryzae.* It is a fungus that causes "plague" in rice crops. It was developed by the U.S. military. Existing stocks were destroyed in 1972.

Rice water diarrhea Diarrhea caused by cholera.

Ricin Poison derived from the beans of the castor oil plant that was developed as a toxic weapon during World War II. The NATO military code name for ricin is Compound W.

Ricinus communis The castor bean plant, which is the source of castor bean oil and ricin. The seeds from the castor bean plant are poisonous to people, animals, and insects.

Ricinus communis **agglutinin (RCA)** One of the main toxic proteins is "ricin", named by Stillmark in 1888 when he tested the beans extract on red blood cells and saw them agglutinate. The agglutination was due to another toxin that was also present in his sample, called RCA (*Ricinus communis* agglutinin). Ricin is a potent cytotoxin but a weak hemagglutinin, whereas RCA is a weak cytotoxin and a powerful hemagglutinin. *See also* Ricin

Rickettsiae Class of biological agents that are obligate intracellular parasites. This class includes *Coxiella burnetii, Rickettsia quintana* (also known as *Rochalimaea quintana*), and *Rickettsia prowazeki.*

Rickettsia prowazekii Rickettsial agent that causes endemic typhus. Typhus is characterized by fever, aches, headaches, weakness, and pain. Followed by stupor, delirium, and death (about 30 percent). Spread by lice.

Rickettsia rickettsii Causative agent for Rocky Mountain spotted fever. Characterized by sudden onset of fever, severe headache, fatigue, swollen and reddened eyes, muscle pain, and chills. Within 2 to 6 days a maculopapular rash spreads from wrists, hands, feet, and ankles to the rest of the body. This rash may herald a hemorrhagic fever. About 25 percent of untreated cases are fatal.

Rickettsia typhi Rickettsial agent that causes murine typhus. Murine typhus is characterized by gradual onset of fever, aches, severe headaches, weakness, dry cough, and generalized pains. A macular rash appears by about the fifth day. Transmitted by fleas or lice, the natural hosts are rats and mice.

Rictus sardonicus The "sardonic grin" typically seen in tetanus infections.

Rift Valley fever (RVF) virus An acute, fever-causing virus that affects domestic livestock (e.g., cattle, buffalo, sheep, goats, and camels) and humans. RVF is most commonly associated with mosquito-borne epidemics during years of unusually heavy rainfall. The virus is a member of the genus *Phlebovirus* in the family Bunyaviridae. River Valley Fever was first reported among livestock by veterinary officers in Kenya in the Rift Valley in the early 1900s, hence the name.

Risk (1) The chance of being exposed to an infectious agent by its specific transmission mechanism. (2) The chance of becoming infected if exposed to an infectious agent by its specific transmission mechanism.

RNA Acronym for *ribonucleic acid.*

Rochalimaea quintana Also called *Bartonella quintana,* this agent causes trench fever, which was a significant medical problem during World War I. *Rochalimaea quintana* is a rickettsial disease.

Rocky Mountain spotted fever Fever caused by *Rickettsia rickettsii* that is characterized by sudden onset of fever, severe headache, fatigue, swollen and reddened eyes, muscle pain, and chills. Within 2 to 6 days a maculopapular rash spreads from wrists, hands, feet, and ankles to the rest of the body. About 25 percent of untreated cases are fatal.

Roentgen equivalent in mammals (rem) Unit for the biological dose of radiation.

RT-PCR (reverse transcriptase polymerase chain reaction) Powerful technique for producing millions of copies of specific parts of the genetic code of an organism so that it may be analyzed more easily. Specifically, RT-PCR produces copies of a specific region of complementary DNA that has been converted from RNA. The technique is often used to help in the identification of infectious agents.

Ruby laser A laser that consists of a flash tube (like those found on cameras), a ruby rod, and two mirrors (one half-silvered).

Russian Spring-Summer encephalitis virus Tick-borne virus that causes inflammation of brain tissue.

RVX Russian V-gas.

S-330 A choloramide that has been shown to provide further protection from mustard when added to skin barrier creams.

SA NATO military designator for arsine. The chemical formula is ASH_3. Exposure results in hemolysis and kidney failure. It is a true blood agent. CAS Number 7784-42-1.

SAH Acronym for *sub-arachnoid hemorrhage.*

San Joaquin Valley fever An infection caused by coccidioidomycosis. Also called *desert fever* or *valley fever.*

Sarin NATO military designator for nerve agent with the chemical name isopropyl methyl phosphonofluoridate. The NATO military designator is GB. This is one of the original German nerve agents. CAS Number 107-44-8.

Saxitoxin A poison derived from shellfish that ingest dinoflagellates. The NATO military designator for saxitoxin is SS. This toxin is among the most lethal toxins known.

Scintillation counter A device that detects and measures radiation by means of tiny visible flashes produced by the radiation when it strikes a sensitive substance called a *phosphor.*

SEA Staphylococcal enterotoxin A.

SEB The causative agent of food poisoning derived from *Staphylococcus aureus.* The NATO military designator for this agent is PG.

SEB disease The disease cause by staphylococcal enterotoxin B.

SEC Staphylococcal enterotoxin C.

SEE Staphylococcal enterotoxin E.

Seivert A unit of the biological dose of radiation.

Selective serotonin reuptake inhibitors (SSRIs) A class of antidepressants that act on the brain to increase the amount of the neurotransmitter serotonin (5-hydroxytryptamine or 5-HT) in the synaptic gap by inhibiting its reuptake.

Self-contained breathing apparatus (SCBA) A respirator with an independent air supply that is used to enter toxic and otherwise dangerous atmospheres.

Self-limited A disease that limits itself rapidly and causes no permanent damage.

Semiquantitative assay A term for numerical results from immunoassay technology that is an approximation of the true quantitative result produced by gas chromatography (GC) and GC/mass spectrometry (MS) techniques.

Sera Plural of *serum.*

Sergiyev Posad A Russian Ministry of Defense biological weapons facility located northeast of Moscow.

Seroconversion The development of detectable, specific antibodies to microorganisms in a serum as a result of infection or immunization. Prior to seroconversion, the blood tests seronegative for the antibody; after seroconversion, the blood tests seropositive for the antibody.

Serologic studies Tests on blood or serum that look for specific antibodies resulting from infection or immunization.

SERPACWA (Skin Exposure Reduction Paste Against Chemical Warfare) SA protective ointment developed by the U.S. military as a supplement to reduce or delay the absorption of chemical warfare agents through the skin. It contains a PTFE component.

Shedding The release of infectious particles (e.g., bacteria, viruses) into the environment; for example, by sneezing, excretion of fecal matter, or oozing from an open lesion.

Sheep pox virus An animal pathogen that is related to smallpox. A member of the Poxviridae, the viron contains one molecule of linear double-stranded DNA.

Shelf life The length of time that an item or material may be stored and remain suitable for use. Usually an estimation.

SIPRI Acronym for the *Stockholm International Peace Research Institute.*

Slaman Pak An Iraqi biological weapons facility.

SLE (systemic lupus erythematosus) Acronym for *systemic lupus erythematosus,* a collagen-vascular disease that often affects young women.

Smallpox A highly contagious transmitted disease that is passed person-to-person. The disease is caused by a variola virus. Although wild smallpox was eradicated worldwide in 1977, laboratory samples continue to exist.

SO_3 Sulfur trioxide, a noxious gas. Sulfur trioxide-chlorosulfonic acid is a standard smoke mixture for aircraft spray tanks. When dispersed in the air, it absorbs moisture to form a dense white fog consisting of small droplets of hydrochloric and sulfuric acids. In moderate concentrations, it is highly irritating to the eyes, nose, and skin. The NATO Designator is FS. CAS Number 7446-11-9.

Sodium nitroprusside Compound that breaks down in the blood and releases nitric oxide (NO). Nitric oxide enters the muscle cells in the walls of the blood vessels and causes them to relax. The chemical name is sodium nitroferricyanide dihydrate. CAS Number 13755-38-9.

Soman NATO military designator for nerve agent having the chemical name pinacolyl methyl phosphonofluoridate. The NATO military designator is GD. One of the original German nerve agents. CAS Number 96-64-0.

Sonography A noninvasive diagnostic technique, also known as ultrasonography, in which high-frequency sound waves are aimed at a body area or organ. The resulting echoes are converted to images.

Spastic paralysis A form of paralysis in which the part of the nervous system that controls coordinated movement of the voluntary muscles is disabled.

Spectrophotometry The quantitative measurement of the reflection or transmission properties of a material as a function of wavelength.

Spirometry Measurement of pulmonary functions, such as vital capacity, tidal volume, and forced expiratory volume.

Spores The dormant form of a bacterium or fungus.

SS The NATO military designator for saxitoxin, a paralytic shellfish toxin.

SSRIs (selective serotonin reuptake inhibitors) A class of antidepressants that act on the brain to increase the amount of the neurotransmitter serotonin (5-hydroxy-tryptamine or 5-HT) in the synaptic gap by inhibiting its reuptake.

St. Louis encephalitis virus A virus that causes swelling of the brain tissue.

Staphylococcus enterotoxin B Causative agent of food poisoning derived from *Staphylococcus aureus*. Also called SEB or PG.

State Research Center for Applied Microbiology A Russian biological research facility where it is suspected that scientists worked on biological weapons, particularly bubonic plague.

Sternutators A substance that causes irritation of the nasal and respiratory passages and causes coughing, sneezing, lacrimation (tearing of the eyes), and possibly vomiting.

Subclinical Without clinical signs or symptoms; sometimes used to describe the early stage of a disease or condition before symptoms are detectable by clinical examination or laboratory tests.

Substance 33 Synonym for V-gas developed by the former Soviet Union.

Substance 35 Synonym for Sarin developed by the former Soviet Union.

Substance 55 Synonym for Soman developed by the former Soviet Union.

Sulfhydryl group Also called a *thiol group*. A functional group composed of a sulfur and a hydrogen atom (-SH). It is the sulfur analog of the hydroxyl group -OH found in alcohols. Organic compounds containing a sulfhydryl group are known as *thiols* or *mercaptans*.

Sulfur mustard A clear, yellow, or amber oily liquid with a faint sweet odor of mustard or garlic that may be dispersed in aerosol form. It causes blistering of exposed skin. The chemical name is bis (2-chloroethyl) sulfide. CAS Number 505-60-2.

Superinfection An infection that occurs in an area of damage or distress. A common term for a pneumonia that follows from inhalation of a chemical agent that damages the lung.

Survey meters General purpose radiation detection instruments. A common survey meter is the Geiger-Mueller survey meter.

Sympathomimetic effect Causing an effect similar to that caused by stimulation of the sympathetic nervous system.

Sympathomimetics Drugs which mimic the stimulation of the sympathetic nervous system.

T The NATO military designator for a blister agent with the chemical name bis-2-chloroethylsulfide. It is closely related to mustard and similar in effect. CAS Number 693-07-2.

T-2 One of the trichothecene complexes. T-2 mycotoxin is a skin necrosis agent.

Tabun The NATO military designator for nerve agent having the chemical name ethyl N,N-dimethyl-phosphoroami-docyanidate. CAS Number 77-81-6.

Tacaribe complex The arenaviruses are divided into two groups: the New World, or Tacaribe, complex and the Old World, or LCM/Lassa, complex. Several New World (Tacaribe complex) arenaviruses (Arenaviridae) are known to cause severe hemorrhagic disease in humans.

Taliban The Taliban (Pashtun and Persian: "students of Islam"), also transliterated as "Taleban," is an Islamist and Pashtun nationalist movement that ruled most of Afghanistan from 1996 until 2001.

Tear gas. *See* Lacrimator agents.

Tenesmus The constant feeling of the need to empty the bowel, accompanied by pain, cramping, and involuntary straining efforts often associated with diarrhea.

Teratogenic A substance that produces birth defects.

Tetanus toxin Toxin secreted by *Clostridium* species that is similar to botulinum. It causes effects at extremely low concentrations, is irreversible, and, like botulism, requires activity of the nerve to cause toxicity to that nerve.

Tetrodotoxin A biological toxin produced by the puffer fish, among animals.

TG Thiodiglycol.

TLD Acronym for *threshold limit dose.*

Torsade de pointes (TDP) An uncommon variant of ventricular tachycardia (VT). Torsade is defined as a polymorphous VT in which the morphology of the QRS complexes varies from beat to beat.

Toxemia The presence of toxins in the blood stream.

Toxidrome A toxic syndrome that indicates a type of poisoning.

Toxin A poison derived from plants, animals, or microbes that causes disease.

Toxin weapons Noncontagious biological weapons that are generally odorless, tasteless, and invisible.

Toxoid A vaccine that prevents a disease process by inducing an immune reaction to a denatured toxin.

TP Triphosgene or trichloromethyl carbonate. A pulmonary agent similar to phosgene. Has the chemical formula $C_3Cl_6O_3$. CAS Number 32315-10-9.

Tracheal-bronchial mucosa The mucosa that lines the trachea and bronchial tubes of the respiratory system.

Tracheobronchitis Inflammation of the trachea and bronchus.

Transmission of infectious agents Any mechanism through which an infectious agent, such as a virus, is spread from a reservoir (or source) to a human being.

Transthoracic impedance devices Devices that use changes in transthoracic impedance to monitor respiratory effort. Variations in thoracic pressure cause variations in air volume within the lungs, which, in turn, result in variations in transthoracic impedance.

Trichothecenes mycotoxin A fungus-based toxin, allegedly used by the former Soviet Union as "yellow rain" in Vietnam and the Lao People's Democratic Republic.

Triphosgene Also called *trichloromethyl carbonate*. A pulmonary agent that is similar to phosgene with NATO designator TP. Its molecular formula is $C_3Cl_6O_3$. CAS Number 32315-10-9.

Tularemia Also called *rabbit fever*, tularemia is a plague-like infectious disease that causes chills, fever, muscle aches, fatigue, and pneumonia-like symptoms. It is an infection common in wild rodents caused by the organism *Francisella tularensis* and is transmitted to humans by contact with animal tissues or ticks.

Typhoid fever A life-threatening illness caused by the bacterium *Salmonella typhi*. *Salmonella typhi* lives only in humans.

Tyvek A fabric made from high-density polyethylene fibers by Dupont. Tyvek is an extremely versatile material, offering a balance of physical characteristics that combine some of the properties of film, paper, and cloth.

Umbilicated Having an umbilicus or stalk.

Undifferentiated fever Fever without an identified source.

Unit 731 The Japanese biological warfare unit. During World War II, this unit carried out experiments on local Chinese and on Allied prisoners of war. The unit used fleas to spread plague in several Chinese cities.

UNSCOM Acronym for *United Nations Special Commission.*

Urban typhus Synonym for murine typhus caused by *Rickettsia typhi.*

Urticant A substance that causes burning or itching of the skin such as that caused by nettle stings. Often classified with the blister or vesicant agents. An example is phosgene oxime.

Urushiol A sticky, clear oil containing catechols and other phenolic resins that acts as a powerful hapten (a substance that does not stimulate antibody formation but reacts selectively in vitro with an antibody).

USAMRIID Acronym for the *United States Army Medical Research Institute for Infectious Diseases.*

V agents The NATO military designator for persistent, highly toxic nerve agents developed in Britain in the mid-1950s that are absorbed primarily through the skin. V agents are generally colorless and odorless liquids that do not evaporate rapidly. The standard V agent is VX; others include V gas, VE, VM, and VX-2.

Vaccinia Causative agent for cowpox; used by Jenner to vaccinate for smallpox.

Variola major Causative agent for the most common form of smallpox. In populations that have not been inoculated, the mortality from smallpox ranges from 30 to greater than 70 percent. It can be prevented by vaccination.

Variola minor Causative agent for a mild variant of smallpox that has a 1 to 2 percent fatality rate in unvaccinated individuals. It can be prevented by vaccination.

Vascularization The process whereby body tissue becomes vascular and develops capillaries.

VE Military designator for a V-series nerve agent, phosphonofluoridic acid, ethyl-, 1-methylethyl ester, that was developed, but never produced. CAS Number 1189-87-3.

Vector (1) The Russian virology research institute near Novosibirsk in western Siberia. Vector developed virus weapons for the USSR. (2) A carrier that transmits an infective agent from one host to another. The delivery system of a disease or bioweapon (eg, birds, insects, or other animals).

Venezuelan equine encephalitis virus Biological agent that causes inflammation of the brain in horses and human beings. Disseminated by mosquitoes or aerosol. The NATO military designator is NU. It is a member of the family Togaviridae, genus Alphavirus. It is closely related to Eastern and Western equine encephalitis viruses.

Vesicant A substance that causes blister formation (bullae). This is the proper name for a blister agent. *See also* Blister agent.

Vesicles A small fluid-filled blister ranging in size from a pinpoint to 5 or 10 millimeters in diameter. As a rule, the term *vesicle* is used to describe a small blister, whereas the term *bulla* is used to describe a larger blister.

Vestibular system The body system that keeps tabs on the position and motion of the head in space.

VG The NATO military designator for a V-series nerve agent that was developed, but never produced. It was originally developed as an insecticide and was to be marketed as Amiton. CAS Number 78-53-5.

V-gas NATO military designator for the V-series nerve agent having the chemical name methylphosphonothioic acid, S-[2-(diethylamino)ethyl] O-2-methylpropyl ester. It was produced by the former Soviet Union.

Vibrio cholera Biological agent that causes cholera. The genus *Vibrio* consists of gram-negative straight or curved rods. They are motile by means of a single polar flagellum.

Viral hemorrhagic fever (VHF) A virus that causes hemorrhagic fever. One of several that was developed as a weapon by the US and several other countries.

Viron The smallest replicating particle of a virus.

Virulence factors Factors produced by an organism that increase its ability to infect. Viral virulence factors determine whether infection occurs and the severity of the resulting viral disease symptoms.

Virus The smallest reproducing microorganism, this class of biological agents includes the Ebola, Dengue, Marburg, and smallpox viruses.

VM A V-series nerve agent having the chemical name o-ethyl S-(2-diethylaminoethyl) methylphosphonothiolate. It is considered to be a persistent agent. CAS Number 21770-86-5.

Volatility The tendency of a substance to produce vapors.

Vomiting agent A nonlethal chemical warfare agent specifically designed to cause vomiting. These are generally not used, because the dose that causes vomiting may be unacceptably close to that that causes fatalities. *See also* Adamsite.

Vozroshdeniye Island A major biological warfare testing site in the former Soviet Union.

VR Russian V-gas, a Russian variant of V-series nerve gas.

VV The NATO military designator for *thickened mustard*.

VX NATO military designator for V-series nerve agent having the chemical name o-ethyl-S-(2-diisopropylaminoethyl) methyl phosphonothiolate. Considered to be a persistent nerve agent.

VX-2 VX in binary form.

West Nile Virus (WNV) An arbovirus that is transmitted by mosquitos. Can cause encephalitis in infected humans and horses and can result in wild and domestic bird mortality. First discovered in a woman from the West Nile District of Uganda in 1937. It spread across areas of Africa, Eastern Europe, West Asia, and the Middle East. First detected in the Western Hemisphere in 1999 and has since spread rapidly across the North American continent into all 48 continental states, seven Canadian provinces, and throughout Mexico.

Western equine encephalitis virus A member of the family Togaviridae, genus Alphavirus. Closely related to Eastern and Venezuelan equine encephalitis viruses.

WGE-6 A NATO term for a *Working Group of Experts*. Includes three groups: PG-31, PG-32, and PG-33 that specialize in defense against biological weapons.

Wheat stem rust (*Puccinia graminus triciti*) A biological anticrop agent that makes infected grain unfit for human consumption.

WHO Acronym for the *World Health Organization*.

WMD Acronym for *weapons of mass destruction*. Includes chemical, biological, and nuclear weapons. Technically in-accurate, because most chemical weapons and almost all biological weapons are designed to cause casualties, not destruction.

Woolsorter's disease Another name for naturally caused inhalation anthrax.

Worm A destructive program that replicates itself throughout a computer's disk and memory, using up the computer's resources and eventually taking the system down.

WP The NATO military designator for White Phosphorus. Chemical name: white or yellow phosphorus. Chemical formula: P4. Used as incendiary, antipersonnel, and smoke munition.

X The NATO military designator for botulinum toxin.

YE The NATO military designator for endemic typhus.

Yellow fever virus Biological agent that causes yellow fever. A classic feature of yellow fever is hepatitis, which is the reason for the yellow coloring of the skin (jaundice) and the name of the disease. Belongs to the Flaviviridae family.

Yersinia pestis (Pasteurella pestis) The bacteria that causes the plague ("black death"). It is named after its discoverer, A. Yersin. Considered to be one of the more lethal bioweapons.

Yersinia pseudotuberculosis The least common of the three main *Yersinia* species that infect humans. Primarily a zoonotic infection, but has been transmitted to humans. Has been evaluated as a bioweapon.

Yperite A synonym for *mustard gas*. Its chemical name is bis(2-chloroethyl) sulfide. CAS Number 505-60-2.

Zoonotic disease or infection An infection or infectious disease that may be transmitted from vertebrate animals (such as a rodent) to humans.

C

PHOTO CREDITS

Chapter 1

1-1 Courtesy of Library of Congress, Prints & Photographs Division, FSA-OWI Collection [LC-USW3-004800-D DLC]; 1-2 Courtesy of U.S. Department of Defense; 1-3 © United Nations; 1-4 © Chikumo Chiaki/AP Photo; 1-5 © Shailendra Yashwant/Greenpeace; 1-6 Courtesy of Trent Bollinger, CCWHC - Saskatoon

Chapter 2

2-1 Courtesy of Pratap Chatterjee and The Rainforest Information Centre; 2-2 © Clinton Harman/istockphoto

Chapter 3

3-1 Courtesy of Library of Congress, Prints & Photographs Division, FSA-OWI Collection, [LC-USW3-004802-D DLC]; 3-5 © Mitretek Systems. Used with permission.; 3-8 © Mitretek Systems. Used with permission.; 3-9 Courtesy of Astra Tech.; 3-10 Courtesy of Meridian Medical Technologies®, Inc., a wholly owned subsidiary of King Pharmaceuticals®, Inc. Used with permission.; 3-11 Courtesy of Lasse Svensson/Swedish Defence Research Agency (FOI); 3-12 Courtesy of U.S. Army

Chapter 4

4-1 Courtesy of U.S. Army Research, Development and Engineering Command, Aberdeen Proving Ground, MD

Chapter 5

5-1 © Mitretek Systems. Used with permission.

Chapter 6

6-1 © Elaine Thompson/AP Photo; 6-2 © Alan Diaz/AP Photo; 6-4 © Susan Weems/AP Photo; 6-5 Courtesy of Cpl. Megan L. Stiner/U.S. Marines

Chapter 7

7-1 Courtesy of ICC: The Compliance Center, Inc.

Chapter 9

9-3 Data extracted from M. Meselson, J. Guillemin, M. Hugh-Jones, et al. *The Sverdlovsk anthrax outbreak of 1979.* 1994. *Science* 266: 1202-1208. © AAAS; 9-4 Courtesy of Professor Emeritus Martin Hugh-Jones, Environmental Studies Department, School of Coast & Environment, Louisiana State University; 9-5 Courtesy of the Western Front Association; 9-6 Courtesy of CDC; 9-7 Courtesy of CDC; 9-8 © National Library of Medicine; 9-9 Courtesy of CDC

Chapter 10

10-2 © National Library of Medicine; 10-3 Courtesy of WHO/CDC

Chapter 13

13-1 © 2001, American Medical Association. All rights reserved.; 13-2 Courtesy of Forest & Kim Starr/USGS; 13-3 Courtesy of Forest & Kim Starr/USGS; 13-4 © Gary Nafis

Chapter 14

14-2 Courtesy of Ludlum Measurements, Inc.; 14-3 Courtesy of Ludlum Measurements, Inc.; 14-4 Photograph by Robert Del Tredici, The Atomic Photographers Guild; 14-6 Courtesy of Charles Stewart, MD - Respective Penetration Characteristics of Radiation.; 14-10 © National Library of Medicine; 14-11 Courtesy of U.S. Air Force Base

Chapter 15

15-1 Courtesy of Dr. Carlo Kopp, Melbourne, Australia; 15-3 Courtesy of Dr. Carlo Kopp, Melbourne; Australia; 15-4 Courtesy of Holland Shielding Systems (www.hollandshielding.com); 15-8 © Northrop Grumman Corporation 2003. All rights reserved. Published with permission of Northrop Grumman.

Chapter 16

16-1 © Jones and Bartlett Publishers. Courtesy of MIEMSS.; 16-2 © Jones and Bartlett Publishers. Courtesy of MIEMSS.; 16-3 © Jones and Bartlett Publishers. Courtesy of MIEMSS.; 16-4 © Jones and Bartlett Publishers. Courtesy of MIEMSS.; 16-5 © Jones and Bartlett Publishers. Courtesy of MIEMSS.; 16-6 Courtesy of Tyco Fire & Security. Used with permission.; 16-7 Courtesy of Lance Cpl. Keith Underwood/U.S. Marines

Chapter 17

17-1 © MIEMSS

Color Plates

2-1 Courtesy of Akorn, Inc. Used with permission.; 2-2 Courtesy of Perry Baromedical Corporation; 2-3 Cyanokit® is a registered trademark of Merck Santé (France), an affiliate of Merck KGaA, Darmstadt, Germany. The product is not yet approved by the FDA in the U.S.; 2-4 Cyanokit® is a registered trademark of Merck Santé (France), an affiliate of Merck KGaA, Darmstadt, Germany. The product is not yet approved by the FDA in the U.S.; 3-2 Courtesy of the U.S. Army; 5-1 Based on photograph, Courtesy of LIBRARY AND ARCHIVES CANADA/C-080027; 5-2 Courtesy of Dr. Saeed Keshavarz/RCCI (Research Center of Chemical Injuries)/IRAN; 5-3 Courtesy of Dr. Saeed Keshavarz/RCCI (Research Center of Chemical Injuries)/IRA; 5-4 Courtesy of James W. Steger, CAPT, MC, USN/Department of Dermatology at Naval Medical Center San Diego; 5-5 Courtesy of James W. Steger, CAPT, MC, USN/Department of Dermatology at Naval Medical Center San Diego; 9-1A Courtesy of James H. Steele/CDC; 9-1B Courtesy of CDC; 9-2 Courtesy of Dr. P.S. Brachman/CDC; 9-3 Courtesy of CDC; 9-4 Courtesy of Renelle Woodall/CDC; 9-5 Courtesy of World Health Organization/CDC; 9-6 Courtesy of Margaret Parsons and Dr. Karl F. Meyer/CDC; 9-7 Courtesy of Dr. Jack Poland/CDC; 9-8 Courtesy of Dr. Jack Poland/CDC; 9-9 Courtesy of Richard Jacobs, MD; 11-1 © Wellcome Trust Library; 11-2 Courtesy of CDC; 11-3 Courtesy of CDC; 11-4 © Pat Roque/AP Photo; 11-5 Courtesy of Alethia Productions; 11-6 A/B Courtesy of Andy Crump/WHO/TDR; 11-7 Courtesy of CDC; 12-1 Courtesy of CDC; 12-2 Courtesy of Andy Crump/WHO/TDR; 15-1 Stuck, B. E., Zwick, H., Molchany, J., Lund, D. J., and D. A. Gagliano. *Accidental human laser retinal injuries from military laser systems. SPIE, Proceedings of Laser-Inflicted Eye Injuries: Epidemiology, Prevention, and Treatment.* 1996. 2674: 7-20.; 15-2 © Chris Barry/Phototake; 15-3 © Chris Barry/Phototake

Unless otherwise indicated, photographs and illustrations are copyright of Jones and Bartlett Publishers, Inc.